Small Animal Surgery

J. B. Lippincott Company
Philadelphia
Grand Rapids   New York   St. Louis   San Francisco
London   Sydney   Tokyo

Small Animal Surgery

Edited by

Colin E. Harvey, BVSc, FRCVS

Professor of Surgery
School of Veterinary Medicine
University of Pennsylvania
Philadelphia, Pennsylvania

Charles D. Newton, DVM, MS

Professor of Orthopedic Surgery
School of Veterinary Medicine
University of Pennsylvania
Philadelphia, Pennsylvania

Anthony Schwartz, DVM, PhD

Professor of Surgery
School of Veterinary Medicine
Tufts University
North Grafton, Massachusetts

With 21 Contributors

Acquisitions Editor: Nancy L. Mullins
Developmental Editor: Richard Winters
Project Editor: Kathy Crown
Copy Editors: Wendy Walker and Jennifer Mintzer
Indexer: Victoria Boyle
Art Director: Susan Hess Blaker
Design Coordinator: Ellen C. Dawson
Interior and Cover Design: Ellen C. Dawson
Production Manager: Carol A. Florence
Production Coordinator: Pamela Milcos
New Illustrations: David Factor and Sandra Sevigny
Compositor: Tapsco, Inc.
Text Printer/Binder: Murray Printing Co.
Cover Printer: Murray Printing Co.

6 5 4 3 2 1

Library of Congress Cataloging-in-Publication Data

Small animal surgery/edited by Colin E. Harvey,
   Charles D. Newton, Anthony Schwartz
      p. cm.
      Bibliography: p.
      Includes index.
      ISBN 0-397-50852-2
      1. Veterinary surgery.   2. Pets—Surgery.   I. Harvey, Colin E.
   II. Newton, Charles D.   III. Schwartz, Anthony.
   SF911.S52   1990
   636.089'7—dc20   89-12553
                                                                    CIP

The authors and publisher have exerted every effort to ensure that drug selection and dosage set forth in this text are in accord with current recommendations and practice at the time of publication. However, in view of ongoing research, changes in government regulations, and the constant flow of information relating to drug therapy and drug reactions, the reader is urged to check the package insert for each drug for any change in indications and dosage and for added warnings and precautions. This is particularly important when the recommended agent is a new or infrequently employed drug.

Contributors

Dale E. Bjorling, DVM, MS
*Diplomate, American College of Veterinary
    Surgeons*
Associate Professor and Chairman
Department of Surgical Sciences
School of Veterinary Medicine
University of Wisconsin—Madison
Madison, Wisconsin

Ronald M. Bright, DVM, MS
*Diplomate, American College of Veterinary
    Surgeons*
Professor and Director of Surgical Services
Department of Urban Practice
College of Veterinary Medicine
University of Tennessee
Knoxville, Tennessee

Dennis D. Caywood, DVM, MS
*Diplomate, American College of Veterinary
    Surgeons*
Associate Professor and Head of the Division
    of Small Animal Surgery
Department of Small Animal Clinical Sciences
College of Veterinary Medicine
University of Minnesota
St. Paul, Minnesota

Jonathan N. Chambers, DVM, MS
*Diplomate, American College of Veterinary
    Surgeons*
Professor of Orthopedics
Department of Small Animal Medicine
College of Veterinary Medicine
University of Georgia
Athens, Georgia

Steven W. Crane, DVM
*Diplomate, American College of Veterinary
    Surgeons*
Professor and Head
Department of Companion Animal and
    Special Species Medicine
College of Veterinary Medicine
North Carolina State University
Raleigh, North Carolina;
Associate in Clinical Nutrition
Mark Morris Associates
Topeka, Kansas

Dennis Crowe, Jr, DVM
*Diplomate, American College of Veterinary
    Surgeons*
Associate Professor of Surgery
Department of Small Animal Medicine
College of Veterinary Medicine
University of Georgia
Athens, Georgia

Colin E. Harvey, BVSc, FRCVS
*Diplomate, American College of Veterinary
    Surgeons*
Diplomate, American Veterinary Dental College
Professor of Surgery
School of Veterinary Medicine
University of Pennsylvania
Philadelphia, Pennsylvania

H. Jay Harvey, DVM
*Diplomate, American College of Veterinary
    Surgeons*
Associate Professor of Surgery
New York State College of Veterinary
    Medicine
Cornell University
Ithaca, New York

Donald A. Hulse, DVM
*Diplomate, American College of Veterinary
    Surgeons*
Professor of Surgery
College of Veterinary Medicine
Texas A & M University
College Station, Texas

Charles D. Newton, DVM, MS
*Diplomate, American College of Veterinary
    Surgeons*
Associate Dean for Student Affairs
Professor of Orthopedic Surgery
School of Veterinary Medicine
University of Pennsylvania
Philadelphia, Pennsylvania

Gert W. Niebauer, DVM, MS
Assistant Professor of Surgery
School of Veterinary Medicine
University of Pennsylvania
Philadelphia, Pennsylvania

John E. Oliver, DVM, MS, PhD
Diplomate ACVIM, Neurology
Professor and Head
Department of Small Animal Medicine
College of Veterinary Medicine
University of Georgia
Athens, Georgia

Marvin L. Olmstead, DVM, MS
*Diplomate, American College of Veterinary
    Surgeons*
Professor of Small Animal Surgery
Veterinary Teaching Hospital
The Ohio State University College of
    Veterinary Medicine
Columbus, Ohio

Michael Pavletic, DVM
*Diplomate, American College of Veterinary
    Surgeons*
Associate Professor
Section Head of Small Animal Surgery
School of Veterinary Medicine
Tufts University
North Grafton, Massachusetts

Marc R. Raffe, DVM, MS
*Diplomate, American College of Veterinary
    Anesthesiologists*
Associate Professor of Anesthesia and
    Critical Care
Department of Small Animal Clinical Sciences
College of Veterinary Medicine
University of Minnesota
St. Paul, Minnesota

Cheryl J. Mehlhaff Schunk, DVM
*Diplomate, American College of Veterinary
    Surgeons*
Staff Surgeon
Hillsborough County Veterinary Hospital
Amherst, Massachusetts

Anthony Schwartz, DVM, PhD
*Diplomate, American College of Veterinary
    Surgeons*
Associate Dean and Chairman
Department of Surgery
School of Veterinary Medicine
Tufts University
North Grafton, Massachusetts

Elizabeth Arnold Stone, DVM, MS
Diplomate, American College of Veterinary Surgeons
Professor of Surgery
Department of Companion Animal and Special Species Medicine
Veterinary Teaching Hospital
College of Veterinary Medicine
North Carolina State University
Raleigh, North Carolina

Tommy L. Walker, DVM
Diplomate, American College of Veterinary Surgeons
Staff Surgeon
Southern California Veterinary Surgical Group
Newport Beach, California

Walter E. Weirich, DVM, PhD
Diplomate, American College of Veterinary Surgeons
Professor of Surgery
Department of Veterinary Clinical Sciences
School of Veterinary Medicine
Purdue University
West Lafayette, Indiana

Milton Wyman, DVM, MSc
Diplomate, American College of Veterinary Ophthalmologists
Associate Dean of Student and Academic Affairs
Professor of Comparative Ophthalmology
The Ohio State University College of Veterinary Medicine
Columbus, Ohio

Preface

Small animal surgery has grown at a staggering rate in the last 15 to 20 years. Textbooks that attempt to provide a comprehensive account of the topic now require at least two hefty volumes; yet much of this material is necessary only for the small animal surgical specialist.

The editors of *Small Animal Surgery* believe that the time is right for a different approach. The veterinary student and the small animal practitioner need an accessible, useful textbook of small animal surgery that will tell them not all there is to know, but what they *need* to know in a modern small animal practice. Our goal, therefore, has been to provide a textbook that will describe what procedures are available, provide in-depth descriptions of those procedures that the practitioner is likely to perform, and include enough detail about the more complex procedures to allow the practitioner to make an informed referral.

The textbook begins with a preliminary section describing the mechanical and cellular events surrounding a surgical procedure. This section encompasses the material of a "Surgical Principles" course in a veterinary school.

The following types of procedures are described in such depth that the reader could perform them without referring to any other source:

- Common, relatively simple techniques that every practitioner can be expected to perform, such as cystotomy, enterotomy, pinning or wiring simple fractures, and lateral ear canal resection.
- Less frequently used techniques that may be required in an emergency, such as tracheotomy, gastric decompression, and conjunctival flap, as well as emergency management techniques,

such as wound care and stabilization of fractures, that will allow an animal to be sent on for definitive care.

• Certain more complex but very commonly performed procedures, such as feline perineal urethrostomy and cruciate ligament repair.

"Middle level" procedures that are performed commonly, but may require more sophisticated equipment for diagnosis and surgery, are discussed in sufficient detail for the reader to understand the concepts, and advantages and disadvantages, but without a suture-by-suture description. Readers interested in using these procedures are directed to other sources for specific technical descriptions. Examples are more complex fracture repair techniques, such as plating, closure of patent ductus arteriosus, and endodontic and dental restorative procedures.

Procedures that require special instrumentation and expertise, or that for other reasons should be performed only by individuals with advanced training, are described only with regard to indications and prognosis, with no more than a few sentences or a paragraph about the technique itself to orient the reader. Examples are intraocular procedures, orthodontic procedures, total hip prostheses, and cardiac surgery requiring heart-lung bypass.

Authors contributing to a "concise" textbook face special demands. The contributors to this book were selected for their acknowledged expertise and for their willingness to write concisely rather than to let the world know how much they know. For this, as well as for their enthusiasm, the editors thank them all. The progress that has led to the need for a text such as this has been made due to the efforts of many dedicated and talented veterinary surgeons, to whom the editors acknowledge their debt. We hope that you, the reader, find this book of interest and value.

Colin E. Harvey, FRCVS
Charles D. Newton, DVM, MS
Anthony Schwartz, DVM, PhD

Contents

Small Animal Surgery

1

Stephen W. Crane

Principles of Companion Animal Surgery

Veterinary surgery is a combination of biological and medical science and clinical art, the latter in the form of planning and judgment skills and psychomotor craft. The veterinary student who develops the skills, techniques, knowledge, and requisite compassion for patients and clients will have the opportunity to participate in one of the most therapeutically useful areas of our healing profession.

The history of veterinary surgery is rich and colorful: ancient Mesopotamian, Phoenician, Greek, Hindu, and African cultures describe surgical procedures on domesticated animals kept as companions or for food, transportation, or draft. Although few of these procedures would be acceptable by current medical or husbandry standards, they were based on the desire to improve the animal's utility, efficiency, or quality of life.

Since the discovery of anesthesia (1848) and the advent of aseptic principles and techniques (late 19th century) in human surgery, the clinical science of surgery has emerged to replace superstition and tradition. The intent of surgical science is to systematically and objectively test, by statistical comparison, hypotheses about patient care and operative techniques against control populations. The scientific method has transformed surgery from a primitive to a highly efficacious therapy. Because much of the physiologic data and operative techniques allowing these advances in surgical biology and operative methods were learned from animal models, a great deal of basic data exists for application in animal patients.

This information was of tremendous importance in the development of modern veteri-

The author acknowledges the contribution of Stephen Gilson, D.V.M.

nary surgical sciences in the 1920s. In the 1930s, the standards of veterinary surgery for companion animal clinical practice improved and began to approximate the standards for human surgical practice in a few institutions. This growth was assisted by the examples and standards set by the American Animal Hospital Association. This group grew rapidly and promulgated continuing education and standards for small animal hospital practice. After World War II, clinical internships became more widely available and companion animal practice emerged as an economically viable option for an increasing number of graduate veterinarians. By the 1950s, further growth in surgery was available when veterinary curricula continued to acknowledge small animal medicine and surgery and the scientific method, as applied to surgical clinics, was used on a wider scale.

In 1965, the American College of Veterinary Surgeons was founded; one of its main objectives was to establish formats for veterinary surgical residency training and requirements consistent with those in human general surgery. The birth of the certified veterinary surgical specialist system has facilitated the development of a second opinion and referral system in both institutional and private specialty practices; this, in turn, has improved patient care, has benefited both general veterinary practitioners and specialists, and has stimulated advances in techniques.

Changes in attitudes toward companion animals have increased the demand for veterinary surgical care. With the growth of cities and the relative "anomie" of much of modern society, cats, dogs, and other small animals have assumed an important position in many families.

Because it is possible to approach almost all anatmic areas surgically, surgeons must have a comprehensive knowledge of the basic medical sciences, particularly biochemistry, anatomy, biomechanics, physiology, pathology, pharmacology, microbiology, and internal medicine.

Objectives of Veterinary Surgery

The purpose of operating on an animal is to restore the anatomic integrity of an injured area, to remove or reconfigure normal or abnormal structures to allow their functional or cosmetic improvement, or to neuter the animal. Surgery may be needed if an organ or region has been compromised by displacement, malpositioning, obstruction, neoplastic invasion, hyperplasia, hypoplasia, atrophy, derangement, fracture, scarring, or other deformation.

Preoperative Care

Preoperative History and Physical Examination

In the patient's preoperative evaluation, it is extremely important for the surgeon to gain a complete overview of the animal's medical and husbandry status. Both the history and physical examination should explore all body systems, with a secondary focus on the signs of injury or perturbation on a regional or local basis. Data from the complete history and physical examination are the cornerstones of diagnosis.

Preoperative Ancillary Diagnostic Testing

Indirect Diagnostic Methods

In using tests, the clinician should keep in mind the relationship between testing and treatment and should not use tests in a "shotgun" or "make-no-mistakes" approach. The latter approach means higher client bills and lower benefit/cost ratio. Ancillary tests of structure and/or function should be used to support the history and physical examination and to confirm initial impressions. Well-known clinical pathology function tests include the hemogram, serum biochemistries of metabolic substrates and waste products, electrolytes, gases, enzymes, hormones, antibodies, the complete urinalysis, and diagnostic microbiology. Fortunately, advances in laboratory technology have made a wide range of office-based tests efficient and accurate. Affordable and reliable commercial laboratory services are also available in most geographic areas.

Radiographs can delineate many morphological abnormalities and are widely used to confirm both obvious and occult lesions. Radiographs enhanced by the addition of contrast media are especially useful and are sometimes suggested from suspicious signs in plain radiographs. The most common contrast radiographs are those of the gastrointestinal and urinary tracts and of the subarachnoid space. Contrast studies of certain diarthrodial joints, the heart and great vessels, selective angiograms, and contrast medium delineation of draining fistulae and sinuses are sometimes performed. Less frequently done contrast studies are of the pleural and peritoneal spaces, airways, salivary glands, and lymphatic system.

Ultrasonographic imaging of the heart and abdominal viscera is very helpful and growing in usefulness and availability. Ultrasonography is particularly well suited to delineating subtle boundary relationships between and within soft tissues and can be more specific and sensitive than plain radiographs in some situations. For example, differential absorption and reflection of acoustic energy may produce an image that clearly separates normal tissue from metastatic or cavitary foci in the liver. Computerized tomography and magnetic resonance imaging are now being used in some veterinary teaching hospitals.

Direct Diagnostic Methods

Viewing body cavities, joints, and the luminal surfaces of hollow viscera is a subset of surgery, and these endoscopic procedures can be immensely valuable in reducing the need for open exploratory surgery. A wide range of rigid speculae, and flexible or rigid-lensed scopes are available for endoscopy. Although it takes practice to master the capabilities of internal viewing scopes, directly visualizing lesions can often be more useful than indirect information from radiographs or laboratory tests. In small animals, flexible pediatric or adult endoscopic instruments are particularly valuable because they can be used to examine many cavities, including the external ear canal, nasal cavity, pharynx, larynx, trachea, esophagus, stomach, colon, and rectum.

Other semi-invasive ancillary diagnostic techniques are laparoscopic and arthroscopic examinations, in which rigid lensed instruments penetrate a body cavity or joint. In laparoscopy, the abdomen is trocarized through a stab wound and the abdominal cavity insufflated with carbon dioxide or room air to the point of distention. This allows visceral borders to fall away from each other so that organ surfaces and aspects can be seen as the scope is moved, and permits guiding of a biopsy needle by direct vision.

Arthroscopic examination is possible in the stifle and shoulder of larger companion animals. After trocarization of the joint and distention of the capsule with fluid, most of the cartilaginous joint surfaces and synovium can be seen well.

Biopsy and Cytology

Direct assessment of tissue and cell specimens by histopathologic microscopy is time proven and cost effective. If available, frozen section biopsy is also time efficient. A lesion should be completely removed by excisional biopsy when possible. If only a portion of the lesion is removed or complete removal is impossible, the procedure is termed an incisional biopsy. With incisional biopsy, it is important to obtain a width and depth cross-section of the lesion so that normal and abnormal tissue and the junctional zone between the two are present. A properly collected, fixed, and processed specimen is critically important if the clinician is to receive maximum diagnostic and prognostic assistance from a pathologist.

In most cases, biopsy allows a specific diagnosis to be reached or confirmed. The most diagnostic information is usually available from the interface between normal and abnormal tissue. Because the center of larger or rapidly growing lesions may be full of hemorrhage or necrotic debris, these areas should be avoided. Incisional tissue specimen slices may be taken by a sharp scalpel, from tissue cores via a cutting biopsy punch, from pinches of mucosal surfaces taken by grasping forceps passed through an endoscope, and by needle biopsy devices designed to cut and retrieve tissue specimens (see "Biopsy Techniques and Equipment," Chap. 3).

Cytologic examination of exfoliated cells, properly stained for microscopic examination, is also a practical diagnostic method. Cells may be obtained for examination by the "touch-prep" of tissue slices or fragments, from fine-needle aspirates of masses, lesions, or lymph nodes, or from centrifuging the fluids from body cavity aspirates and lavages into a cytologic pellet before making smears. Endoscopically obtained brushings of airway mucosa are also used in obtaining cells. After collection, cell specimens are smeared and stained to delineate cytologic morphology. Some cytopathologic and histopathologic diagnoses can be easily reached, but others may require the skilled interpretation of a specialist. Fortunately, such expertise is usually available at regional veterinary biomedical laboratories.

Staging of Pathology

The progression or resolution of a disease or injury must often be identified to produce a rational prognosis. Especially in the case of tumors, further testing by radiography, ultrasonography, endoscopy, additional biopsy, or exploratory surgery may be required to place the lesion into biological progression catego-ries ("stages") by a scheme that takes into account the size, growth, and invasive characteristics of the tumor in its primary location (Tumor), whether local spread to regional lymph nodes has occurred (Node), and whether distant metastasis has occurred (Metastasis). This scheme, sanctioned by the World Health Organization, unifies the description of the tumor's biological insult to the host. When TNM staging is coupled with the histopathologically established cell type, a specific prognosis can usually be provided to the animal's owner with documentation for or against surgery or another form of treatment. Biopsy and histopathologic examination can also be important in diagnosing and staging other pathologic disorders, including degenerative and immune-mediated diseases.

Surgical Indications

The value of the history, physical examination, and direct and indirect testing is to achieve diagnosis and to plan therapy. Therapy by surgery would result from an indication, a mandate for action. Surgical indications are based on a sign, syndrome, diagnosis, or clinical circumstance that suggests the action of a specific operative treatment be taken for the best outcome. Several factors must be carefully considered in evaluating the patient to develop a surgical indication. This process of gathering information and making decisions is strongly aided by a problem-oriented medical record (POMR) system. This approach to medical record information is designed to place all definable abnormal elements of an animal's health status on organized lists of problems. A level of resolution is then described for each problem listed until all problems are inactive or resolved. Recently, the POMR has been widely adopted throughout veterinary medicine because of its power and efficiency in planning care for the total needs of the patient, and for the structure the system imparts in assessing objective and subjective sources of information.

Making the Decision for Surgery

Once a disease or injury has been diagnosed and staged and the surgical indication identified, the next question is whether the procedure is the correct one for the patient. Selecting an available and indicated technique or procedure for a patient is one of the most critically important tasks in veterinary medicine. This is because once the operation is undertaken, a commitment to the indication has occurred; the decision cannot be undone and many risks have already been taken. Therefore, consistency and reliability in arriving at surgical indications and the surgical judgment used in patient/treatment matching says much about the clinician's therapeutic maturity.

The first step in surgical judgment is to appreciate the natural course of a diagnosed disease or injury if left untreated. The option of allowing nature to take its course should be considered, even if rapidly discarded. Secondly, it is vital to stage clinical signs at presentation against the natural progression of the disease or injury: Are the signs shown consistent with early, late, or intermediate manifestations? What is the rate of progression? Staging decisions are sometimes difficult and error prone, but can be improved with accumulation of detailed experience. Dealing with a nonverbal patient only makes these evaluations more difficult. Second opinions and/or referral should be considered in instances of significant doubt.

Personal and local factors also need to be considered as a part of surgical judgment. These factors include the skill and experience of the veterinarian as an anesthetist and surgeon, the availability of equipment and supplies for the primary procedure, the ability to deal with contingencies or complications, and the ability of the hospital's nursing staff and/or the pet owner to provide postoperative monitoring and supportive care.

Of course, owner input is essential to the final surgical decision. Owners usually feel an obligation to the pet to understand in advance the effect that the diagnosis, prognosis, surgery, and pre- and postoperative care being proposed will have on the animal's utility, lifestyle, cosmetic appearance, and the human/animal bond. Many clients seeking veterinary surgery are sophisticated consumers of medical information and services, and they often have particular concern about the transient or permanent loss of function and the level of pain the pet may experience postoperatively. During the discussion with the owner, the subject of fees, risk of complications, pain, death, and timing of the operation must be raised and always deserve frank discussion. *Client education always is best done before the surgery.* Postsurgical recovery expectation and rehabilitation timetables should also be presented before making a final decision. For example, no owner should leave a discussion of the surgical options for an acutely paralyzed dachshund with the idea that the animal will be walking immediately after decompressive surgery for an extruded intravertebral disc.

Failure to mention the options and implications regarding the prognosis, surgical risk, and negative postoperative possibilities or expectations is the most important single cause of owner dissatisfaction and lawsuits. The essence of informed consent is that the client understand all the factors involved, and the effective veterinarian is one who can list and clearly describe the menu of options for care and the advantages and disadvantages of each. However, the wise veterinarian will also avoid making value judgments as an owner's surrogate about the options available. This is especially true if euthanasia or a salvage procedure such as amputation is introduced by either party as a "treatment" possibility. The exception is when an owner is unaware of or denies a high level of suffering in the pet or has impossible or improbable expectations. True compassion for the animal and unhurried empathy for the owner, who often must weigh several options and make difficult choices, is surely a description of the best possible "bedside manner."

Surgical Biology

Response to Injury

Injury, accidentally or surgically induced, produces major and rapid changes in mammalian physiologic homeostasis. These rapid response alterations have evolved to allow the maximum chance for survival. Initially, pain, tissue injury, and loss of circulating blood volume are stimuli that trigger sympathoadrenal neuroendocrine responses. The adrenal medulla responds quickly with epinephrine and norepinephrine to elevate cardiac output and to activate both α and β agonist receptors in the smooth muscle of the precapillary arteriolar sphincters. This causes reduced blood flow to splanchnic viscera and skin, but increases circulation in skeletal muscle and the heart. With a significant loss of blood volume, a pronounced and generalized peripheral vasoconstriction acts to divert most of the remaining circulatory volume to the "critical core" organs, which include the brain, liver, and myocardium. Powerful renal sodium and fluid conservation responses are activated through release of aldosterone and antidiuretic hormone. Glucocorticoids are secreted from the adrenal cortex in response to ACTH release.

Energy metabolism is markedly affected during response to injury. Primarily, the ratio and cellular effects of insulin:glucagon are altered, and levels of glucocorticoids, growth hormone, and triiodothyronine increase. These and other endocrine and cellular changes induce a temporary and relative "insulin resistance" in the cell. This state of pseudodiabetes forces conversion from carbohydrate to protein and fat for energy substrates. Therefore, lipolysis and catabolism of lean muscle mass, with a negative nitrogen balance, are characteristic features of host response to significant injury. These catabolic changes are obligatory and reversible and are regulated up to a finite maximal response by the degree of injury. This can be the case even if nutrition is being provided, because the insulin resistance at the cellular level is in force.

The changes in energy metabolism persist until the neuroendocrine signals for their activation cease. At that point, gluconeogenesis diminishes and a transition occurs back to the anabolic rebuilding of the volume and strength of skeletal muscle. As carbohydrates again become available as the primary fuel substrate, fat deposits can also be restored. The clinical effect of these processes varies from virtually unnoticeable in minor injury or surgery to profound body wasting in severe trauma injury or surgery (Figs. 1-1, 1-2). It is important to keep these stress response relationships in mind during diagnostic work-up and planning for surgery. Planning for perioperative care should be designed to reduce stress and optimize nutritional intake.

Evaluation for Anesthesia

A complete preoperative evaluation of all organ systems must be done before elective anesthesia, with special attention given to the effect of the lesion or injury on the conduct of safe anesthesia. Blood volume and cardiopulmonary, hepatorenal, and cerebral function must be confirmed as adequate, or corrected.

Ventilation of the lungs by an adequate minute volume is critical. Gas exchange that arterializes the venous blood occurs in alveolar respiratory units, a functional entity distal to the conducting airways. Respiration, the delivery and exchange of oxygen for carbon dioxide, occurs at the cellular level via conversion of oxyhemoglobin to carboxyhemoglobin. Obvious dyspnea or ventilatory distress, insufficient velocity and volume of air flow through the nostrils, cyanotic blood and mucous membrane color, and abnormal radiographs of the thorax are all useful indicators of improper ventilation.

Additional requirements for gas exchange and cellular respiration are physiologic levels of hemoglobin and cardiac output. The latter can be indirectly assessed by the pulse rate, pulse pressure, and the pulse wave profile, detected by a finger on the femoral artery. In addition to indirect clinical assess-

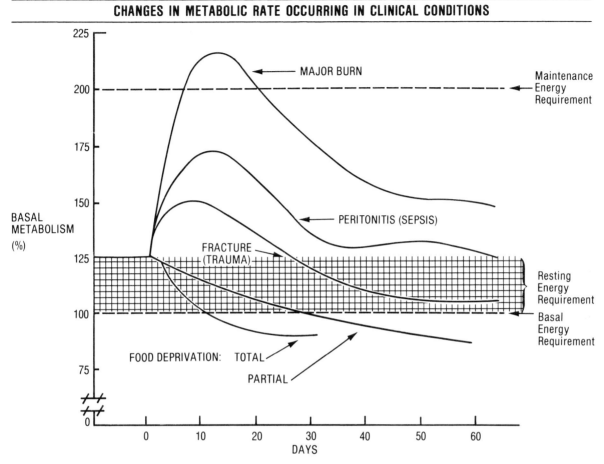

Figure 1-1. *Changes in basal metabolism secondary to partial or full starvation and in response to various levels of injury. (Lewis L, Hand M, Morris M. Small animal clinical nutrition III. Topeka, KS: Mark Morris & Associates, 1987:5)*

ment, invasive and noninvasive measurements of blood pressure are available. The noninvasive Doppler or oscillometric flow devices indicate flow and pressure in vessels and are useful and practical monitoring devices, but can be unreliable under conditions of low cardiac output. The appearance of the gingival, buccal, or conjunctival mucosa is also useful for detecting signs of capillary vasoconstriction or vasodilatation.

Management of pain is a priority in the preoperative period and in planning for anesthesia. Pain control must be considered before the induction of anesthesia because pain pro-

duces stress and distress. The physical distress of acute pain and the mental anguish and fatigue accompanying chronic pain leads to animal suffering. A clinician must alleviate pain and suffering not only to provide humane treatment, but also because pain will further drive, and ultimately compromise, the capacity for compensatory sympathoadrenal responses at a time when they are most needed. Therefore, pain has a negative physiologic effect. Some signs of animal pain are listed in Table 1-1.

Unfortunately, several well-known and knotty dilemmas exist in recognizing and alle-

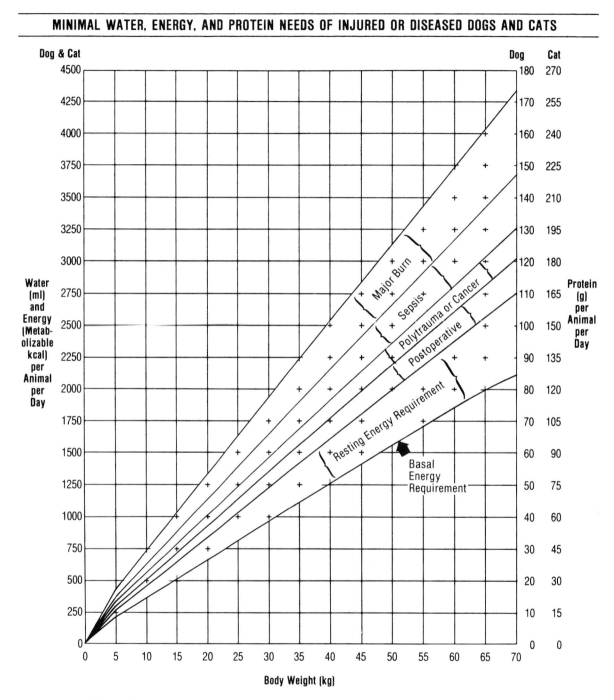

MINIMAL WATER, ENERGY, AND PROTEIN NEEDS OF INJURED OR DISEASED DOGS AND CATS

Figure 1-2. *Effects of injury on protein, calorie, and water requirements for dogs and cats between 1 and 70 kg. (Lewis L, Hand M, Morris M. Small animal clinical nutrition III. Topeka, KS: Mark Morris & Associates, 1987:5)*

viating animal pain. How can a veterinarian or owner tell if an animal is really in pain, when the animal cannot communicate in words? Does stress-induced analgesia occur at injury? Are non-human animals inherently more stoic than humans? Does a species- or breed-specific stoicism exist? If so, to what degree and in which species or breeds? If significant tissue injury exists, but the patient does not appear to be in obvious pain, should the significance of the injury be dismissed by a clinician on the basis of animal stoicism?

Because no objective pain measurement index exists for the nonverbal patient, the alternatives are limited. I believe that when there is significant acute or chronic tissue trauma, but little expression of the behavioral elements of pain, one must estimate the pain likely for a human with that condition, and project that estimate to the animal patient. Providing analgesia by immobilizing a fracture, draining an abscess, or giving pharmacologic analgesia is a very practical method of optimizing patient care by reducing stress. Fortunately, modern agonist-antagonist analgesic drug combinations allow safe analgesia, even in severe physiologic compromise (Table 1-2). The only other option is to ignore the possibility that occult pain exists or that pain has deleterious physiologic consequences. This latter course is not recommended, for both humane and homeostatic reasons.

Management of Anesthesia

Anesthesia, the reversible and controlled production of analgesia, hypnosis, amnesia, and immobilization, is an essential aspect of modern surgical practice. The main techniques used in companion animal practice are intravenous, intramuscular, and inhalation administration of chemicals that selectively depress the cerebral cortex. Local and regional infiltration and nerve-blocking procedures can also be useful, but most companion animal patients will be more safely and efficiently managed under general anesthesia. It is important to realize that there are no safe anesthetics, only safe anesthetists, and it is essential to formulate a customized anesthetic plan for each patient.

Planning for anesthesia includes considering the anatomic location and potential duration of the surgery, the patient positioning required, and the possibility of intraoperative changes in positioning. All anatomic and physiologic impairments should be taken into account, along with the injury or disease, in classifying patient risk. While the concept of relative anesthetic risk will guide the selection of the drugs, airway management, fluid management, and monitoring requirements, emergency drugs and equipment should always be kept close to *any* anesthetized patient, regard-

Table 1–1.   Signs of Animal Pain

Physical Signs	Behavioral Signs
Tachypnea/panting	Vocalization—wide variety of changes
Tachycardia inappropriate to physical status	Aggression on touching a painful area
Mydriasis	Demeanor changes; expression of fear
Extremity nonuse or limping	Reclusive or attention-seeking behavior atypical for the individual
Postural change to "rest" body part or region	Catatonia
Rigidity of neck, back, or abdomen	
Rolling and thrashing	

less of the preoperative anesthesia risk classification.

If the procedure will be anything but brief, body temperature management and special padding for areas of local pressure should be considered. Temperature loss is faster in smaller patients, and damage to pressure-sensitive areas more probable in heavier patients.

In emergency procedures, dehydration, anemia, acid-base imbalance, cardiopulmonary and respiratory distress, and hepatorenal dysfunction all become active problems on the POMR for assessment and resolution. Except in an emergency, food should be withheld for at least 12 hours before surgery. If there is an emergency and the patient has recently eaten, the possibility of occult or overt intraoperative regurgitation or vomiting should be anticipated, especially if the surgery is an abdominal procedure such as a cesarean section.

Physiologically well patients (Class I) intended for routine procedures should be screened for suitability for general anesthesia by packed cell volume, total protein by the re-

fractometer method, urinalysis, and an examination for the ova of intestinal parasites. Control measures for ectoparasites are taken as necessary. Classes II through V require increased preoperative testing, intraoperative monitoring, and postoperative care (Table 1-3).

Anesthesia Induction and Maintenance

The induction procedure for general anesthesia in both dogs and cats is typically the intravenous administration of a thiobarbiturate or neuroleptanalgesic through an indwelling venous cannula. The former uses 2% thiopental given intravenously as a bolus at 12 to 20 mg/kg to rapidly induce unconsciousness. The latter is achieved by combining narcotics and tranquilizers (Table 1-2). After the induction of hypnosis, analgesia, and immobilization, endotracheal intubation with a flexible, cuffed

Table 1-2. Preoperative Analgesic or Antianxiety Agents

Classification	Drug	Preanesthetic Tranquilizer	Post-traumatic Postoperative Analgesic
Major tranquilizer	Acetylpromazine	0.05–0.1 mg/kg IM	Tranquilizers are NOT analgesics
Minor tranquilizer	Diazepam	0.1–0.2 mg/kg IV	
Opiate agonists	Morphine		0.1–0.2 mg/kg IV
	Oxymorphone		0.001–0.05 mg/kg*
	Meperidine		0.1–0.25 mg/kg IV (Dog)**
Opiate agonist-antagonists	Pentazocine (0.1× morphine potency)		0.05–0.1 mg/kg IV (Cat)
	Butorphanol (3× morphine potency)		0.4 mg/kg IV (Dog)†
Neuroleptoanalgesia	Combine acetylpromazine and oxymorphone OR Diazepam 0.3 mg/kg Ketamine 5.5 mg/kg		
Anticholinergic	Glycopyrrolate	0.01 mg/kg SQ	

* Contraindicated in cats without concurrent use of tranquilizer.
** Half-life is about 20 minutes.
† Doses above or below this value do not give optimum analgesic action.

endotracheal tube protects the patency of the larynx and prevents aspiration of liquids from the pharynx or esophagus.

Inhalation agents are elected to maintain general anesthesia if the procedure is to be longer than the effective duration of two administrations of short-acting thiobarbiturates. Inhalation agents commonly used in veterinary surgery are methoxyflurane, isoflurane, and halothane. Isoflurane is a particularly good inhalation anesthetic because it yields exceptional stability of cardiac rhythm and output, even if myocardial electrical irritability and high circulating levels of catecholamines exist.

Halothane and isoflurane produce rapid anesthetic induction because their blood/gas partition coefficients are much lower than that of methoxyflurane. This means that these agents are less soluble in blood and higher concentrations of drugs are transported more quickly to the brain. The brain is rich in both blood supply and lipids, which promote distribution and drug uptake respectively. Because there is very little metabolism of the inhaled agents, especially isoflurane, depth of anesthesia may be rapidly increased or decreased by adjusting the alveolar concentration of the inhaled gas.

The addition of nitrous oxide to oxygen will act as an adjunct to the analgesic effects of the primary inhalation anesthetic. The concentration of nitrous oxide is regulated because it must be delivered in concentrations above 50% for any analgesic effect. However, it does not achieve enough analgesic effect at even a 75% concentration to be used as the only anesthetic agent. Nitrous oxide does not produce significant hypnosis or muscle relaxation. Because of its high diffusibility, it should be avoided when gas is trapped in a closed viscus or cavity. When nitrous oxide is used as an adjunct to a primary inhalation agent, its administration can commence after nitrogen washout has occurred. This may be done by preoxygenating the patient with 100% oxygen for 10 minutes before anesthesia induction, or by turning the nitrous oxide on after initial

skin preparation and positioning of the patient on the operating table. However, nitrous oxide can be used immediately in circle systems if an oxygen flow is maintained at 30 ml/kg/min or greater. Because nitrous oxide may diffuse from the blood back into the alveoli, its use should be discontinued 10 minutes before returning the patient to breathing room air.

Inhalation anesthesia is generally recommended for veterinary surgery and is delivered by one of three categories of breathing circuits: closed, semiclosed, and semiopen. The totally closed rebreathing circuit system requires a flow rate of fresh gas that only replaces the animal's minute oxygen consumption of 11 ml/kg/min. The closed-circuit system has the advantage of reducing waste-gas pollution in the operating room and retarding the progression of intraoperative hypothermia after the first hour of surgery. Hypoventilation and hypercapnia, caused by the imperfect removal of CO_2 from the circuit, or a gradually progressive imbalance of the O_2:N_2O ratio are potential hazards in closed systems.

A semiclosed system needs oxygen flow rates above minute oxygen consumption; it is intended to "pop off" the excess anesthetic gas mixture. This system is less economical and releases anesthetic agents into room air if they are not removed by a scavenging system. A semiclosed circle has improved theoretical safety; there is an increased "forgiveness" of gas ratio imbalance and a lower chance of hypercapnia and respiratory acidosis. The semiclosed system works quite well and is recommended for general use in animals heavier than about 8 kg, because patients this size will have adequate ability to propel their exhaled breath against the resistance of the circuit. Oxygen flow rates should be 15 to 20 ml/kg/min, or 30 ml/kg/min if nitrous oxide is also being used.

For patients lighter than about 8 kg, several configurations of the semiopen, nonrebreathing systems can be used. The advantage of this apparatus is that it presents a fresh anesthetic gas supply at the endotracheal tube. This reduces the functional dead space of the

Table 1–3. Preoperative Patient Classification, Workup, and Monitoring

Patient Risk Classification	Suggested Preoperative Workup	Intraoperative Monitoring	Postoperative Monitoring
I. (Excellent) Normal animal. Excellent previous health.	1, 2, 3	Basic = A–F, L	All categories evaluated upon awakening and at appropriate intervals thereafter
II. (Good) Mild systemic disease. Elective procedures in geriatric animals or very young puppies and kittens.	1, 2, 3, 5, 6a (6a omitted in puppies and kittens)	Basic = A–F. Add G in geriatrics or long, difficult procedures. Add H, I, L, as appropriate. Prolonged cases in puppies and kittens require glucose monitoring or glucose administration.	All categories evaluated upon awakening and at appropriate intervals thereafter
III. (Fair) Major systemic illness or trauma. Tumors with early TNM staging. Advanced aging changes in geriatric patients.	3, 4, 6b, 7, 9, 10 Other tests as indicated	Basic = A–G. Add H, I, L, as appropriate.	All categories evaluated upon awakening. Continuous monitoring recommended.
IV. (Poor) Major systemic illness with or without secondary complications. Polytrauma. Chronic debilitation.	3, 4, 6b, 7, 8, 9, 10, 11, 12 Other tests as indicated	Basic = A–I. J, K if indicated and available. L as needed. J, K left indwelling.	All categories evaluated upon awakening. Continuous monitoring recommended.
V. (Critical) Shock, of all etiologies. Patient in process of dying for any reason with surgical intervention mandatory.	3, 4, 6b, 7, 8, 9, 10, 11, 13 Serialized studies of 8, 10, 11, 12	Basic = A–I. Add glucose monitoring. Add J, K, if indicated and available. L as needed. J, K left indwelling.	All categories evaluated upon awakening and at appropriate intervals thereafter

Preoperative Workup
1. PCV (Microhematocrit)
2. Total protein (refractometer)
3. Internal and external parasites (including microfilaria if needed)
4. CBC
5. Screening dipsticks of blood or urine
6a. Mini urinalysis; specific gravity and dipsticks
6b. Complete urinalysis with sediment exam
7. Full biochemical panel

Intraoperative Monitoring
A. Adequate minute volume
B. Depth of anesthesia: Analgesia, hypnosis, immobilization, palpebral reflex, jaw tone, pupil size and reaction
C. Body temperature
D. Blood loss (sponges and suction)
E. Blood color and pulse pressure
F. Mucous membrane color; capillary refill time
G. Urine output (0.25–0.5 ml/kg/hr)

Postoperative Monitoring
Adequate ventilation and minute volume? Cardiac output? Anemia?
State of consciousness?
Need for analgesia?
Ability to stand, focus, and walk?
Need for immobilization of body region or need for restraint of mouth or paws?
Ability to eat, drink, and eliminate without assistance?
Systemic changes? TPR. Lab. and x-ray diagnostics?

Table 1–3. Preoperative Patient Classification, Workup, and Monitoring (*continued*)

Patient Risk Classification	Suggested Preoperative Workup	Intraoperative Monitoring	Postoperative Monitoring
	8. Electrolyte panel with anion gap 9. Thoracic radiographs 10. Electrocardiography 11. Central venous pressure 12. pH and total CO_2 with base excess 13. Full blood gas panel with base excess	H. Central venous pressure I. Indirect blood pressure measurement by Doppler or oscillometric techniques J. Intraarterial line for serial, direct, pressures, and blood gases K. Blood gas, pH, or total CO_2 determinations L. Sponge count	Wound changes? Separation, discharge, induration, edema, automutilation? Does animal need contact with owner or vice versa? Physical therapy? Follow-up evaluations?

system and eliminates the work of exhaling against the resistance of a circuit. Because of its simplicity, the Norman Mask Elbow is recommended, using flow rates of 2.5 to 3.0 times the minute volume. Minute volume is calculated as the tidal volume times respiratory rate, or about 180 ml/kg/min. A simple rule of thumb in using these systems for smaller dogs and cats is to provide 0.5 to 1 l/kg/min of at least 30% oxygen. The disadvantages of a semiopen, non-rebreathing system include the continuous presentation of cold dehumidified gases, which can potentiate hypothermia. Also, increased waste anesthetic gases are vented into the room, unless reduced by an absorptive canister or removal to the outside atmosphere.

Patient Monitoring

Before inducing anesthesia, patient monitoring should be started. The purpose of monitoring is to provide a base of comparison for subsequent changes in selected physiologic observations as anesthesia and surgery continues. Monitored items vary but always include the rate and depth of ventilation, because hypoventilation is the most common precursor of anesthetic death. Hypoventilation, persisting over time, produces hypercapnia and respiratory acidosis; hypoxemia develops and the combined acidosis and hypoxemia potentiate the

depressant and arrhythmia-producing effects of the general anesthetic agent on the myocardium. The primary reduction in cardiac output provokes compensatory sympathoadrenal discharge with endogenous releases of catecholamines. The resulting sinus tachycardia predisposes to the development of more severely perturbing arrhythmias such as runs of premature ventricular contractions. The falling cardiac output can lead to further catecholamine release and, eventually, serious or fatal arrhythmias such as ventricular fibrillation. Therefore, simple monitoring of the rate and depth of ventilation, and awareness that cellular respiration is occurring through gas exchange at the tissue level, are vital features of anesthesia evaluation.

Monitoring cardiac activity for changes in rate and output is similarly important. An esophageal stethoscope monitors both ventilatory and cardiac sounds, which are amplified into the operating room by an audiosonic amplifier or a radiostethoscopic transmitter/receiver device. Some esophageal stethoscopes also have channels for core temperature measurement and electrocardiographic display. Pulse wave and pressure measurements and peripheral perfusion and hemoglobin saturation are determined by periodic vessel palpation and inspection of mucous membrane color and capillary refill time. These observations indicate perfusion pressure and peripheral vasoconstriction. Perfusion, and the normal pink color of that perfusion, should return in less than 1.5 seconds following digital blanching. Prolonged capillary refill time indicates systemic vasoconstriction, possible volume depletion, and excess sympathoadrenal discharge. Red or muddy-red colors mean vasodilatation and microcirculatory distress. Cyanosis (blue coloration) means lack of oxyhemoglobin. Pale mucous membranes indicate anemia or profound volume depletion. Gray mucous membranes are a combination of pale and cyanotic changes and frequently indicate a generalized cardiopulmonary collapse or ventilatory failure.

Monitoring cardiopulmonary status by mucous membrane color and perfusion has the advantage of simplicity, accessibility, and convenience. Disadvantages are that it is an indirect, subjective method and, therefore, open to various interpretations. It is also difficult to recognize trends in subtle changes in color, which may delay identification of the onset of serious problems.

Arterial pressure is directly or indirectly measurable, and central perfusion to the body core is measured by urinary output. Monitoring urine output is easy and important because the leading cause of anuria in an anesthetized patient is reduction of mean blood pressure below 60 mmHg. It is uncommon in veterinary surgery to measure cardiac output as a monitoring method.

Another important observation is the depth of anesthesia. Pupil size is only moderately useful as an indicator with modern inhalation agents. After loss of consciousness, the palpebral touch/blink reflex is the first involuntary response to disappear with the newer anesthetic agents. Next, there is a progressive loss of jaw tone, and progressive muscle relaxation is an important indicator of an increasing depth of anesthesia. For example, a light plane of anesthesia is indicated by a loss of the palpebral reflex, but the presence of considerable jaw tone. Monitoring more items and systems, such as blood pressure and central venous pressure, produces information that com-

pounds itself because the *in vivo* responses of one system are often linked to changes in another. However, in making the decision to proceed with more sophisticated and/or invasive monitoring, the surgeon must weigh the need for the information against the threat of complications from invasive monitoring. Table 1-3 summarizes recommended monitoring practices by patient risk category.

Fluid Balance in Surgical Patients

Alterations in fluid balance and in electrolyte, acid-base, and blood-gas homeostasis are closely related. These items are often in nonphysiologic ranges after trauma or shock and in response to acute or chronic illness. In veterinary medicine, patients typically are presented later rather than sooner after onset of clinical signs, and derangements of water, electrolyte, and acid-base imbalances may be so profound at initial presentation as to jeopardize the patient's life. This is particularly true with urinary or gastrointestinal obstruction, sepsis, and shock. Although the best approach is to identify the abnormalities in water volume and the composition and concentration of electrolytes, an emergency may require an empirical approach. The following sections summarize only the principles of fluid balance, electrolyte, and acid-base abnormalities because excellent reviews of the subject are widely available.

Dehydration

Dehydration is the loss of the normal quantity of total body water. The normal compartmentalizations of body water between extracellular, intracellular, and interstitial areas can shift in response to oncotic and osmotic gradients between the compartments. A common clinical example is hemorrhage that acutely "dehydrates" the intravascular space. In response, a transcapillary refill of water occurs from the interstitial and extravascular space to the intravascular space. The most common conditions associated with dehydration are anorexia, the inability to eat or drink, or fluid loss through vomiting, diarrhea, wound exudation, or hemorrhage.

The degree of dehydration of the extracellular compartment is clinically assessed by skin turgor changes. Dehydration above 4% is noted by the progressively increasing loss of skin elasticity when the skin is pinched into a tent by the fingers. Six percent dehydration is detected by very significant reductions in skin turgor and elasticity. At 8% dehydration, the tented skin pinch will not return to its normal position; mucous membranes are dry, urine production is scant, and the ocular globes are sunken into their bony orbits. Elevations in hematocrit and total protein can reflect intravascular dehydration and hemoconcentration. However, they are most useful when compared to baseline status , or when serial samples are taken to expose a trend.

Electrolytes

In addition to maintaining intravascular volume, it is important during stress to preserve the osmolality and electrolyte compositions of the blood and central nervous system. All cations and anions have direct or indirect homeostatic importance, and wide departures from normal concentrations may provoke serious functional disturbances. The first step in evaluating electrolytes is to suspect an abnormality, based on the history, and to confirm the suspicion by tests. Electrolyte quantitation is widely available from commercial clinical pathological laboratories.

The major circulating cationic electrolytes are sodium and potassium; chloride and bicarbonate are the major circulating anions. Concentrations differ considerably between the extracellular and intracellular compartments for some of these cations and anions (see Table 1-4). While water movements are primarily passive to maintain osmotic equality, the electrolyte gradients across cell membranes are maintained by selective permeabilities and active ion pumping processes. Both are energy-consuming processes. Because the total body quantities of an electrolyte and the intracellular electrolyte fractions are not measured clinically, electrolytes are quantified by taking a "snapshot" through the "window" of the extracellular fluid compartment. The clinician must extrapolate from these data to the state of intracellular ion concentration.

Sodium
The normal range for extracellular sodium is 137 to 150 mEq/L, and sodium accounts for more than 90% of the normal serum osmolality.

Table 1–4. Composition of Common Replacement Fluids

	Extracellular Fluid	Intracellular Fluid	D5W	NaCl	D2.5% in .45 NaCl	Lactated Ringer's	LRS in D5W	K+ supplemented Restricted Na+ Isolyte-R® D5W	K+ supplemented D5W in 0.45 NaCl with 40 mEq/KCl
Na+	144.0	10.0		154	77	130	130	41	77
K+	5.0	141.0				4	4	16	40
Ca++	5.0	0				3	3	5	
Mg++	3.0	60						3	
Cl−	107	4.0		154	77	109	109	40	117
HCO3−	27	10.0							
HPO4−	4	23.0							
Acetate								24	
Lactate						28	28		
Calories			170		85	9	179	170	170

Osmolality receptors at various locations in the central nervous system and volume stretch receptors in the cardiovascular system and kidney serve as independent but integrated sensors for water, sodium, and osmolality balance. Effector arms of this control loop are aldosterone, antidiuretic hormone, and natriuretic hormone, which are potent regulators of water and salt retention by the kidney.

Hypernatremia usually results only from serious pure water losses, such as from central or nephrogenic diabetes insipidus or from iatrogenic overdose with sodium-containing solutions (for instance, 0.9 N NaCl or sodium bicarbonate). Therefore, hypernatremia is not commonly encountered as a primary entity, but may well be a complication of well-intentioned but inappropriate fluid therapy.

Hyponatremia, defined as a sodium level of less than 137 mEq/L, results from the loss of sodium and/or the sequestration of sodium-rich fluid outside the vascular compartment. Clinically, this results from chronic vomiting, diarrhea, wound drainage or suction, small-bowel obstruction, burns, peritonitis, hydrothorax, and the diuresis after postobstructive uropathy. Primary or secondary renal tubular diseases may also account for high sodium loss. Mild hyponatremia from sodium extravasated from the intravascular compartment can result from the prominent ascites concurrent with congestive heart failure, hepatic cirrhosis, or severe hypoproteinemia. Treatment will improve surgical homeostasis and is achieved by correcting the cause of water excess or the sodium deficit. In cases of sodium loss to outside the body, with normal cardiopulmonary hepatic and renal functions, sodium deficits are calculated using the formula:

Equation 1)

$$Na^+ \text{ deficit mEq/L} = 0.6 \times \text{body weight (kg)} \times (140 - \text{plasma } Na^+)$$

The normal sodium level is best restored by the intravenous or subcutaneous administration of 0.9 N NaCl solution or the oral administration of salt or sodium bicarbonate tablets.

Potassium

About 30 times less potassium is found in the extracellular fluid than in the intracellular fluid. Therefore, the serum potassium concentration is a poor and delayed indicator of the total body and intracellular potassium levels, and small alterations in serum potassium may reflect serious disruptions between intracellular and extracellular concentrations and distributions. In addition, potassium and hydrogen are exchangeable between the cell and extracellular fluid during acidosis and alkalosis. Serum potassium concentration abnormalities are clinically important because they occur in many sick animals and have a profound effect on the electrical properties of cell membranes.

Hypokalemia, defined as a serum potassium level below 3.5 mEq/L, manifests by generalized weakness of the skeletal and smooth muscle. Cardiac arrhythmias can also be observed. Causes of hypokalemia include protracted anorexia or tissue catabolism, chronic use of non-potassium-sparing diuretics, metabolic alkalosis (H^+ exits the cell to buffer alkalosis in exchange for entering K^+), insulin overdose, and dilutional hypokalemia from the overadministration of potassium-free fluids. Vomiting and diarrhea are major primary or secondary factors in causing hypokalemia (Table 1-5).

For example, a 6-year-old female dog with chronic, copious exudative drainage from an "open" pyometritis was examined. Other than cachexia and the drainage, the dog appeared well and was afebrile. Laboratory values for blood and urine tests were unremarkable except for moderate leukocytosis. Electrolytes were not measured. Surgery was recommended to remove the reproductive tract and intraoperative status was uneventful as she received a polyionic, isotonic solution (lactated Ringer's) during ovariohysterectomy. At 14 hours postoperatively, the animal became profoundly weak from muscle hypotonia and could not stand, even with assistance. The serum potassium level was 1.9

mEq/L. With potassium replacement therapy marked clinical improvement was noted.

Hyperkalemia exists when serum potassium is greater than 5.5 mEq/L; it becomes clinically important above 7.0 mEq/L because of the sustained depolarization of muscle cell membranes. As in hypokalemia, the initial sign of potassium intoxication is muscle weakness. Progressive hyperkalemia affects cardiac Purkinje tissue and causes bradycardia. Eventual third-degree heart block, with severe compromise of cardiac output, is a well-known feature of hyperkalemia. The causes of perioperative hyperkalemia include acute and chronic renal failure, acute obstructive uropathy, and the overuse of potassium-sparing diuretics with water and sodium overexcretion.

The treatment of hyperkalemia depends on the degree of immediate threat to life; the primary cause must be determined as rapidly as possible. Fluid therapy with isotonic saline can be used to dilute the excess potassium in moderate hyperkalemia. More severe cardiotoxicity with an idioventricular cardiac rhythm may require alkalinization with 0.5 mEq/kg of $NaHCO_3$ in 0.9 N NaCl given slowly. If response is poor, more aggressive resuscitation is a combined infusion of regular crystalline insulin and 50% dextrose. The rate for this mixture is 0.5 unit insulin/kg, with 2 ml of 50% dextrose/0.5 unit of insulin. In the absence of an obvious cause for hyperkalemia, acute adrenocortical insufficiency should be considered. This endocrinopathy is confirmed by a lowered Na^+:K^+ ratio, hypovolemia, and a rapid clinical response to fluid, glucocorticoid, and mineralocorticoid administration. It also is confirmed by a low plasma cortisol level in a blood specimen taken before hormone replacement therapy.

Chloride and Bicarbonate

The major circulating anions are chloride and bicarbonate. Chloride is quantitatively the major anion, but bicarbonate is critically important because of its immediate buffering capacity that helps protect a physiologic blood pH.

Acid-Base Balance in the Surgical Patient

Acid-base balance and blood-gas partial pressures are important because in surgical patients there often is primary or secondary injury or compromise to tissues and organs responsible for the maintenance of normal blood pH and oxygen and carbon dioxide transport. Reduced erythrocyte numbers and/or hemoglobin content, inadequate cardiac output or ventilation of the lungs, compromised alveolar/capillary gas exchange for the arterialization of venous blood, and renal oliguria or anuria may all contribute to acid-base or gas transport disorders.

An acid is any substance that can donate a hydrogen ion to a chemical reaction. Acidemia is a blood pH of less than 7.35. Acidosis is the clinical state resulting from pathologic accumulation of H^+ from acidemia. Metabolic acidosis results from a primary gain of H^+ or a loss or consumption of bicarbonate from extracellular fluid. Respiratory acidosis is an accumulation of H^+ resulting from primary reduction in alveolar ventilation relative to CO_2 production by tissues.

A base is a substance that accepts a hydrogen ion in a chemical reaction. Alkalemia is a pH of greater than 7.45. Alkalosis is a pathologic accumulation of hydrogen receptors. Metabolic alkalosis is a pathologic gain of bicarbonate or loss of acid from the extracellular fluid. Respiratory alkalosis results from a primary increase in alveolar ventilation relative to the rate of CO_2 production.

The role of the lung in maintaining normal pH is critical: it is the "quick response" organ to changes in blood pH.

Two essential equations are:

Equation 2)

$$CO_2 + H_2O \rightleftarrows H_2CO_3 \rightleftarrows H^+ + HCO_3^-$$
$$\text{(lung)} \qquad \text{(blood)} \qquad \text{(cell)}$$

Equation 3)

$$pH \sim \frac{[HCO_3]\ (base)}{[CO_2]\ (acid)} = \frac{20}{1}$$

Table 1–5. Guidelines to Fluid Selection

Lesion	Requirement	Suggested Best Fluid(s)	Comments
Dehydration, hemoconcentration	Water replacement	D5W	Insignificant number of calories from this concentration of carbohydrate
Hypovolemia	Rapid expansion of intravascular space. Isotonicity and physiologic balance of electrolytes desirable.	Lactated Ringer's or lactated Ringer's in D5W	Low-volume hypertonic IV solutions may have beneficial role in shock resuscitation.
Vomiting	Vomitus = 60 mEq/L Na$^+$, 15 mEq/L K$^+$, 120 mEq/L Cl$^-$, 0 mEq/L HCO$_3$$^-$. Replace water loss and metabolic alkalosis.	0.9 N NaCl. 0.45 N NaCl and D5W. 0.9 N NaCl + 20 mEq/L KCl	Add KCl if hypokalemic. K$^+$ supplementation requires controlled infusion rate.
Diarrhea	Diarrhea = 115 mEq/L Na$^+$, 18 mEq/L K$^+$, 70 mEq/L Cl$^-$. Correct metabolic acidosis if present.	Lactated Ringer's in D5W + 20 mEq/L KCl	K$^+$ solutions require controlled infusion. HCO$_3$$^-$ is not compatible with lactated Ringer's solution.
Burns	Same as diarrhea. May need colloid oncotic pressure supplementation.	As for diarrhea	May add buffer with HCO$_3$$^-$ precursors per base deficit. K$^+$ solutions require controlled infusion.
Severe metabolic acidosis	Add base buffer. Confirm renal function and liver perfusion.	Lactated Ringer's. 0.6 M Na lactate.	Bicarbonate therapy, if elected, should be slow and controlled.
Hypernatremia	Dilute sodium hypertonicity	D5W	
Hyponatremia	Na$^+$ replacement	0.9 N NaCl	Hyperchloremic metabolic acidosis can result from too-rapid administration of NaCl.
Hyperkalemia	Dilute potassium. Confirm renal function. Measure acid-base balance.	0.9 NaCl or 0.45 NaCl in D5W.	See text for use of alkalinization or insulin:dextrose infusion.
Hypokalemia	K$^+$ replacement	Lactated Ringer's with KCl added.	K$^+$ solutions require controlled infusion rates.
Hypocalcemia	Ca^{++} replacement	Calcium gluconate	Evaluate dietary intake of Ca^{++} or vitamin D. Endocrine and lactation status are considered.
Anemia	Erythrocytes/hemoglobin	Whole blood. Packed cells, fresh or banked.	—
Hypoproteinemia	Plasma proteins	Stored plasma	—
Clotting factors	Plasma procoagulant factors and platelets	Fresh whole blood Fresh plasma Fresh frozen plasma Cryoprecipitate	—

Table 1–5. Guidelines to Fluid Selection (*continued*)

Lesion	Requirement	Suggested Best Fluid(s)	Comments
Reduction in colloid oncotic pressure	Elevation of oncotic pressure	Albumin, canine or human Plasma Low molecular weight dextran Hetastarch	Upper dose limits of dextran and hetastarch must be strictly observed.
Postoperative fluid maintenance after major surgery; fasting or anorexia	Meet water requirements. Balanced replacement of electrolytes. Potassium supplementation frequently needed.	Lactated Ringer's with K$^+$ supplementation. Potassium-enriched commercial maintenance solutions.	Formula for "homemade" fluid: 1 L lactated Ringer's plus 2 L D5W plus 20 mEq KCl
Disseminated intravascular coagulation	Reestablish perfusion of microcirculation. Arrest spontaneous clotting.	Lactated Ringer's. Low molecular weight dextran.	Subcutaneous "mini-dose" heparin for antithrombin activity.
Deliver intravenous drugs	Carrier must be compatible with the drug.	Consult drug compatability table or package insert.	

In equation 2, it can be seen that acids from cellular metabolism are buffered by combining with bicarbonate. A weakly dissociated carbonic acid is immediately formed in the blood stream for transport of the metabolic acid to the lung. At the lung, carbon dioxide is released from carbonic acid and is exhaled. Upon release of carbon dioxide, the reformation of HCO_3 replenishes the buffer supply so the cycle of hydrogen ion pick-up, neutralization, and elimination may continue. In this way, carbon dioxide exhalation is the primary means for removing metabolic acids, and the lung excretes about one thousand times more acid than any other organ.

Equation 3 indicates that a *fixed* ratio exists between the metabolic and respiratory control components. This ratio is fixed because it is based on the physical dissociation constant for carbonic acid; changes in one component will affect the other. These interchangeable yet independent compensatory mechanisms between respiratory and metabolic buffering are of major importance in compensating for pH changes that are beyond physiologic ranges. This is because *either* the respiratory or metabolic component can be activated through *retention* or *excretion* of CO_2 or

HCO_3^- to keep the 20:1 ratio and, therefore, the pH intact. As an example, if carbon dioxide is lost in excess through hyperventilation, the kidney compensates by eliminating bicarbonate into the urine.

Figure 1-3 provides a summary of primary pH abnormalities and compensations. When interpreting the results of a pH and blood-gas analysis, it is important to remember that mixed respiratory and metabolic disorders and compensations can exist.

Interpretation of Blood-Gas Studies

A rapid qualitative interpretation of pH and blood-gas values can be done as follows. Obtain an arterial or venous blood specimen collected anaerobically. Venous pH and bicarbonate are adequate for acid-base status; however, arterial samples are preferable and are required for blood oxygen tensions. Percutaneous arterial puncture in the dog is often performed where the femoral artery can be palpated directly over the femoral diaphysis. With the artery firmly immobilized against the bone by the finger and the overlying skin pulled taut, the artery is entered with a 22- to

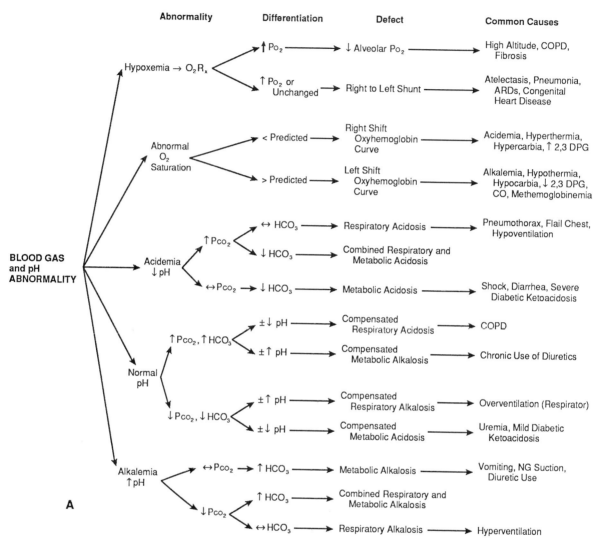

Figure 1-3.

A, *Primary and compensatory changes in blood gas and acid-base disorders and a partial list of etiologic agents (Otto C. Surgical decision making. 2nd ed. Philadelphia: W.B. Saunders, 1986:3)* (continued)

25-gauge needle. One to two ml of blood is collected into a glass or plastic syringe, the barrel of which has been rinsed with heparin. During aspiration, no air should enter the syringe. The cranial tibial artery can also be used in dogs over 20 kg.

During abdominal surgery, it is possible to take a specimen directly from any major abdominal artery, such as the splenic. During neck surgery, the carotid arteries are immediately available. During orthopedic surgery, concern about the patient's acid-base or blood-gas status may require deviation from the fracture fixation to identify an adjacent artery or vein. If a suitable artery is not available, venous blood from a lingual vein may be substituted. The sample is capped with a rubber stopper and processed as soon as possible.

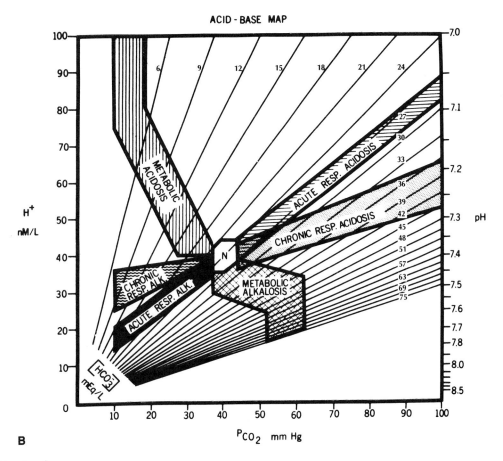

ACID - BASE MAP

Figure 1-3 (*continued*)
B, *An acid-base map is a useful aid in determining the primary classification and chronic compensations for blood pH changes. (Levine RD. Anesthesiology. Philadelphia: JB Lippincott, 1984:79)*

The following steps allow a rapid qualitative interpretation of the returned information:

1. Determine if the pH is acidic or alkaline. This is the most important value in determining the animal's acid-base status and serves as the base point for a trend line. The further the deviation from pH 7.40 ± 0.05, the greater the need for intervention.
2. Determine the $PaCO_2$. Respiratory alkalosis exists if the $PaCO_2$ is less than 35 torr; respiratory acidosis exists if it is greater than 50 torr.
3. Determine the bicarbonate levels. Metabolic alkalosis exists if the bicarbonate

level is greater than 27 mEq/L; metabolic acidosis exists if it is less than 23 mEq/L.

4. From the values of the pH, $PaCO_2$, and bicarbonate, the primary metabolic or respiratory contributions to the primary pH change can be determined. From these values, it is further determined if a mixed disturbance or chronic compensation exists for the primary problem. Acid-base maps are of assistance in this process of determining acute versus chronic (compensated) lesions.

5. If blood oxygen has been measured, a PaO_2 of less than 60 torr is defined as hypoxemia.

If a blood-gas machine with a blood pH electrode is unavailable, clinically useful information can be obtained by determining total blood CO_2. This value is less expensive to determine. Serum CO_2 less than 18 mEq/L is by itself suggestive of metabolic acidosis or respiratory alkalosis.

An adjunct to the interpretation of the blood–gas information is the calculated *base excess*. The base excess value, available from the blood–gas nomogram, is an index expressing the buffering contribution from bicarbonate and other blood-buffering components and relating them to the pH. The degree of the negative or a positive-base "excess" indicates the buffering capacity deficit or surplus. A base "excess" in negative numbers implies a base deficit, lack of buffering capacity, and true nonrespiratory acidosis.

An additional adjunct to the interpretation of acid-base disturbances is the *anion gap*, which is calculated as follows:

Equation 4)
$$\text{Anion gap (mEq/L)} = (\text{sodium} + \text{potassium}) - (\text{chloride} + \text{bicarbonate})$$

The word "gap" is used in this relationship because the normal sum of the measured anions is less than the sum of the measured cations (even though the total of all cations and anions must be equal to maintain electrical neutrality). The normal anion gap, using the

electrolytes mentioned above, is 10 to 14 mEq/L. Increases in the anion gap often represent metabolic acidosis, and a "high anion gap" acidosis will further confirm a negative base excess and indicates a primary consumption of bicarbonate. However, acidosis with a normal anion gap often indicates hyperchloremia.

Correction of Dehydration, Electrolyte, and Acid-Base Disturbances

Perioperative fluid therapy is very important in total patient management. Correction of volume, compositional, and concentration disturbances always yields better surgical homeostasis. Even if the animal is a Class I or II risk patient with normal or near-normal physiologic fluid balance before surgery, fluids are given to replace blood loss and evaporation from exposed surfaces, to deliver drugs if needed, to provide an immediate access to the vascular system, and to keep the circulation in a state of slight volume expansion. The latter is important because maintaining cardiac preload helps negate the depression of myocardial contractility that occurs under anesthesia. The generalized vasodilatation of anesthesia also leads to hypotension.

Oral fluid replacement is preferred, but is frequently an unavailable route in acute medical and surgical conditions. Subcutaneous administration of an isotonic hydrating and/or electrolyte solution is convenient and effective if the required quantities are not too large. An individual "bleb" of hypodermoclysis should not exceed 75 ml in a medium-size dog. Intravenous therapy is required for large volumes of fluid, as in resuscitation from shock, in severe degrees of dehydration, or when hypertonic fluids will be required.

Selection of Fluid

Because the sugar in 5% dextrose in water (D5W) is metabolized, leaving pure water, this fluid is selected for simple rehydration. Unless other specific deficiencies exist, hyperventilating patients and those with fever should receive D5W. However, hyperventilation may also be in response to metabolic acidosis or hemorrhage.

Balanced, polyionic, isotonic, crystalloid solutions are the replacement fluids of choice for isotonic fluid losses such as from hemorrhage or wound transudate. Lactated Ringer's solution is popular for this purpose and provides lactate anion, an HCO_3^- precursor, to maintain buffer capacity. Normal saline is substituted for lactated Ringer's when metabolic alkalosis is associated with acute severe vomiting and other causes of hyponatremia and/or hypochloremia. When the patient is hyperkalemic, sodium chloride or sodium chloride in dextrose is the fluid of choice. When cardiotoxic levels of serum potassium and urea (obstructive uropathy) are present, 0.9 N or 0.45 N sodium chloride or 0.6 M sodium lactate is selected.

Sodium lactate provides a significant level of bicarbonate precursor and is safer than direct administration of bicarbonate. Table 1-5 presents additional information on fluid selection.

Rate of Fluid Replacement

Daily maintenance volume for water in dogs and cats is 40 to 60 ml/kg/day. In dehydration, the replacement volume for water deficit is calculated in the following manner:

Equation 5)
Replacement volume (L) = wt (kg) $\times$ dehydration (%)

For example, for a 20-kg dog with 6% dehydration, 20×0.06 equals 1.4 liters, or 1,200 ml.

For the total daily fluid dose, the maintenance volume is added to the replacement dose requirements. Fluid losses from exudation, transudation, or diuresis are then added to this sum for a guideline to the quantity of fluid administration.

Baseline postoperative fluids are given at 40 to 60 ml/kg/24 hours daily for maintenance requirements if the animal has not returned to oral alimentation. In the presence of normal cardiopulmonary status, the rate of fluid administration should repair acute volume and electrolyte deficits rather rapidly, up to one third of the calculated dose over the initial two to three hours. The remainder of the repair and maintenance volume is then given over the next 24 hours, unless immediate surgical intervention is required. In the latter case, more of the total volume will be provided before anesthesia is induced. For patients with a history of mitral insufficiency, congestive heart failure, or clinical signs of cardiac compromise such as murmurs or arrhythmias, the rate of volume replacement must be more conservative. In these instances, 75% of the total estimated correction should be provided in the first 24 hours, with complete correction by 48 hours after therapy is initiated. Alternatively, a "fluid challenge" with central venous pressure (CVP) monitoring may be used to correct the fluid deficit more quickly.

A true syndrome of *volume excess,* particularly in the older postoperative patient with a compromised cardiovascular system, does exist. Although the otherwise normal animal can tolerate an acute volume overexpansion extremely well, the less compliant or efficient cardiovascular system may decompensate into pulmonary edema due to excess fluid volume, fluid rate, or sodium administration. To help prevent iatrogenic waterlogging, a "mini-drip" (60 drops/ml) drop counter is used to regulate more precisely the delivery of fluids in small dogs and cats and in those with a compromised cardiovascular system. Sodium-restricted fluids are also used. For the patient in Classes III to V and with heart disease, the CVP may guide the rate of fluid administration. After placing a central venous catheter near the right atrium, two baseline CVP measurements are taken and averaged. During the rapid volume expansion of a patient with suspected or confirmed cardiovascular disease, a rise of 5 cm of water or more above the baseline value is an indication to stop the infusion and wait until the CVP returns to within 2 cm of water of the initial CVP. Then the infusion is resumed, but more slowly. Improving cardiac performance with dobutamine or other ionotropic agents may allow rapid volume expansion by alleviating the risk of overloading the cardiovascular system.

Administering fluids through an intravenous catheter during surgery is important, with fluid dripping at 10 ml/kg/hr. Fluid is given to replace blood losses at a 3:1 ratio. For the estimate of blood loss, a saturated 4×4 gauze sponge contains about 15 ml of blood. If the fluid in a surgical suction jar is opaque, the PCV is greater than 5%.

Surgery in the Medically Compromised Patient

Shock and Multiple Organ Failure

The clinical and experimental study of hypovolemic, cardiogenic, and endotoxic shock is a fascinating aspect of surgical history. The currently unifying concept of shock is that the various etiologies and causative agents of shock converge to a final common pathway that produces cell and organ devitalization. This final common pathway is the hypoperfusion of microcirculation, which leads to tissue hypoxemia and cellular organelle and membrane dysfunction. At the biochemical level, aerobic ATP production in the cytochrome oxidase-electron transport chain fails to meet cell energy requirements under hypoxic conditions. The lack of ATP results in disruption of cell housekeeping functions such as maintaining electrochemical gradients via active ion pumps, enzyme and protein synthesis, membrane porosity and selectivity, and loss of cell reproduction. If intervention does not occur to restore oxygen substrate for aerobic energy metabolism, there can be broad-scale homeostatic failure of the cell.

A working definition of shock, then, is the devitalization of energy production and other metabolic dysfunction on a cellular and organ system basis secondary to hypoxemic injury from any cause.

Etiologies of Shock

Hypovolemic Shock

Hypovolemia can occur from hemorrhage to outside of the body or within the body but out of the vascular compartment. An acute 35% hemorrhage produces shock; an acute 60% hemorrhage is usually fatal. Frequently seen clinical examples of hypovolemia result from the circulating blood volume lost into the hematoma surrounding most comminuted fractures, or hemothorax or hemoabdomen from a traumatically disrupted viscus. Other causes of hypovolemia include volume depletion through dehydration and "third space sequestration" of fluid into compartments that are removed from the *effective* circulation. As mentioned previously, a large number of compensatory volume preservation responses, such as reduced glomerular blood flow and oliguria, transcapillary refill from the extracellular space into the intravascular space and retention of Na^+, will help to preserve the circulating volume. These compensatory mechanisms are aided by the intense splanchnic vasoconstriction at the precapillary arterioles and postcapillary venules. After vasoconstriction and hypoxemic injury, visceral pooling occurs as the precapillary arterioles relax, but the postcapillary venules remain constricted. At this point, the hypoperfusion and hypoxemia in the now engorged and sluggish microcirculation is even worse than before. Further deterioration of perfusion occurs with the subsequent opening of arteriovenous shunts around the engorged capillary beds. Unfortunately, this bypass of the capillary bed may persist even if cardiac output is returned to normal. During this process, endothelial integrity is lost and protein-rich fluids begin to leak from small vessels. This event further compounds hypoperfusion by the loss of volume and colloid oncotic pressure from the intravascular space.

The terms "reversible" and "irreversible" shock have been historically used to describe the possibility of resuscitation from shock. Following the creation of a standardized, experimental shock model, the demarcation between the two was previously based on the period of time after which a given infusion of blood or crystalloid fluid could restore circulation and prevent death. The definition of irreversibility would be that point after which cell devitalization was so complete that repair of the enzyme systems and organelles necessary for normal energy production could not occur, even with a restoration of normal oxygen substrates.

Cardiogenic Shock

Inadequate cardiac output, despite normal blood volume and cardiac-filling pressures, is termed cardiogenic shock. Because coronary artery disease is infrequent in companion animals, cardiogenic shock due to myocardial infarction is uncommon in veterinary medicine. However, persistent low cardiac output for a variety of other reasons is a potential cause of shock and is quite common in animals. In assessing "pump failure," one should consider the degree of ventricular filling (preload), the contractility forces that the ventricular myocardial fibers can develop, and heart rate and rhythm. Management of the condition is by removing or reducing the cause of the low cardiac output. This may require therapy for arrhythmia control, positive inotropic pharmaceuticals, or removal of the obstruction to venous return to the heart.

Septic Shock

Infection is common in veterinary patients and takes many forms: extensive skin pyoderma, cellulitis/abscess, osteomyelitis, dental infection, endocarditis, urinary tract infections, peritonitis, pyothorax, etc. The many factors leading to wound contamination, the transition from tissue contamination to established aerobic and anaerobic infection, and the characteristics of gram-positive exotoxemias and gram-negative endotoxemias, are covered in Chapter 3, The Surgical Wound.

In infection, the host defenses must neutralize the microorganisms and their endotoxic or exotoxic products. If host defenses such as complement, antibodies, and phagocytes do not destroy bacteria and neutralize exotoxins and/or endotoxins, these toxins cause primary structural and metabolic cell damage. The effect of endotoxins on the circulation is also profound, with loss of tone, resistance, and integrity in small vessels of the splanchnic circulation in particular. This results in peripheral pooling and loss of effective circulatory volume. Microcirculatory hypoxemia, microthrombosis, hypoxia, acidosis, and release of vasoactive substances can occur within minutes after the onset of endotoxemia, setting the stage for multiple organ failure.

Septic, endotoxic shock typically begins with an initial, transient, "hyperdynamic" response phase, characterized by increased cardiac output, hyperventilation and its associated respiratory alkalosis, and low peripheral vascular resistance. At this stage, however, onset of impaired cellular metabolism prevents the normal utilization of oxygen and energy substrates for the production of ATP. A "hypodynamic" phase ensues shortly thereafter, with increased vascular pooling, hypoperfusion, and the onset of capillary fluid leakage. With fluid loss, decreased cardiac output and circulatory stasis occurs, perpetuating the destructive cycle.

Vasculogenic Shock

Trapped blood within the vascular space causes hypoperfusion and decreased cardiac return. This maldistribution of circulatory volume caused by peripheral pooling may be seen after central nervous system trauma and epidural anesthesia, which may cause vasodilatation. In the dog, anaphylactic reactions release vasoactive substances that cause hepatic venules and veins to constrict, leading to sequestration of blood in the portal circulation. Obstruction of pulmonary venous return occurs from air emboli or thromboemboli in the pulmonary circulation. Obstruction of the vena cavae by heartworms, pericardial tamponade or effusion, gastric dilatation-volvulus, too long an inspiratory cycle and/or too high an intrathoracic pressure during positive-pressure ventilation also inhibit filling of central veins and the right atrium.

Combined Shock

In some clinical conditions, several etiologies combine to produce shock. For example, generalized peritonitis due to gastrointestinal tract leakage manifests as both endotoxemia and hypovolemia. In the gastric dilatation-volvulus syndrome, vasculogenic shock will occur from the obstruction of the caudal vena cava; chances are very high that additional endotoxic, cardiogenic, and hypovolemic shock will occur. Clinical and laboratory features of shock are summarized in Table 1-6.

Management of Shock

Management of Hypovolemic Shock

Management of shock is individualized and depends on the cause and duration. The adequacy of the circulatory volume and pressures at initial examination, laboratory findings, and evidence of single or multiple organ failure are of major concern. If the cause of shock is unknown, a physical examination and diagnosis should be performed as resuscitative treatment is initiated. A flow chart that tracks several observations simultaneously on a time line is an essential tool for organizing and analyzing observations and therapy, because information gleaned from response to therapy and monitoring trends becomes important in determining overall response and prognosis. Such therapy and monitoring requires considerable attention from professional and paraprofessional staff and is frequently very expensive in terms of costs for professional services, drugs, and supplies.

If simple isotonic fluid losses have resulted in hypovolemia and hypoperfusion, ex-

Table 1–6. Classification/Features of Shock in Dogs and Cats

	Venous Return	Central Venous Pressure	Blood Pressure, Urine Output	Cardiac Output	Peripheral Vascular Resistance	Capillary Refill Time
Hypovolemic shock (Blood/fluid loss)						
35% Acute blood loss → shock	↓	↓	↓	↓	↑	↑
60% Acute blood loss → fatality						
Endotoxic/Septic shock (Uncontrolled infection)						
(Early stage)	↓	↑ or (N)	↑	↑↑	↓	↑
(Late stage)	↓	↓	↓	↓	↑	↑
Cardiogenic shock (Prolonged, substantial reductions of cardiac output)	↓	↑ or ↑↑	↓	↓↓	↑	↑
Vasculogenic shock with sequestration of fluid. Opening of capacitance vessels. Obstruction of caval return	↓	↑ or ↑↑ (Elevated in caval obstruction syndrome)	↓	↓	↓	↑

A = Abnormal
N = Normal
E = Early
L = Late
V = Variable

pansion of the intravascular space is the *first and most essential* step in returning volumes, pressures, flows, and microcapillary perfusion to normal. In acute shock, except for cardiogenic shock, bolus administration of crystalloid fluids is provided at 90 ml/kg in 20 to 30 minutes. In the cat, this volume is limited to 50 ml/kg. Recent clinical research has also suggested benefit from 5 ml/kg of hypertonic (7%) NaCl in initial resuscitation. However, this alternative has not been extensively tested or employed clinically.

After the rapid volume expansion, pharmacologic doses of synthetic glucocorticoids are indicated because they relax postcapillary venular sphincter constrictions. This step may reduce capillary pooling and improve flow and perfusion. Stabilizing the membranes of intra-cellular lysosomes and other organelles is an additional effect of glucocorticoids in high doses. Combined bactericidal antibiotics are begun by intravenous drip for wide-spectrum coverage against both aerobic and anaerobic species. Concurrent with these resuscitative efforts, first aid or definitive treatment for the original cause of the shock is begun and monitoring is initiated.

If severe acidosis is present due to prolonged hypoperfusion, blood pH, bicarbonate, or total carbon dioxide values are desirable to allow calculation of the base excess. Therapy for buffer deficit is based upon the formula:

Equation 6)
$$\text{Buffer needed mEq/L} = 0.5 \times \text{body weight} \times \text{base excess}$$

Color of Mucous Membranes	Respiratory Minute Volume	Erythrocyte Packed Cell Volume	Plasma Protein Concentration	Urinalysis	Blood pH	PaO₂
Pink (E) Pale (L)	Tachypnea (E) ↑	↑ or (E) ↓ (L)	↓	N	→ (E) ↓ (L)	↓
Red "injected" "muddy"	↑	N	→ or ↑	N Unless primary sepsis in urinary tract	↓	↓
Pale, cyanotic or gray	↑ or → Breathing rapid but shallow	↑ or (N)		A	↓	↓
Pink, pale or gray (V)	↑	N	N	N	↓	↓
Usually pale (V)	↑	(N) or ↓	(N) or ↓	V	↓	↓

This dose of bicarbonate or bicarbonate precursor is added to a separate drip so that only half the calculated dose of bicarbonate is provided at the initial resuscitation; the remainder is given over the next 12 hours or as guided by blood pH and base deficit trends. Giving sodium bicarbonate too rapidly, especially in bolus form, can have the undesirable side effects of producing iatrogenic alkalosis, hypokalemia, hypernatremia, and paradoxical acidosis of the cerebrospinal fluid.

A favorable resuscitation from hypovolemic shock clinically shows a reduction in tachypnea and tachycardia, the return of an improved pulse wave, and resumption of urine output. Vasoconstriction in the superficial capillary beds of the gingiva decreases and mucous membrane color improves, indicating that hemodynamic perfusion is returning to normal. Because catecholamine-induced splenic contraction causes the release of large quantities of erythrocytes into the circulation (PCV about 70%), and due to the lag phase in transcapillary refill of extracellular water into the vascular spaces, the true erythrocyte quantity lost as hemorrhage may not be measurable for an hour or more. Initial PCV measurements may be normal, or even elevated, in an animal bleeding to death! Therefore, serialized PCV measurements are essential to avoid a false sense of security about the magnitude of the hemorrhage. If the PCV acutely falls to 15 to 25 percent, whole blood transfusion therapy is usually indicated.

Blood Transfusion

Providing fresh whole blood, banked whole blood, concentrated erythrocytes, and fresh frozen plasma is well within the capability of most veterinary hospitals; it requires the maintenance of donor animals and blood-storage facilities.

The ideal blood donor is large, tractable, in good health, and free of any blood-borne disease or parasite. The animal's blood may be repeatedly harvested from the jugular vein, but at least two weeks should elapse between donations. Ideally, donors can maintain packed cell volumes between 45 and 55 percent before their next donation, and donor blood should be used for fresh transfusion purposes only when the hematocrit of the donor is 40% or higher. Blood grouping is of some importance, and antigenic factor A should be confirmed as negative for a prospective donor animal. These tests are available at some commercial veterinary laboratories. Harvesting of blood is by a 15-gauge needle into prepackaged blood collection packs; siliconized needles, tubing, and acid-citrate dextrose solutions contained in collapsible plastic pouches are ideal.

The blood can be used immediately as a fresh transfusion, can be refrigerated for use as fresh blood within 20 to 25 days, or processed into blood components. The most common components are plasma and "packed" (concentrated) erythrocytes. These two components are separated by centrifugation or, less desirably, by gravity sedimentation. The supernatant plasma is transferred to a separate storage bag through a transfer tubing system designed for the purpose. This process is assisted by a simple flat device that squeezes the plasma fraction toward the top of the bag and the transfer tubing. The result is fresh plasma, which can be given to improve oncotic pressure, expand volume, treat hypoproteinemia, and provide passive antibody protection and, perhaps, clotting factors. It can also be frozen and used up to one year later. The concentrated packed cell fraction is available to replace cells when volume expansion is not a concurrent requirement. Unfortunately, fresh whole blood is a reliable carrier for oxygen for only 24 hours, during which time the enzyme 2,3 DPG undergoes rapid degradation. However, 2,3, DPG can be regenerated within the erythrocytes after their transfusion for up to 20 to 25 days. Therefore, the useful life of banked fresh blood is about three weeks, after which plasma can be harvested and frozen.

Before transfusing a patient, the donor erythrocytes are tested for compatibility with the serum of the intended recipient by crossmatching. In this test, the patient's serum is mixed with washed erythrocytes from the prospective donor and samples are incubated at 4°, 25°, and 37°C for at least 30 minutes. The mixture is then centrifuged into a cell button that is resuspended by gentle shaking. The mixture is observed for clumping or agglutination; absence of clumping suggests that the transfusion will be compatible. In gross incompatibility, the agglutination may occur rapidly. Subtle blood group and immune incompatibilities may be detected only by more sophisticated testing.

After confirming cross-matched compatibility of fresh whole blood or packed erythrocytes, the transfusion is best administered intravenously through a large-bore intravenous cannula to reduce hemolysis. If banked blood is used after refrigeration, it should be gently warmed before use and administered through an in-line filter to remove the large number of platelet/erythrocyte/fibrin microaggregates that accumulate during storage.

In addition to erythrocytes and plasma fractions, it is also possible to prepare cryoprecipitate and platelet-rich fractions that are specific for treatment of coagulation defects. The reader is referred to the references for details of these techniques.

Management of Cardiogenic Shock

In cardiogenic shock, fluid loss is not the problem; the heart needs more effective pumping rather than more preload. Thus, if adequate volume exists, much practical information can be gained by serially examining the pulse rate and characteristics, blood pressure, central venous pressure, and the electrocardiogram. Low cardiac output can often be improved dramatically if it is due to a correctable cardiac arrhythmia or if there is myocardial compromise that will respond to positive inotropic therapy. For the former, a bolus of lidocaine (1 to 2 mg/kg IV) is required for serious ventricular arrhythmias. For the latter, the positive cardiac inotropic effect of dobutamine infusions (5 to 10 μg/kg/min) is considered useful.

Management of Septic Shock and Multiple Organ Failure

Four primary goals in managing septic shock are to remove the source of the sepsis, maintain nutritional support for any failing organ(s), correct acidosis, and restore tissue perfusion by vascular volume expansion. Removing the source of sepsis often requires emergency surgery in very nonoptimal circumstances. Providing intensive intravenous antibiotic therapy with broad-spectrum bactericidal agents and using supraphysiologic doses of water-soluble dexamethasone phosphate (2 mg/kg IV) or prednisolone sodium succinate (10 mg/kg IV) early in treatment after volume expansion are also useful to combat bacteremia and to support the failing intracellular metabolic and protein synthetic processes.

In addition to glucocorticoids, positive inotropic agents such as dopamine or dobutamine are considered adjuncts to intravascular volume expansion to support the circulation during hypodynamic phases of septic shock. Volume expansion is initiated with crystalloids, but colloid oncotic pressure maintenance, with fresh plasma or canine-origin albumin, may be needed as colloid intravascular oncotic pressure drops through capillary leakage of protein-rich fluid. The rationale for using colloids is that they maintain oncotic pressure and, thus, tend to retard fluid loss through endothelia. Human-origin albumin solution can be substituted for canine albumin and is cheaper. Synthetic plasma expansion agents maintain intravascular oncotic pressure, are large enough molecules not to be readily lost through leaky endothelium, and are nonantigenic/hypoallergenic. They include carbohydrate polymers (starches such as Hetastarch) and low and high molecular weight dextrans. The upper dose limits of 30 ml/kg synthetic colloids such as low molecular weight dextran should not be exceeded.

Monitoring should be frequent and focused because the deleterious effects of septic shock can progress quickly (in minutes) once the bloodstream is septic with bacteria and/or endotoxins. Support of an effective cardiovascular system and circulation is extremely important in maintaining the delivery of oxygen and carbohydrate substrates. This is especially true once the hyperdynamic phase is replaced by hypodynamic perfusion.

In the dog, the primary "shock organ" is the gastrointestinal tract, and manifestations include mucosal distress and sloughing. Unfortunately, another organ prone to failure after endotoxic shock is the lung. This usually occurs after the episode of gastrointestinal system distress. Ideally, respiratory support would include taking thoracic radiographs for the initial radiographic appearance of the lung fields and the monitoring of blood gases if possible. The onset of the respiratory distress syndrome (RDS) is seen as part of generalized injury responses. Features of RDS that make it difficult to manage include the loss of surfactant production from alveolar macrophages and the loss of pulmonary compliance and efficient ventilation.

As alveolar and capillary injury progresses, alveoli fill with proteinaceous transudate. These deposits "hyalinize" the blood-exchange surface to inhibit gas transport across alveolar and interstitial membranes to the capillaries, thereby reducing blood arterialization. The first sign of pulmonary failure is tachypnea. Oxygen therapy by nasal catheter, frequent changes in the patient's position, and antibiotics and steroids should be given at this time (Table 1-7). Progressive alveolar fluid infiltration, determined by thoracic radiographs, is characteristic of RDS pneumonia. If progressive alveolar and interstitial consolidation of the lung increases, the mismatch between aerated alveoli and perfused capillaries in the lung leads to further deterioration of arterialization with increased hypercapnia and hypoxemia. If circumstances permit, referral for tracheostomy and ventilator management with intermittent or continuous positive end expiratory pressure could be considered. Maintaining both a central venous pressure at 8 to 10 cm of water and adequate hemoglobin concentrations, perhaps by administering packed cells, will also be needed to ensure adequate oxygen delivery to peripheral tissues. The essential concepts are to prevent this syndrome from developing by early, adequate support and to act early and aggressively if multiple organ failure or RDS appears.

Management of Vasculogenic Shock

Obstruction to caval venous return by gastric dilatation-volvulus, acute pericardial tamponade, restrictive pericarditis/epicarditis or "caval syndrome" due to heartworm emboli can cause severe splanchnic and peripheral pooling. Correcting the mechanical obstruction is more important than any other treatment. Functional vasculogenic shock occurs from anaphylactic reactions, which in dogs usually respond to pharmacologic therapy and volume expansion with crystalloid solution. Consolidated suggestions for drug therapy in shock are presented in Table 1-7.

Surgical Hemostasis and Coagulopathy

Normal flow of blood through all sizes of arteries, veins, and capillary beds is made possible by the equilibrium between thrombin-mediated reactions, which cause blood to clot, and plasmin- mediated reactions, which maintain blood fluidity and lyse fibrin polymer. Spontaneous intravascular thrombosis would clearly be fatal, yet coagulation of blood is an essential survival mechanism in injury and trauma. Both intrinsic and extrinsic factors can initiate the final normal common pathway of blood coagulation, shown in Figure 1-4.

The intrinsic system is activated by traumatic exposure of the subendothelial layer of the vessel wall. This initiating event leads to a series of integrated reactions between the vessel wall, plasma procoagulant factors of the intrinsic cascade, and platelets. Platelets become activated and a platelet plug forms, enlarges, and stabilizes at the end of the transected vessel. Later, the platelet plug is replaced with a fibrin seal. When hemostasis is no longer needed, the process continues with subsequent fibrinolysis and angiogenesis in the injured area.

Clotting can be initiated not only by processes associated with the vessel wall, but also by products released from damaged tissue outside the vessel. Activated tissue thromboplastin, a tissue protein, can initiate the final clotting cascade in the injured area. The surgical importance of normal hemostasis is that for every vessel tied or cauterized by the surgeon, literally thousands of smaller ones will be transected, but will spontaneously clot and then repair themselves. In abnormal hemostasis, however, many of these small vessels will

not stop bleeding and will contribute to excessive blood loss.

Causes of abnormal hemostasis include qualitative and quantitative platelet disorders, lack of circulating procoagulant factors such as fibrinogen, and inappropriate overactivation of the plasmin-mediated fibrinolytic system. The lack of circulating procoagulant factors is usually due to liver disease. Platelet function disorders and thrombocytopenia can seriously inhibit surgical hemostasis, and platelet deficiency is the most frequent cause of surgical coagulopathy. The normal platelet count is 150,000 to 400,000/ml, or 3 to 5 megakaryocytes per HPF on the CBC's blood smear. Platelet counts below 50,000/ml are associated

Table 1–7. Pharmacologic Treatment of Shock

Category	Drug	Dose	Comments
Colloid oncotic pressure expander	10% LMW dextran in D5W	10–30 ml/kg/IV	May cause bleeding. Respect upper dose limit.
Antibiotics	Gentamicin Kanamycin Na⁺ Penicillin Ampicillin Cefoxitin	4 mg/kg/QID IM 10 mg/kg/QID IM 10,000 units/kg q 2h IV 22 mg/kg/QID IV 22 mg/kg/TID IV	Confirm renal function first.
Corticosteroids	Dexamethasone phosphate Prednisolone sodium succinate	2 mg/kg/IV >10 mg/kg IV	
Positive ionotropic agents	Dopamine Dobutamine	2–15 µg/kg/min IV drip 3–10 µg/kg/min IV drip	AVOID DIGOXIN.
Ventricular antiarrthmia therapy (PVC's)	Lidocaine Procainamide	2–4 mg/kg/IV 4–8 mg/kg/5 min IV	Bolus therapy 2× only in 30 min. Lidocaine or procainamide drip may be needed for refractory arrhythmia.
Metabolic acidosis	Sodium bicarbonate or lactate	See Table 1–5.	
Osmotic diuresis	20% mannitol	0.5–2.0 mg/kg IV	
Tubular diuretic	Furosemide	1.0–2.0 mg/kg IV	
Hypoxemia	Oxygen	100–125 ml/kg/min yields inspired O₂ concentration of 40%.	Delivered by nasal catheter placed in nasopharynx. Assisted ventilation, controlled ventilation may be needed.*

* Consult appropriate reference texts.

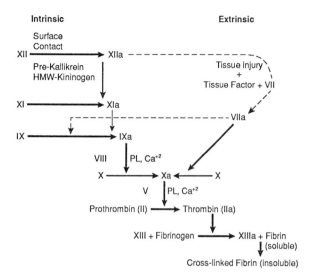

Figure 1-4. *The normal blood coagulation pathway. Once activated by either extrinsic (tissue factor) or intrinsic (surface contact XIIa) triggers, the coagulation cascade proceeds by activation of circulatory procoagulants proteins and cofactors. Factor Xa to the final fibrin polymer is considered the final common pathway. (Sabiston DC, ed. Essentials of surgery. Philadelphia: WB Saunders)*

with increased surgical bleeding; platelet counts less than 20,000/ml are associated with spontaneous bleeding. These platelet numbers are encountered in dogs with medically unresponsive autoimmune hemolytic anemia (AIHA), severe bone marrow megakaryocyte hypoplasia, and generalized aplastic anemias. However, some patients with chronic AIHA and platelet counts around 50,000 ml may still show adequate operative hemostasis because the platelets that are present are very young and hemostatically competent. Conversely, patients treated with prostaglandin inhibitors (aspirin or flunixin) and those with uremia or primary platelet function disorders may have normal platelet numbers but may experience deficient hemostasis.

Low platelet numbers are also seen as a component of the disseminated intravascular coagulation (DIC) syndrome, a common disorder of hemostasis characterized by inappropriate intravascular thrombosis. DIC is a very serious threat to the patient's health because the thrombosis compromises microvascular perfusion of organs, and the aberrant coagulation consumes clotting factors, making them unavailable for appropriate hemostatic requirements elsewhere. Paradoxically, the patient is afflicted with generalized intravascular clotting and microvessel thrombosis, yet often bleeds freely into body cavities, wounds, or surgical incisions.

The cause of DIC is the unregulated formation of active thrombin from prothrombin. The possible precipitating clinical events for thrombin activation are multiple; thromboplastic substances are released from tissue necrosis as in acute hemorrhagic pancreatitis, gastric dilatation-volvulus syndrome, local or generalized peritonitis with or without bacteremia, serious prolonged infections, polytrauma, heat stroke, extensive neoplasia, poisonings and envenomations, shock of any etiology, and other injury. Prolonged and difficult orthopedic operations and obstetrical labors have also precipitated the syndrome in animals. It is also important to realize that DIC can "smolder" in a chronic, subclinical form. Lowered fibrinogen and platelet levels, prolonged clotting times, and the presence of fibrin degradation products are characteristic clinicopathologic features of the syndrome.

Von Willebrand's disease is an inherited coagulopathic defect caused by the lack of von Willebrand's factor, a protein found in the subintimal portions of the vessel wall that augments the adhesion of the forming and stabilizing platelet plug to the damaged vessel. The level of the protein can be determined in selected laboratories. Von Willebrand's disease occurs with some frequency in purebred Doberman pinschers and less frequently in other breeds. Bleeding defects range from mild to quite serious, depending on the level of protein depletion.

A practical way to screen for a coagulopathy is to measure the bleeding time, a test that evaluates the total hemostatic capability in general and platelet function in particular. The bleeding time is measured by amputating a toenail at midpoint to initiate cuticle bleeding. Normal duration of bleeding in the dog is 5 to 7 minutes. If performed after anesthesia but before surgery, this time can elapse while the patient is being clipped and scrubbed. The activated clotting time (ACT), another easy and reliable laboratory procedure, measures the effectiveness of the final coagulant cascade. Normal duration for this test is about 80 seconds. Other tests include the activated partial thromboplastin time and the prothrombin time to measure intrinsic and extrinsic function, respectively, but these are not indicated as screening tests.

Surgery in the Immunologically Impaired Patient

The immune system should recognize antigens from living foreign tissue, dead tissue, bacteria, and other microbes and bacterial toxins. These elements can activate the cellular, humoral, and phagocytic components of the immune system. Surgery in patients with known circulating antigen-antibody complexes or autoimmune antibodies, as in rheumatoid arthritis, systemic lupus erythematosus, glomerulonephritis, or mixed immune-mediated collagen diseases, represent no particular surgical problem. However, respect for the compromised tissue in terms of supportive care is important. If thrombocytopenia is present in AIHA, immunosuppression is continued through surgery, even though drug-induced cytotoxicity may cause postsurgical difficulty.

Iatrogenic immunosuppression sometimes occurs when chronic glucocorticoid therapy has been used as a substitute for flea control or, chronically, to control the pain of degenerative joint disease. Cytotoxins may be used to control antigen-antibody complex formation in autoimmune diseases and in antitumor chemotherapy. Glucocorticoids and cytotoxins potentially predispose to infection by decreasing normal humoral and cellular inflammatory defenses and inhibiting fibroplasia. Therefore, a surgical procedure performed on an immunosuppressed patient is considered similar to a known contaminated procedure, and prophylactic antibiotic coverage is elected, consisting of intravenous administration of a bactericidal antimicrobic such as cephazolin starting when anesthesia is induced. The antibiotic infusion continues throughout the operation and recovery, but ends on the same day of the surgery. This technique ensures that blood levels of antibiotics are high when local and systemic microbe contamination is most likely to occur. Low doses of chronic postoperative antibiotics are discouraged for prophylaxis, because this practice does not optimize control of surgical contamination when it occurs and encourages the development of antibiotic-resistant bacterial strains. The use of glucocorticoids, cytotoxics, and antineoplastics also prolongs wound healing. Therefore, when selecting sutures and pattern, the surgeon should bear in mind the delayed acquisition of tensile and bursting strength in wounds and organs and should recognize that the suture will be the primary coaptation for the wound for longer than normal.

Surgery in the Nutritionally Compromised Patient

Sick and injured animals often have anorexia or other nutritional compromise that must be actively appreciated and managed for best surgical results. As mentioned previously, an obligatory gluconeogenesis, negative nitrogen balance, and increased basal metabolic rate accompany injury. Unfortunately, patients must fast before elective surgery and some diagnostic tests. Pre- and postoperative feedings are also often omitted or modified, especially with oral, pharyngeal, and gastrointestinal tract procedures. Anorexia from illness or disruption of feeding schedules can also be problems in hospitalized patients. Preoperative estimates of the patient's protein, calorie, and trace element nutritional status is important, but not as critical as fluid, electrolyte, and

Table 1–8. Methods of Perioperative Nutritional Maintenance

A. Anorexia
1. Manual force feeding
2. Orogastric tube feeding
3. Indwelling nasogastric tube feeding
4. Pharyngostomy or gastrostomy tube feeding
B. Requirement for oral bypass
1. Indwelling nasogastric feeding tube
2. Pharyngostomy or gastrostomy feeding tube
C. Requirement for esophageal bypass
1. Indwelling nasogastric feeding tube
2. Indwelling pharyngostomy feeding tube
3. Gastrostomy feeding tube
D. Requirement for gastric bypass
1. Jejunostomy feeding catheter (via open surgical placement)
E. Nonfunctional gastrointestinal tract
F. Total parenteral nutrition*

* May be available at tertiary care centers.

acid-base balance on a short-term basis (see Fig. 1-2). Methods of perioperative alimentation are listed in Table 1-8.

Suggested Readings

Authement JM, Wolfsheimer KJ, Catchings S. Canine blood component therapy: Product preparation, storage, and administration. J Am Anim Hosp Assoc 1987; 23:483.

Crane SW. Perioperative analgesia: A surgeon's perspective. J Am Vet Med Assoc 1987;191: 1254.

Crowe DT. Clinical use of an indwelling nasogastric tube for internal nutrition and fluid therapy in the dog and cat. J Am Anim Hosp Assoc 1986: 22:675.

Gilroy BA, Crane SW. Parenteral fluid therapy, resuscitation from low flow states and cardiopulmonary resuscitation. In: Betts CW, Crane SW, eds. Manual of small animal surgical therapeutics. New York: Churchill Livingstone, 1986: 141.

Green RA. Bleeding disorders. In: Ettinger S, ed. Textbook of veterinary internal medicine. 2nd ed. Philadelphia: WB Saunders, 1986:2076.

Jones RL. Control of nosocomial infections. In: Kirk RW, ed. Current veterinary therapy IX. Philadelphia: WB Saunders, 1986:19.

Mark Morris Associates. Anorexia. In: Lewis L, Morris M, Hand M, eds. Small animal clinical nutrition III. Topeka: Mark Morris Associates, 1987:515.

Otto C. Blood gas and pH abnormalities. In: Norton LW, Eiseman B, eds. Surgical decision making. 2nd ed. Philadelphia: WB Saunders, 1986:3.

Pestona C. Fluids and electrolytes in the surgical patient. 3rd ed. Baltimore: Williams & Wilkins, 1985:3.

Polzin DJ, Osborne CA. Anion gap—diagnostic and therapeutic applications. In: Kirk RW, ed. Current veterinary therapy IX. Philadelphia: WB Saunders, 1986:52.

Riviere JE. Antibiotic therapy. In: Betts CW, Crane SW, eds. Manual of small animal surgical therapeutics. New York: Churchill Livingstone, 1986:35.

Schaer M. The diagnosis and treatment of metabolic and respiratory acidosis. In: Kirk RW, ed. Current veterinary therapy IX. Philadelphia: WB Saunders, 1986:59.

2

Stephen W. Crane

The Operative Procedure

Surgical Environment

The physical aspects and features of an appropriate veterinary operating room are listed in Table 2-1. The operating room should be used only for that purpose and should be well equipped, lighted, ventilated, and maintained at the highest sanitary standards. Amortization and upkeep expenses on a per-square-foot basis will be significant and should be passed through to surgical bills without apology. This room is important for conducting major, "clean" operative procedures; when possible, clean procedures are always scheduled before "contaminated" ones. Dentistry, bandage changes, abscess drainage, and other grossly contaminated procedures should be done elsewhere.

Surgical Instruments and Supplies

The purpose of surgical instruments and supplies is to allow an efficient, effective operation. Surgical instrument packs for both soft tissue and orthopedic procedures should be liberally equipped with basic instruments such as scalpels, hemostats, and tissue forceps. These basic packs can be modified depending on the needs of the practice and the preferences of the surgeon.

Surgical instruments are made from chrome-plated carbon steel or solid stainless steel. The body of the instrument is hot-stamp forged; after the instrument part has cooled, machine-shop operations create teeth and

35

Table 2–1. Physical Aspects and Features of the Veterinary Operating Room

Essential

- Adequate size, >144 ft²/table.
- No through traffic. Sole purpose and physically isolated.
- Proximity to instrument decontamination area.
- Immediate proximity to scrub sink, gowning, and gloving area, which are outside the room.
- Proximity to x-ray and treatment areas.
- High ambient lighting (ceiling recessed lighting desirable).
- Smooth, hard, impervious surfaces and paints. Surfaces should permit damp dusting with dilute hypochlorite, detergents, or phenolic cleaning compounds daily.
- HVAC cold air return from floor level.
- Surgical light(s) fully positionable. Prefer pod to track mounts.
- Built-in cabinets to minimize dust gathering.
- Ground fault interruption on all electrical service.
- Radiograph illuminator.
- Source of emergency lighting.

Desirable

- Pass-through window or cabinet to outside.
- Oversized (44–50″) swinging door.
- Hands-free communication or signalling system.
- Vacuum service for waste anesthetic gas evacuation and surgical suction.
- Hanging "sky hook(s)" fastened to substantial ceiling support.
- Separate HVAC circuit to attain positive pressure.
- Wall oxygen service.

Debatable

- Observation windows.
- Floor drains.
- Music system.
- Telephone service.

grooves, box locks, and ratchets. After assembly, the instrument is polished and ground with fine abrasives to make it completely smooth and free of imperfection. Next, chemical baths in strong acids produce a metallic oxide "passivation" of the instrument's surface to inhibit surface corrosion. Solid stainless steel instruments may be further treated to dull the finish, to avoid distracting reflections. After finishing, the finest instruments are manually adjusted for "feel" (such as the closing characteristics of a needle holder).

Care of Surgical Instruments

Surgical instruments should be protected by proper use and care. The main cause of premature instrument demise is abuse by the surgeon. While improvisation in the use of instruments is certainly possible, a purpose-specific instrument, used properly, will usually be more efficient for the procedure and safer for the patient with less wear and breakage of the instruments. Classic examples of instrument misapplication are using delicate hemostatic forceps to hold and manipulate bone fragments and using needle holders to twist and pull steel pins and wires.

The second most common cause of premature wear is pitting, corrosion, and rusting. After an operation, instruments should be separated by size and scrupulously cleaned by removing gross debris and blood with a surgical scrub brush. The instruments are left open and placed in a high-energy ultrasonic cleaner (with a specific ultrasonic detergent) that produces cavitation bubbles in the water to break and remove remaining proteinaceous debris. Next, the instruments are rinsed in hot (80°C) distilled water and bathed in an "instrument milk" emulsion that displaces water from inaccessible locations and lubricates moving parts. Petroleum-based lubricants for box locks are avoided because they will not permit steam penetration. Other than the initial gross washing, all phases of instrument cleaning are done in deionized or distilled water because chloride anion, in particular, rapidly attacks "stainless" steel. Even the finest instruments will begin to show surface pitting and will corrode at a faster pace if regular water is used as an instrument rinse or in autoclaving. Before packing, the tips of delicate instruments are inserted into rubber or plastic sleeves to protect the points and cutting edges from collision.

Preparation of Surgical Instruments

Methods for the layout, packing, and wrapping of the surgical pack or individual instruments range from simple to elaborate. The simplest system is to assemble the instruments by group on a flat tray or in a ventilated instrument pan. The instruments are kept grouped by a stringer device, and a heat- and pressure-sensitive autoclave indicator tape strip is placed on a towel lining the bottom of the instrument panel. Four towels are enclosed in the pack, and the instruments are then double wrapped. Specific muslin or crepe papers with the required porosity for admitting and releasing steam and moisture are available for wrapping surgical packs. The wrap is closed with autoclave tape, which is labelled with the pack's contents and the sterilization date. Another popular method is using a rigid, ventilated metal case containing the instruments in a removable tray.

Packaging systems for small instrument groups or individual instruments or accessories include transparent plastic pouches or transparent plastic-and-paper containers whose open end may be sealed with a heated pressure bar. With all packs and packaging systems, whether the covers are double wrappings of cloth, double wrappings of crepe paper, or plastic wrappers, shelf-life is significantly extended by applying an outer plastic dust cover to prevent dampness or disturbance of the wrapper during storage. For example, applying an outer polyethylene film dust cover after the instruments have been removed from the autoclave extends the shelf-life for double-wrapped muslin instruments from 7 weeks to 1 year.

Sterilization of Surgical Supplies

Sterilizing routines for surgical instruments must be reliable and consistent. Cold disinfection is achieved by immersing an instrument, or a rubber or plastic item, for a prolonged period in a bactericidal, virucidal, and sporicidal solution. Examples of such solutions are quaternary ammonium detergents, alcohols, phenolic derivatives, aldehydes, and halogens. A 2% aqueous solution of buffered glutaraldehyde is considered an effective instrument disinfectant. When used as directed, and if kept fresh, these solutions are generally effective in reducing microbial counts. But when the solutions are not used or replaced as directed, they may become contaminated and lose effectiveness. Also, instruments are not literally sterilized (the total absence of any life form) in cold disinfection.

Total sterilization is achieved by heating the instruments with pressurized steam or by poisoning the microorganisms with heated ethylene oxide gas. Either way, sterilization is achieved only after minimum conditions of temperature, pressure, and time of contact with the sterilizing agent are met, even in the most inaccessible area of each pack and in the most inaccessible portion of each individual instrument within that pack.

An autoclave is the usual equipment used for total sterilization by steam. Time and temperature requirements for total sterilization are 121°C at 15 pounds per square inch (psi) for 15 minutes, or 126°C at 20 psi for 10 minutes. "Flash" instrument sterilization is obtained by 134°C at 30 psi for 3 minutes. Vacuum-displacement autoclaves are superior to gravity-displacement models and are a cost-effective investment for the larger veterinary practice because of faster sterilizations and drying cycles. Because autoclaves use high pressure, they can explode; periodic inspection and service by a qualified autoclave mechanic should be performed at the manufacturer's recommended intervals. As mentioned previously, only distilled or deionized water is used in an autoclave so that salts do not deposit on instruments, autoclave valves, steam lines, or the chamber lining.

Instrument trays and individually wrapped small items must be properly positioned. Instrument trays or pans should be arranged vertically, not horizontally, and should be loosely packed within the autoclave cavity to facilitate air displacement and full circulation and penetration of steam through the entire load. Steam must penetrate to the depths of each instrument pack. Linen packs such as towels and drapes should be loosely bundled, without excess compression by an overly tight outer wrapper. These items should also be arranged loosely so that steam can circulate, displace air, penetrate fabric, and dry out promptly.

Ethylene oxide is the sterilizing agent of choice for surgical equipment and supplies such as vinyls and plastics, rubber goods, endoscopes, power equipment, and delicate instruments. In delicate or ophthalmic instruments, even minor heat damage or steam-induced corrosion may affect cutting surfaces, plastic flexibility, or optical surfaces of endoscopes. Ethylene oxide penetrates plastic and rubber materials quite well and kills all forms of microorganisms. Criteria for sterilization are 40% humidity in the presence of 500 mg/l ethylene oxide gas, and 54°C temperatures for a 4-hour sterilizing period. Packaging films of polyethylene, polypropylene, polyvinyl chloride, or autoclavable nylon transmit ethylene oxide; cellophane, mylar, and butyl plastic wrappers do not. Efficient, self-contained ethylene oxide sterilization kits of modest capacity are commercially available and are practical for the veterinary practice. Full aeration is required to expel the toxic gas and to make the materials safe for use. This time period ranges from 3 days for general-use instruments to 15 days of passive aeration for plastic intended for implantation.

Occupational Safety and Health Act (OSHA) regulations must be followed for potentially harmful substances used in the surgical preparation or procedure areas.

Selection of Surgical Instruments

The best way to become familiar with the range of surgical instruments and their applications is to peruse the catalogue of a major surgical-instrument manufacturer, but specific handbooks on veterinary instrument selection are available. Basic instruments used in veterinary surgery include the following.

Tissue Forceps

Tissue forceps are essential for grasping, holding, and moving tissue with traction in all procedures. As with most categories of surgical instruments, there are numerous sizes and configurations (Fig. 2-1). Important differences are the length and the presence or absence of interlocking teeth on the grasping surface of the instrument. Toothed forceps are advocated on the principle that it is better to penetrate tissue and kill a few cells rather than to disseminate excess pressure with nontoothed forceps and devitalize a larger volume of tissue. Obviously, the need for grasping and traction in an operation is a major factor in choosing a toothed or nontoothed forceps. The 1×2 toothed Adson, the Adson-Brown, and the Russian are among the most popular general-use forceps. "Atraumatic" tissue forceps such as the DeBakey and the untoothed Adson forceps are also popular and should be used when delicate, noncrushing grasping is required; applications include holding arteries and veins, tendons, and any structure where compromising blood supply or puncturing an organ capsule or sheath would have undesirable consequences. Tissue forceps are always held with a "pencil grip," not in the palm of the hand. Holding them between first two fingers and the opposing thumb offers better control and pressure sensitivity at the instrument tip.

Needle Holders

As the extension of the surgeon's arm, wrist, hand, and finger movements, a good needle holder is essential for the precise placement and driving of the suture needle. Therefore, a needle holder should fit the hand comfortably. Numerous styles, configurations, and sizes are available depending on the need for deep or superficial access and the size and strength of the needle to be held. Jaw inserts of extremely hard tungsten carbide can be installed on the

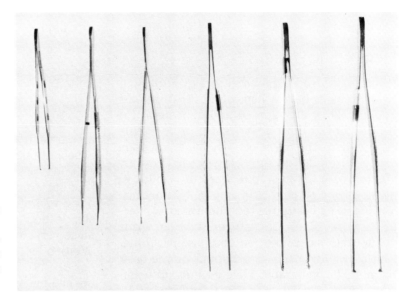

Figure 2-1. *Tissue forceps, both toothed and nontoothed varieties, are needed in various surgical procedures.* **Left to right:** Iris; 1 × 2 tooth Adson; Adson-Brown; DeBakey; Russian; toothed dressing forceps.

closing surface of the needle-holder jaws. While initially more expensive, the inserts greatly prolong the life of an instrument and can be replaced. Some smaller needle holders do not have locking ratchets, using pressure from the surgeon's palm to hold the needle in the jaws. However, most styles have ratchet locks so the needle can be positioned and clamped (Fig. 2-2). The Olson-Hegar needle holder is notable because of its built-in scissors that may speed the cutting of sutures. While popular, the instrument's drawbacks are that the grasping jaws are small, the scissors and box locks are not noted for long wear, the distance from instrument tip to hinge is long (making needle twisting more likely), and su-

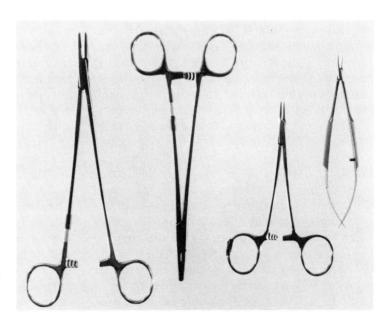

Figure 2-2. *Needle holders of various sizes.* **Left to right:** *Crile-Wood; Mayo-Hegar; Derf; Castroviejo.*

ture material may be cut prematurely when the instrument is closed on a needle.

Hemostatic Forceps

Hemostats are designed to grasp and close blood vessels before hemostatic ligatures are applied. They are tapered and delicate at the tip so that the blood vessel can be easily clamped and the tissue near the bleeding point can be excluded from the ligature. They are applied with the tips up (toward the ceiling or open portion of the incision) so that suture material can be easily passed underneath. There are several sizes, curvatures, and serration configurations on the various forceps, representing useful or trivial variations on the basic theme. The venerable Halsted mosquito forceps is the most frequently used hemostatic forceps in companion animal surgery. Larger-jawed instruments such as Kelly hemostats are useful when some fibrous tissue is included with the vessel, as for ovarian pedicles.

Organ-Handling Instruments

Numerous instruments exist for grasping, retracting, manipulating, and crushing both solid and tubular organs. Skin hooks are useful for the atraumatic traction and movement of skin flaps. Allis tissue forceps have opposing rows of grasping teeth and, when used singly or in groups, can provide coordinated traction. Since the Allis forceps closes with a crushing pressure, it should not be used on skin unless that area of skin is to be removed. The Carmalt forceps has tips with deeply serrated longitudinal grooves and is specifically designed to be placed perpendicularly across the long axis of a tubular organ or vascular pedicle. Since the parallel, interdigitating ridges of the instrument are placed transversely to the long axis of the organ, there is very secure grasping and crushing to prevent slippage. These features make the Carmalt popular and widely applicable to numerous surgical situations, including cross-clamping vascular/ligamentous pedicles such as uterine pedicles, or ovarian pedicles in large dogs. Use of specific noncrushing instru-

ments for gastrointestinal surgery is described in Chapters 12 and 13 and for cardiovascular surgery in Chapter 10.

Retractors

Adequate exposure is a requirement for safe, efficient surgery. Because veterinarians often operate alone, traction and countertraction are especially important, and exposure can be facilitated by self-retaining retractors. These retractors are usually packaged apart from the basic operating pack and are brought to the sterile field only when needed. Among the most versatile self-retaining retractors is the Weitlander, a ratcheted, adjustable, dual-opposed rake retractor that is positioned and opened for wound-edge separation. The Beckman retractor is similar, but has articulating hinges on both retractor arms that allows it to be "draped" onto or into a wound. Because the fit of the retractor blades to the wound is better, the body of the instrument is less obtrusive in the operative field. The Gelpi retractor is suitable for wound applications requiring minimal exposure (Fig. 2-3A). The Balfour or a similar retractor is used in extensive celiotomies; with or without the attachable retraction spoon, this type of instrument is essential in retracting the abdominal wall for complete exposure of all portions of the abdominal cavity. For the same reason, rib spreaders are needed in an intercostal thoracotomy; either the Burford or the Finochietto style is satisfactory for companion animal practice. Three sizes are needed: the premature infant model, and sizes with 15- and 25-cm spreads of the blades.

Hand-held retractors are useful when operating with an assistant. The most versatile are the Senn, US Army-Navy, Parker, and malleable "ribbon" retractors (Figs. 2-3B & C). The latter are available in various widths and can be bent into the shape required. The malleable ribbon retractors function especially well to move or deflect large visceral structures or sheets of tissue away from a surgical area in a deep cavity. Examples of use would be in exposure of the diaphragm by a caudal

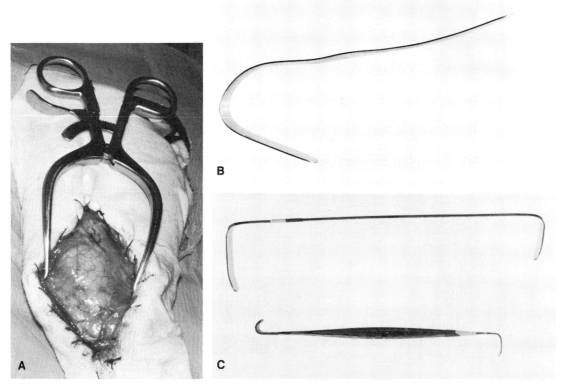

Figure 2-3. *Self-retaining retractors **(A)** are useful when operating alone. In addition to many other styles of hand-held retractors, the malleable ribbon retractor **(B)** is practical because of its versatility and low cost. The U.S. Army-Navy and the Senn retractors **(C)** are also useful for a wide variety of applications.*

retraction of the liver or the cranial retraction of the stomach to reveal the mesenteric root. Senn retractors work very well for limited-length incisions; the blade portion of the retractor is especially useful for deep exposures through limited, "keyhole" incisions. The Army-Navy retractor is multipurpose and is often used to retract muscle bellies during orthopedic procedures.

Several specialized orthopedic and neurosurgical retractors also have important veterinary applications (see Chaps. 18–24). Sterile latex Penrose drains and rubber bands are used to isolate, protect, and retract delicate structures such as nerves and blood vessels. These soft retractors are preferred to cotton umbilical tape for this purpose.

Scissors

Scissors are available in many sizes, shapes, and point patterns. The basic surgical pack should have a pair of sharp-sharp straight scissors for cutting sutures, heavy straight tissue scissors such as the Mayo scissors for cutting fascia, and a delicate curved, blunt-pointed soft tissue dissection scissor such as the Essrig or Metzenbaum. Surgical scissors are available with straight or curved blades. Curved scissors are designed to allow the wrist to remain in a comfortable position while the blade tips are at the correct angle for dissection. The instrument is turned over in the hand to position the tip for dissection in the opposite direction. Scissors are manipulated with the thumb and fourth finger in the rings and the index finger used near the hinge to stabilize and control the cutting surface.

Scalpels

Except for a few special applications (*e.g.*, ophthalmic surgery), scalpel blades are standardized to #10 and #15 for companion animals. Blades are disposable and applied to two #3 Bard-Parker handles at the beginning of the procedure. One blade is used for skin and will be contaminated with the resident bacterial flora of the skin during incision of dermis and epidermis. The other blade is reserved for deep dissection. To reduce the risk of injuring the operator, a scalpel blade is loaded onto the handle by grasping the back of the blade with a needle holder and locking the blade to the handle, with the sharp edge pointed away from the surgeon. As with all other sharp and potentially contaminated disposable devices, scalpel blades are disposed of in a rigid hazardous waste container.

Other Instrumentation

Equipment of nearly universal utility are electrosurgical machines and their accessories for delivering cutting, coagulation, or fulguration current to target tissue. Using electrosurgical technique in veterinary surgery is excellent practice if guidelines for its atraumatic application are followed. All electrosurgical equipment must be in perfect working order and the patient grounded, with a wide area of contact between the grounding pad and patient to preclude burning. Cutting, coagulating, and ''blended'' settings have distinct uses that must be understood: for instance, attempting to cut tissue with a coagulating current will result in excess burning, tissue trauma, and delayed wound healing.

Current is delivered to the target tissue through monopolar or bipolar application devices. In bipolar cautery, the current travels only a short distance from one electrode to another, directly through the tissue to be coagulated. An example is bipolar forceps, which are used to grasp a smaller bleeding vessel close to a delicate structure. The vessel is directly heat-sealed by the passage of the current, without local tissue heating or muscle or nerve stimulation.

In monopolar cautery, the more common situation, current is applied to the intended area for cutting or coagulation. The circuit to dissipate the current is provided through a large electrode, placed a distance away from the surgical site. Thus, the current originates at the electrosurgical generator, passes into tissue at the monopolar electrode, travels through the tissues in a path to the grounding electrode, and exits the patient with the current spread over the area of the electrode contact. Therefore, current densities sufficient to heat tissues or burn the patient are avoided, if there is a very good electrical contact to the patient's body over a wide area. Monopolar electrodes come in several configurations including needles, blades, loops, and balls.

To remove blood and lavage fluid from the wound, suction is preferred to blotting with sponges, although it increases the volume of blood lost during surgery. The volume of fluid in the suction bottle should be examined periodically. Suction equipment is desirable in all but routine elective procedures where the blood loss and duration of exposure are expected to be minimal.

Cryosurgical instruments and surgical lasers use thermal effects to ablate unwanted tissue. Cryosurgical ablation results from local freezing that causes intracellular ice-crystal formation, metabolic death, and expansion and rupture of the cell organelles. When the frozen area thaws, cell membranes also rupture. To freeze tissue, the surgeon may use a probe with circulating refrigerant or may directly apply a cryogen (Freon, carbon dioxide, nitrous oxide, or liquid nitrogen). Prefrozen probes can also be used. The temperature of the base of the tissue undergoing freezing must be monitored by needle thermistors to optimize the freezing process.

In spite of the theoretical elegance of this approach, controlling the volume of tissue undergoing the freezing-thawing cycle can be difficult, and thus the extent of tissue death is unpredictable. The result can be that pathologically involved tissue remains viable or, conversely, that normal tissues and structures are damaged by unnecessary freezing.

Surgical lasers are emerging as important tools and dissection devices. They work by interacting an intense beam of laser-generated light with target tissue to cause thermal effects. The laser wavelength determines the effects on tissue. With the argon ion laser (514 nanometers), hemoglobin will selectively absorb the green light, causing intravascular hemostatic effects. If the YAG laser is selected, near-infrared light of 1,060 nanometers will scatter through tissue, be absorbed by tissue proteins, and heat a three-dimensional volume of tissue. Light from the carbon-dioxide laser has a frequency in the very far infrared range of 10,600 nanometers that will be totally absorbed by surface intracellular water under the light beam. The absorption of the energy will superheat intracellular water and will cause the cell to explode with vaporization of water into steam and the carbonization of protoplasm as smoke. Since the beam can be finely focused, precision incisions as well as vaporization of volumes of tissue are possible. The disadvantages of laser use are the cost of the equipment and the special training required for the safe and efficient use of the equipment.

Other instrumentation of specialized application includes nitrogen- or electric-powered instruments to improve the efficiency of many operative steps in orthopedics (high-speed burring drills, and drills and saws for cutting or sculpting bone), low- or high-speed dental handpieces, dermatomes, pneumatic tourniquets, vision magnification instruments, and hydraulic wound lavage devices. Specialty equipment and instrumentation will be further considered in appropriate chapters.

Aseptic Technique

It is a myth that animals are more resistant to infection than humans. Operative invasion of normal tissue should be undertaken only if postoperative infection will not threaten the patient's well-being or life. The basic principle of aseptic technique is that microbiological contamination cannot occur if microorganisms are totally excluded from the wound. The reality of aseptic technique is a working set of complementary and interdependent technologies and operating-room protocols designed to prevent or minimize microbiological contamination in the surgical wound.

Aseptic technique begins with sterilized surgical instruments, implants, linens, and supplies. The total environment for the operative procedure is designed and maintained to minimize microbiological contaminants. This includes the patient's skin, and particulate and microbial exposure from the surgical team and operating room. Movement of people in and out of the room is discouraged; excess numbers of people are prohibited.

Because most particulate and bacterial contamination comes from the surgical team, operating-room personnel should be diligent in covering themselves. Hair is the primary source of particulate contamination, so a surgical mask and cap should cover all of the head, except the eyes. This may require a bouffant hood and/or beard covers designed for the purpose. Disposable paper masks are more effective than cloth masks for filtering particles. Street clothes are replaced with freshly laundered scrub suits to reduce dirt and dust contamination.

The external skin surfaces of both the patient and operative team are prepared so that, as much as possible, they are not a source of wound contamination. Although skin cannot be made sterile, skin-preparation techniques attempt to eliminate the transient bacterial flora on the skin surface and reduce the resident bacterial population of deep dermis and dermal adnexa. This process starts by removing the patient's hair with electric clippers or a depilatory cream (shaving causes varying degrees of epidermal damage that can become colonized with bacteria). Gross skin dirt and epidermal debris are removed with soap and water. Next, a surgical scrub soap is applied, starting with scrubbing strokes at the proposed incision line and centrifugally expanding to the circumference of the hairline (Fig. 2-4). Several scrub-sponge changes will be needed. Based on a controlled, prospective, microbiological culture study at a veterinary hospital, a suggested skin-preparation technique includes a 6-minute scrub of chlorhexidine gluconate followed by a 1-minute rinse with 70% isopropyl alcohol. On the operating table, the surgical preparation of the patient is completed with one more 3-minute soap scrub of chlorhexidine, a 1-minute alcohol rinse, and the spray application of povidone-iodine solution.

Ancillary Steps in Surgical Preparation

The surgeon is responsible for checking the patient and environment before final skin preparation and toweling and draping. This should include a final check for all emergency supplies, lighting, radiographs, patient positioning (including contingency needs for repositioning during surgery). The surgeon also should check that the correct anatomic area is prepared and exposed. The grounding pad of the electrosurgical unit, if used, should be coated with conducting electrolyte jelly and

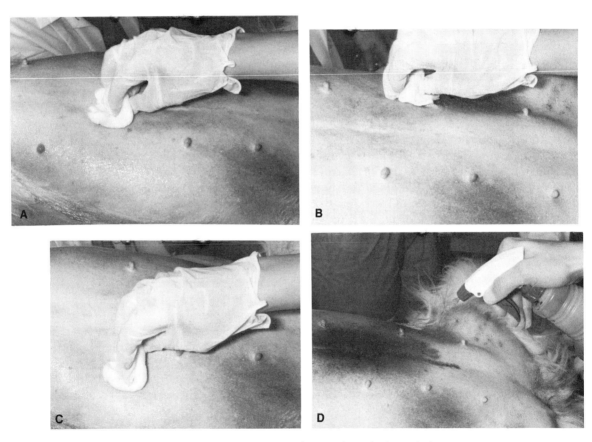

Figure 2-4. *A, The skin preparation scrubbing pattern is begun along the intended line of incision. The principle is to scrub from the clean central area toward the periphery without returning to the center (**B, C**). D, Skin preparation is completed by spray application of an organically complexed iodine surgical preparation solution, which is allowed to dry before toweling. Care is taken to avoid iodine staining of white-haired animals.*

placed under a broad, thinly haired portion of the patient's body to ensure excellent contact.

Precaution against intraoperative hypothermia is usually taken in most small animals. The most effective means of preventing heat loss is a circulating warm-water blanket. The second most effective means is to insulate the patient from the "heat sink" of the steel table by using insulation. The disposable plastic "bubble wrap" used for shipping packages is ideal for the purpose and is available at paper supply and freight companies. Another means is placing hot-water bottles or water-filled rubber gloves around the patient, with an initial water temperature no higher than 106°F.

An electric heating pad should *never* be used to maintain or restore patient body warmth due to the likelihood of superficial or deep burning.

Once the patient is positioned, secured, instrumented for monitoring, and physiologically stable, the surgeon or operative team prepare themselves with a 6-minute scrub with chlorhexidine (Fig. 2-5). A closed gowning and gloving procedure is practical and reliable (Fig. 2-6). Next, the gowned and gloved operative team place quadrant towels around the operative site. The operative site is always surrounded by double-folded, sterilized cloth towels or disposable impervious (plastic-coated) paper drapes to exclude the prepared

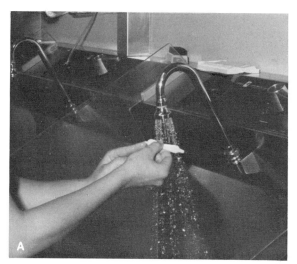
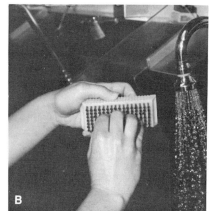
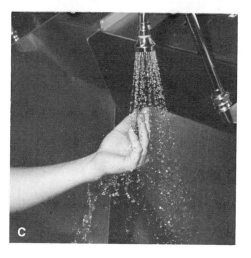

Figure 2-5. ***A,*** *Hand and arm scrubbing sequence prior to gowning and gloving. A chlorhexidine scrub detergent is recommended.* ***B,*** *The hands, forearms, and elbows are vigorously washed with surgical scrub soap. The fingernails are cleaned with soap and water.* ***C,*** *At all times during scrubbing and rinsing, the wrists are kept higher than the elbows so that water drains off the elbows, not the fingers. The principle is to scrub from the cleaner toward the dirtier areas, with the hands and wrists receiving the longest duration of scrubbing.*

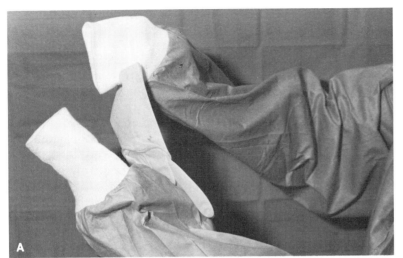

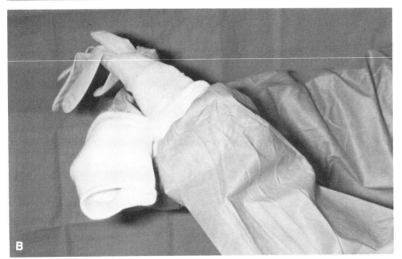

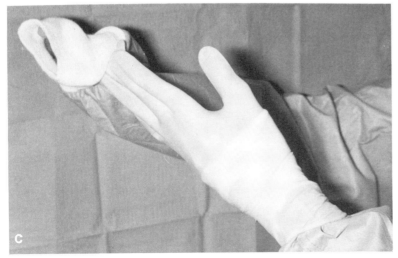

Figure 2-6. *A "closed" gloving sequence begins with the gown and gloves opened by an assistant after scrubbing. The gown is first only partially pulled on so that the hands remain within the cuff portion of the sleeves **(A).** One glove is picked up through the fabric of the gown and pulled over the opposite sleeve cuff. Thumb/finger orientation of the glove must be correct **(B).** The glove cuff is then pulled up and unfolded over and onto the gown's sleeve. Next, the glove's fingers are distracted and aligned so that fingers are insertable **(C).** (continued)*

Figure 2-6. *(continued)*
*Then, the sleeve and glove cuff are
pulled toward the elbow as a unit to
complete the glove donning process
on the first side (**D**). Taking care that
the bare hand is retained well within
the cuff, the gloved hand picks up
the remaining glove and feeds it over
the cuff (**E**). The sequence of above
is repeated so that both hands are
gloved (**F**). Using this method, the
chance of touch contamination
breaks is reduced when compared to
an "open" gloving sequence.*

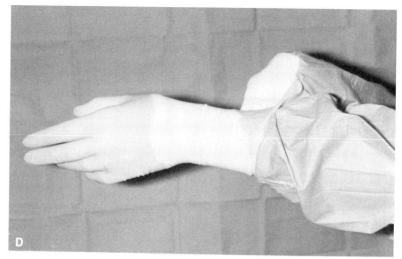

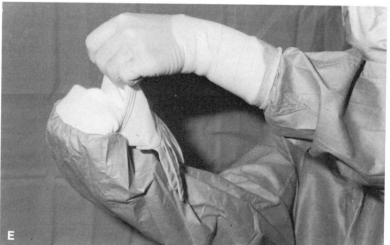

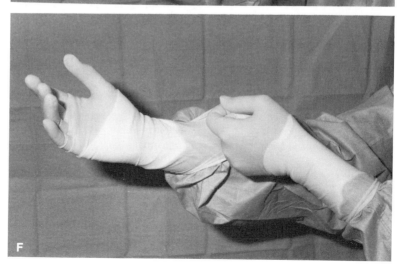

site from the rest of the patient. Toweling is an especially vulnerable time for breaks in aseptic technique that can occur by brushing against exposed surfaces. A sterile "fanfolded" overdrape is then opened to cover the patient and create a sterile working surface. If the drape is prefenestrated, the fenestration is situated to expose the incision site.

Basic Surgical Techniques

The four points of good technical surgery are maintaining asepsis, obtaining hemostasis, producing adequate exposure, and operating with gentleness to tissue.

Asepsis is maintained by having a well-prepared environment and preventing breaks in aseptic technique (Tables 2-2, 2-3). One of the major characteristics of good surgery is that each step has a definite purpose and is accomplished efficiently and effectively. A "flow" results from preplanning and minimizing wasted motion. Efficiency is important because increased operative times lead to disproportionately increased levels of mechanical trauma, drying, contamination of tissue and risk of arrhythmias, anesthesia, and hypothermia. Every procedure, including exploratory surgery, should have a definite, predetermined plan for its conduct and progress. Indeed, having plans A and B makes sense and improves

Table 2–2. Procedures to Control Nosocomial Infection

Environment Related	Patient Related	Hospital Policy Related
Sanitation of surfaces and cages	Aseptic surgical technique	Identify endemic resistant strains
Sanitation of operating room daily or as needed	Aseptic catheterization of bladder and central and peripheral veins	Isolate patients with resistant infections
Sanitation of operating table between cases	Avoid pathway contamination for IV fluids	Alternate patterns of antibiotic selection
Sterile instruments and supplies	Limit antibiotic use	Minimize hospitalization duration
	Limit drain use	
	Change wet dressings and bandages	

Table 2–3. Common Infractions of Operating Room Protocol

Operating Team	Scrub Procedure	Touch Contamination Breaks	Technique Breaks
Exposed hair	Rings and bracelets	Sterile team member having front-to-back contact with another sterile member	Protect drapes from saturation
Active respiratory infection	Long or dirty fingernails	Any contact with any unsterile surface or individual (usually during draping)	Opening of contaminated viscus
Dermatitis	Improper scrub sequence, duration, or technique	Hands below table level	Unnecessary conversation
Loose-fitting mask	Gowning, gloving with wet hands	Torn glove	Unsterile person leaning over operative field or instruments
Soiled scrub suit			

confidence and versatility. For example, the surgeon should have two strategies for a fracture repair, and the equipment and implants for both should be available so that one can serve as a back-up for the other. Stopping an operation is legitimate if the surgeon or operative team need to study a lesion, wait for laboratory data, or make a decision; otherwise, they should keep moving.

Gentleness in surgical technique is exceptionally important in minimizing the trauma associated with a procedure. Gentleness and speed are not mutually exclusive and frequently go hand-in-hand. Conversely, a plodding or slow approach does not automatically mean high-quality dissection or minimal overall trauma.

Operative Technique
Skin Incisions

Skin incisions made with the scalpel are the least traumatic, heal most rapidly, and produce the finest postoperative scar. Skin incisions made or extended with scissors are crushed, and those created with heated scalpels, electrosurgical current, or laser beams

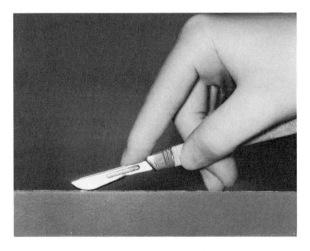

Figure 2-7. *When used to make skin incisions, the scalpel is held in the palm grip and drawn cleanly, with even speed and pressure. The belly of the blade rather than the point is the functional surface.*

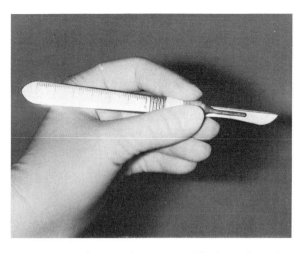

Figure 2-8. *The pencil grip is used for fine, sharp dissection in limited spaces.*

will be devitalized from thermal injury, resulting in delayed wound healing and, perhaps, less attractive scars. When using the scalpel to cut skin, it should be held by the palm grip and cleanly and evenly drawn across the tissue to be incised (Fig. 2-7). For fine dissection in a limited area, the pencil grip should be used (Fig. 2-8).

Tissue Dissection

After completing the skin incision, tissue dissection is continued with sharp or blunt dissection. Generally, sharp dissection is quicker and produces minimal trauma, but also causes increased hemorrhage. The advantages and disadvantages of blunt dissection are just the opposite. Sharp surgical dissection using scalpel, scissors, or electrosurgical cutting is preferred, but should follow the normal connective tissue cleavage planes between vital structures whenever possible. For example, surgical approaches to the long bones should never dissect through muscle bellies. The preferred method is to sharply incise the binding fascial envelopes of the extremity, then separate intermuscular connective tissue so that muscle bellies, with their blood and nerve supplies intact, can be retracted away from the bone.

Intraoperative Hemostasis

If the patient's blood-coagulation system is normal, hemostasis of the smaller vessels is secured by direct pressure with a moistened gauze sponge. The tissue should be compressed, not rubbed or wiped. Hemostasis of larger bleeding points is achieved by applying permanent or absorbable hemostatic clips, ligatures, or electrocoagulation. Ligature placement is traditional and is preferred for larger vessels, but means leaving suture material, a foreign body, in the wound.

To ligate a vessel, the surgeon or assistant applies the tips of the hemostatic forceps directly to the bleeding vessel, with the tips up. The hemostat handle is then lowered nearly parallel with the tissue plane, and the ligature material is placed under and around the upturned tips. The first throw of a square-knot ligature is thrown tightly onto the vessel; as the first throw is set, the vessel is momen-tarily released to allow the first throw to tighten completely. Then the square knot is completed and the hemostat released. The three-clamp method of ligating a vascular pedicle for hemostasis is summarized in Figure 2-9. A basic technique for the secure ligation of a large vessel is the transfixation ligature shown in Figure 2-10.

To electrocoagulate a vessel, a tissue forceps or a hemostatic forceps is applied to secure the bleeding vessel and the electrode is touched to the instrument to send coagulating current directly to the vessel. The vessel should desiccate and quickly seal by coagulation if under 1.0 mm in diameter. Electrocoagulation of vessels without first applying hemostatic forceps requires pinpoint application directly to the vessel. Contact between the electrode and a volume of tissue or a pool of blood disseminates the current over a wide area, causing damage to healthy tissue and failure to seal the bleeding vessel.

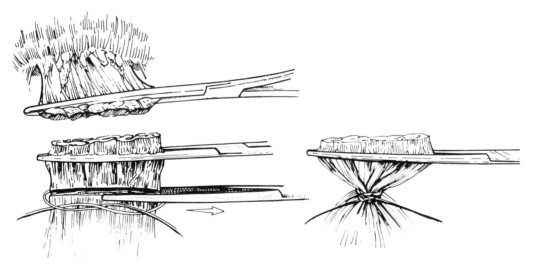

Figure 2-9.   *Three-clamp technique. The three-clamp method is used to ligate a pedicle containing vessels, connective tissue, and variable quantities of fat. A ligature is placed under the clamp closest to central circulation and is tightly tied in the tissue indentations left by the clamp after it is removed. (Note: For extremely broad, fat-filled pedicles, the second clamp may have to be momentarily loosened to allow full tightening of the ligature). The most distal clamp is to prevent backflow of blood and fluids from the transected pedicle.*

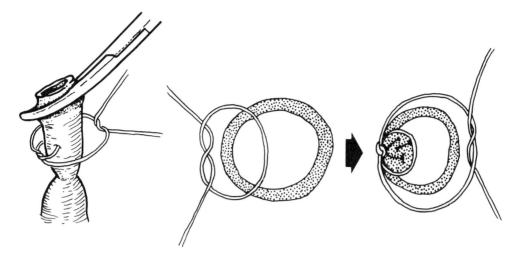

Figure 2-10. *Transfixation suture ligatures are an essential technique and are created when a needle with suture material is first passed through a vessel or pedicle to subdivide it prior to tying over each half. As this ligature cannot be dislodged, it is recommended on larger vessels where security of ligation is critically important.*

Suction and Lavage

For all difficult or extended procedures, and in instances where exposure will be limited in a deep cavity, the use of irrigation and lavage is important to improve visibility. Irrigation also prevents drying and devitalization of tissue. Lavage (pressure washing) allows hydraulic debridement of bacterial and particulate contamination during the procedure. For either technique, warm sterile isotonic electrolyte solution is delivered to the incision by bulb syringe. Spilling fluid onto drapes is to be discouraged to avoid a break in sepsis. Lavage fluid is removed by suction.

Suturing Technique

It is obvious, but frequently forgotten, that a curved needle cannot be driven through tissue in a straight line. The arc of the needle passage is determined by the curve of the needle. Not following the needle by attempting straight-line passage of the suture can only result in excess tissue laceration, bent needles, or both. The curved passage of a curved needle is achieved by rotating the needle in an arc by wrist motion.

Suture Materials

Placing suture material within a wound always results in delayed wound healing, foreign body reaction, and predisposition to infection, although these results vary in degree. The surgeon should be aware of the trade-offs made between the need for a suture or ligature and its negative effect on wound healing. It is best to restrict the number and size of sutures, and thus the bulk of suture material, to the minimum needed to coapt the wound.

Considerations in selecting suture material are the tensile strength requirements for coapting the host tissue, the allowable rate of loss of tensile strength, and the material's physical and chemical characteristics. The duration of a suture's tensile strength determines whether the suture is absorbable or nonabsorbable at an arbitrary period of 60 days. For extended or permanent tensile strength, nonabsorbable suture material should be selected.

Physical Characteristics of Suture Materials

Diameter per unit of strength, total tensile strength, and the coefficient of friction are important physical features of suture material, and vary widely. Braided suture material harbors tissue fluid and bacteria within interfiber interstices if the material becomes contaminated, and thus serves as a potential nidus for infection. While monofilament materials cannot hold fluid, they usually are slippery and handle more poorly than a braided, multifilament suture. Knot security is obviously important to safe surgery, and material that is larger, stiffer, hygroscopic, and more slippery will generally produce less secure knots or require additional throws on the knot (Table 2-4).

Chemical Characteristics of Suture Materials

Biological reactivity to the suture material is an important consideration because excessive inflammatory response increases pain and delays wound healing. Usually, natural fibers such as collagen, surgical gut, cotton, and silk provoke more intense inflammatory responses than synthetic fibers such as steel, nylon, polyester, polypropylene, or polydioxanone. A suture made of carbohydrate-based material, such as polyglycolic acid, will be removed by hydrolysis. Otherwise, the body removes absorbable sutures by inflammatory phagocytosis. One of the degradation products following dissolution of nylon suture is bacteriostatic and may inhibit, rather than facilitate, the onset of infection in an area contaminated by a break in aseptic technique. Selecting particular suture materials and sizes for particular tissues is described in the relevant chapters.

Suture Needles

Common needle configurations are tapered noncutting for soft and/or friable tissue and cutting or reverse cutting points and edges for use in dense connective tissue and skin. De-

grees of curvature range from straight to $\frac{5}{8}$ of a circle. The strongly curved needles are best used in limited-access situations where the wound is much deeper than it is wide. In contrast to the bulk and drag of suture material threaded onto a multi-use needle, a swaged-on needle passes with less tissue disruption, though swaged-on needles are more expensive. A needle that requires little energy to pass and allows the wrist to follow its arc permits optimized atraumatic technique. Such ease of needle passage can be extremely important in small places or in delicate or friable tissue.

To thread an eyed needle, hold the suture material vertically and motionless. Approach the material by lowering the needle, thread the eye from the inside (concave) portion of the needle toward the outside, and pull a length of the suture material through the needle. Suture material threaded this way will pull out of the eye less easily than if threaded from the outside (convex) aspect. Threading a needle and then rethreading it a second time to prevent the material from becoming unthreaded is unwise because it increases the bulk of material dragged through tissue by the needle.

Metallic staple systems for closing hollow organ and skin incisions are available. Advantages are speed of application, evenness of apposition, security of closure, and bioinertness. Disadvantages of stapling are cost, training requirements, and the possibility of staple migration.

Selection of Suture Patterns

The surgeon must decide how many sutures to use and how they should be placed. The most basic concern is the number of sutures to be placed per unit of incision length. In normally taut skin, the distance between sutures will be about twice the distance of the suture placement from the wound edge, and the distance of suture placement from the wound edge is equal to the thickness of the skin. These placements will usually bring the skin edges into an accurate coaptation.

Full- or split-thickness suture placement through skin is another consideration. Split-thickness placement gives the best apposition of the dermal and epidermal layers, but full-thickness is faster and stronger.

Another primary consideration is the tensile strength and suture holding power of the tissue to be sutured. There is no point in using a strength of suture that exceeds the holding power of the area sutured. In choosing

(text continues p. 57)

Table 2–4. Features of Suture Materials

Suture Description	Trade Name(s)®	Size-to-Strength Ratio or Knot-Pull Tensile Strength	Relative Knot Security	Handling Ease	Tissue Reactivity
"Plain catgut"	—	Relatively low	Knots may loosen when wet	Very good	Very high
"Chromic catgut"	—	Relatively low	Knots may loosen when wet	Very good	High
Polyglycolic acid	Dexon-S	High	Good	Fair	Initially moderate, but low during absorption
Coated, braided, polyglycolic acid	Dexon-Plus	High	Good	Very good	Initially moderate, but low during absorption
Coated, braided polyglactin 910	Vicryl	High	Good	Fair	Initially moderate, but low during absorption
Monofilament polydioxanone	PDS	Very high	Good	Good	Initially moderate, but low during absorption
Silk	—	Moderate	Good	Excellent	Moderately high
Polyester, Dacron	Mersilene Polydek	Very high	Fair	Poor	Low
Coated polyester	Ethibond Tevdek Ticron	Very high	Fair to good, requires proper technique	Fair	Low
Silicone treated, braided nylon	Surgilon	High	Fair to good	Very good	Very low
Monofilament nylon	Dermalon Ethilon	High	Fair (poor in large sizes)	Fair to poor (stiff in large sizes)	Very low
Monofilament polypropylene	Prolene Surgilene	Very high	Good to poor (stiff in large sizes)	Fair (stiff in large sizes)	Extremely low
Monofilament polyethylene	Dermalene	High	Good	Good	Low
Monofilament stainless steel wire	—	Very high	Excellent	Poor	Low
Twisted multifilament stainless steel wire	Flexon	Very high	Excellent	Fair to poor	Low
Polyfilament polyamide polymer encased in outer tubular sheath of caprolactum	Suprylon Vetafil Braunamid	High	Good	Very good	Low (high if outer envelope breaks)
Stainless steel and tantalum clips	Hemoclip Versa-Clip	N.A.	N.A.	Excellent	Very low

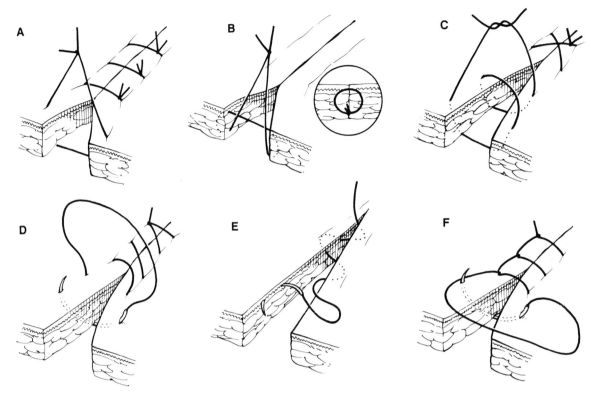

Figure 2-11. *Appositional suture patterns.*

A, Simple interrupted skin suture. Suture lines created from these sutures are more secure than continuous suture line. The removal of one interrupted suture is tolerable, but in a continuous line, the entire suture line is subject to failure upon breakage in any location.

B, Technique for inverting the knot in subcutaneous tissue closures. This is recommended for the second layer of abdominal closures or when overlying skin is thin.

C, The cruciate suture doubles the distance covered per suture compared to the simple interrupted pattern. This pattern causes less eversion and compromise of blood supply than the horizontal mattress.

D, Continuous suture patterns are quickly placed and appose tissue well. As it is being placed, the suture line should be examined and adjusted at frequent intervals for tightness. The major disadvantage of any continuous suture pattern is the potential for partial to total dehiscence if the suture breaks in any location.

E, Continuous, intradermal sutures provide anatomic skin layer apposition. Externally exposed sutures or suture sinus tracts associated with penetrating the epidermis are eliminated. This suture is recommended for the most cosmetic-appearing skin scars.

F, The Ford interlocking suture pattern keeps continuous suture lines flat and opposed.

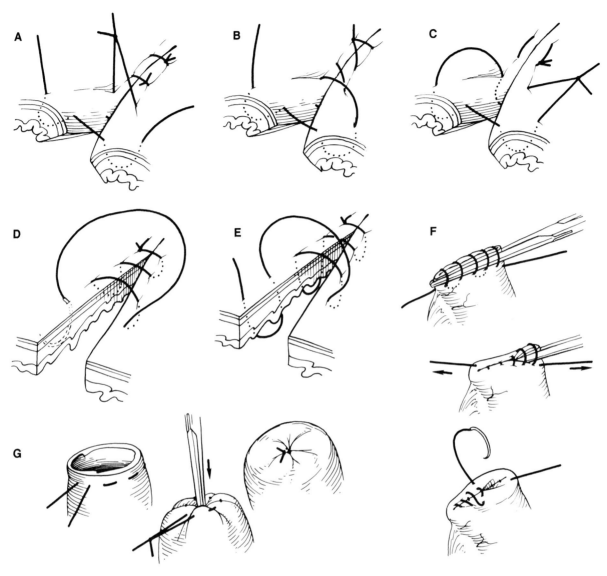

Figure 2-12.

A, Inverting seromuscular sutures can be used in closing hollow abdominal viscera to a watertight closure. The submucosal layer of hollow viscera must be incorporated into each suture bite for adequate strength of closure because all other layers have very little tensile strength. The exception is the esophagus.

B, Simple interrupted or continuous patterns of seromuscular inversion sutures, also called Lembert sutures.

C, A simple interrupted horizontal mattress inverting seromuscular pattern is also known as the Halstead pattern.

D, A continuous, horizontal, mattress pattern with suture advancement parallel to the suture line is known as the Cushing suture.

E, The above suture is termed the Connel pattern if it penetrates the mucosa. One must be aware of the effect of organ contents on the suture if it penetrates into the mucosa.

F, Inversion of a transected, hollow visceral organ is an essential surgical skill. The Parker-Kerr oversew is a two-layer closure that aseptically inverts a clamped viscus with a contaminated cavity.

G, A second useful suture pattern for closing a tubular viscus is the "pursestring" suture. The pursestring suture also can be used when a watertight, circular closure is needed around a tube entering an organ or cavity.

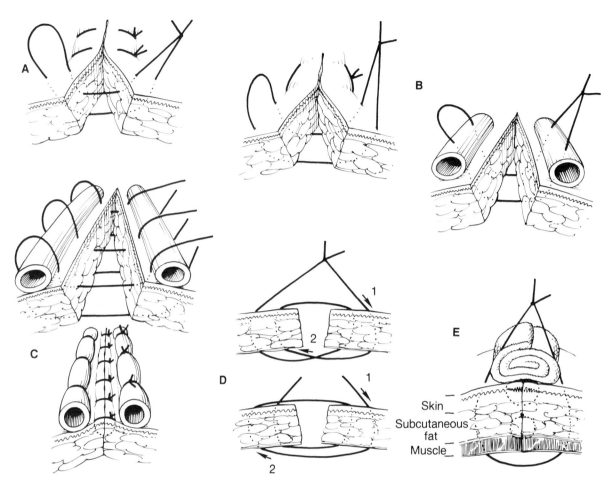

Figure 2-13. *Various suture placement strategies when wounds are under considerable distractive tension.*

A, *Vertical mattress. Note that the far arm of the suture relieves distractive tension
forces, while the near arm causes the skin edges to be in apposition or slight
eversion.*

B, *Horizontal mattress sutures. Stents can be made from various materials to help
distribute local pressure from suture material over a wider area to help prevent
pressure necrosis and the cutting through of the suture.*

C, *Deep through-and-through vertical mattress sutures placed over rubber surgical
tubing to relieve tension. The skin wound has been closed with simple interrupted sutures.*

D, *Two variants of an interrupted "pulley" suture that concurrently bring the skin
edges together and relieve local tension.*

E, *Through-and-through suture incorporates all closure layers for wide relief of
tension. This suture also creates compression and immobilization.*

absorbable or nonabsorbable suture, the basic consideration is whether permanency or extended duration of strength are needed. Motion or fatigue are important considerations, too. Diaphragm, stomach, bladder, intestine, tendons, muscle, and bone have severe stretching or cyclic loading stresses that frequently test both the material and the pattern. Additionally, the presence of gastric juice, bile, or urine may predispose the suture to premature weakening, infection, or calculus formation.

After selecting the suture material and the number and spacing of sutures, the suture pattern must be selected. Suture patterns are classified according to whether they are continuous or noncontinuous and whether they appose ("edge-to-edge"), invert, or evert the wound edges. Common suture patterns are presented in Figures 2-11 to 2-13. In apposing

(text continues p. 63)

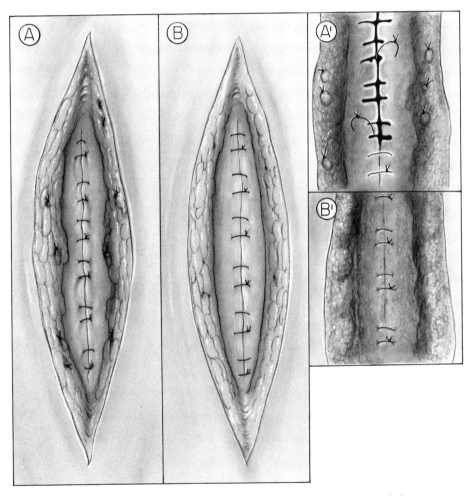

Figure 2-14. *The appearance and aftermath of sutures placed too tightly* **(A)** *versus the correct degree of gentle apposition of the wound edges* **(B)**. *(Redrawn from Reid MR. Some considerations of the problems of wound healing. N Engl J Med 1936;215:753.)*

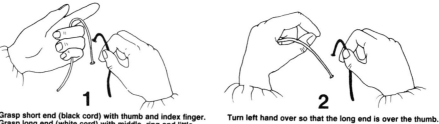

1 Grasp short end (black cord) with thumb and index finger. Grasp long end (white cord) with middle, ring and little fingers of left hand.

2 Turn left hand over so that the long end is over the thumb.

TWO HAND TIE

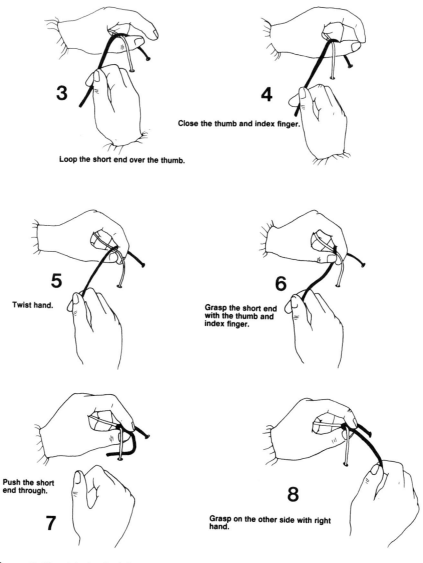

3 Loop the short end over the thumb.

4 Close the thumb and index finger.

5 Twist hand.

6 Grasp the short end with the thumb and index finger.

7 Push the short end through.

8 Grasp on the other side with right hand.

Figure 2-15. *Method of the two-hand tie using a left-hand lead. Either hand may be used as the primary hand. This is the usual means of knot-tying in general surgery.* (continued)

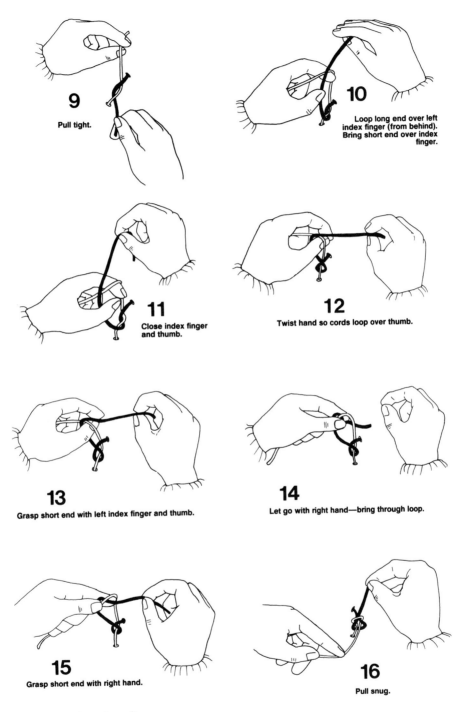

9
Pull tight.

10
Loop long end over left index finger (from behind). Bring short end over index finger.

11
Close index finger and thumb.

12
Twist hand so cords loop over thumb.

13
Grasp short end with left index finger and thumb.

14
Let go with right hand—bring through loop.

15
Grasp short end with right hand.

16
Pull snug.

Figure 2-15 *(continued)*

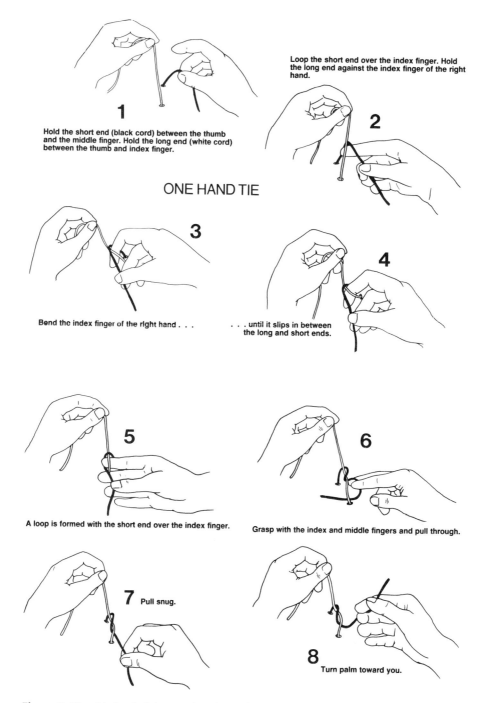

ONE HAND TIE

1 Hold the short end (black cord) between the thumb and the middle finger. Hold the long end (white cord) between the thumb and index finger.

2 Loop the short end over the index finger. Hold the long end against the index finger of the right hand.

3 Bend the index finger of the right hand . . .

4 . . . until it slips in between the long and short ends.

5 A loop is formed with the short end over the index finger.

6 Grasp with the index and middle fingers and pull through.

7 Pull snug.

8 Turn palm toward you.

Figure 2-16. *Method of the one-hand tie. This is an alternative method of hand tie and is useful when deep or limited access to the wound prevents use of the two-hand tie.* (continued)

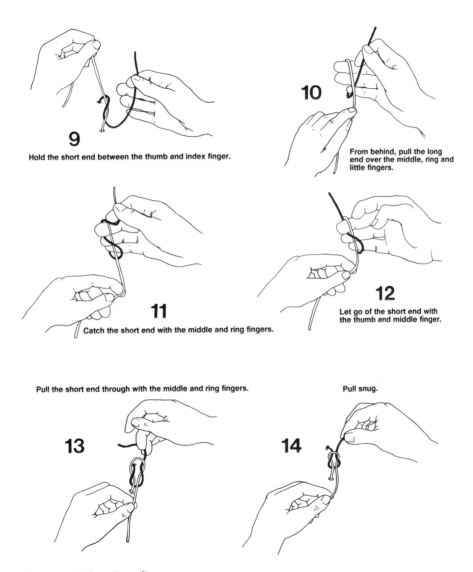

9 Hold the short end between the thumb and index finger.

10 From behind, pull the long end over the middle, ring and little fingers.

11 Catch the short end with the middle and ring fingers.

12 Let go of the short end with the thumb and middle finger.

Pull the short end through with the middle and ring fingers.

13

Pull snug.

14

Figure 2-16 (*continued*)

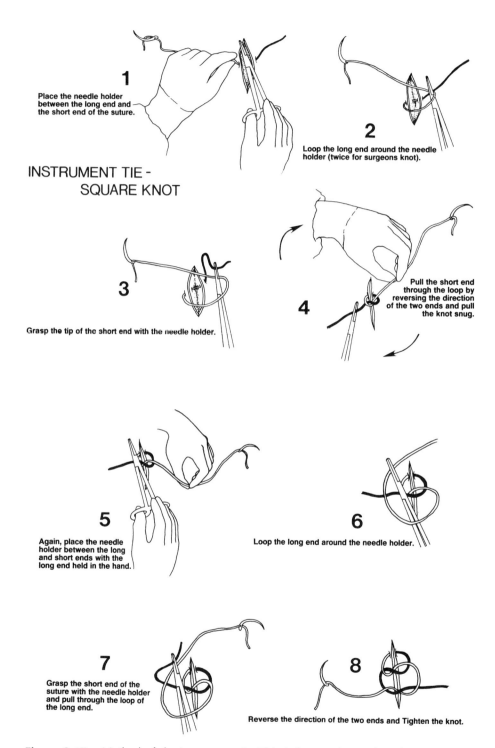

INSTRUMENT TIE - SQUARE KNOT

1. Place the needle holder between the long end and the short end of the suture.

2. Loop the long end around the needle holder (twice for surgeons knot).

3. Grasp the tip of the short end with the needle holder.

4. Pull the short end through the loop by reversing the direction of the two ends and pull the knot snug.

5. Again, place the needle holder between the long and short ends with the long end held in the hand.

6. Loop the long end around the needle holder.

7. Grasp the short end of the suture with the needle holder and pull through the loop of the long end.

8. Reverse the direction of the two ends and Tighten the knot.

Figure 2-17. *Method of the instrument tie. This is frequently employed in skin closures because it can be used rapidly and can conserve suture materials.*

any tissue type, sutures must not be placed too tightly (Fig. 2-14), because overly tightened sutures tend to strangulate blood supply and cause local necrosis. The sutures then "cut through," with dehiscence of the suture line.

Patterns and materials of sutures and ligatures recommended for particular applications are found in the relevant chapters.

Surgical Knots

Once an interrupted suture or continuous suture line is placed, it must be knotted. The surgical knot is a weak link in the ligature or suture because as tension forces are converted to shearing forces, internal stress is created on the suture. There is also the danger that the material may slip or the knot may come untied due to hygroscopic swelling or poor knot-tying technique.

Knotting is a fundamental surgical skill. There are several ways to tie several different knots, but the basic skills are the creation of the square knot, slipped square knot, and the surgeon's knot. A basic two-hand tie, one-hand tie, and the instrument method are illustrated in Figures 2-15 to 2-17.

Suggested Readings

Hurov L. Handbook of veterinary surgical instruments and glossary of surgical terms. Philadelphia: WB Saunders, 1978:94.

Knecht CD, et al. Fundamental techniques in veterinary surgery. 3rd ed. Philadelphia: WB Saunders, 1987:40.

3

Colin E. Harvey

The Surgical Wound

Wound Healing

The process of wound healing is the same whether the wound is of surgical or traumatic origin. The first phase is the *inflammatory phase,* in which debris is cleared from the wound. The local inflammatory response creates the environment for the *repair phase* that follows. The inflammatory phase takes longer to become established if the wound is severely disrupted or contaminated. Clean, uncontaminated wounds heal more rapidly than dirty, disrupted ones. Surgical techniques, therefore, are designed to minimize wound contamination and disruption. This can be done in the following ways:

- Using sterile instruments and supplies.
- Employing gentle direct surgical technique.
- Minimizing the time a surgical wound is open to suspended particle contamination.
- Selectively debriding a traumatic wound to

create a clean wound with a minimum of traumatized tissue.

Wound healing requires an adequate combination of local and systemic physiological functions. To proceed optimally, these factors must be present in appropriate ratios.

Healing tissues are very active metabolically. Without adequate blood flow to the wounded tissues, there will not be enough oxygen and nutrient substrate to support cell metabolism or to remove carbon dioxide and other metabolic byproducts. Local defense mechanisms are suppressed, and contamination with bacteria introduced during the traumatic incident may lead to infection.

Conditions in different parts of a large wound may differ significantly. However, if one area of a wound loses its ability to fight infection, the entire wound may become infected, with potentially disastrous consequences (*e.g.,* abdominal wound dehiscence).

65

The Inflammatory Phase

The first response to injury locally is vasoconstriction, which has the immediately essential purpose of reducing or preventing further hemorrhage. Hemorrhage has two major consequences for wound healing. First, reduced blood flow and local tissue perfusion, as a result of hypovolemia and hypotension, causes reduced oxygen-carrying capacity. If severe enough, this can cause anaerobic conditions locally. The other consequence is that clotted blood may physically separate viable tissues. Blood clots must be removed before the separated tissues can unite, and the clotted blood forms an ideal culture medium for bacteria that have found their way into the wound.

Preventing and controlling hemorrhage, thus, is an important step in optimizing wound healing. In a surgical wound, hemorrhage should be controlled as it is observed. In a traumatic wound, the first step in management is to control hemorrhage. The events in and around the torn or cut ends of the vessel that cause and clear the clot are described below (see "Hemostasis").

In a minimally traumatized wound, such as a clean surgical incision, local vasoconstriction lasts only a few minutes and is followed by vasodilation, both arteriolar and venous. Local vasodilation results in increased vascular permeability and thus leakage of fluid into the wound spaces. This is due to the endothelial cell-rounding effect of histamine, serotonin, and kinin release, creating gaps between cells. Another source of rapid wound fluid leakage is the disruption of lymphatics. The leaked fluid initially contains no cells, but does contain fibrinogen and other constituents that form fibrin clots to plug lacerated blood vessels, limiting the spread of the fluid produced. As healing progresses, the fibrin plugs in the lymphatics are removed by fibrinolysis, and local lymphatic flow resumes.

The endothelial surface of blood vessels in the injured area becomes coated with white blood cells within about an hour of injury. Initially, polymorphonuclear leukocytes (PMNs),

but later monocytes, move through the endothelial cell gaps into the extravascular wound spaces. The PMNs phagocytize bacteria. As they degenerate and die, intracellular enzymes that work on wound debris are released. The PMNs are thus the first wave of damage-clearance cells. Their importance during this phase can be appreciated by watching the rapid and significant increase in circulating PMNs in the first several hours after injury.

Monocytes (macrophages) continue the clean-up work by phagocytizing necrotic tissue and debris and disruption products of dead PMNs. In a clean wound, this process does not take long, because once vascular-wall integrity is restored, cells can no longer easily pass into the wound fluid. However, in a large wound or one with much necrotic debris, mononuclear cell infiltration may persist, and sometimes multinucleated giant cells may be seen.

Although there is some overlap between the inflammatory (clean-up) and repair (fibroblastic) phases of healing, the tissue debris must be removed to a large extent and the vascular-wall permeability restored toward normal before significant active cell proliferation can proceed. Macrophage activation within a wound increases lysosomal enzyme activity, secretion of proteases, complement components, interferon, thromboplastin, and probably many other substances that have specific local effects in hastening the clearance of wound debris, bacteria, and necrotic tissue from the wound area. These products also trigger the next phase of healing by releasing a chemotactic factor that attracts mesenchymal cells and promotes their differentiation into fibroblasts. Increased numbers of lymphocytes (both B- and T-cell) are usually found only in more chronic wounds and are particularly associated with the continuing presence of bacterial contamination.

In a clean wound in a healthy animal, the inflammatory stage clears the way for the start of the repair phase within 3 to 5 days, depending on the size of the wounded area.

The Repair Phase

Within 24 hours of the time a surgical wound is made, assuming local control of hemorrhage, the wound edges are held closed by an acellular fibrinous clot that provides the architecture for subsequent cellular healing. The connective tissue and epithelial tissue repair phases occur in different ways and at different rates; epithelial healing is more rapid.

Epithelial Repair

Healthy epithelial cells immediately adjacent to a wound edge start the healing process by becoming mobile, particularly as a result of activity at the marginal basal cell layer. They enlarge and start to migrate down and across the wound by sliding over adjacent cells. Migration occurs over exposed connective tissue surfaces or fibrinous deposits; it stops when the migrating epithelial cell comes into contact with another epithelial cell ("contact inhibition"). In a clean narrow wound, restoration of epithelial continuity can occur by cell enlargement and migration, without an actual increase in cell numbers from mitosis. The latter, which does not occur for 1 to 2 days, is responsible for reforming the normal epithelial thickness rather than restoring epithelial continuity. In a clean surgical wound with epithelial edges brought into apposition with sutures, epithelial continuity usually occurs in 24 to 48 hours. Epithelial migration and subsequent mitosis together are referred to as "epithelialization."

Epithelial mitosis increases the thickness of the epithelium at the defect and provides additional cells for covering defects too wide to be covered by migration alone. Mitosis of epithelial cells is stimulated either by a "wound hormone" or by the lack of chalone, the normally present epithelial mitosis inhibitor.

A skin wound that is covered by an intact epithelial surface is weak for several days, because no significant amount of collagen joins the two sides of the wound until about 5 to 7 days after injury. Until then, the wound edges are held together by fibrin and a thin layer of epithelial cells. Epithelial wounds in other tissues heal at slightly different rates, depending on the rate of epithelial turnover of that particular tissue; oral squamous epithelium heals more rapidly than skin, and alimentary canal epithelium heals very rapidly. During the "sealed but weak" period, the role of surgical sutures in providing mechanical strength across a wound is paramount in preventing dehiscence.

Connective Tissue Repair

Repair can occur optimally only when the inflammatory or clean-up phase is well under way. The progress of wound contamination to wound infection must be halted, which requires the presence of large numbers of PMNs. However, a sterile wound does not require PMNs for the repair process to move ahead. Similarly, lymphocytes are not essential for the progress of healing in an uncontaminated wound. Macrophages are needed to initiate the repair phase because they stimulate angiogenesis, fibroblast migration, and collagen formation. Generally, the rate of connective tissue healing does not differ between tissues, although there may be a greater intrinsic blood supply in some areas than in others.

Fibroblasts are basic to the healing process. They are thought to originate from local mesenchymal cells, often from vessel walls. These mesenchymal cells become migratory fibroblasts, entering wounded areas that have a reestablished blood supply and that have been cleared of wound debris. The fibroblasts use the fibrin network laid down during the inflammatory process as a scaffold, moving about by extending a cytoplasmic ruffled membrane that adheres to adjacent structures and pulls the rest of the cell in that direction. Contact between two migrating fibroblasts causes migration to cease in that direction, and the cytoplasmic extensions are thrust in other directions. Capillaries, formed by endothelial budding, follow the fibroblasts to nurture them and the adjacent tissues and to provide endothelial cells that are able to secrete plasminogen activators to break down the fibrinous network, which otherwise would interfere with the progress of wound repair.

Fibroblasts secrete ground substance that permits the synthesis and orientation of collagen, starting from about the fourth or fifth day in a healthy wound. Collagen formation and conversion to fibrils requires hydroxyproline and hydroxylysine and endopeptidase enzymes. Bonding of collagen fibrils into bundles causes them to become less soluble, eventually resulting in the dense collagen bundles that maintain adhesion of the edges of the wound. This process takes 2 to 4 weeks in a healthy wound. The wound tensile strength increases slowly from 1 to 5 days, then significantly from 5 to 15 days, coinciding with the period of maximum collagen synthesis and maturation. By the fourth week, the connective tissue aspect of the wound is maturing: fibroblasts, glycoproteins, mucopolysaccharides, and capillaries are starting to regress, and the rate of collagen synthesis is in approximate balance with normal destruction and replacement of mature collagen.

The wound healing process does not stop once there is epithelial continuity and collagen bridging across a defect. Tensile strength continues to increase slowly for several months after injury as a result of collagen cross-linkage. The connective tissues are reformed and shaped in response to tissue tension, resulting in laying down of more specifically oriented collagen fibers.

Healing of bone and cartilage follows a similar pattern, though the process takes longer because of the need for specific orientation of connective tissue and mineralization of ground substance that together provide the strength necessary for weight bearing. Bone healing is described in Chapter 21, Principles of Fracture Management.

Healing of Open Wounds

Healing of open wounds (wounds in which the epithelial edges are not apposed) takes much longer because of the large surface area that must be covered, though the processes that result in healing are the same. Healing of the surface of an open skin wound begins with coverage by a blood clot and development of granulation tissue. If hair follicles or skin glands with viable epithelium are scattered over the surface of the defect, epithelial healing occurs from these sites as for a closed wound, with cell enlargement and migration. From the edges of the defect or from hair follicle islands, epithelialization occurs; the migrating epithelium secretes a proteolytic enzyme that separates the clot from the underlying tissue, allowing the epithelium to migrate across the tissue surface in a protected position beneath the clot. The advancing epithelium is thinner than the epithelium at the edge of the defect, and may even be a monolayer in a large defect.

If this were the only epithelial coverage, it would produce a thin, easily traumatized surface. Fortunately, another healing phenomenon also is at work in large epithelial defects: *contraction*. Contraction results in the coverage of large defects with epithelium of normal thickness and with hair follicles and other features of normal epithelium. It results from movement of existing skin from the wound edges.

Contraction is caused by the action of myofibroblasts around the edge of the granulation tissue bed; these cells, which probably originate from the same progenitor cells as the fibroblasts involved in the usual healing process, have cellular attachments and are able to contract, so that the epithelial edge and adjacent full-thickness skin is pulled over the granulation tissue bed over a period of several days or weeks, depending on the size of the defect. Contraction ceases when the epithelial edges come into contact or when the adjacent skin is under tension higher than the tension that can be produced by the myofibroblasts.

Initially, the wound surface enlarges because the wound edges retract. The wound is covered by a clot; then, PMNs and macrophages from the exposed connective tissue clean up the surface, and capillary budding, fibroblast migration, and proliferation occur.

At the wound edges, the epithelial cells start the enlargement, migration, and mitosis processes. Thus, the normal healing processes are set in place for approximately the first 7 days. After this "lag phase," enough fibroblast proliferation has occurred that contraction commences.

In the dog and cat, the loose skin and perhaps the well-developed panniculus muscle layer assist contraction. The result is that even very large defects can be covered. The process works very successfully on open surfaces such as the neck, thorax, and abdomen, but is of more limited usefulness in areas with little loose skin, such as distal limbs. It may create contractural tension that may limit the range of motion of joints or may cause other defects, such as distortion of eyelid margins.

Categories of Wound Healing

Healing is often described as being of first or second intention, depending on whether the wound is closed or left open to granulate.

First-Intention Wound Healing

This is achieved when healthy and relatively uncontaminated tissues with an adequate blood supply and cleanly incised or lacerated edges are brought into and held in apposition until collagen formation has occurred across the wound. This type of healing is usually the goal when a surgical wound is created. Sutures are used to maintain the wound edges in apposition. Healing is rapid, restoration of full function is expected, and minimal scar tissue formation is anticipated. Epithelial migration and closure occurs as the first repair stage; connective tissue repair does not occur until fibroblasts have been activated a few days later. As noted above, the wound is relatively weak during the early phase of healing, despite complete epithelial coverage. Sutures assist the healing process by keeping the epithelial edges and supporting connective tissues apposed during the initial several days. However, sutures can interfere with healing if

placed too tightly, resulting in incorrect apposition of tissue layers. In addition, the deeper layers must be healthy: first-intention healing will not occur in the presence of subepithelial wound fluid and gross contamination, even if the epithelial edges are apposed correctly. Sometimes, the epithelial edges are apposed and temporarily create epithelial coverage, but become disrupted if infection ensues, causing dehiscence. The client sees only the external wound, but the surgeon must ensure that the deeper hidden tissues are treated with equal or more respect and care.

Second-Intention Wound Healing

This occurs when there is a significant epithelial defect that cannot be closed by epithelial migration within a few days. The exposed connective tissue surface (which may be subepithelial tissue, fascia, muscle, or bone) granulates and the epithelium adjacent to the defect covers the defect by contraction to the extent that it can be pulled by the myofibroblasts. The wound may go on to heal completely, the final epithelial coverage occurring by epithelial migration over the narrowing defect, or a residual defect may result.

Delayed Primary Closure

This method is used for extensive or contaminated wounds that cannot be closed primarily, or for an area where extensive debridement is not practical. The wound is allowed to develop a granulation tissue surface so that the clean-up phase of healing is performed by the local tissues without sequestration of contamination or fluid beneath the epithelium. Then the wound edges are closed, by undermining if necessary, to achieve epithelial apposition. The advantage of this technique is that it avoids the need for anesthesia for extensive debridement, yet significantly speeds the final healing process and circumvents the need to manage a large open wound for long periods during the contraction process.

The closure procedure is performed when the healing connective tissues are at their most active, usually 5 to 7 days after injury. At that time, healing is particularly rapid because the apposed edges of the wound do not have to go through the clean-up/inflammatory phase preparatory to connective tissue repair. Thus, a wound closed by delayed primary closure develops significant wound strength sooner after closure than does a first-intention closure wound. A similar benefit is seen when a wound dehisces and is resutured: healing appears to be more rapid because the inflammatory response is well established and tissues necessary for repair are mobilized. Of course, wounds that have dehisced can go on to heal rapidly only if the conditions that caused the dehiscence (such as inadequate suture technique, inadequate local blood supply, or excessive tension on tissues) are corrected.

The observation that dehisced wounds seem to heal more rapidly led to suggestions that a second wound made several days later on the same body might heal more rapidly than the first wound as a result of the release of a systemically active "wound healing hormone" from the first wound. This is, in fact, not so. The "advantage" of repair of a dehiscence or use of delayed primary closure is localized to within 1 or 2 cm of the wound, the area of the inflammatory response itself.

For both second-intention healing and delayed primary closure, the healing process is greatly assisted by effective external management of the wound. Techniques are described later in this chapter and in Chapter 4.

Requirements of a Healing Wound

Many factors, both systemic and local, affect the rate of wound healing. Recognizing and avoiding conditions that have a deleterious effect are major considerations when evaluating a surgical patient. When the condition impairing healing cannot be avoided, other steps may be possible, such as protecting or supporting the wound externally; or, it may be appropriate to postpone the surgery until the complicating factors have been resolved.

The "ideal" wound is one that is freshly made, without contamination, in a healthy animal. Any other circumstances will delay healing to some extent. For this reason, large open wounds often are best managed by closing them to form long but narrow closed wounds (wounds heal across the defect, not along the length of the defect). Similarly, when feasible, wounds with necrotic or severely traumatized tissue that is likely to have a reduced blood supply are best managed by resecting the dead or damaged tissue back to normal healthy tissue ("debridement"), followed by closure as a simple clean wound. Anatomic factors or the sheer size of the wound may prevent using these techniques. This topic is discussed further in Chapter 4, The Skin: Wound Closure and Reconstructive Surgery.

Factors Affecting Wound Healing

Local Vascularity

For the first several minutes after injury, the vessels at the site constrict. However, they soon dilate, and the dilation and generation of neovascular channels continues during the third to twenty-first days, when the wound is healing rapidly. Factors that affect the ability of the local vascular channels to respond appropriately include anatomical derangement in adjacent tissues (such as a crushing injury or hematoma or edema formation), pressure from continued abnormal position of the body part due to lack of function or from weight of adjacent body parts, ligation of major vessels as a means of controlling severe hemorrhage, and extensive injury and shock, where the circulating blood volume may be insufficient to fill all the dilated vessels in the injured parts.

Blood loss itself is a common but usually temporary cause of reduced perfusion, because of mobilization of extravascular fluids into the vascular compartment. This may be more serious if the blood loss is severe enough to result in shock, and can be an ongoing problem in wounds such as those due to severe extensive burns, where loss of blood or serum continues at significant rates for prolonged periods.

Local Tissue Perfusion and Oxygenation

Ensuring adequate blood flow may not be enough to optimize healing. Other factors that will have an effect include the following:

Edema. May result from hypoproteinemia.

Anoxia. This can be caused by inadequate vascular oxygenation from blood loss or anemia or by respiratory distress due to pulmonary edema ("shock lung") or pulmonary or thoracic injury.

Hypovolemia and hypotension (shock, cardiovascular injury). Associated effects are local sludging of blood or even microvascular coagulation from the local release of clotting factors as a result of the injury. Arteriovenous shunting occurs in some tissues, with similar local effects.

Vasoconstriction. Several conditions mentioned above cause local vasoconstriction, particularly in nonessential tissues such as skin, connective tissue, and some muscles. This causes local tissue temperature to drop, and the combination of local vasoconstriction and reduced tissue temperature causes further reduction in cellular metabolism. In superficial tissues, ambient temperature will have an effect on wound healing: raising or lowering the temperature to 10°C above or below the normal ambient temperature will speed or slow, respectively, the gain in wound tensile strength, although the effect is short-lived.

Presence of necrotic debris and secondary infection.

The effect of all of these local circumstances is to delay rather than permanently interfere with wound healing. All these factors hinder the provision of oxygen and essential nutrients to and clearance of carbon dioxide and other metabolic byproducts from the wounded and healing tissues. Inflammatory or reparative cells in healing wounds often are exposed to a low oxygen tension; the diffusion gradient from the capillaries to the actively metabolizing cells is very steep. Active metabolism (seen as fibroblast replication or collagen formation) will cease beyond the zone of adequate oxygen tension. Budding capillaries will slowly extend the area of active healing, but this takes time.

Correcting the factors listed above allows healing to proceed at an optimal rate, but often with a lag period between correcting the problem (e.g., restoring cardiovascular volume in hemorrhagic shock) and clearing the local effects (e.g., sludging or microvascular coagulation).

Providing supplemental oxygen in an otherwise normal animal increases early wound strength slightly, but this finding has no clinical usefulness.

Systemic Conditions Having Local Effects

In addition to the cardiovascular and oxygen delivery effects noted above, the following systemic conditions have deleterious or delaying effects on wound healing:

Immune system abnormalities. Because immune-suppressed animals are less able to deal effectively with contamination, they are more likely to develop overt wound infections.

Uremia. Poor kidney function results in increased levels of circulating protein degradation products. These act as tissue toxins, slowing metabolic activity. Healing is delayed or poor-quality collagen is formed.

Hypoglycemia and diabetes. Rapidly metabolizing cells require energy. The stress of trauma, surgery, and inappropriate fluid therapy or insulin dosage during and immediately after surgery may slow the rate of healing by reducing the availability of energy substrates, although this usually is a short-term effect.

Malnutrition. Several deleterious effects on wound healing can be attributed to malnutrition. Gross protein malnutrition leads to hypoproteinemia, with local wound edema and delayed cellular activity and substrate for tissue repair. Gross calorie malnutrition also has a delaying effect. Specific nutritional abnormalities causing abnormal wound healing include the following:

Vitamin A. Vitamin A stimulates fibroblasts and collagen production, and in high doses counters the inhibition of wound healing caused by high doses of corticosteroids. While a normal level of vitamin A is required for optimal wound healing, there is no advantage to feeding high doses of vitamin A. However, in an animal that is receiving corticosteroid or vitamin E therapy for treatment of a condition unrelated to the wound, supplementary vitamin A can be given to counter the inhibitory effects associated with these medications.

Vitamin C. Vitamin C deficiency (scurvy) delays wound healing because of a specific function of vitamin C in the hydroxylation of proline and lysine in the production of collagen. Dogs and cats normally do not require exogenous sources of vitamin C.

Vitamin E. Vitamin E stabilizes cell membranes and at high doses retards wound healing and collagen production. Therefore, diets or vitamin supplements containing higher-than-recommended levels of vitamin E should not be fed to animals with healing wounds (also see above under Vitamin A).

Minerals. Enough trace minerals are present in the usual diets of dogs and cats that particular concern is not necessary, unless the animal is being fed artificially for prolonged periods (intravenously or by gastrostomy, enterostomy, or pharyngostomy tube). An appropriate calcium-phosphorus ratio is essential to rapid bone healing (see Chap. 21, Principles of Fracture Management). Zinc-deficient diets disrupt or delay epithelialization and collagen formation, but at high levels zinc has a deleterious effect on macrophage function and collagen formation. Zinc supplementation is best avoided.

The Effects of Drugs on Wound Healing

Corticosteroids

Corticosteroids have several effects on healing. They suppress the inflammatory process, the driving force behind the initial stages of healing, and inhibit macrophage migration; this may allow contamination to progress to infection. Later effects are inhibition of capillary budding, fibroblast proliferation, and collagen formation, and a reduced rate of epithelialization.

Both exogenous and endogenous corticosteroids hinder wound healing; however, administration for at least several days is necessary before a clinically obvious effect is noticeable. Endogenous corticosteroid release results from diseases such as hyperadrenocorticism (Cushing's disease) or from continued or intermittent stress. The effects of single or short-duration dosage of corticosteroids on wound healing are short-lived and should not preclude their use, even in very high doses, for treatment of shock. Low-dose steroid therapy designed to stabilize an animal with hypoadrenocorticism should not be discontinued during wound healing.

The effect of corticosteroids on slowing the connective tissue aspects of wound healing is more pronounced than its effect on epithelial healing. This difference can be useful when suppression of granulation tissue and collagen formation, but with continued epithelialization, is required, such as when managing ulceration or scar tissue in tubular structures such as the larynx and esophagus. This lathyrogenic effect can be achieved more specifically by other drugs such as beta-aminoproprionitrile; however, prednisolone (1 mg/kg daily in divided doses for 3 to 4 weeks) is often used because other lathyrogenic drugs have potentially toxic side effects.

Other Therapies

In very large doses, drugs such as aspirin, phenylbutazone, and indomethacin suppress healing, but these effects are not clinically obvious at the usual doses.

Cytotoxic drugs suppress cell metabolism and replication. If given locally in high doses (*e.g.*, by intra-arterial perfusion), they can have clinically obvious effects on wound healing, but if given at the systemic doses used in veterinary practice they do not have deleterious effects on local wounds.

Radiation has a similar effect, particularly if used for the first time a day or two after wounding. Radiation therapy should be started before surgery or delayed until there has been some fibroblast proliferation and collagen formation. In practical terms, starting radiotherapy at the time of suture removal is recommended, because the animal has recovered from the prolonged anesthesia and blood loss associated with the procedure, and local vascularity has been restored to near-normal levels so that replication of malignant cells (and thus sensitivity to radiation) has recommenced.

External Effects

Pressure from recumbency and inability to change position reduces blood flow to superficial areas. This effect is aggravated if a paralyzed animal is incontinent, as the wound may be bathed continuously with urine; this inhibits epithelial migration and proliferation and is a common cause of dehiscence in recumbent animals.

Wound vasculature, particularly superficial tissues such as skin and nonessential muscle, is affected by vasoconstriction designed to reduce heat loss when body temperature is low. This is particularly likely when an animal is recovering from anesthesia; fortunately, this period usually is short. The normal rate of increase in wound strength (particularly for skin) slows in animals subjected to abnormally cold conditions or animals with cranial trauma or other disease that interferes with the normal homeothermic mechanism.

The technique and materials used for superficial wound care should be selected carefully; many cleansing agents and antiseptics are toxic to tissue and can thus encourage deeper penetration by bacteria into contaminated wounds. Recommended techniques and cleansing solutions are described in Chapter 4.

Wound Infections

Infection develops only when a large number of organisms overwhelms the inflammatory response or when the animal is unable to mount a normal inflammatory response due to local or systemic factors. The four factors inherent in any infection are the host's defense mechanism, the number and types of organisms, the length of time during which contamination is allowed to occur, and the local environment in which the organism finds itself.

Ideally, a surgical wound contains no bacteria; however, some microorganisms gain access to the wound during all procedures. The environment in which veterinary surgical procedures are performed is never sterile; it ranges from grossly clean, with provision of filtered and controlled airflow, to frankly contaminated and open to the external environment. Equipment may add significantly to the environmental contamination; for example, ultrasonic teeth scaling pollutes the environment with bacteria-laden water droplets that can remain suspended for a considerable time.

Despite this very high contamination rate, the rate of infection of surgical wounds is low in most veterinary hospitals. The initial inflammatory phase of healing commences with flooding of the surgical wound with PMNs, followed by macrophages. The result is that the vast majority of surgical wounds do not develop infection, even though they are not sterile at the end of the procedure. The reason is that for most animals, a critical number (approximately 10^5 to 10^6/ml) of bacteria must be present in a wound before infection develops. With one or two exceptions, the type of organism present is less important than the number.

The longer the surgical wound is open to suspended particle contamination, the higher the number of bacteria in the wound will be at the end of the procedure, and the more likely an infection will develop. In human studies, infections were found to be much more common in procedures with a mean duration of 5 hours or more.

The distinction between contamination and infection is blurred. One wound may be able to handle very efficiently a bacterial inoculum of 10^5 potentially pathogenic organisms, if wound conditions are ideal. In another, an inoculum of 10^3 similar organisms may result in a disastrous infection if the organisms are protected amongst necrotic debris or if phagocytosis is inadequate.

Infection is sometimes defined as the growth of microorganisms within tissues; in many wounds, however, microorganisms grow without producing the clinical signs associated with infection. While difficult to define, an infection implies at least a temporary overwhelming of the local antimicrobial defense mechanisms.

Detecting Infection

The initial signs of infection are similar to those of an inflammatory response, which is expected in any wound; thus, there is a period during which it is difficult, if not impossible, to determine if a wound is infected.

Measuring body temperature, combined with careful inspection and palpation of the surgical wound, is the best means of diagnosing wound infection.

Fever may develop earlier, reach a higher level, and last longer in an animal with an infected wound than in an animal with an uninfected wound. This may be a useful response, because increased temperature inhibits the growth of many microorganisms. Fever that develops 3 to 5 days after wounding is especially likely to indicate incipient wound infection.

Inflammatory changes should be expected in the first day or two in any wound. Some swelling, redness of incised skin edges, and discomfort are common, but leakage of fluid from between the wound edges is not. Increase in volume of leaking fluid and a change in consistency from a clear serous or slightly bloody fluid to a turbid or frankly purulent discharge indicate infection; wounds of this sort also are more painful on palpation than would be expected.

Assessing deeper wounds is more difficult, particularly incised wounds in intra-abdominal or intrathoracic structures, because the discharges from these wounds collect in the body cavity rather than exiting through the skin incision. Incisions in intra-abdominal structures are best assessed by careful abdominal palpation and by observing return of function to the operated organ if the gastrointestinal or urinary systems were wounded.

Body temperature and periodic white-cell counts are other aids in detecting infection. For monitoring intrathoracic incisions, thoracic auscultation and observation of respiratory rate and effort are used to supplement body temperature and white-cell counts. Abdomino- or thoracocentesis should be performed if palpation, auscultation, or radiographic examination suggests the presence of fluid in an animal with fever or an increasing white-cell count.

Peripheral white-cell counts are useful monitors of wound infection, particularly if serial measurements are available. Presurgical patient assessment by leukocyte count is strongly recommended. A significant rise (to between 20,000 and 35,000/dl) is to be expected in the first 24 to 48 hours after surgery. A further increase in white cells or a decrease in the ratio of mature to band PMNs suggest that infection is present. White-cell counts and differential counts also are useful indicators of how treatment for infection is progressing and how well the animal can respond to the microbial challenge. When significant wound drainage is found, wound infection can be distinguished from other causes of fluid drainage, such as leakage from an inadequately closed urinary tract incision, by examining a smear of the fluid for bacteria. Paired serum and fluid creatinine concentration measurements also help differentiate urinary tract rupture from infection.

Bacteria can arrive in a wound from the animal itself (adjacent contaminated surfaces, hematogenous spread), the surgeon, the instruments and supplies, and by gravitational movement of suspended particles from the environment. The latter is the most difficult to control. Using a laminar airflow, particle-absorbing filters, and ultraviolet light in the operating room results in only a moderate drop in the infection rate in human hospitals, compared to clean surgical suites without these refinements. Movement of operating-room personnel is the major source of suspended particles. Methods to significantly reduce or eliminate the bacteria present on the animal's skin, the surfaces of the surgical team presented to the patient, and the instruments and supplies are described in Chapter 2, The Operative Procedure.

The standard procedures for animal, surgeon, and instrument preparation are of little use if the significance of the procedure is not appreciated. To assess the likelihood that contamination will reach a critical level, surgical procedures have been divided into the following four categories*:

1. *Clean wound.* A surgical (nontraumatic) wound. No inflammation or infection encountered. No break in aseptic technique. No hollow organ opened. (Includes hysterectomy and castration if no inflammation of the genital tract is found.)
2. *Clean-contaminated wound.* A hollow organ is opened but minimal spillage of

contents occurred. Noninflamed oropharynx, vagina, or biliary tract is entered. Minor break in aseptic technique occurred.
3. *Contaminated wound.* Hollow muscular organ is opened with gross spillage of contents, or acute inflammation without pus is encountered. A traumatic (nonsurgical) wound less than 4 hours old. A clean or clean-contaminated procedure in which a major break in technique occurred.
4. *Dirty wound.* Pus is encountered at operation, or a perforated hollow organ is found. A traumatic (nonsurgical) contaminated wound more than 4 hours old.

In surgical history, frequent mention is made of "laudable pus." This refers to the fact that before the understanding of antisepsis and asepsis, a surgical wound that was able to respond to the massive contamination that was unknowingly present was associated with a better prognosis; the lack of any drainage was associated with overwhelming infection, toxin production, and rapid death. Now that bacteria's role in infection is understood, pus is no longer laudable, because it indicates the presence of significant contamination that must be eliminated before the wound can heal.

Sources of Infection

Traumatic wounds with gross contamination, and penetration of hollow viscera containing bacteria, are the most obvious sources of infection because the bacteria are present at the surgical site itself. Less obvious sources are the skin of the animal adjacent to the surgical site (particularly as a result of secretions from hair follicles and skin glands that are squeezed up during surgical manipulation), and distant sites, from which bacteria travel by hematogenous or lymphatic routes.

The distant site need not be an area of obvious infection; all that is needed is a source of bacteria able to enter the body. The oral cavity is a common source, particularly if the teeth are cleaned or even examined during the

* From Recommendations of the Committee on Control of Surgical Infections and of the Committee on Pre- and Post-operative Care of the American College of Surgeons

procedure, because a bacteremia results. Other epithelial surfaces that may be inflamed and manipulated during surgery are the ear or other skin areas with dermatitis, the rectum, and the lower urinary tract. In a normal uninjured animal, the resulting bacteremia is cleared very rapidly (usually within 20 minutes) by the reticuloendothelial system, with no long-term consequences. In an area of injury, bacteria can adhere to pockets of hemorrhage and other extravasated fluids or damaged vessel walls, and hypoxic or anoxic conditions may persist for several hours, preventing the PMNs and other defense mechanisms from clearing the bacteria. This protected period allows rapidly growing bacteria to reach the critical bolus concentration, even if the inoculum was small to begin with.

Defenses Against Infection

Bacteria and other disease-causing organisms are everywhere, but a normal uninjured animal is protected in several ways. The primary method is by preventing organisms from entering deeper tissues. Every body surface open to the environment is covered with an epithelium that is generally impermeable to most microorganisms and that replicates itself. (The major exceptions are the teeth, which are covered with a nonrenewable enamel coating, and the toenails; these two areas are troublesome with regard to controlling entry of bacteria, particularly the teeth because of the moist bacteria-laden environment surrounding them.) Epithelial surfaces secrete fluids that are bactericidal, and some are equipped with mechanisms (such as the ciliary ladder in the respiratory tract, and peristaltic activity in the gastrointestinal tract) that remove material before it has time to permit bacterial penetration of the epithelial surface.

Thus, disease conditions that affect these normal clearance mechanisms (such as intestinal obstruction or ileus) or that may overwhelm the clearance system (such as aspiration of material into the airway during anesthesia) increase the possibility of wound infection by increasing the bacteremic load. Organisms that do manage to penetrate the epithelial barrier are dealt with by phagocytosis in the subepithelial tissues or by the reticuloendothelial filtration system. They may also stimulate an immune response that results in humoral (antibody) or cellular protection mechanisms.

In both surgical and traumatic wounds, tissues such as connective tissue are penetrated, exposed, and contaminated. Because these tissues are rarely exposed to bacterial contamination under normal circumstances, the protection mechanisms take longer to become established. Thus, bacterial growth has more time to reach the critical concentration that may overwhelm the tissues locally and produce infection. The so-called "golden period" of 4 to 6 hours is generally regarded as the time during which, if definitive wound treatment is applied, an infection is unlikely to develop. However, this period varies from one tissue to another depending on the local vascularity and the extent to which that tissue is routinely exposed to invading bacteria. Thus oral tissues, with a greater blood supply and "experience" with contaminating organisms, are able to manage a higher bacterial burden more successfully than can skin.

The most important mechanism available in connective tissues that have been invaded by bacteria is the inflammatory response. After the initial short period of vasoconstriction, local blood vessels dilate as a result of histamine release from degranulating mast cells and serotonin release from damaged platelets. As a result, the wound area is flooded with vascular and tissue fluids that are chemotactic for white blood cells. Initially, the intravascular leukocytes marginate in the area of injury, then penetrate through the gaps between swollen endothelial cells. Delivery of phagocytes to the area of injury is the key step in neutralization and clearance of bacteria. The fluid leaked into the injured area contains antigen-specific immunoglobulins that react with antigenic sites on the cell walls of the microorganisms. Activation of the complement cascade and opsonization permit the phago-cytes to recognize and engulf the bacteria. Within the phagocyte, the bacterium is killed and digested by lysosomal activity.

Host Defense Mechanism Failures

Some causes of reduced or absent host defense mechanisms are obvious. Congenital abnormalities include neutrophil dysfunction (such as in collies with gray collie syndrome) or, on the humoral mechanism side, lymphocyte dysfunction and agammaglobulinemia.

Many acquired diseases also affect an animal's ability to prevent or fight existing infections. Generalized conditions that affect wound healing such as malnutrition or chronic untreated diseases such as kidney failure, diabetes, and pancreatitis lower resistance to infection. Uncontrolled infection itself will consume white blood cells, and some bacteria produce toxins that depress formation of additional leukocytes.

Mechanical factors at the site of infection can have a potentially devastating effect. These may include the following:

- Reduced blood flow, tissue perfusion, and oxygenation, whether temporary due to blood loss or shock or more permanent due to chronic heart failure or anemia.
- Volume of infection, which prevents inflammatory cells from penetrating throughout the infected mass.
- Anatomic factors, such as presence of necrotic tissue, and fascial planes that direct wound fluids away from the original site.

Prevention of Wound Infection

The major method of reducing the likelihood of wound infection is by using the principles of good surgical technique. Aseptic technique, hemostasis, minimal dissection, sharp incision, gentle handling of tissue, avoidance or obliteration of dead space, and accurate apposition of sutured tissues without tension will go a long way to ensure that conditions within the wound are optimal for controlling contamination and speeding healing.

Rarely can we arrange to build a custom-designed surgical suite, and state-of-the-art human surgical suites are beyond the financial resources of even major veterinary institutions. As noted above, the actual reduction in suspended particle contamination that results from extensive design considerations is minor. A clean, smooth- and washable-surfaced room with minimal open shelves and stored unused equipment is satisfactory. Recommendations for cleaning the surgical room are described in Chapter 2, The Operative Procedure.

Instruments, supplies, surgical personnel, and patient preparation also are described in Chapter 2. Surgical procedures should be scheduled so that contaminated procedures are performed after clean procedures; they should be followed by cleansing of the entire room. Ideally, two or more surgical rooms or suites should be provided so that contaminated procedures such as teeth cleaning, ear cleaning, lancing of abscesses, and treatment of perianal fistulae or anal sac disease can be performed in an area that has an airflow away from the clean surgical area.

Specific recommendations for preparing the surgical site for particular body structures are given in the individual organ system chapters. Preparation and debridement of traumatic wounds is described in Chapter 4.

Antimicrobial Prophylaxis and Treatment

Since antimicrobials have become generally available, surgical infections have become significantly fewer, and management of infections has become much more successful. There is, therefore, a temptation to use routine antibiotic coverage, but as a result of this tendency resistant bacteria and fungal superinfections have become much more common in hospitalized patients (nosocomial infection). During this same 30- to 40-year period, because of significant advances in wound preparation techniques, antiseptic materials, and improved surgical supplies, foreign body responses that may predispose to surgical infection have become less likely. In general, studies designed to evaluate the effectiveness of an antibiotic drug on the likelihood of development of a surgical infection show that there is little correlation between the two.

Therefore, it is not necessary to use antibiotic coverage routinely for veterinary surgical patients; excellent results and a very low infection rate can be anticipated if the general principles of surgery, correct technique, and appropriate supplies are used. Antibiotic administration should not be used to cover for inappropriate or inadequate techniques or materials. The indiscriminate use of antibiotics, particularly prophylactically, can do more harm than good. Some antibiotics can cause toxic or anaphylactic reactions, although these are uncommon. The major reason for limiting usage of antibiotics is to decrease the likelihood that resistant strains will develop.

Use of the terms 'prophylaxis' and 'antibiotic cover' suggests that some contamination can be managed without serious consequences to the patient. The result is that attention to the other, more important aspects of surgical practice, such as maintaining aseptic technique, may slip. If contamination occurs, and an antibiotic suppresses growth of the more easily controlled, less pathogenic bacteria, the field is clear for growth of the resistant pathogens. Judicious use of technique cannot be overemphasized as the major means of reducing the likelihood of infection. This is one area where the surgeon is in absolute control.

Surgical drains are helpful in allowing egress of wound fluids and are indicated in wounds expected to produce more than a minimal amount of fluid. They are contraindicated when minimal wound fluid is anticipated, because they can result in retrograde flow of bacteria into a wound and subsequent infection. The use of surgical drains is described below.

Antibiotic coverage is indicated when a particular surgical wound seems significantly likely to develop an infection. Several factors should be considered, including the following:

1. *Procedure.* In general, clean and clean-contaminated wounds should not require antibiotic administration. Contaminated and dirty wounds may benefit from antibiotic administration, although debridement, local flushing of an antibiotic or antiseptic agent, and surgical drainage may be more definitive as management of the circumstances causing the wound to be placed in these categories. If the contaminated wound will be drained onto an accessible epithelial surface such as the oral or nasal cavities, gastrointestinal tract, or the skin, antibiotic treatment generally is not necessary. Factors such as the length of the procedure, extent of dissection necessary, and extent of debridement possible also must be considered. Procedures that will result in implantation into the wound of foreign material with a large surface area, such as orthopedic plates and screws, carry a higher risk of infection. If the decision is between extensive debridement with considerable risk of loss of function, or conservative debridement and antibiotic administration with the hope that some damaged tissues will heal and remain functional, the conservative approach is indicated, at least until clinical evidence shows that infection is present and is not controlled by the conservative treatment regime. Procedures such as cranial vault or spinal surgery in which even minimal infection may cause severe and possibly permanent disability are indications for antibiotic treatment.

2. *Tissue.* Tissues differ in both the local blood supply and the anatomical position relative to recumbency (and thus venous return and tissue fluid stagnation). Dependent tissues with poor intrinsic blood supply are more at risk of infection; however, antibiotic penetration is also likely to be less satisfactory in these tissues. Even in tissue with an excellent intrinsic blood

supply, a traumatic wound that is grossly contaminated has a bacterial burden that will at least temporarily overwhelm the defense mechanisms. Using an antibiotic in this circumstance must again be tempered by consideration of the likely penetration of the drug into the wound environment.

3. *Animal.* In general, medically compromised patients (those with shock, cardiovascular and respiratory disease, immunopathies, hyperadrenocorticism, or other diseases that will affect adversely tissue perfusion or local defense mechanisms) should be treated with an antibiotic when undergoing clean-contaminated, contaminated, or dirty wound procedures. Animals with concurrent injuries that may become seeded with bacteria or may be a source of bacteria during surgery should be treated with an antibiotic, as should animals treated with immune system- or inflammatory response-suppressive drugs (such as corticosteroids or cytotoxic drugs).

4. *Special circumstances.* An animal undergoing two procedures, one of which is likely to cause bacteremia and the other that will normally result in a clean or clean-contaminated closed wound, should be treated with an antibiotic. A common example is surgical treatment of a neoplasm or pyometra combined with teeth cleaning, as this is more likely to be indicated in an older dog in which avoidance of multiple anesthetic episodes is desirable. Teeth cleaning of itself is not necessarily an indication for antibiotic treatment (see Ch. 6).

A second special circumstance is liver surgery. If any damaged liver tissue is likely to be left in place without a viable blood supply, growth of *Clostridium spp.* (present in normal liver tissue of dogs) can result in toxin production and rapid death of the patient. Other examples of such special circumstances are given in appropriate chapters.

These four factors should be considered as a package: a questionable need for antibiotic therapy based on one factor may be strengthened if another factor also suggests a possible need.

Choice of Antibiotic, Dosage, Route, Timing, and Duration

If an antibiotic is indicated, the next considerations are the drug, dosage, route of administration, and timing and duration of administration.

Drug and Dosage
The choice of drug depends on the bacteria most likely to cause infection in that tissue and on the ability of a particular drug to penetrate the target tissue in high concentration. Because of the wide variation among tissues, specific recommendations for particular drugs and dosages are included in the individual organ system chapters. Recommended drugs and dosages for animals in shock are listed in Table 1-7. The choice of drug may be affected by the need for intravenous administration, and the time taken to achieve effective tissue concentrations by the intravenous route, if there is not enough time before surgery for oral or intramuscular administration. The general health of the animal must be considered when selecting a drug, particularly one with nephrotoxic or gastrointestinal disturbance effects.

The surgeon also must consider the relationships between the antibiotic and agents used during surgery (*e.g.*, general anesthetics, neuromuscular blocking agents) to allow for additive effects when calculating anesthetic or ancillary drug dosages. When a broad spectrum of microorganisms is expected, a combination of drugs may be indicated; the surgeon must ensure that the drugs selected are not antagonistic.

Route
Ideally, the drug should be available in bactericidal concentration in the wound fluid at the time of surgery. Because this requires administering the drug before creating the wound, this is possible only for elective (nontraumatic)

surgical wounds. For existing wounds that will be extended by debridement or for repair of tissue defects, administration should be intravenous, because this route gives the most rapid and reliable penetration of the drug into the wound fluid. However, even intravenous administration will not produce effective concentrations if local tissue perfusion is inadequate. Beginning fluid therapy at the time of or before intravenous antibiotic treatment is indicated in severely traumatized animals or animals that are in shock. If continuing treatment is indicated, intramuscular or oral administration is acceptable if the drug will be absorbed satisfactorily. This requires restoration of normal cardiovascular function and tissue perfusion for satisfactory intramuscular use, and good appetite without vomiting or diarrhea for satisfactory oral administration.

Timing and Duration of Administration

In elective procedures, antibiotic treatment generally is started about 24 hours before surgery to ensure an effective tissue concentration at the time of surgery. For particular organ systems such as the gastrointestinal tract, 24 hours may be insufficient; specific recommendations for antimicrobial preparation of the gastrointestinal tract are given in Chapter 12, The Esophagus and Stomach, and Chapter 13, The Small and Large Intestines. In nonelective procedures, the decision is not the time of initial administration, but rather the route to be chosen to obtain an effective tissue concentration most rapidly.

There is no standard period of administration. In some circumstances such as teeth cleaning or gingival surgery in an animal that is medically compromised, a single intravenous dose at the time of preanesthetic medication (thus achieving a high concentration for the duration of the bacteremia associated with the procedure) is sufficient. When a surgical wound with dissected tissue planes is created, antibiotic therapy should continue until the inflammatory phase of healing is well established; 3 to 4 days is appropriate. For severe wounds with considerable tissue destruction,

the clean-up and inflammatory phases of healing will take longer. Antibiotic treatment should continue for 6 to 7 days, with close monitoring of the wound for signs of infection. There is no necessary correlation between the duration of antibiotic treatment and continuing presence of a surgical drain.

Using antibiotics at the time of and following surgery does not reduce the need for vigilance in clinical assessment of the patient and surgical wound. Infections can develop in spite of, and occasionally because of, antibiotic treatment. If signs of infection develop, exploration of the wound and a culture of the organisms present, and a possible change in antibiotic treatment, may be indicated.

Management of Infected Wounds

Exudate must be drained by removal of one or more sutures, if necessary. Necrotic debris within the wound may require debridement, as described under management of traumatic wounds (see Chap. 4). The cause of infection should be considered: if there is evidence of bacterial overload of local defense mechanisms, antibiotic treatment may be required to return the tissues to the normal homeostatic state. If the cause of the infection is drainage of contaminated fluid from a dehisced hollow viscus (with the exception of the lower gastrointestinal tract, which is considered grossly contaminated and thus a dirty wound), antibiotic treatment probably is not necessary, and treatment should be directed at closing the dehiscence or providing more direct drainage, with delayed closure subsequently.

Surgical Drains

A *surgical drain* is a device to establish or to maintain an opening from a body part for the exit of fluid. The most commonly used surgical drain is a thin latex rubber tube 1.28 or 2.54 cm in diameter, often referred to as a Penrose drain. Other types used occasionally in clinical veterinary practice are sump, or suction, drains, that allow continuous or intermittent negative pressure to be applied to the end of a semi-rigid tube.

Indications for Use of a Surgical Drain

- In severely contused wounds in which blood and serum will accumulate otherwise.
- In wounds with extensive devitalized tissue or gross contamination, in which infection is likely.
- Following extensive surgical dissection or debridement, when prevention of pockets of dead space by sutures is not practical.
- When fluid may leak from an imperfectly closed incision in a hollow viscus.
- Following incisional drainage of an abscess or cyst, to prevent recurrence of fluid collection.
- For intermittent or continuous suction of a body cavity (see "Thoracic Drains," Chap. 9 and "Peritonitis," Chap. 11).

To be effective, drains must remain in place, must not restrict movement or tightly encircle tubular structures, and must not increase the chance of infection.

To maintain drain positioning, drains can be led from the outside to the inside of the tissue, exiting from a different site, with anchorage at both exteriorizing sites (*e.g.*, drains passed through the ear canal and middle ear cavity, exiting at the external ear canal opening and bulla osteotomy incision; or, drains placed into or next to the prostate, exiting from two different abdominal skin incisions). Alternatively, the end of the drain can be sutured at the deepest point to prevent migration outwards as a result of muscular activity. If this is done, the suture should not encircle the drain, as a section of drain may be torn off and retained as a foreign body when the drain is pulled out.

Drains work by allowing fluid to flow along the surface or through the lumen of the drain. Therefore, it is essential that the drain is placed loosely and that the suture holding it in place at the skin surface does not obstruct the skin opening. Just as fluid can pass to the exterior through a drain, fluid from the exterior can pass along a drain into the body. Bacteria from the skin surface can be drawn in, leading to infection. The risk of infection can be minimized by: 1) Maintaining the drain in place for the minimum period (usually considered to be when the flow of fluid has decreased significantly), and 2) Covering the exit point of drains that lie in a moist contaminated environment. The covering must not be tight, as this will prevent egress of fluid, and must include some absorbent material immediately over the drain. The absorbent material must be changed frequently. As is also true of antibiotic therapy, placement of a drain is not a substitute for good surgical technique. Administration of an antibiotic is not necessary simply because a drain is place.

Hemostasis

Tissues bleed when incised because vessels are transected. A completely bloodless field is not practical or even desirable during surgery because it indicates inadequate local perfusion and, therefore, poor conditions for healing.

Under some exceptional circumstances, it is possible to temporarily prevent all blood flow to an area of surgical interest, either by applying a tourniquet, temporarily occluding or ligating segmental blood vessels, or, for specialized procedures such as open-heart surgery, temporarily stopping cardiac contractions. The period during which flow ceases should be minimized (except when permanently ligating the carotid artery or arteries during major head surgery). After normal blood flow is reestablished and before the wound is closed, it should be examined for obvious areas of bleeding so that severed vessels can be identified and ligated.

Hemorrhage from severed vessels normally ceases from two effects. One is vasoconstriction and retraction of the end of the vessel, which has the sphincter-like effect of closing down the vessel lumen. The other is the coagulation mechanism.

The success of coagulation depends to a large extent on the presence and effective action of platelets. A complete blood count as part of presurgical patient assessment should include at least a subjective evaluation of the number of circulating platelets. If the laboratory reports that the smear examined has an inadequate number of platelets, a platelet count should be performed. If the circulating platelet count is below about 70,000 to 100,000/ml, elective surgery should be postponed until a cause for the thrombocytopenia is found and treated. If the procedure cannot be postponed and may cause considerable blood loss, fresh blood should be obtained for transfusion.

Platelets are responsible for the initial hemostatic plug. They accumulate rapidly at the site of vessel injury, adhere to the vessel wall, and promote intrinsic coagulation that results in formation of the fibrin clot. The effects of platelet action in causing vessel wall adhesiveness and fibrin production are counteracted by some drugs, particularly aspirin and indomethacin. The coagulation pathway ("clotting cascade") is shown in Chapter 1 (see Fig. 1–4). The result is a mass at the severed end of the vessel that consists of platelets and red and white blood cells enmeshed in a fibrinous clot. This process continues while the vessel endothelial cells are damaged, as this is the primary stimulus to platelet adhesiveness and the start of the intrinsic coagulation pathway. As the inflammatory phase of healing progresses, the vessel ends are sealed by adventitial cell closure, or blind-ended vessels in close proximity link up and recanalize. Healthy endothelial cells produce prostacyclin, which inhibits platelet function and causes vessel wall smooth-muscle relaxation. The fibrinous clot is then cleared by activation of plasmin.

These systems work very efficiently on small- and even medium-sized vessels, but are incapable of functioning well without the necessary substrate (platelets, calcium ions, and prothrombin). Thus, conditions that result in congenital coagulation factor deficiencies (*e.g.*, von Willebrand's disease, which is particularly prevalent in Doberman pinschers), that suppress bone-marrow function (*e.g.*, lymphosarcoma or cytotoxic drugs), that cause hypocalcemia (pregnancy, lactation) or abnormal liver function or vitamin K deficiency (*e.g.*, cirrhosis or warfarin poisoning) will make significant hemorrhage more likely.

For larger vessels, the size of the vessel is not the only factor determining its ability to constrict and be closed off by the normal coagulation process. Blood pressure often varies considerably between deep surgical anesthesia and recovery, particularly if the recovery is uncomfortable. A surgical wound with no obvious hemorrhage when the wound is closed may develop hemorrhage during the immediate postoperative period. This a common cause of oozing of fluid from a wound during the first 12 to 24 hours following injury and does not indicate infection, although it creates conditions in the wound that predispose to infection if a critical level of contamination is present. In some tissues, even larger vessels (3 mm in diameter and over) can close down and form hemostatic clots spontaneously. This is generally more likely for vessels running in folds of connective tissue, where the elastic fibers in the vessel wall can have maximal effect on vessel contraction and infolding of the vessel wall. Vessels that run in connective tissue attached to hard structures, such as intercostal arteries and vessels attached to periosteum of long bones, are unable to retract in this way and therefore bleed freely when cut.

To prevent blood loss that may result in hypovolemia and exacerbate the effect of hypotension associated with a surgical plane of anesthesia, bleeding must be controlled. Ideally, this is done by identifying, isolating, and clamping the vessel before transecting it; however, as vessels are cut and identified by oozing or spurting of blood, they should be clamped or coagulated. Techniques and instruments for this purpose are described in Chapter 2, The Operative Procedure. Using suction during surgery improves visualization of the wound significantly; however, it should not be used a a means of dealing with hemorrhage because it will not stop the flow of blood, and the extent of blood loss can only be appreciated by periodically observing the suction bottle.

Where a routine approach has to be made to obtain access to a target organ or area, such as in thoracotomy or laparotomy, the body wall incision often is rather neglected in the natural desire to grapple with the definitive problem. The result is that superficial and deep epigastric vessels during laparotomy, and intercostal or internal thoracic vessel during thoracotomy, may continue to bleed beneath the internal drapes used to delimit or pack off the area of interest. Hemorrhage from these vessels can be considerable and may confuse the surgeon by contributing to the accumulation of blood within the opened body cavity.

Blood transfusion techniques are described in Chapter 1, Principles of Companion Animal Surgery.

Neoplastic Disease— Surgical Aspects

Malignant neoplasms present a special challenge to the surgeon. Treating most other surgical diseases involves interference and reconstruction with an expectation that the tissue left in place consists of normal viable cells that will heal, and that if the tissue heals successfully, the condition requiring surgery will have been corrected. In this sense, tissues that look grossly healthy can be spared and used for reconstruction.

This is not so for malignant disease: the grossly normal tissues at the edges of the lesion may carry the seeds of further destruction because of microscopic invasion by malignant cells. For this reason, surgical management of malignant neoplasms is often frustrating for the surgeon and owner of the animal, because the procedure may go well, the tissues may heal, and function may be restored, only to

have recurrence of the original lesion become clinically obvious weeks, months, or even years later. Distant metastasis presents the same problems in a different way, the frustration being that successful management of the local lesion is of little or no long-term value if the disease has spread.

Compounding this problem is the fact that recognizing microscopic areas of tumor is not possible clinically. Thus, thoracic radiographs taken to examine for lung metastasis are incapable of detecting lesions smaller than about 0.5 to 1 cm in diameter. Radiographic examination and palpation of tissues to determine local limits of affected tissue is notoriously ineffective, particularly with lesions such as fibrosarcoma and hemangiopericytoma.

To minimize these problems, the clinician must obtain as much information about the lesion as possible. In general, histopathological diagnosis from a biopsy specimen is essential because of the differences in biological behavior among tumor types. Biopsy often requires general anesthesia to ensure that representative tissue is obtained; avoiding two anesthetic episodes by combining biopsy and definitive surgery is often a practical necessity. If an apparently neoplastic mass is found during exploratory surgery, the practical limitations of retaining function may dictate the extent of resection that is possible: conservative biopsy, and reexploration once the diagnosis and prognosis have been determined, will permit the owner to be better informed of the likely consequences.

Knowledge of combined therapy options (surgery-radiation, or surgery-chemotherapy) is necessary. Some tumors are much more likely to spread by hematogenous routes to the lungs (*e.g.*, thyroid gland tumors), others are disseminated by lymphatic channels (*e.g.*, tonsillar tumors), and others metastasize by both hematogenous and lymphatic routes (*e.g.*, mammary tumors). Staging of tumors, based on physical and radiographic examination findings and biopsy results, is a way to give accurate prognostic information for an increasing number of canine and feline malignancies; staging schemes set up by the World Health Organization are mentioned in the individual organ system chapters.

The superficially simplistic statements that "the first surgical procedure should be the definitive procedure" (excepting biopsy procedures), and that "a chance to cut is a chance to cure" have considerable application in the surgical management of neoplastic diseases. Although a conservative procedure may be indicated in a nonneoplastic condition as a means of retaining maximum function, to be followed by a more radical procedure if the results are unsatisfactory, conservative surgery on a malignancy invites direct tumor-cell implantation or metastasis into tissue planes that are opened during the procedure, increases the blood supply locally as a result of the healing process (therefore increasing the likelihood of hematogenous spread), and results in physical manipulation of the tumor, delivering a shower of malignant cells into the bloodstream.

Fortunately, small animal patients tolerate radical procedures well and rarely require complex restorative procedures or prosthetic devices to ensure function as an esthetically acceptable companion animal.

Biopsy Techniques and Equipment

The major requirement of any biopsy procedure is to ensure that diagnostic information has been obtained, particularly if the risks and expense of general anesthesia have been taken. For visible or palpable masses, the incision, or direction of penetration of the biopsy instrument, can be planned to avoid areas of necrotic tissue that may be unreadable microscopically. The surgeon should avoid taking tissue that includes only the edges of the mass, which may consist of inflamed but nonneoplastic tissue or, in the case of tumors arising from or attached to bone, periosteal new bone formation ("Codman's triangle"). The surgeon also should avoid taking tissue only from the

middle of the lesion, because this may be necrotic (and thus unreadable microscopically) in a rapidly growing neoplasm.

For deeper masses, a long biopsy needle instrument can be used. This carries the risk of hemorrhage; in some situations, this risk is sufficient that a careful surgical incision should be used instead so that any hemorrhage can be controlled. Examples are masses in the cranial neck/laryngeal area of dogs (which may be thyroid adenocarcinoma) and suspected masses in the spleen and liver (which are likely to be hemangiosarcomas), because these tumors bleed very freely when penetrated and may result in exsanguination. Appropriate biopsy techniques for each organ are described in the organ system chapters.

The tissue biopsied should be placed in fixing solution immediately.

Surgical Resection of Malignant Tumors

Ideally, the entire tumor and a zone around the tumor large enough to include all areas of microscopic invasion are resected. This sometimes requires a procedure that may result in functional impairment. Where possible, the grossly obvious tumor and surrounding zone of possibly infiltrated affected tissue are isolated from normal tissue and resected using a planned process of dissection of known tissue planes, vessel location, identification, and ligation. Defects resulting from removal of the tumor are repaired or reconstructed. In some instances, it is easier to remove more tissue because the control of hemorrhage or closure is simplified; thus forequarter amputation is preferred in dogs and cats to mid-humeral or shoulder amputation.

En bloc resection is a technique whereby a section of tissue is removed without regard for the natural tissue planes. Hemorrhage is thus much more likely during the procedure, and neurological or other functional impairment is likely to be long-term. Examples are nasal or oral resection, where the bone structure prevents the isolation of particular areas of tissue without affecting other areas.

Combination therapy (surgery-radiation, surgery-radiation-hyperthermia, or surgery-chemotherapy) may permit limited resection of lesions, leaving remaining neoplastic tissue to be managed by the subsequent radiation or chemotherapy. This is referred to as debulking surgery. Because tumor tissue is left in place, wound complications are more likely. Debulking procedures are used occasionally as palliative treatment, although they are worthwhile only if the likelihood of complications is low.

Suggested Readings

Dodds WJ. Hemostasis and coagulation. In: Kaneko JJ. Clinical biochemistry of domestic animals. 3rd ed. New York: Academic Press, 1980.

Hunt TK. Wound healing and infection—theory and surgical practice. New York: Appleton-Century Crofts, 1980.

Johnston DE. The processes in wound healing. J Am Anim Hosp Assoc 1979;13:186.

Peacock EE, Van Winkle W. Wound repair. 3rd ed. Philadelphia: WB Saunders, 1984.

Riviere JE, Kaufman GM, Bright RM. Prophylactic use of systemic antimicrobial drugs in surgery. Compend Cont Ed Pract Vet 1981;3:345.

Savlov ED, Dunphy JE. The healing of the disrupted and resutured wound. Surgery 1954;36:362.

4

Michael M. Pavletic

The Skin: Wound Closure and Reconstructive Surgery

Surgical Anatomy of the Skin

The skin is composed of two basic layers: the epidermis and the dermis. The epidermis of hairy skin has three major regions: the stratum cylindricum (stratum basale), the stratum spinosum (stratum malpighii, prickle cell layer), and the stratum corneum. The stratum cylindricum and stratum spinosum are collectively termed the stratum germinativum. Mitotic activity in the stratum germinativum is responsible for the continuous replacement of epidermal cells in healthy skin. Similarly, cells from this layer serve as the source of epithelium for full-thickness skin defects healing by second intention.

The dermis is predominately composed of a mucopolysaccharide ground substance (hyaluronic acid and chondroitin sulfuric acid) and collagen. It contains the important cutaneous capillary network, lymphatics, hair follicles, and glandular structures. Hair follicles, sebaceous glands, and sweat glands are of ec-

todermal origin. The outer root sheath of hair follicles in particular is continuous with the stratum cylindricum and can serve as a major source of epithelium for partial-thickness skin wounds healing by second intention.

The panniculus muscle (panniculus carnosus) is a term collectively describing a layer of thin muscles including the platysma, sphincter colli superficialis, sphincter colli profundus, and cutaneous trunci. The cutaneous trunci is the major cutaneous muscle of the body, and covers most of the trunk in the dog and cat. There is no panniculus muscle layer in the middle and lower regions of the limbs. The circulation to the overlying skin is closely associated with the panniculus musculature.

Circulation to the skin is derived from direct cutaneous arteries in the dog and cat. These arteries and companion veins travel parallel to the skin surface in the subcutaneous tissue. Terminal branches of direct cutaneous arteries supply the subdermal (deep) plexus at the level of the panniculus muscle layer (where present) or in the hypodermis associated with the dermal surface of the skin on the extremities. Branches from the subdermal plexus penetrate the dermis to supply the middle and superficial plexuses. Preserving the skin's circulation is key to the survival of the skin (see "Undermining the Skin" below).

Wound Classification

Wounds should be closely examined and classified into one of four categories according to condition: clean, clean-contaminated, contaminated, or dirty and infected (see Chap. 3, The Surgical Wound, p. 75).

If the veterinarian is unsure of the severity of the wound (*e.g.*, sccms to fit both clean-contaminated and contaminated categories), it should be treated as though it belongs in the more serious category. The age of the wound was once a major criterion in determining whether it could be closed primarily. The so-called "golden period" of 4 to 6 hours after wounding was suggested as a safe time frame for primary closure; after 6 hours, infection was considered more likely. Surgeons experienced in wound management today realize that the severity of contamination, tissue injury, and circulatory compromise are more important than time alone in classifying a wound and selecting the appropriate closure. For example, wounds involving the head often can be closed primarily because of the excellent blood supply to this region, whereas similar wounds to the lower extremities should be handled in a more conservative fashion.

Options for Wound Closure

Classifying the wound enables the clinician to logically decide upon the proper method of management. For a given wound, there may be more than one option for closure. The four basic options for closure of an open wound include: primary closure, delayed primary closure, secondary closure, and healing by second intention.

Primary Closure

Primary closure or healing by first intention is reserved for wounds created under aseptic conditions. Wounds with minor contaminants can be converted to surgically clean wounds with judicious debridement and copious lavage with sterile isotonic solutions.

Delayed Primary Closure

Wounds with borderline contamination may be left unsutured and temporarily covered with a sterile dressing. Delayed closure allows for adequate drainage and time for improved resistance of tissue to infection before suturing. If no devitalized tissue or infection is noted upon wound inspection by the fourth or fifth day, primary closure may be attempted.

Secondary Closure

Secondary closure is generally reserved for wounds with superficial contamination or invasive infection, including wounds that become infected during delayed primary closure. Secondary closure can be attempted between the fifth and tenth days, with two methods—direct suture opposition of the two granulation surfaces (healing by third intention), or granulation tissue excision and primary closure. The latter technique is preferred by many surgeons due to the relative ease in mobilizing the wound edges for closure, improved cosmetic results, and the lower incidence of infection after the granulation tissue is excised.

Closure by Second-Intention Healing

Healing by second-intention contraction and epithelialization is commonly employed in veterinary medicine. It generally is reserved for dirty and infected wounds in which closure by the previous three techniques is unadvisable. Large cutaneous defects that cannot be sutured closed may be left to contract and epithelialize. As noted in Chapter 3, two processes occur in the open wound to promote closure: epithelialization and wound contraction.

Wound healing is incomplete without restoration of the epithelial surface. In the open wound, the epithelial cells from the adjacent skin border become mobilized, proliferate, flatten out, and migrate out and downward over the exposed dermal border and adjacent healthy granulation bed. Migrating epithelial cells travel under any clot or scab present. Epithelial cells secrete proteolytic enzymes to "cleave" a path for their migration. In sutured wounds with a small dermal gap, epithelial cells can bridge the gap within 48 hours.

However, in a moderate-sized wound, epithelial migration may take weeks or may never cover completely the open wound. The surface of epithelialized wounds (scar epithelium) under these circumstances is thin and fragile. On the more protected areas of the animal, this wound covering may be satisfactory, but areas subject to periodic trauma or wear will abrade or split the scar epithelium. In full-thickness skin losses that have healed in this fashion, a limited number of hair follicles and sebaceous glands may regenerate by differentiation of migrated epidermal epithelium. Under these circumstances, a skin flap or durable skin graft would be required.

Most veterinarians have seen large skin wounds heal with surprisingly small epithelialized scars compared to the magnitude of the original defect. Under these circumstances, the normal bordering skin appears to have been pulled toward the center of the wound. This centripetal movement of the skin is termed *wound contraction*. Wound contraction occurs remarkably well in areas of loose skin in the dog and cat, independent of the process of epithelialization previously discussed.

Extensive research has demonstrated that specialized fibroblasts with contractile protein are probably responsible for the stretching or pulling of the normal adjacent skin. These cells, termed myofibroblasts, appear to attach to the underlying dermis of the bordering skin margin and the underlying fascia or panniculus muscle layer in the dog and cat. As these cells contract together, the skin slowly stretches forward. Scarring can lock the overlying skin, preventing skin gliding and offsetting the force of myofibroblastic contrac-

tion. Similarly, skin excessively stretched or areas with limited available loose skin (such as distal extremities) can create counter-tension that neutralizes the myofibroblasts. Interestingly, square wounds contract more readily than circular wounds because the straight sides are drawn inward unimpeded, whereas the force of contraction in a circular wound is not distributed evenly on a linear surface. Open wounds no longer able to contract must rely on epithelialization to complete the closure without surgical intervention. Contraction has been reported to occur between the 3rd and 42nd days in the rabbit. In the dog, a longer lag period of approximately 5 to 9 days occurs. The stretching and thinning of the skin surrounding the contracted wound is termed "intussusceptive growth." New epithelial cells and new connective tissue form to bolster and restore the stretched cutaneous areas.

In many cases, healing by second intention is a practical and economical method of effecting closure, if adequate wound care is administered. However, not all wounds will heal properly by second-intention healing. Some wounds will not contract and epithelialize to completion; other wounds form a fragile epithelialized scar that abrades or splits open. Excessive scarring and contraction may result in restricted motion to a limb or other body region (wound contracture). Cosmetic results may be unsatisfactory. The occasionally prolonged process of healing, combined with the cost of hospital visits, bandage materials, and medications, may end up costing the owner more time and money, and the animal and owner more "aggravation," than early closure with a skin flap or grafting technique.

Healing by Adnexal Reepithelialization

Cutaneous burns and abrasions may be categorized as superficial, partial thickness, and full thickness according to the depth of injury. Superficial cutaneous loss includes loss of the epithelium but preservation of the germinal layer. Reepithelialization originates from this epithelial layer. A partial-thickness loss results in the loss of the entire epithelial layer and a variable portion of the dermis. Reepithelialization in this case arises from adnexal structures (hair follicles, sebaceous glands, sweat glands). Any partial-thickness injury may be converted to a full-thickness loss from infection and improper, abusive wound management.

A full-thickness skin loss results in complete loss of the epidermis and dermis. Ultimate coverage of this cutaneous defect must occur from the viable cutaneous epithelium peripheral to the wound unless surgical intervention or graft coverage is instituted. The donor site from which a split-thickness graft is harvested will heal as a partial-thickness wound. Healing of the donor site, however, has the advantage of minimal tissue injury because the wound is made under aseptic conditions with minimal trauma.

Basic Wound Management

Clean wounds and those with minor contamination received within 6 hours of occurrence pose less of a problem to the surgeon, but wounds with gross contamination or infection can become a major challenge in treatment and closure. In selected areas of the dog or cat, small wounds of this nature can be excised completely and the surgical defect closed primarily. Larger wounds generally require management in a stepwise fashion before closure can be safely accomplished.

The primary goal in managing all wounds is to establish a healthy vascular wound bed free from necrotic tissue, foreign debris, and infection. The six basic steps in managing contaminated, dirty, or infected wounds follow:

1. Prevention of further contamination
2. Debridement of dead and dying tissue
3. Removal of foreign debris and contaminants
4. Adequate wound drainage
5. Promotion of a viable vascular bed
6. Selection of the appropriate method of closure

Preventing Further Contamination

On admission, wounds should be protected temporarily from drying and further contamination with debris and resistant strains of hospital organisms by temporarily applying a sterile dressing with an antimicrobial agent. Water-miscible ointments are preferred to heavier oil-based agents, which are difficult to rinse out of the wound. Wet saline dressings (sterile gauze soaked with saline) that include an antibiotic or nonirritating antimicrobial agent are useful. In one study, a povidone-iodine solution of 0.5%, a benzalkonium chloride solution of 1:2,500, and a chlorhexidine solution of 0.5 to 1.0 percent proved to be useful in reducing bacterial populations, with the chlorhexidine solution the most effective for wound irrigation. These agents also could be incorporated into wet dressings. In general, the more serious infected wounds should be cultured (aerobic and anaerobic) before instituting systemic antibiotic therapy.

Ideally, animals should be anesthetized for optimal wound preparation and debridement. Upon removal of the bandage, the open wound should be covered with sterile gauze pads impregnated with sterile K-Y Jelly (Johnson & Johnson, New Brunswick, NJ), sterile saline, or an antimicrobial solution, and the skin should be liberally clipped around the defect for surgery. Waterproof drapes are used to drape the surgery site and the wound cover is removed.

Debridement

Necrotic tissue should be excised, along with areas of questionable viability if the tissue is not essential to healing or function. However, staged (daily) debridements may be advisable over a single aggressive surgical debridement. Contaminated and injured fat overlying exposed skeletal muscle can be excised safely to remove debris. However, aggressive excision of subcutaneous fat and portions of panniculus muscle attached to exposed skin segments should be avoided to preserve the skin's blood supply (subdermal plexus and associated direct cutaneous vessels). Skin can be excised liberally in areas where ample loose skin prevails; a more conservative "wait-and-reassess" approach is justified when skin of questionable viability is on the extremities, where skin is at a premium.

Although bleeding along the skin margins is considered a desirable intraoperative clinical sign of adequate cutaneous arterial circulation, it does not give any information about venous return. Vasospasm may cause a temporary drop in local cutaneous circulation, with a misleading decline in bleeding from the wound edge. The presence of bleeding from the subdermal plexus is no guarantee that blood is not being shunted from the nutrient circulation of the skin. Furthermore, the presence of circulation within a skin area also is no assurance that trauma, edema, infection, venous compromise, or progressive thrombosis will not destroy the circulation present at the time of the initial examination.

Various enzymatic debriding agents are available and can be employed successfully. Agents on the market include trypsin-chymotrypsin, fibrinolysin-desoxyribonuclease, collagenase, sutilains, and streptokinase-streptodornase. They vary in strength and effectiveness when used topically. The author restricts their use to small areas or pockets where surgical debridement is likely to cause unnecessary trauma and bleeding. However, these agents generally are not a substitute for surgical debridement of larger areas of necrosis.

Removal of Debris and Contaminants

Dirt, clay particles, and organic debris promote infection and delay wound healing. Manual removal of gross debris, followed by pressure lavage with an isotonic solution, can remove most contaminants remaining after initial debridement. Moderate-sized wounds generally are lavaged with 500 to 1,000 ml of saline or lactated Ringer's solution. More lavage solution can be used if necessary. Adding chlorhexidine, povidone-iodine solution, and benzalkonium chloride can reduce significantly the bacterial count of the wound, as discussed above.

Excellent clinical results follow the use of isotonic solutions in contaminated wounds under pressure using a 19-gauge needle attached to a 35-ml syringe. Full force of the plunger will effectively deliver 8 pounds per square inch (psi) to the wound surface when the needle is placed immediately perpendicular to the surface. Adding a three-way stopcock attached to a sterilized intravenous fluid line will enable the surgeon to refill the syringe rapidly. Cupping a hand around the area minimizes overspray.

It is important for the surgeon to carefully separate and elevate the wound edges and explore adjacent fascial planes that may harbor debris. However, indiscriminant dissection should be avoided to prevent additional tissue trauma and contamination in uninvolved areas.

Drainage

Wound drainage is critical to the treatment of grossly contaminated wounds. Unless the surgeon is confident that necrotic tissue and all debris has been removed, and bacterial contamination has been minimized, primary closure is best avoided. Even then, a Penrose drain should be inserted to drain tissue fluid to reduce the risk of postoperative infection. When possible, the drain should be covered with a sterile protective bandage to minimize the danger of an ascending infection.

Delayed primary closure is a more conservative approach to postoperative wound care. The author's current preference is to pack the wound open with a wet dressing, using several layers of gauze pads soaked in saline solution with or without a nonirritating antimicrobial agent, followed by layers of adherent roll gauze and an outer elastic tape covering. Packing the wound open maximizes wound drainage, while the saline bandage maintains tissue hydration, thins any thick or tenacious discharge, and absorbs and stores drainage material. In difficult areas, a "tie-over" dressing can be used by placing a series of interrupted suture loops around the edge of the wound and lacing suture material through the loops to retain the underlying dressing. Bandages are changed under aseptic conditions one to three times daily, allowing the surgeon to reinspect the wound for additional necrotic tissue requiring debridement. In 3 to 5 days, the wound is generally healthy enough that an appropriate closure technique can be selected.

Promoting a Viable Vascular Bed

The veterinarian's major goal in managing a dirty, infected wound is to promote a healthy vascular (granulation) bed. Granulation tissue forms a barrier that discourages bacteria from invading underlying tissues, fills in defects, and provides a vascular scaffold capable of supporting epithelialization and grafts, if necessary.

Removing necrotic tissue, debris, and contaminants minimizes infection and the hazards of delayed healing. Similarly, adequate postoperative drainage provides an escape route for debris and discharge, further reducing the likelihood of abscessation. Postoperative wound bandaging and support protects the wound from additional contaminants and trauma. Under these circumstances, circulation to the remaining viable tissues can improve and support the development of a granulation bed. Although exposed bone stripped of periosteum cannot support a granulation bed, the adjacent viable soft tissue often will form healthy granulation tissue that creeps over its surface.

Selecting the Method of Closure

The true magnitude of the defect is best determined once tissue swelling subsides and the wound is devoid of necrotic tissue. At this stage (generally 7 to 10 days after the initial injury), the surgeon may note that the wound is considerably smaller than originally ascertained and may heal by contraction and epithelialization without further surgical intervention. Such wounds may be closed secondarily if there is adequate skin. Similarly, the clinician may promote second-intention healing and reserve surgical intervention when contraction and epithelialization slows or early complications are recognized (*e.g.,* a contracture).

Local or distant flap techniques or free grafts should be considered for larger defects, especially when second-intention healing may take a long time (if it occurs at all) or when they can economically bypass the prolonged wound care required. Pedicle grafts and free-grafting techniques also are advisable when excessive scarring or wound contraction may restrict function (contracture) in the area involved. If the veterinarian elects to promote wound closure by wound contraction and epithelialization after formation of a healthy granulation bed, wet dressings are discontinued in favor of topical ointments and protection of the wound with a bandage if necessary. Petroleum jelly and antibiotic ointments can be used successfully. A spray medication containing trypsin, balsam of Peru, and castor oil (Granulex-V, Dow B. Hickam, Inc., Houston, Texas) can be used to protect the granulation tissue and epithelial border from dessication, to remove any remaining necrotic tissue, and to stimulate wound closure. This medication is easy for an owner to apply and eliminates the need to apply creams or other products with an applicator or fingers. Warm compresses should be applied to larger open wounds before applying the medication to remove accumulated crusts and tissue debris.

Wound Healing Complications

The surgeon can minimize or eliminate many complications noted in wound healing by adhering to the basic surgical principles outlined by Halsted and Esmarch (see Chap. 1).

Healthy tissue is surprisingly resistant to infection. The surgeon can significantly reduce the incidence of infection simply by excising necrotic tissue and preserving the circulation of the bordering viable tissue. Injuries heal more slowly when destruction of the blood supply is a primary feature. Hypoxic wounds more readily become infected.

Infection

Although a laceration and a puncture wound may have the same degree of tissue injury, the environment of each wound is vastly different. Open wounds rarely are the source of invasive infection. A puncture wound lacking drainage forms a closed pocket, providing an ideal environment for bacterial proliferation. As a result, puncture wounds (such as bite wounds) should be incised, gently explored, debrided, lavaged, and allowed to heal as an open wound, unless the surgeon can be sure that treatment has converted the wound into a surgically clean one that will tolerate closure.

Abscess formation is more common in the cat, usually as a result of previous bite wounds from other cats. The small puncture holes readily seal and promote abscessation. *Pasteurella multocida* is a common oral contaminant in small animals and often is responsible for bite wound infections. Areas of cellulitis eventually coalesce to form the abscess cavity. Abscesses are drained ventrally once they have "pointed," and warm compresses can facilitate such formations. Many abscesses in small animals readily respond to this regimen followed by gentle exploration, flushing, debridement, and systemic broad-spectrum antibiotic support for 7 to 10 days. Large abscess cavities occasionally are packed open for 2 or 3 days with moistened medicated gauze packs, changed once or more daily. Partial drying of the pack facilitates the absorption of the discharge and helps to strip out necrotic tissue that adheres to the cotton fibers. Thereafter, warm compresses and nonirritating topical agents are applied to protect the developing granulation bed from dessication until second-intention healing is complete. Culture and sensitivity testing and gram stains usually are not warranted for many of the smaller abscesses seen in small animal practice. Deep abscesses, recurrent infections, persistent or recurrent draining tracts, and potentially life-threatening infections do warrant their use. These clinical observations should alert the clinician that the condition is not a minor local infection, and warrant a detailed clinical workup, examination, and any necessary surgical exploration.

Draining Tracts

Persistent or intermittent draining tracts have occurred in the presence of large pockets of necrotic tissue that the body cannot expel; underlying bone infection, bone sequestra, or bone chips harboring bacteria; bacterial or fungal organisms resistant to the current treatment regimen; foreign bodies, especially plant material (*e.g.,* grass fragments, wood, grass awns); surgical foreign bodies such as implants or braided nonabsorbable suture material (*e.g.,* silk, Vetafil, cotton, polyester); and neoplastic conditions (with or without the presence of microorganisms) that mimic infection or foreign bodies. Immunosuppression by various therapeutic measures or underlying disease (*e.g.,* feline leukemia, feline infectious peritonitis) may explain the patient's susceptibility to infection and poor healing and should be investigated.

Radiographs of these draining areas occasionally reveal radiopaque objects amenable to removal. Fistulograms sometimes are useful to highlight foreign bodies, determine the magnitude of the tract(s), and examine their relationship with neighboring structures. Cannulation and injection of dyes such as sterilized methylene blue can stain the tracts, facilitating their surgical removal. Deep wound cultures should be obtained for aerobic, anaerobic, and fungal culture. Small foreign bodies can be elusive by migrating through tissue planes or can be hidden by layers of scar tissue and necrotic debris. Whenever reasonably feasible, the author cannulates each tract and dissects around the tracts and associated granulomatous tissue *in toto*, avoiding the spillage of contaminated material into neighboring tissues. After surgery, the excised tissue is opened and examined, culture samples are taken, and the tissue is submitted for histopathologic examination.

The Non-Healing Wound

The debilitated patient with poor nutritional status or serious underlying disease is naturally prone to healing problems. The veterinarian must remember that an open wound requires more circulation and energy to heal than does a primary closed wound, a factor that must be considered in the patient on anti-inflammatory medication. After a careful clinical workup on the patient and correction of any underlying disorders, closure of the wound with skin flaps or free grafts often can eliminate the slow healing process or stagnant open wound.

Open wounds occasionally fail to heal by second intention. Inflammation is needed for wound healing; if too little occurs, repair slows. However, if the inflammation process is exaggerated, the inflammatory cells compete with fibroblasts for vital nutrition, also slowing repair.

Chronic low-grade infection usually leads to excessive scarring. An exposed healthy pink vascular granulation bed will in time progress to a bed laden with collagen with a decline in capillaries and fibroblasts. This bed is a poor surface for epithelial cells to survive.

Among the factors that can stop the process of wound contraction are restrictive scars, offsetting peripheral skin tension that impedes myofibroblastic activity, anti-inflammatory agents, the elevation and separation of the skin borders from the underlying tissues and bed, and repeated shearing forces applied to the wound surface. Indeed, repeated trauma to the area can damage local circulation, exaggerate the inflammatory response, and rub off the epi-

thelium attempting to migrate over the wound surface. The foot pads, elbow, hock, and skin over other bony prominences are susceptible to continuous rubbing, pressure, and exposure to moisture and contaminants unless good nursing and proper closure techniques are used.

Topical vitamin A can restimulate a suppressed anti-inflammatory reaction as a result of a steroid-suppressed immune system. Vitamin A systemically should be used sparingly when steroid-suppression of inflammation is desirable. Under these circumstances, topical vitamin A may be preferable. Zinc is necessary to mobilize vitamin A from the liver, but steroid therapy suppresses the zinc serum level. Some surgeons will supplement human patients with zinc and vitamin A under these circumstances, although proof of its efficacy is lacking. Vitamin A can restimulate wound epithelialization but not steroid-retarded contraction. However, the total nutritional status of the patient must be maintained for optimal healing (see Chaps. 1 and 3).

Scarring

Scar tissue is a normal response to healing. Scarring is beneficial in some injuries but undesirable in others. For example, the formation of granulation tissue and collagen deposition is desirable for many shearing injuries involving the carpal or tarsal points to improve joint stability and close the defect. Excessive scarring in other areas, however, may restrict motion or function.

To minimize scar tissue, meticulous atraumatic surgical technique, physical therapy, traction, pressure, and control of infection is essential. Infection has the added undesirable effect of diverting components required for healing and promoting the unsatisfactory deposition of scar tissue to wall off the microorganisms.

The term "wound contracture" implies a loss or restriction of motion to an area, usually as a result of excessive scarring. Excessive wound contraction may contribute to contracture formation. Positioning the affected area in a more comfortable flexed position by the injured patient can favor collagen deposition, which locks the area into this position. Preventing wound contracture requires early recognition of the developing problem and appropriate steps to combat it. In veterinary medicine, early appropriate coverage of open wounds with skin flaps and related Z-plasty techniques or by free grafts followed by physical therapy can prevent contracture development. Once contracture has developed, scar excision, partial myotomies, flap or free-graft coverage, and physical therapy may be required. Traction to the area may be required temporarily to combat recurrence until healing is complete and physical therapy can be implemented. Physical therapy can be effective in modifying collagen deposition and cross-linking to improve mobility.

Seromas

Seromas may form beneath the skin in areas traumatized accidentally or surgically. Inflammation and lymphatic injury result in the formation of serum pockets in areas where dead space prevails. Traumatic surgical techniques, harsh wound cleansing techniques, the presence of foreign debris and irritants, and constant movement of an area also contribute to seroma formation. The serum separates tissues and discourages adjacent surfaces from healing.

Small seromas beneath skin are of no major consequence, but larger pockets usually require drainage. Aspiration of large seromas generally is unrewarding, although applying a firm compression bandage after aspiration may help eliminate dead space to promote healing of the separated tissue planes. However, the insertion of a Penrose drain for 2 to 5 days generally is necessary with an overlying compression bandage, when possible. Any foreign debris or irritants should be removed to discourage recurrence. Compression bandages, Penrose drains, closed suction units, or a combination of bandages and a drain may be used

when the surgeon suspects that the fluid accumulation is likely in an area where dead space is present.

Buried "tacking" sutures are used to discourage seroma formation in small sterile dead space areas. However, large areas of dead space may be impossible to tack down completely. Excessive use of buried sutures may promote wound infection and cannot be recommended for routine use in contaminated wounds. Buried sutures also may result in loculation (formation of smaller seromas that do not communicate with one another for simple drainage).

Primary Closure

Undermining the Skin

The loose elastic skin over the neck and trunk in the dog and cat permits the surgeon to close many skin defects by undermining alone. The key to the successful surgical elevation of skin is preserving its blood supply. This requires the preservation of the direct cutaneous arteries and associated subdermal (deep) plexus. The following six points can serve as general guidelines for undermining skin in small animals:

1. Skin should be undermined below the panniculus muscle layer when present to preserve the subdermal plexus and associated direct cutaneous vessels.
2. Skin without an underlying panniculus muscle layer (middle and distal portion of the extremities) should be undermined in the loose areolar fascia beneath the dermis to preserve the subdermal plexus.
3. Direct cutaneous arteries and veins should be preserved when possible during undermining.
4. Skin closely associated with an underlying muscle should be elevated by including a portion of the outer muscle fascia with the dermis rather than undermining between these structures. This may help minimize

injury to the subdermal plexus. The close relationship of the superficial pectoral muscle to the overlying skin is an example of this anatomic consideration.

5. Direct injury to the subdermal plexus can be avoided by using atraumatic surgical technique.

6. Surgical manipulation of skin recently traumatized should be avoided or minimized until circulation improves as noted by the resolution of contusions, edema, and infection.

Simple Geometric Designs

Primary wound closure is facilitated by converting irregularly shaped skin defects into a simple geometric design. Similarly, irregular masses can be excised using square, rectangular, triangular, elliptical, or circular incisions (Fig. 4-1). Large skin puckers called "dog-ears" can be excised to improve the cosmetic results of the closure. Small dog-ears generally flatten and disappear without excision. However, the surgeon also must evaluate the magnitude of the skin wound in relation to the skin tension. Lax or loose skin adjacent to large defects should be surgically elevated and stretched toward to the areas of the defect when wound closure and postoperative tension are primary concerns.

Tension-Relieving Techniques

Relaxing Incisions

Relaxing incisions are skin incisions of variable length created parallel to a wound that cannot be closed without excessive tension. As a result, relaxing incisions are perpendicular to lines of tension and vary in length and placement according to the area in question. A relaxing incision may be little more than a stab incision, or may parallel the length of the primary closure site, in effect creating a bipedicle advancement flap (see "Local Flaps," below). The secondary defect that forms generally is

allowed to heal by second intention. This "exchange" of open wounds is justified when:

1. Primary closure of the wound is necessary to protect underlying vital structures.
2. Complications associated with wound dehiscence are greater than managing the secondary defect.
3. Creating a secondary defect in a "sheltered" area enables the surgeon to close the wound with full-thickness skin in areas subject to chronic physical abuse (e.g., bony prominences, areas subject to self-mutilation).
4. Creating a secondary defect in a healthy vascular area permits wound closure of a poorly vascularized area incapable of healing by second intention (e.g., irradiated areas, non-healing ulcers).

Multiple stab incisions created in staggered rows (skin meshing) have been used clinically in the horse and reported experimentally in the dog. The skin on each side of the defect is meshed, resulting in a cumulative gain. However, skin necrosis is possible with this technique and with long parallel relaxing incisions. Because direct cutaneous arteries and the subdermal plexus of the skin travel parallel to the skin, indiscriminate placement of the incisions may compromise circulation to the skin being used for closure.

Z-Plasty

Z-plasty is used to lengthen scar contractures, alter or relieve tension on an incision, and make a scar less conspicuous and, therefore, more cosmetically acceptable. In companion animals, this technique is most commonly used to lengthen restrictive scars involving flexion surfaces. Z-plasty generally involves creating two equilateral triangular flaps adjacent to a scar and transposing them to their opposing donor bed. The rotation of each flap transplants adjacent loose skin into the previously restricted area. Although a variety of Z-plasty designs are reported in human reconstructive

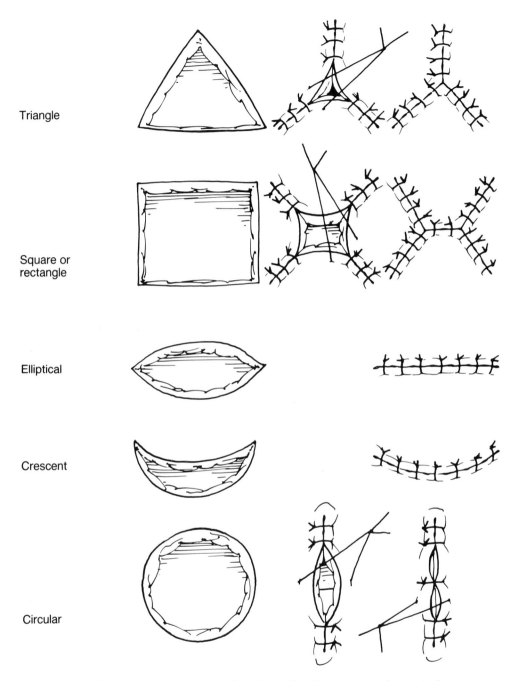

Triangle

Square or
rectangle

Elliptical

Crescent

Circular

Figure 4-1. *Closure of simple geometric defects. Small tumors can be excised using one of these patterns as long as adequate tissue margins are obtained. Similarly, irregular skin wounds can be trimmed with a scalpel to the geometric pattern that will facilitate closure of the defect.*

textbooks, the 60° Z-plasty is considered optimal in small animal surgery. Single or multiple Z-plasties may be used (Fig.4-2).

Skin Flaps (Pedicle Grafts)

A pedicle graft or skin flap is a portion of skin and subcutaneous tissue with an intact vascular attachment that is transferred from one area to another. Properly developed flaps survive because of their intact circulation. Flaps are very versatile and can be used to cover defects with poor vascularity, improve regional circulation to an area, cover areas difficult to immobilize, cover holes overlying body cavities, provide a full-thickness skin surface over areas where padding and durability are essential, give immediate protection to nerves, vessels, tendons, and other structures susceptible to exposure and injury, and provide a skin surface with hair growth comparable to the donor area from which it was harvested.

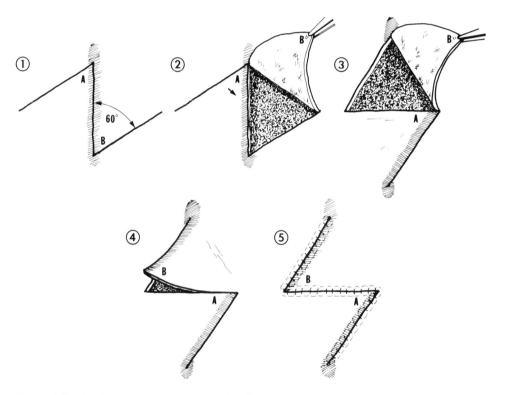

Figure 4-2. *Z-plasty in wound closure. The three incisions forming the letter "Z" are equal in length. In this example, the central limb of the "Z" overlies a restrictive scar. The two arms of the "Z" are placed at a 60-degree angle to the central limb incision, in effect creating two equilateral triangular flaps A and B. Each undermined flap is rotated in opposite directions and sutured into their new positions. The transposed flaps contribute skin to the previously scarred region, resulting in an overall gain of 75% in the length of the restricted area. Z-plasty is occasionally employed to relieve tension on an incision line by placing the central limb of the "Z" in direct alignment to the line of tension. (Pavletic MM. Surgery of the skin and management of wounds. In: Sherding RG, ed. Diseases of the cat: diagnosis and management. New York: Churchill Livingstone, 1989)*

Pedicle grafts can be classified according to their circulation, location, or composition (compound or composite flaps).

Pedicle grafts that incorporate a direct cutaneous artery and vein are termed axial pattern flaps. Axial pattern flaps have an excellent blood supply and enable the surgeon to create flaps of considerable dimension in the dog and cat, using the general guidelines established. Variations of the axial pattern flap include the island arterial flap and the secondary axial pattern flap (Fig. 4-3). Although island arterial flaps can be transferred as free flaps, using microvascular or surgical techniques to anastomose the direct cutaneous artery and vein at the recipient site, at present they have limited clinical practicality over the other reconstructive techniques discussed in this section. Flaps elevated without including direct cutaneous vessels primarily rely upon circulation via the deep or subdermal plexus and are termed subdermal plexus flaps.

As noted, flaps are also classified as *local* or *distant* according to their location in respect to the recipient bed. Local flaps are elevated adjacent to the defect and are advanced or rotated (pivoted) into place. Distant flaps, on the other hand, are created in another body region and are used more often to close defects involving the limbs.

Distant flaps are generally transferred as delayed tube flaps (indirect flaps) to the defect (Fig.4-4) or by elevating the affected limb to a flap developed on the lower lateral thorax or abdomen (direct flaps) (Fig. 4-5). Distant flaps have several disadvantages when used for extremity defects in small animals. Many animals, especially cats, may not tolerate having their limbs bound to their trunk. In addition, the time and care required for distant flap transfer preclude their routine use, except for isolated instances. Because free grafts, axial pattern flaps, and myocutaneous flaps are more effective and less costly, distant flaps are rarely needed.

Compound or *composite* flaps are pedicle grafts that incorporate skin and other tissues, including muscle, fat, bone, or cartilage. *Myocutaneous* flaps, one such group of flaps, are created by the submuscular elevation of a muscle segment with the overlying skin as a unit. Myocutaneous flaps have been effectively used in the human clinically and employed in the dog primarily on an experimental basis. Clinical use at present is limited for defects in the cat and dog because the loose skin available in small animals enables the veterinarian to close wounds with more conventional reconstructive techniques.

Surgical Considerations

The size, location, shape, and condition of the wound will generally dictate the technique required to close the defect. The simplest method of satisfactorily closing a skin defect prevails

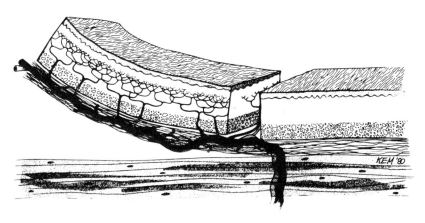

Figure 4-3. *Island arterial flap in the dog and cat. The island of skin is nourished solely by a single direct cutaneous artery and vein. Vessels have the potential to be severed and reanastomosed with microvascular surgical techniques to a recipient site a considerable distance from the donor area. (Pavletic MM. Canine axial pattern flap using the omocervical thoracodorsal, and deep circumflex iliac direct cutaneous arteries. Am J Vet Res 1981;42:391)*

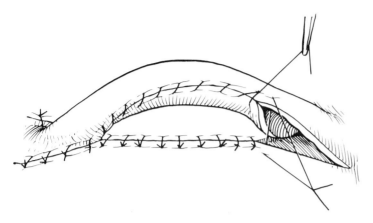

Figure 4-4. *Tubed (indirect) flap in the dog. Completion of the tubed flap and closure of the underlying donor bed. The flap should be created 2 or 3 cm longer and wider than measured to offset flap shrinkage during the period.*

in veterinary medicine because of cost considerations.

The surgeon must consider all possible flap designs and combinations when choosing the method for closure. Skin tension and pliability can be evaluated by manually lifting or

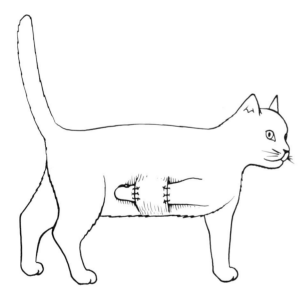

Figure 4-5. *Distant bipedicle direct flap. Two incisions equal to the width of the skin defect are made. The flap is undermined below the panniculus muscle. The affected limb is secured beneath the pedicle graft and the edge of the recipient bed is sutured to the edges of the flap. When the flap "takes," the two pedicles are severed in four stages (one-half is severed every two days) to avoid vascular compromise.*

pushing the adjacent skin towards the center of the wound. Ideal donor areas have ample skin available to elevate a flap without creating a secondary defect (donor bed) unamenable to simple closure. To avoid wound dehiscence or compromise to local mobility, donor sites subject to excessive motion or tension should be avoided. However, it is occasionally preferable to close a wound for the protection of exposed structures even though a secondary defect is created. The second defect, in turn, can be closed by a second flap, a free graft, or healing by second intention.

Factors that maximize the circulation to a pedicle graft should be considered during flap planning. Increasing the width of a pedicle graft will *not* increase its total surviving length. Flaps created under the same conditions of blood supply survive to the same length, regardless of flap width; the only effect of increasing the width of the pedicle graft is to include direct cutaneous vessels in the flap. Moreover, the cutaneous circulation differs regionally and a set length-to-width ratio does not apply. Narrowing a pedicle can reduce the perfusion to the body of the flap and increase the likelihood of necrosis. Axial pattern flaps are an exception to this rule, as long as the direct cutaneous artery and vein are preserved. Creating unduly long subdermal plexus flaps can also result in necrosis.

With these facts in mind, the author generally designs flaps with a base slightly wider than the width of the flap body to avoid inadvertent narrowing of the pedicle, and limits the flap length to the size required to close the defect bed without tension.

The recipient bed should be free of debris, necrotic tissue, and infection. Local flaps properly developed and transferred can survive on avascular beds. However, distant flaps require the establishment of circulation from the defect in order to eventually divide the pedicles for completion of flap transfer. Vascular tissue, such as healthy muscle, periosteum, and the paratenon, can vascularize an overlying skin flap. Chronic granulation tissue should be excised to reestablish a healthy granulation bed, and a few days before closure epithelialized borders on the wound should also be removed to cover the entire wound with full-thickness skin.

Local Flaps

Local flaps are the most practical method of closing wounds that cannot be adequately closed primarily. Their effective use generally requires loose elastic skin adjacent to the wound. Local flaps are simple, economical, and more likely to maintain a similar color and hair-growth pattern than is skin transplanted from a distant location. Local flaps are subdivided into advancement flaps and rotating flaps. Not every local flap option will be discussed in this chapter, but the three flap techniques considered most versatile will be reviewed.

Advancement Flaps

The single pedicle advancement flap (sliding flap) is probably the most common local flap used in veterinary medicine because its design is simple and it does not create a secondary defect requiring closure. Forward advancement of the pedicle graft is accomplished primarily by using the elasticity or stretching of the skin. Paired single pedicle advancement flaps can be used to close square or rectangular defects, resulting in a "H" closure design (H-plasty) (Fig. 4-6). In fact, two short single pedicle advancement flaps may be more effective than elevating one long advancement flap, which may have a greater likelihood of partial necrosis along its tip.

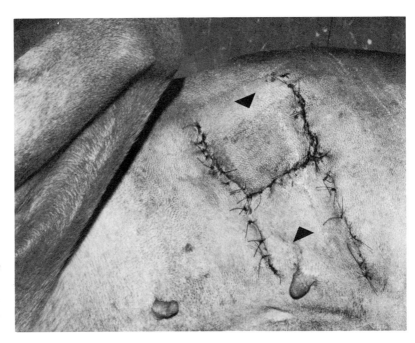

Figure 4-6. *Clinical example of the use of two single pedicle advancement flaps (H-plasty) employed for the closure of a rectangular skin defect.*

To create a single pedicle advancement flap, two skin incisions equal to the width of the defect are made in progressive fashion. The distant edge of the flap borders the defect. As noted, the two incisions are designed to diverge slightly to ensure that the flap pedicle is not inadvertently narrowed as the flap is developed. The flap is undermined and advanced into the defect. Monofilament nylon or polypropylene (3-0) simple interrupted suture are used.

A single pedicle advancement flap should not be used where postoperative skin tension must be avoided, such as around the eyelids. A 90° transposition flap would be preferable there because it carries loose skin into the defect; the advancement flap primarily relies upon stretching to cover the wound.

Bipedicle Advancement Flaps

Bipedicle advancement flaps are easily constructed by making an incision parallel to the long axis of a defect, with the flap's width equal to the width of the adjacent defect. Advancement may be eased if the relaxing incision is curved, with the concave side toward the defect. The flap is undermined and sutured into the defect. The secondary defect is usually closed by undermining and suturing the adjacent skin edge.

Two pedicles allow the creation of longer flaps, but necrosis can occur at the vascular interface between the two pedicles. This does not necessarily correlate with the center of the flap unless the circulatory perfusion pressure from each pedicle is equal. As discussed, the relaxing (release) incision, occasionally used to reduce tension to facilitate wound closure, is a bipedicle advancement flap in design (Fig. 4-7).

Transposition Flaps

The transposition flap is the most useful of the local flap designs for wound closure. The transposition flap is a *rotating* rectangular pedicle graft usually created within 90° of the long axis of the defect. An edge of the defect

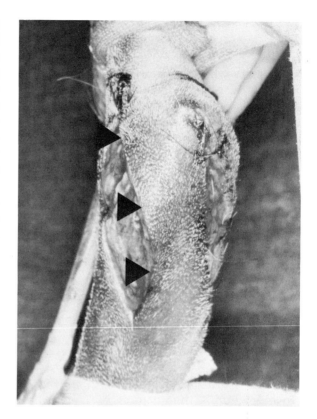

Figure 4-7. *A bipedicle advancement flap used to cover a large granulation bed overlying the calcaneal tuber. The remaining open wounds medial and lateral to the flap healed by second intention. Relaxing incisions by design are similar to bipedicle advancement flaps.*

serves as part of the flap border. The width of the flap normally equals the width of the defect. The flap length, from the pivot point of the flap to the most distant point of the flap, should equal the distance between the pivot point and most distant point of the defect (Fig. 4-8).

Transposition flaps decrease in length as the arc of rotation increases. A dog-ear also is more likely to develop as the rotation of the flap is increased, although the increased rotation will result in less tension on the primary area of repair. Any secondary defect created is usually closed by direct apposition. A second local flap may be used to close the donor bed, if necessary. Mild tension along the line of greatest tension can be relieved with a small perpendicular stab incision.

Figure 4-8. *Transposition flap created at 90 degrees to the long axis of skin defect. The width of the flap is equal to the width of the defect. Note that the length of the flap* **(A),** *measured from the pivot point of the flap, equals the ruler measurement taken from the pivot point to the most distant border of the defect* **(B, C).** *The secondary defect created is sutured closed after undermining of the skin edges.*

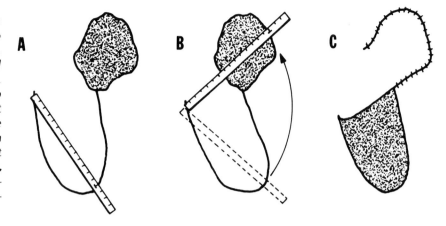

Axial Pattern Flaps

Not every flap elevated on the patient can include a direct cutaneous artery and vein. However, axial pattern flap development can enable the surgeon to transfer large skin segments in a single stage safely without a delay procedure. The five major direct cutaneous arteries of the dog used for axial pattern flap development are the caudal superficial epigastric artery, the cervical cutaneous (superficial cervical) branch of the omocervical artery, the thoracodorsal artery, the deep circumflex iliac artery, and the genicular branch of the saphenous artery. The patient must be carefully positioned before outlining the proposed flap onto the skin with a felt-tipped marking pen. Skin distortion or shifting in relation to the anatomic landmarks may result in failure to include the direct cutaneous vessels in the pedicle graft. Table 1 summarizes the five axial pattern flaps described in the dog.

Axial pattern flaps can be rotated into adjacent defects or to distant sites of the lower trunk and extremities. Part of the flap can be tubed to traverse the skin between the donor and recipient beds, or a bridge incision may be made in the skin between the donor/recipient site. The flap is sutured to the edges of the bridge incision, eliminating the need to tube the flap. The flap body can be elevated as the standard (peninsular design) or the ''L'' (hockey-stick) design, depending on the shape and size of the cutaneous defect (Figs. 4-9 to 4-12).

Island arterial flaps are dependent on a single direct cutaneous artery and vein. They can be developed in each of the canine axial pattern flaps by dividing the cutaneous pedicle below the entry of the respective direct cutaneous artery. Although island arterial flaps are more mobile than conventional axial pattern flaps, they have limited clinical use on a routine basis.

The similar survival area of axial pattern flaps and island arterial flaps indicates that a ''backcut'' procedure at the pivot point of a skin flap can be performed to improve flap mobility with a considerable degree of safety in an axial pattern flap, as long as the direct cutaneous artery and vein are preserved.

Reverse Saphenous Conduit Flap

A variation of the axial pattern flap is the reverse saphenous conduit flap. This flap incorporates the cranial and caudal branches of the saphenous artery and medial saphenous vein after division of their femoral vascular connections. Blood flow is maintained in reverse by distal anastomotic arterial and venous connections between:

1. The cranial branch of the saphenous artery and superficial branch of the cranial tibial artery, as well as the cranial tibial artery;

Table 4–1. Anatomical Landmarks, Reference Incisions, and Uses for Axial Pattern Flaps

Artery	Anatomical Landmarks	Reference Incisions	Potential Uses*
Cervical cutaneous branch of the omocervical artery	Spine of the scapula Cranial edge of the scapula (caudal shoulder depression) Dog in lateral recumbency, skin in natural position, thoracic limb in relaxed extension Vessel originates at location of the prescapular lymph node	Caudal incision: spine of the scapula in a dorsal direction Cranial incision: parallel to the caudal incision equal to the distance between the scapular spine and cranial scapular edge (cranial shoulder depression) Flap length: variable; contralateral scapulohumeral joint	Facial defects Ear reconstruction Cervical defects Shoulder defects Axillary defects
Thoracodorsal artery	Spine of the scapula Caudal edge of the scapula (caudal shoulder depression) Dog in lateral recumbency, skin in natural position, thoracic limb in relaxed extension Vessel originates at caudal shoulder depression at a level parallel to the dorsal point of the acromion	Cranial incision: spine of the scapula in a dorsal direction Caudal incision: parallel to the cranial incision equal to the distance between the scapular spine and caudal scapular edge (caudal shoulder depression) Flap length: variable; can survive ventral to contralateral scapulohumeral joint	Thoracic defects Shoulder defects Forelimb defects Axillary defects
Deep circumflex iliac artery	Cranial edge of wing of ilium Greater trochanter Dog in lateral recumbency, skin in natural position, pelvic limb in relaxed extension Vessel originates at a point cranioventral to wing of the ilium	Caudal incision: midway between edge of wing of ilium and greater trochanter Cranial incision: parallel to caudal incision equal to the distance between the caudal incision and cranial edge of the iliac wing Flap length: dorsal to contralateral flank fold	Thoracic defects Lateral abdominal wall defects Flank defects Lateral/medial thigh defects Defects over the greater trochanter
Caudal superficial epigastric artery	Midline of abdomen Mammary teats Base of prepuce	Medial incision: abdominal midline In the male dog, the base of the prepuce is included in the midline incision to preserve the adjacent epigastric vasculature. Lateral incision: parallel to medial incision at an equal distance from the mammary gland teats Flap length: variable; may safely include the last four mammary glands and adjacent skin	Flank defects Inner thigh defects Stifle area Perineal area Preputial area
Genicular artery	Patella Tibial tuberosity Greater trochanter	Base of the flap: 1 cm proximal to the patella and 1.5 cm distal to tibial tuberosity (laterally) Flap borders: extend caudodorsally parallel to the femoral shaft and flap terminates at the base of the greater trochanter	Lateral or medial aspect of the lower limb from the stifle to the tibiotarsal joint

* Major defects only.

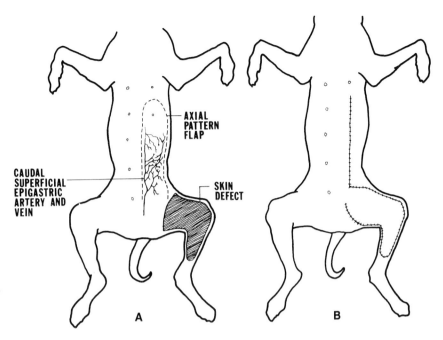

Figure 4-9. *A,* *Extent of the vascular supply to the skin from the caudal superficial epigastric artery and vein. B, Example of one potential application of such an axial pattern flap. The flap can be rotated 180 degrees if care is taken to avoid undue twisting or kinking of the direct cutaneous vessels. (Pavletic MM, Peyton LC. Skin. In: Bojrab MJ, ed. Current techniques in small animal surgery II. Philadelphia: Lea & Febiger, 1983)*

2. The caudal branch of the saphenous artery and the perforating metatarsal artery via the medial and lateral plantar arteries;
3. The cranial branch of the medial saphenous vein and the cranial branch of the lateral saphenous vein; and
4. By other venous connections with the cranial and caudal branches of the medial sa- phenous veins distal to the tibiotarsal joint.

Circulation to the overlying skin is maintained via direct cutaneous vessels branching off the saphenous vasculature.

The resultant flap can be used for major cutaneous defects at or below the region of the

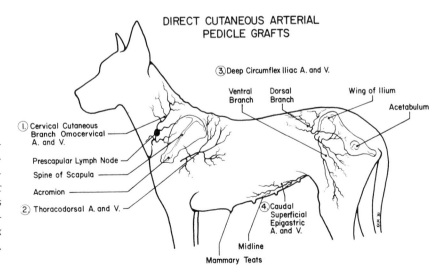

Figure 4-10. *Four major direct cutaneous arteries are illustrated in relation to their anatomic landmarks. (Pavletic MM. Canine axial pattern flaps using the omocervical, thoracodorsal, and deep circumflex iliac direct cutaneous arteries. Am J Vet Res 1981;42:391)*

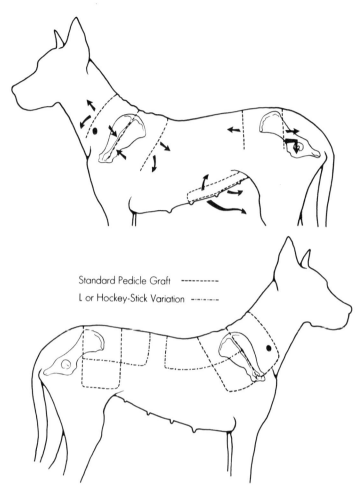

Standard Pedicle Graft ----------
L or Hockey-Stick Variation --·--·--

Figure 4-11. *Reference lines for the omocervical, thoracodorsal, deep circumflex iliac and caudal superficial epigastric axial pattern flaps. Flaps may be created in the standard peninsula (dashed lines) or "L" or hockey-stick (dashed and dotted lines) configuration. Note the flaps extend completely to the opposite side of the dog. (Pavletic MM. Canine axial pattern flaps using the omocervical, thoracordorsal, and deep circumflex iliac direct cutaneous arteries. Am J Vet Res 1981;42:391)*

tibiotarsal joint, as long as the saphenous vessels and the collateral circulation are preserved. When the reverse saphenous conduit flap is considered for use on skin defects secondary to extensive trauma, angiography should be performed to ensure that anastomotic connections are intact and that the saphenous artery and medial saphenous vein are not the major routes of circulation for the lower limb.

Measurements are taken to determine the length of the flap needed to reach and cover the lower limb defect. The flap width is tapered distally, owing to the limited skin available for flap development. A skin incision is made across the central third of the inner thigh, at or

slightly above the level of the patella. Metzenbaum scissors are used to expose the underlying saphenous artery, medial saphenous vein, and nerve before they are ligated and divided. Two incisions are extended distally in converging fashion, 0.5 to 1 cm cranial and caudal to the borders of the cranial and caudal branches of the saphenous artery and medial saphenous vein, respectively. The flaps are undermined beneath the saphenous vasculature. To avoid injuring the caudal branch of the saphenous artery and medial saphenous vein during progressive raising of the pedicle graft, part of the medial gastrocnemius muscle fascia is included with the flap. Below this point, the tibial nerve merges with the de-

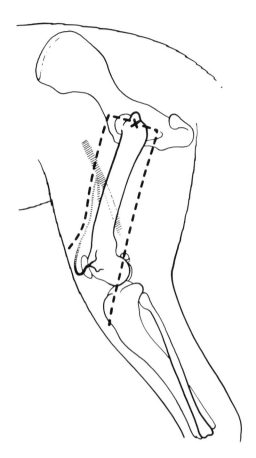

Figure 4-12. *Outline of the genicular axial pattern flap. (See Table 4-1 for anatomic landmarks.)*

scending caudal branches of the saphenous artery and medial saphenous vein and is preserved by meticulous dissection between these structures. Ligation and division of the peroneal (fibular) artery and vein are necessary for flap mobility. Flap raising is completed proximal to the anastomosis between the cranial branch of the medial saphenous vein and the cranial branch of the lateral saphenous vein. The donor bed is initially closed with interrupted subcuticular sutures, then with simple interrupted skin sutures at the end of the transplantation. The transfer pedicle can be tubed or sutured to a bridge incision connecting the donor or recipient beds. Care should be taken that the tubed transfer pedicle is not under undue tension with extension of the tibiotarsal joint.

Compound and Composite Flaps

Compound flaps created by the submuscular elevation of a muscle segment and overlying skin unit are called myocutaneous or musculocutaneous flaps. They have been effectively used in human reconstruction surgery. Musculocutaneous flaps based on the submuscular elevation of the gracilis muscle and a portion of the latissimus dorsi muscle with the overlying skin have been used for microvascular studies in dogs. The latissimus dorsi myocutaneous flap and cutaneous trunci myocutaneous flap recently have been developed for potential clinical use in the dog (Fig. 4-13). Secondary or revascularized musculocutaneous flaps have also been developed in dogs by suturing skin to portions of the adductor and sartorius muscles. Vascularization subsequently occurs between the muscle-dermal interface, allowing the successful transfer of the muscle and attached island of skin to another region as a second procedure.

Other examples of composite flaps in the dog include the labial advancement flap for full-thickness rostral labial defects and the composite mucocutaneous subdermal plexus flap for complete lower eyelid reconstruction. By strict definition, skin flaps elevated in the dog and cat with subcutaneous fat and panniculus muscle could be considered composite flaps. Fortunately, the routine elevation of major skeletal muscles to transfer the overlying skin is unnecessary in the dog and cat. The ample amount of loose, elastic skin available and the comparable ease of elevating axial pattern flaps preclude their routine clinical use.

Free Skin Grafts

Free skin grafts lack a vascular attachment upon transfer to the recipient graft bed. Free grafts must survive the initial transfer by ab-

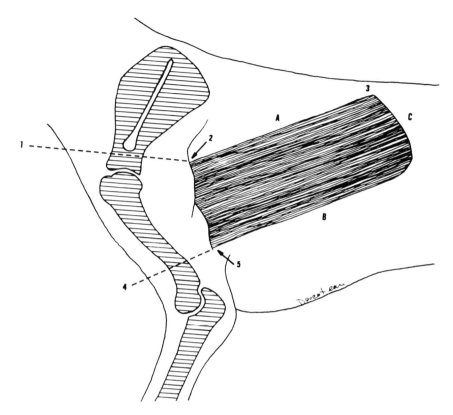

Figure 4-13. *Anatomic landmarks for the latissimus dorsi and cutaneous trunci myocutaneous flaps including the: (1) lower border of the acromion and (2) adjacent caudal border of the triceps muscle; (3) head of the last rib; (4) lower third of the humerus, which corresponds to the (5) axillary skin fold. The flap is drawn onto the skin with a marking pen by connecting landmarks 2 and 3 to form (A) the dorsal flap border. A second line is drawn from landmarks parallel to line "A" to the border of the last rib forming (B) the lower flap border. A third line (C) is drawn along the caudal border of the last rib, connecting lines A and B. The latissimus dorsi myocutaneous flap is initially incised along the lower border and the latissimus dorsi muscle is identified. The muscle's border is elevated and the incision is extended along line C and A. The latissimus dorsi muscle flap is elevated with a width at least equal to the overlying skin flap. (Pavletic MM, Kostolich M, Koblik, Engler S. A comparison of the cutaneous trunci myocutaneous flap and latissimus dorsi myocutaneous flap in the dog. Vet Surg 1987;16:283)*

sorbing tissue fluid from the recipient bed by capillary action during the initial 48 hours after transplantation. During this period, capillaries from the recipient bed unite with the exposed graft plexuses to reestablish vital circulation. New capillaries later grow into the graft, and the vascular channels remodel. In addition, fibrous connective tissue forms to hold the graft securely in place. Grafts assume a pink color in 48 hours if circulation is adequate. Viable grafts with poor venous return have a cyanotic hue until circulation improves.

Any accumulation of material, such as pus, serum, blood, or foreign matter, between the graft and recipient bed will delay or prevent graft revascularization. This delay often results in graft necrosis. Motion between the graft and the recipient bed has a similar effect. Fibrinolysis secondary to bacterial infection can destroy the early fibrin "glue" between the graft and the bed, resulting in motion and graft necrosis. Improper contact between the graft and the recipient bed prevents proper surface-to-surface interdigitation and incomplete graft revascularization. This improper contact may occur if the graft is stretched over the bed like a "drum skin" or if an excessively large graft is applied to form graft folds that lack proper contact with the recipient bed.

Although grafts require a vascular recipient bed for survival, granulation tissue is not necessary before a graft is applied. Healthy pink granulation tissue, however, is an excellent recipient bed for skin grafts. Pale, collagen-laden chronic granulation tissue has a poor vascular supply and should be excised to promote formation of a healthy granulation tissue. Contamination and infection should be controlled, and the granulation surface must be free of any epithelial cover before graft application.

Free grafts can be classified according to the source of the graft, the graft thickness, and the graft shape or design. Whereas autogenous grafts are used for permanent free graft coverage in the dog and cat, allografts (homografts) and xenografts (heterografts) are used as a temporary biologic dressing until an autogenous graft can be successfully applied. Free grafts can be harvested as full-thickness or split-thickness skin grafts. Graft thickness varies according to the amount of dermis included with the overlying epidermis. Split-thickness grafts are harvested with razor blades, graft knives, or a dermatome. The donor bed of a split-thickness graft bed can be excised and closed, or it may be left to heal by adnexal regeneration and epithelialization. Thin split-thickness grafts are reported to "take" more readily than full-thickness grafts, but lack the durability and hair growth of full-thickness grafts. Full-thickness grafts are preferred by many veterinarians for these reasons.

Free grafts can be applied as a sheet over the entire recipient bed or they may be divided into various shapes or patterns. Pinch (punch) grafts (Fig. 4-14), strip grafts (Fig. 4-15), stamp grafts, and mesh grafts (Fig. 4-16) are commonly used as partial-coverage grafts to increase the total recipient surface area that a small graft harvest can cover.

Open spaces between the graft perimeters allow for drainage until the granulation tissue bed is covered by the advancing epithelial cells originating from the graft. As a result, partial-coverage grafts are useful for recipient beds with low-grade infections. Small grafts also conform to irregular recipient beds, are simple to apply, and are economical to perform. Unfortunately, the resulting epithelialized surface lacks the functional and cosmetic results achieved with full-thickness graft coverage. The author prefers to use full-thickness mesh grafts to close wounds of the lower extremities, restricting the use of punch or strip grafts for smaller wounds that are not located over areas where durability is essential. Use of thin split-thickness mesh grafts, harvested with a dermatome, is reserved for extensive body defects, usually resulting from burns.

Postoperative Care

Proper protection is essential for survival of a skin graft. The animal should be confined to a cage and sedatives should be administered if the patient is excitable. The type of bandage, the dressing, and the sequence of bandage changes may vary. The author prefers to cover grafts postoperatively with an Adaptic pad (Johnson & Johnson, New Brunswick, NJ) or a Telfa pad (Kendall Corp., Boston, MA) and a bland antimicrobial ointment, followed by a flat layer of gauze pads. Alternate layers of adherent gauze and cotton are applied snugly. A layer of elastic tape completes the bandage. Such bandages are bulky and restrict motion to the graft. Additional external supports, such as splints, casts, slings, and reinforcement rods, are used if necessary. Shroeder-Thomas splints are ideal for immobilizing grafts overlying the elbow, carpus, knee, or tibiotarsal joints. Spica splints may be advisable when Shroeder-Thomas splints cannot be used.

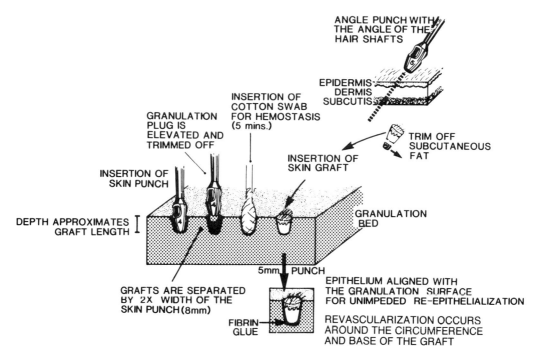

Figure 4-14. *Punch graft technique (pinch grafts). A sharp 5- or 6-mm biopsy punch is used to harvest the graft plugs from a suitable donor site. The donor area is clipped, leaving the hair shafts exposed. Subcutaneous fat is trimmed off the graft base. A single stitch is used to close the donor bed. The grafts are placed between two moistened saline pads until needed. A 4-mm biopsy punch is used to remove cores of granulation tissue. Holes are spaced 8 mm apart (twice the width of the biopsy punch). Fine scissors are required to remove the granulation core. A sterile cotton swab is inserted into each hole for five minutes. The graft plugs are then inserted in the direction of natural hair growth. A firm dressing is applied post-surgically to maintain the position of the grafts. The following advantages may be noted with this procedure: 1) 4-mm granulation holes compensate for graft shrinkage and allow the grafts to fit more snugly; 2) the epithelial surface of the graft is level with the granulation bed, and reepithelialization is unimpeded; 3) as many hair follicles as possible are included into each graft to promote hair growth; 4) reepithelialization is possible despite partial graft necrosis from surviving hair follicles and skin adnexa deep in the graft; and 5) graft revascularization occurs around the circumference as well as through the base of the graft plug, a comparatively large surface area. (Pavletic MM, Peyton L. Plastic and reconstructive surgery in the dog and cat. In: Bojrab MJ, ed. Current techniques in small animal surgery II. Philadelphia: Lea & Febiger, 1983)*

The bandage is changed 3 to 5 days post-surgically with the patient under light anesthesia or sedation. Earlier bandage changes risk graft motion during the critical 48-hour period of graft revascularization. The veterinarian must resist the tremendous temptation to "check" the graft in the early stages. To remove the bandage, the outer layers are cut away and the dressing is removed carefully. Any bandage materials sticking to the graft should be left alone because "bandage picking" and "scab pulling" may move or remove the graft in the early healing stages. Warm saline, however, can be applied to soften the dressing and facilitate its removal.

The graft is inspected for signs of infec-

Figure 4-15. *Strip grafts. Application of strip grafts is similar to that of punch grafts. Linear strips of skin are laid in granulation troughs cut with a scalpel blade. Granulation tissue between the strips is eventually reepithelialized from the grafts. (Pavletic MM, Peyton L. Plastic and reconstructive surgery in the dog and cat. In: Bojrab MJ, ed. Current techniques in small animal surgery II. Philadelphia: Lea & Febiger, 1983)*

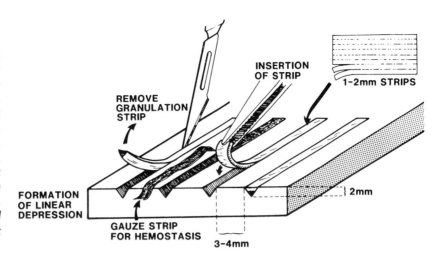

tion, necrosis, or elevation from the graft bed. Cultures can be taken if the graft appears to be in serious jeopardy, followed by treatment with an appropriate topical antimicrobial. Early signs of graft necrosis are discouraging but not always catastrophic, because hair follicles and cutaneous adnexa in the deep portion of the graft may survive and serve as a source for wound epithelialization. Subsequent bandage changes are repeated every 2 to 4 days, depending on the graft condition. This routine is continued for about 2 weeks, followed by application of a lighter bandage for another 10 to 14 days if necessary.

The veterinarian must always keep in mind the potential adverse effects of bandages. Excessive pressure or wrinkled bandage materials can abrade the graft if the affected area is inadequately immobilized.

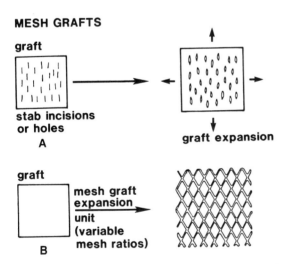

Figure 4-16. *Mesh grafts. Both full-thickness and split-thickness grafts may be used. **A,** Multiple stab incisions or holes are cut into the graft to allow the graft to expand and to provide adequate drainage. The graft is sutured to the periphery of the recipient bed. **B,** Mesh-graft expansion units have been developed to expand the graft into a uniform mesh. A graft can be expanded 1.5 to 9 times its original surface area to cover extensive skin defects. Most surgeons use a 3:1 ratio. (Pavletic MM, Peyton L. Plastic and reconstructive surgery in the dog and cat. In: Bojrab MJ, ed. Current techniques in small animal surgery II. Philadelphia: Lea & Febiger, 1983)*

Dressings and Bandages

A dressing is a protective covering in contact with a wound. A bandage is a wrap used to hold dressings in place, to support or immobilize a body part, or to apply pressure to control hemorrhage or obliterate cavities. Both terms are occasionally used interchangeably, although "dressing" is used most often to describe that portion of a bandage directly contacting the wound surface.

Bandages have three basic layers: the primary (contact dressing) layer, the secondary (intermediate) layer, and the tertiary (outer) layer. A nonadherent dressing is generally applied over wounds to facilitate bandage removal without disturbing the underlying tissue. Telfa nonadherent strips (Kendall, Boston, MA) and Adaptic dressings (Johnson and Johnson, New Brunswick, NJ) are the most useful nonadherent dressings.

Adherent dressings are useful in wound debridement. Dry, coarse or wide-mesh gauze can be applied over moist wounds with loose necrotic tissue. The dry gauze absorbs exudate and adheres to pieces of dead tissue. The gauze is removed "dry." Lifting off the "dry-to-dry" bandage strips the necrotic tissue from the underlying viable tissue. A variation of this technique is the "wet-to-dry" dressing. Gauze pads soaked with sterile saline or water can be applied to wounds to soften tenacious necrotic tissue and thin the viscous exudates on the wound. The gauze is allowed to dry; removal of the "dry" gauze facilitates debridement. The author has occasionally used a nonadherent dressing in combination with an overlying wet dressing to prevent dessication of an otherwise healthy open wound for 3 to 5 days, until a granulation bed forms for further reconstructive procedures. Wet-to-wet dressings are periodically moistened until the next bandage change, flushing or bathing the wound and accelerating the softening of necrotic tissue.

Adherent dressings are not advisable for healthy wounds, because bandage removal can strip off epithelial cells attempting to migrate over the wound surface. Soaking the gauze with saline can facilitate its removal because removal of adherent dressings can be painful to the animal. Sedation may be necessary during subsequent bandage changes.

The secondary layer of a bandage is an absorptive layer, usually composed of cotton fiber and/or gauze. The secondary layer wicks fluids and exudate from the wound surface. Moisture in this intermediate layer can evaporate, depending on the composition of the outer tertiary layer of the bandage. The frequency of bandage changes depends in part on the volume of wound discharge and the storage capacity of the absorptive layer. For this reason, wounds in the early stages of healing generally require more frequent bandage changes, one to three times daily. As a healthy granulation bed forms, the bandage replace-

ment can generally be reduced to a bandage change every 2 to 4 days, depending on the nature of the wound.

The outer or tertiary layer serves as a binding or security layer for the contact and absorptive layers of the bandage. Stretch gauze, followed by a layer of tape or elastic bandage, is commonly used. Porous surgical tape facilitates aeration and moisture passage from the absorptive layer; however, moisture from the environment also can pass into this layer and contaminate the bandage. Occlusive (nonporous) tapes may be advisable if this is a significant problem, but the veterinarian must remember that the tape will also restrict evaporation from the secondary layer, necessitating more frequent bandage changes to avoid tissue maceration from prolonged moisture contact. In general, the use of occlusive tape should be limited to those bandage areas prone to fluid contamination, with porous tape for the remaining bandage area.

Elastic or self-adhering tapes have the advantage of strength, support, and ease of conformity to the underlying bandage area, but they are much more expensive than surgical tape. They can be used when a bandage requires a durable support covering and when infrequent bandage changes are anticipated.

Protecting the Wound

Bandaging is the most common method of protecting and supporting the affected area. However, inappropriately applied bandages can be detrimental to wound healing. Tight bandages can restrict circulation, but loose-fitting bandages may abrade the wound surface, especially wounds involving the joints and mobile areas (e.g., flank, axilla, neck). These circumstances call for alternate methods of immobilization. Partial casts, Mason metasplints, tongue-depressor splints, and heat-malleable plastics such as Orthoplast (Johnson & Johnson, New Brunswick, NJ) are effective for immobilizing lower limb wounds when applied to the outside of the bandage. Shroeder-Thomas splints provide excellent immobilization to limbs, using aluminum rods on sturdy coat hangers. The Shroeder-Thomas splint will immobilize the elbow, carpus, knee, and tibiotarsal joints and allow the veterinarian to change the bandage without having to remove the entire splint. Spica bandages or splints are also effective in immobilizing the upper extremities. The spica bandage envelops the limb and trunk, restricting motion to the shoulder and hip joint. To increase bandage rigidity, the spica bandage can be reinforced with an aluminum bar or a thin plywood silhouette of the affected limb.

"Tie-over" dressings or stents are useful for maintaining coverage of wounds when it would be difficult to maintain a conventional bandage. A series of loose interrupted sutures is placed outside the skin margins of a wound, then a dressing is placed over the open wound and suture material or umbilical tape is laced over the bandage through the suture loops. Dressings are easily changed by cutting the lacing and replacing the dressing in the same fashion. The bandage is usually abandoned once a healthy granulation bed forms.

Elizabethan collars are tolerated by most dogs and cats to prevent self-mutilation. Tape hobbles on the pelvic limbs of cats are occasionally useful to prevent cats from licking wounds involving the perineum.

The use of hydroactive dressings is a newer concept in wound management. Occlusive pad dressings (Dermaheal, Squibb, Princeton, NJ) have been developed with a hydroactive layer that contacts the wound surface. This layer absorbs wound fluid and forms a moisture-laden gel that promotes wound epithelialization. The pad may require one or two strips of tape to secure it on the body part. The bandages are changed every 3 to 5 days. The pad is useful for smaller wounds on the limbs with a healthy granulation bed.

One study, however, suggested that hydroactive pads can restrict wound contraction while promoting epithelialization. These dressings seem to be more useful for wounds in the reparative stages of healing, once fluid production from the wound has considerably de-

creased. Because occlusive bandages can promote tissue maceration and infection, these dressings should be watched closely and used on uninfected wounds free of necrotic tissue and debris. The veterinarian should compare the convenience and cost of hydroactive dressings with conventional bandaging techniques.

A hydroactive paste has also been used to manage open wounds (Hydron, Bioderm Sciences, Oceanside, NY). The paste limits wound contamination and creates an environment unfavorable for microbial proliferation. This product may have promise for the management of deep ulcers or wounds in small animals.

Undoubtedly, new products will be presented, claiming effectiveness in promoting wound healing and controlling infection. The efficacy, cost, and convenience of these products must be evaluated carefully. The use of newer products, however, does not change the basic principles established in surgery.

Suggested Readings

Amber EI, Henderson RA, Swaim SF, Gray BW. A comparison of antimicrobial efficacy and tissue reaction of four antiseptics of canine wounds. Vet Surg 1983;12:63.

Hunt TK, Dunphy JE. Fundamentals of wound management. New York: Appleton-Century-Crofts, 1979.

Johnston DE. The healing process in open wounds. Compend Contin Ed Prac Vet 1979;1:789.

Pavletic MM: The integument. In: Slatter D, ed. Textbook of small animal surgery. Philadelphia: WB Saunders, 1985.

Pavletic MM, Peyton LC. Small animal plastic and reconstructive surgery. In: Bojrab MS, ed. Current techniques in small animal surgery III. Philadelphia: Lea & Febiger, in press.

Peacock EE. Wound repair. 3rd ed. Philadelphia: WB Saunders, 1984.

Swaim SF. Surgery of traumatized skin: management and reconstruction in the dog and cat. Philadelphia: WB Saunders, 1980.

Swaim SF, Wilhalf D. The physics, physiology, and chemistry of bandaging open wounds. Compend Contin Ed Pract Vet 1985;7:146.

5

Milton Wyman

Ophthalmic Surgery

Each animal presented to you must be evaluated critically before surgery is attempted. Indications for surgery are given for each procedure. The procedures described do not include all the methods available, but they do lend themselves to a multitude of lid and adnexal surgeries.

Proper instrumentation is important. Each section or general topic contains a list of recommended instruments. You may wish to modify them for your particular likes or dislikes; however, you must have small, delicate instruments for these procedures.

The preparation of the surgical site is done gently but thoroughly. Basic principles of skin preparation do not apply to periocular tissues because they are much more sensitive and unforgiving. Overzealous clipping, espe-

cially with a #40 blade, shaving, scrubbing, and irrigating can produce severe inflammatory lesions that often are more irritating than the surgery. For this reason, the periocular region should be adequately and gently scrubbed with povidone iodine and irrigated with sterile saline, or other eye wash, beginning at the eye and widening the area concentrically. This should be done gently and in a circular motion rather than a scrubbing motion. This is repeated three times.

Clipping long hair from the area to minimize contamination is important. The immediate surgical site is shaved with a Schick injector blade without a handle, a technique that requires practice. This is accomplished by lathering the site with povidone iodine, tensing the skin by digital pressure, laying the bare blade almost flat, and shaving the hair in the direction of hair growth. This procedure can be done between one of the three scrubs previously described.

The opposite eye must not be ignored and

Portions of this chapter have been modified from Dr. Wyman's paper, "Ophthalmic Surgery for the Practitioner," in *Veterinary Clinics of North America: Small Animal Practice,* 1979;9:311.

the head should be positioned to elevate the "down" eye from the table surface. This will eliminate the pooling of soap and eye wash in the unoperated eye. Although ointments have been advocated to prevent soap injury to the eye, it has been shown that ointments retain the soap longer than nothing at all and give the surgeon a false sense of security. For this reason, ointments are contraindicated, and proper attention is given to the removal of soap from both eyes by thorough irrigation.

Postoperative care depends on the type of surgery and the extent of ocular involvement. When the condition is limited to the lids and adnexa (not conjunctiva, cornea, or inner eye), no topical medication is necessary. If infection is present, systemic antibiotics are indicated. When overt corneal or conjunctival disease is manifest, treat for these specific lesions.

Procedures for Correcting Entropion

Entropion is a turning in of the lid toward the eye in such a way that the hair of the lid apposes the cornea and bulbar conjunctiva. This condition predisposes the conjunctiva and/or cornea to irritation, ulceration, and, if complicated, corneal perforation.

Diagnosis
Congenital Entropion

This is a common type. Predisposed breeds include, but are not limited to, the chow chow, bloodhound, Labrador retriever, English bulldog, Doberman pinscher, Chesapeake Bay retriever, St. Bernard, rottweiler, poodle, Irish setter, and sharpei. The lower lid is commonly involved; however, entropions of the temporal half of both the upper and lower lid, as well as medial entropion, are not infrequent. Most animals are presented as pups or young adults with bilateral entropion. Redundant skin growth in the bloodhound, English bulldog, and St. Bernard predisposes to entropion. Im-

proper function of the lateral palpebral ligament (which, in the dog, is the lateral retractor muscle) causes a rounding of the palpebral fissure, resulting in lateral entropion. Enophthalmos resulting from an abnormally large orbit also may predispose to entropion, especially in the Doberman, Irish setter, Great Dane, and possibly the St. Bernard. The etiology of other congenital entropions is unknown, although heredity undoubtedly plays a role.

Congenital entropion can be surgically corrected in predisposed breeds very early in life. Indeed, when a sharpei puppy, for example, presents with minor entropion, it may be more prudent to operate then rather than to wait until more serious inversion results. If allowed to persist, tissue tensions produced by lid spasms add to the deformity, resulting in the need for more complex procedures.

Acquired Nonspastic Entropion

Previous trauma is a possible cause of acquired entropion. Trauma can cause atrophy of periorbital and retro-orbital fat, thereby causing enophthalmos, which allows the free lid margins to fall in toward the enophthalmic eye. Characteristically, acquired nonspastic entropion is a unilateral condition and needs to be differentiated from spastic entropion. Other predisposing lesions include phthisis bulbi and atrophy of the masseter muscle.

Acquired Spastic Entropion

Unilaterality is the rule. The lids previously were clinically normal, and during or after some corneal or conjunctival disease they appear to have turned inward. The inversion is caused by spasms of the orbicularis oculi muscle, predisposed by ocular irritation such as chronic conjunctivitis, foreign bodies of the external ocular tissues, keratoconjunctivitis sicca, distichiasis, trichiasis, and ablation of the membrana nictitans. Spastic entropion is sometimes present with congenital and acquired entropion since primary entropion irritates the external ocular tissues, thereby inducing orbicularis oculi muscle spasms.

Because surgical treatment is not recommended under some circumstances, a thorough examination to identify the cause should be performed. Proper medical or corrective management is necessary until a prime surgical period is reached or the entropion is ameliorated. The disease that incites spasms must be treated if detected. Medication may include lubricants, such as artificial tears and antibiotic ointments, to help prevent corneal erosions caused by lid inversion. Topical corticosteroids may be used if corneal erosions or other epithelial defects are not present. Artificial tears should be applied as often as six to eight times per day, depending on the cause and severity. It is imperative that the specific disease be identified and properly treated.

The severity of the signs sometimes makes diagnosis of congenital and acquired spastic entropion difficult. Rather than correcting spastic entropion immediately, the veterinarian can gain some time by performing a temporary tarsorrhaphy and treating the eyes with lubricants and antibiotic ointments until the signs abate. Reevaluation of the etiology must then be accomplished if recurrence is to be avoided. Once surgical intervention is elected, several questions should be answered. Where on the lid should surgery be done? How much tissue should be removed? What technique would best accomplish the job? The first two questions should be answered before anesthesia, and the answers will define the technique of choice. Surgery should encompass the entire involved portion of the lid. The amount of tissue removed is judged by inspection before anesthesia since the lid droop and muscle relaxation caused by anesthesia does not appropriately define the extent of entropion.

Corrective Procedure

Modified Hotz-Celsus Technique

This is the simplest technique and is used on entropions confined to one lid that do not involve either canthus. An incision is made in the skin with a #15 scalpel blade parallel to

and 2 to 4 mm from the free lid margin. The first incision should be as close to the tarsal glands as possible without invading them. Keeping as close to the tarsal glands as possible provides rigidity to the lid, which enhances surgical eversion. The length of the incision extends 1 mm on either side of the inverted portion of the lid. A second skin incision is made in the form of an arc distal to the first incision and joining at either end of the first incision (Fig. 5-1).

The width of skin between the incisions necessary to correct the entropion was predetermined before anesthesia. This assessment is made by placing the thumb on the lid skin adjacent to the entropic lid and, by applying digital pressure, pulling the lid away from the eye (see Fig. 5-1B). The distance the thumb moves is the width of tissue at the widest aspect of the two incisions. The two initial incisions are made perpendicular to the skin surface with a #15 Bard-Parker Beaver blade and handle (Bard-Parker division of Becton Dickinson and Co., Rutherford, NJ). The skin between the incision is removed with tenotomy scissors.

Closure is accomplished (see Fig. 5-1) with simple interrupted sutures placed in an arrow pattern. The incision is bisected by an imaginary line. The first two sutures are placed at an angle (see Fig. 5-1D) on either side of the imaginary line, forming an arrow directed toward the free lid margin. Each additional suture is placed parallel to each of the first two sutures (see Fig. 5-1E). The suture size should be the smallest acceptable suture to close the wound. This is usually no larger than 5-0 and often 6-0 nonabsorbable.

Lateral Canthoplasty

This procedure (Fig. 5-2) is used for entropions involving the lateral canthus, with concomitant weakness of the lateral palpebral ligament. The skin incision is the same as for entropion described above, extending around the lateral canthus (Fig. 5-2A). The skin overlying the zygomatic arch is gently undermined for 1 to 2 cm from the cut edge (Fig. 5-2B).

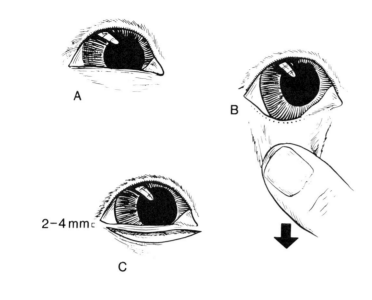

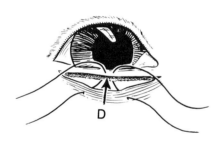

2-4 mm

C

Figure 5-1. *A, The modified Hotz-Celsus technique is used to treat inversion of the lower lid. B, The width of tissue to be removed is determined by digital traction on the adjacent lid skin. C, The distance from the free lid margin to the incision next to the lid margin is 2 to 4 mm. D, Two sutures are placed on either side of the center of the elliptical incision, angling toward the lid in an arrow pattern. E, The suture pattern is complete.*

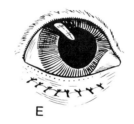

Closure after skin excision will not correct the foreshortened palpebral fissure. This correction is accomplished by fashioning two strips of orbicularis oculi muscle (one on either side of the lateral canthus) approximately 2 by 6 mm (Fig. 5-2C & D). The two strips are freed except at their base and brought into apposition with a cruciate suture using 5-0 biodegradable material with double-armed swaged-on cutting needles. The cruciate suture is completed by firmly seating the stitch through the tissue overlying the zygomatic arch (Fig. 5-2E). Simple interrupted sutures may be necessary to complement the tension and extend the lateral canthus laterally. The skin closure is the same as for lateral entropion. The palpebral fissure should assume the almond shape of a normal eye, and the muscle involved in the new lateral "ligament" will soon become fibrous connective tissue.

Postoperative medical care is restricted to systemic antibiotics unless overt corneal disease is present. When keratitis is manifest, the type of lesion will determine the kind of therapy necessary.

The functional and cosmetic results of these procedures, when correctly performed on the uncomplicated entropion, are excellent. The most important consideration is patient selection, which requires a thorough evaluation of cause and effect. The prognosis is also directly related to the results, and depends on proper patient selection and accurate diagnosis.

Instruments
Two straight mosquito forceps
Blunt-blunt tenotomy scissors
Castroviejo suturing forceps
Castroviejo needle holders

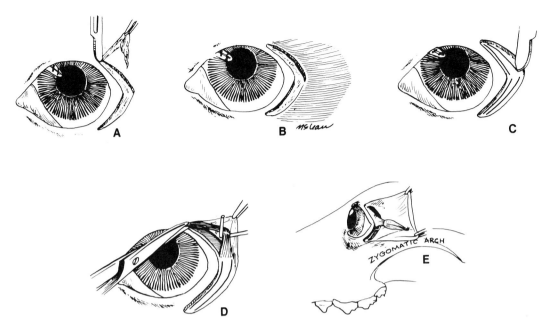

Figure 5-2. *Reconstruction of the lateral canthal ligament using bundles of orbicularis oculi muscle.* **A,** *Lateral skin is excised.* **B,** *Lateral skin (shaded area) is undermined.* **C,** *Orbicularis muscle strip is identified.* **D,** *A pedicle of orbicularis muscle is created.* **E,** *Muscle pedicle is sutured to periosteum.*

Strabismus hook
Bard-Parker handle and #15 blade
Double-armed 5-0 biodegradable suture
Double-armed 6-0 nonabsorbable suture

V-Plasty

This technique is applicable to any full-thickness lesion involving the lid. Approximately one-third of the free lid margin in the dog may be excised without permanent disfigurement. The older cat will not tolerate as much, and alternative procedures will be necessary.

Conditions in the dog that may lend themselves to this procedure include minor ectropion and neoplasms of the tarsal glands such as sebaceous adenoma and adenocarcinoma. Other examples of lid neoplasms are melanomas and papillomas.

The mass may be grossly visible on the external aspect of the lid or easily seen by everting the involved lid. Adenomas are most commonly seen in older dogs, and the inner surface of the lid should be routinely examined in these patients.

The lid skin is prepared routinely, the mass is identified, and two mosquito forceps are placed on either side of the lesion with the tips approaching, but not to, the fornix. The overall configuration is that of a triangle with the apex distal to the free lid margin (Fig. 5-3A). The forceps are removed one at a time, and the lid is cut with tenotomy scissors along the furrow produced by the forceps. This is done primarily to ensure a long straight incision and complete incorporation of the mass within the excised piece of lid.

The triangular defect is closed in two layers, beginning with the conjunctiva and ending with the skin. The first sutures of 7-0 absorbable material are started at the apex. The sutures are placed within the fibrous layer of the conjunctiva and do not penetrate the mucosal surface. A running mattress pattern is used and continued to the free lid margin (Fig. 5-3B).

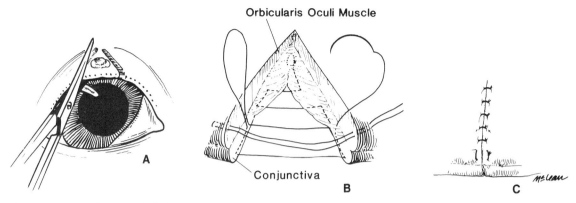

Figure 5-3. *V-plasty.* **A,** *full-thickness triangular piece of lid and conjunctiva is excised.* **B,** *The conjunctiva is closed.* **C,** *A small mattress suture and simple interrupted sutures close the skin.*

The skin is closed with 6-0 nonabsorbable suture material and the first suture, a small mattress, is placed near the free lid margin (see Fig. 5-3B). The small mattress suture is fashioned meticulously so as to reposition the tarsal plate within the lid margin as accurately as possible. The remaining wound is closed with simple interrupted sutures of nonabsorbable material (Fig. 5-3C).

The cosmetic results and prognosis are excellent. The major concern is adequacy of excision and ability to close without excess tension.

Instruments
Two straight mosquito forceps
Blunt-blunt tenotomy scissors
Castroviejo suturing forceps
Castroviejo needle holders
Colibri forceps
Bard-Parker handle and #15 blade
7-0 biodegradable sutures
6-0 nonabsorbable sutures

Permanent Lateral Tarsorrhaphy

Lagophthalmos is a condition observed in the prominent-eyed breeds, such as the Pekingese and Pomeranian. It is usually observed more frequently in older animals, but can be seen in younger ones as well. The animals frequently are presented because of severe axial corneal ulceration of variable degrees, from superficial to ruptured eyes. Some veterinarians erroneously incriminate the nose fold in this disease.

Entropion is frequently seen in dogs with a deeply set eye or "enophthalmos." The lack of support to the lids caused by enophthalmos results in mechanical entropion. One may see a redundant upper lid and deep cul-de-sac that tends to fill with mucopurulent exudate. Conjunctivitis to severe keratoconjunctivitis may be observed. The giant breeds are those most frequently affected; however, it has been recognized in Doberman pinschers, Irish setters, German shepherds (possibly as a sequela to atrophic myosilis), and other breeds.

By permanently shortening the lid, lagophthalmos or entropion secondary to enophthalmos can be eliminated. An efficient technique is a permanent lateral tarsorrhaphy. The procedure is basically a transposition of skin and conjunctiva in two layers (Fig. 5-4). This method is especially useful in breeds in which a prominent eye is the precipitating cause for overt corneal or conjunctival diseases. The overlapping and sliding technique provides a more secure scar with less tendency to spread and recur than does simple shortening by lateral tarsal excision and closure. This simplified method involves excising the dorsal and ventral tarsal glands, skin, and conjunctiva from the lateral canthal region, then closing in two layers. An overlapping

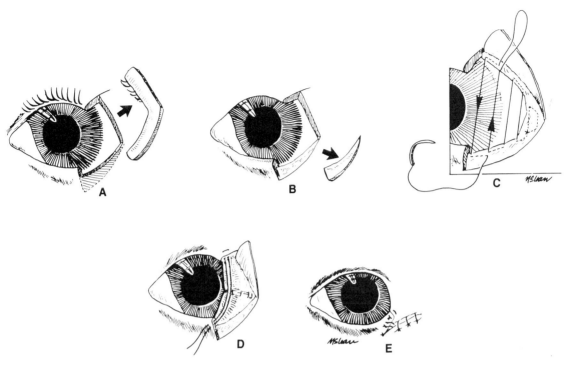

Figure 5-4. *Permanent lateral tarsorrhaphy.* **A,** *The tarsus is excised.* **B,** *A small triangular piece of lower lid skin is excised.* **C,** *The conjunctival layer is apposed.* **D,** *A small tarsal mattress stitch reforms the lateral canthus.* **E,** *The lateral canthal skin is closed with simple interrupted stitches.*

pattern is not indicated when globe pressure is minimal such as when the eye is enophthalmic. Rarely, as much as two-thirds of the lid may need to be removed to correct the defect.

The amount of shortening is determined before anesthesia is induced. The lid is prepared routinely and the tarsal plate is excised in the lateral upper and lower lid margin equal to the extent of shortening (see Fig. 5-4A). This excision is full thickness and extends around the lateral canthus. Closing this defect in two layers completes the simplified method discussed above, which can be used for the enophthalmic eye.

The upper lid skin is retained and the lower lid skin removed (Fig. 5-4B). The upper conjunctiva is removed and the lower retained. Precaution should be taken not to extend to the fornix of the conjunctiva of either upper or lower lid. This is especially true in the upper lid since the lacrimal gland ducts empty in this region and invasion of the fornix

may predispose to occlusion of the lacrimal ducts, predisposing to iatrogenic secondary sicca. An incision is made in the upper lid through skin and muscle to the conjunctiva. The incision should be approximately 4 to 5 mm. The conjunctiva should be dissected and excised from the end of the 5-mm incision to the lateral canthus, forming a triangle-like defect in the upper lateral canthus. The conjunctiva is preserved on the lower lid. The defect in the conjunctiva is closed with a continuous horizontal buried mattress suture of 7-0 biodegradable material started at the apex of the conjunctival defect coursing toward the medial aspect of the wound (Fig. 5-4C). The lateral canthus is reformed with a small intratarsal mattress suture (Fig. 5-4D). This must be done meticulously so as to reestablish the lid margins as accurately as possible (Fig. 5-4E). The upper free apex is sutured to the most ventral angle with simple interrupted sutures, and the wound is closed routinely with 6-0, or smaller, nonabsorbable material (Fig. 5-4*E*). Topical medication is restricted to solutions when they are necessary for the overt corneal or conjunctival disease that often accompanies this type of lid lesion. Blepharitis or other inflammatory lid lesions are preferably treated by systemic medication. Sutures are removed in 7 to 10 days.

The results of this surgery are good to excellent and provide adequate corneal protection to minimize further ulcerative keratitis associated with improper lid closure.

Instruments

Blunt-blunt tenotomy scissors
Bard-Parker handle and #15 blade
Castroviejo needle holders
Castroviejo suture forceps
Colibri forceps
Adson brain forceps
7-0 biodegradable suture
6-0 nonabsorbable suture

Permanent Medial Tarsorrhaphy

The commonly observed epiphora, pannus formation, and corneal vascularization of the nasal cornea may often be attributed to medial entropion. The breeds in which this is observed include the Pekingese, miniature poodle, English bulldog, and pug.

The lesion is frequently overlooked because of the subtle nature of the entropion. Careful examination will reveal minor inversion of both the upper and lower lid adjacent to the medial canthus. Caruncular hair may also contribute to the manifestations of this disease and may similarly be corrected by this surgical procedure.

Technique

The animal is anesthetized and the periocular region routinely prepared. The patient is placed in lateral recumbency with the head at an angle of approximately 45° and the nose pointed toward the ceiling to provide optimal exposure.

The most important consideration of surgical intervention in the medial canthus is the lacrimal drainage apparatus. The structures within this surgical field are the puncta, canaliculi, and the nasolacrimal sac. For this reason, the first few times the surgeon invades this area the puncta and canaliculi should be cannulated for identification and location. This can be done with two tom cat catheters.

When the puncta have been identified, mosquito forceps are fixed to the conjunctiva about 4 to 5 mm laterally from the puncta and 1 to 2 mm from the inner edge of the tarsal plate (Fig. 5-5*A*). The forceps are then used to evert the medial canthus by turning the upper lid out and up and the lower lid down and out. This provides better exposure of the surgical site. By immobilizing the medial canthal skin with an Adson tissue forceps, a mucocutaneous incision is begun at the apex of the canthus and extended 1 or 2 mm past the cannulated puncta on both the upper and lower lids. This incision should be made outside the caruncle.

The next incision is made from the anterior extent of the upper lid incision and carried toward the medial canthus. The degree of this angle will depend on the extent of entropion. A similar incision is made on the lower lid. Completion of this forms a triangular island of skin containing the caruncle. This island of skin is dissected free and discarded (Fig. 5-5*B*).

The resulting defect is closed by joining the mucous membranes, starting at the apex, with a continuous horizontal mattress pattern using 7-0 biodegradable material, burying the knots (Fig. 5-5*C*). The skin edge is reapposed by placing a small mattress suture with 6-0 nonabsorbable material within the tarsus of both lids and closing it as accurately as possible. The remaining defect is closed with simple interrupted sutures (Figs. 5-5*D* & *E*). The skin sutures are removed in 7 to 10 days after surgery.

Treatment after surgery may include systemic antibiotics if presurgical inflammation is diagnosed. Topical antibiotics are not indi-

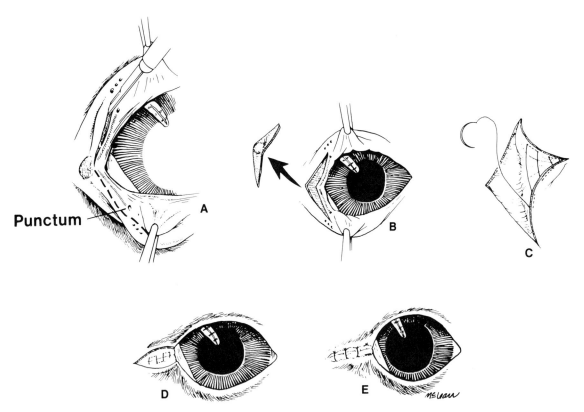

Figure 5-5. *Permanent medial tarsorrhaphy.* **A,** *A mucocutaneous and skin incision is made to include the caruncle.* **B,** *A triangular piece of skin is excised from the medial canthus including the caruncle.* **C,** *Closure of the conjunctiva.* **D,** *The conjunctival suture pattern.* **E,** *The skin is closed with a small mattress suture and simple interrupted sutures.*

cated unless overt keratitis or conjunctivitis is manifest.

The results are cosmetically pleasing and functionally correct. The prognosis is good for minimizing corneal irritation.

Instruments

Adson tissue forceps
#64 Beaver blade and handle
Castroviejo suturing forceps
Castroviejo needle holders
Colibri forceps
Tenotomy scissors
Two straight mosquito forceps
Two tom cat catheters
7-0 biodegradable suture
6-0 nonabsorbable suture

Conjunctival Flaps

Conjunctival flaps are best used when danger of corneal rupture exists, such as in animals with descemetoceles and other deep stromal ulcers. Even after ocular rupture, a conjunctival flap can be used to close the perforation once the edges of the ulcer are cleaned and iris adhesions to the cornea are broken down. Descemetoceles and deep corneal ulcers should be operated on as soon as possible since the results are better and the procedure is easier on an intact globe than on a ruptured one. Corneal, scleral, and conjunctival transposition can also be considered as a corrective procedure. Care must be used in handling these animals, as overzealous restraint may be enough to rupture the thin Descemet's membrane that is keeping the eye intact.

The advantages of a conjunctival flap are that it is a quickly adherent (within minutes to hours) protective covering, the flap provides a rich supply of fibroblasts and blood vessels, and the flap does not shift position on the globe when there is ocular movement, all of which promote faster healing.

The disadvantages of a conjunctival flap are that it is more difficult to apply the flap correctly and it is time consuming. It permanently adheres to the ulcer, which may develop into a heavy opaque scar or leukoma.

There are several types of conjunctival flaps: sling, pedicle, sliding, and the total or 360°. The sliding flap is the most versatile and can be used to cover very large corneal defects. A good blood supply is maintained in the flap. The most important consideration for a successful outcome is to keep the flap thin, which is the most difficult part of the preparation.

The total, or 360° flap, is the most difficult to dissect thinly and is the most traumatic of the conjunctival flaps. The total flap is supposedly useful in very large central ulcers; however, the sliding flap can usually be mobilized sufficiently to cover most of the cornea. Exception may be made in some exophthalmic breeds, such as the Pekingese, in which a great deal of tension on the conjunctiva is required to cover the defect. Then a total flap will distribute the tension more equally over the entire surface.

Technique

Sliding Flap

The periocular region is prepared routinely for surgery. The conjunctival cul-de-sacs are thoroughly irrigated with sterile ophthalmic eye wash or sterile saline. This should be done gently and meticulously so as to remove all the mucus and other debris within the palpebral fissures.

The conjunctiva is gently grasped with a Colibri forceps approximately 2 mm from the limbus. Gentle tension results in tenting of the conjunctiva. The tented conjunctiva is incised with a pair of tenotomy scissors by cutting on the corneal side of the tent. The cut is made perpendicular to the surface of the conjunctiva. The resulting incision is parallel to the limbus and 2 mm from it (Fig. 5-6A). The cut edge is gently elevated with a pair of Colibri forceps and freed by blunt dissection with blunt-blunt curved tenotomy scissors (Fig. 5-6B). When dissecting toward the fornix, it is more difficult to maintain a thin flap. Tenon's capsule is thinnest near the limbus and heaviest as it reaches the insertion of the extraocular muscles and, although the conjunctiva is more adherent to Tenon's capsule near the limbus, it appears to "grow" as you dissect toward the fornix. Therefore, if a few collagen fibers are cut in the initial incision, they retract and cannot be separated from the flap. Subsequent dissection causes more connective tissue to adhere to the flap. In order to minimize this problem, the initial incision is made in the area of the more loosely attached conjunctiva; however, care must be exercised in performing the incision so as to minimize severing fibers of Tenon's capsule.

The length of the incision and breadth of dissection is determined by how much the flap must be stretched to cover the defect, plus a few millimeters. Mobilization is made laterally and medially rather than toward the fornix. Frequently, only two stitches of 6-0 or 7-0 biodegradable material are required. One is placed through the flap and half depth into the limbus (Fig. 5-6C). The flap is then stretched across the cornea and the lesion so that pressure is exerted against the cornea by the flap. Another suture is placed in a fashion similar to the first, at the opposite limbus so as to maintain this pressure. Pressure exerted by two stitches is generally sufficient to maintain the flap over the corneal defect, thereby preventing the flap's natural tendency to withdraw over the sclera. One or two stitches may be placed at the leading edge of the flap and half depth into the cornea if the flap is not firmly

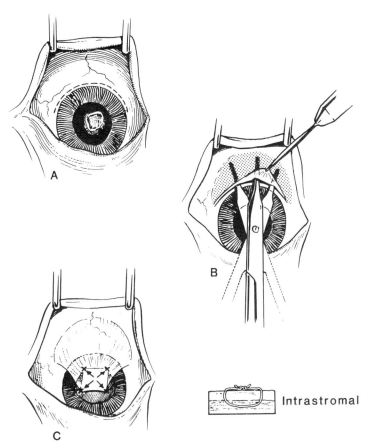

Figure 5-6. *A sliding conjunctival flap is used to cover corneal defects.* **A,** *A dashed line indicates the conjunctival incision.* **B,** *Blunt dissection is performed with tenotomy scissors.* **C,** *Intrastromal sutures hold the conjunctiva firmly to the cornea.*

Intrastromal

tensed over the lesion. An alternative method is to place four sutures equally spaced from the center of the lesion. Conjunctival tension is applied over the corneal lesion (Fig. 5-6C).

Total Flap

The preparation of this flap is the same as for the sliding flap except that the incision extends around the entire circumference of the cornea. After the dissection is complete, the edges are drawn together by a running mattress suture with 6-0 or 7-0 biodegradable material. The cornea is not included in this closure. The running mattress suture is preferred, since puckering and mounding of redundant conjunctiva over the center of the cornea do not occur as with a purse-string suture.

Postoperative Care

No special aftercare is needed except for specific topical antibiotics and 1% atropine sulfate when anterior segmental disease is present. Most animals accept the surgery with little discomfort and consequently do not rub or paw at it. The sutures are removed in 10 to 14 days without freeing the flap. The flap will have adhered only to those areas where a loss of corneal epithelium was manifest and must be freed from the corneal adhesions; however, this should be delayed for several weeks. Do not attempt to trim the flap too close to an adherent area since the injured cornea is thin and predisposed to perforation. The adherent conjunctiva will become smooth and blend into the cornea in a few weeks and the unattached conjunctiva will retract to a normal position. The cornea never regains its normal thickness in this area, but it is adequate. A dense leukoma is the usual expected result of deep stromal corneal lesions that necessitate a conjunctival flap. The prognosis depends on the ocular predisposition towards ulceration. For example, a buphthalmic dog with lagophthalmos is predisposed, and other corrective measures as previously described should be considered.

Instruments

Wire lid speculum
Castroviejo suturing forceps
Castroviejo needle holders
Colibri forceps
Blunt-blunt curved tenotomy scissors
6-0 or 7-0 biodegradable suture material

Corneal, Scleral, Conjunctival Transposition (Modified Parshall Technique)

The incidence of deep stromal ulcerative keratitis with marked keratomalacia is high among prominent-eyed breeds such as the Pekingese and pug. These lesions frequently progress to descemetoceles, staphylomas, or iris prolapses. The etiology is speculative; however, it is believed that the lesion is produced by exposure as a result of lagophthalmos, with epithelial erosion and secondary infection, possibly by *Pseudomonas* spp. with subsequent autolysis.

The primary disease (lagophthalmos) must be kept in mind when correcting the presenting problem, *i.e.*, the deep penetrating ulcer or ruptured eye. The modified Parshall technique is a corneal, scleral, conjunctival transposition.

Surgical Procedure

An animal presenting with an eye that has a descemetocele or iris prolapse should be treated topically and systemically for the corneal and anterior segmental disease. Topical ointments are contraindicated when the cornea is ruptured. However, surgery should be performed as quickly as possible to correct the defect.

The animal is anesthetized routinely. The surface of the eye is carefully irrigated with sterile eye wash and the periocular regions are carefully prepared. Caution must be exercised so the eye is not further injured during this manipulation. A lid speculum is placed in the fissure to provide adequate exposure. The globe is fixed at the limbus with 0.5 mm Castroviejo suture forceps adjacent to but not within the surgical site. Two moderately divergent incisions are made with a #64 Beaver blade encompassing the lesion and extending to the closest limbus (Fig. 5-7A). These incisions should be approximately midstromal in depth and perpendicular to the corneal surface. The next incision should be made outside the lesion, connecting the first two limbs of the incision. This results in a pedicle surrounding the lesion with two limbs extending toward the limbus (see Fig. 5-7A). By careful tissue dissection starting axially and progressing toward the limbus, approximately midstromal deep, a bed is formed over which the lamellar transplant will be placed (see Fig. 5-7B). The tissue around the lesion can be used to manipulate the pedicle without injuring the normal corneal tissue.

The more nearly normal cornea between the limbs of the primary incisions is then dissected midstromally with a #64 Beaver blade or corneal dissector. This lamellar separation is continued past the limbus into sclera, at which time hemorrhage is observed. This is controlled by pressure applied to the area with sponges or cotton applicators. The scleral separation is continued for approximately 3 mm, and the blade is directed toward the conjunctiva, exiting underneath it. A conjunctival flap is then fashioned with the corneal scleral pedicle attached (see Fig. 5-7C). This provides mobilization, which facilitates transposition of the corneal-scleral-conjunctival pedicle over the lesion.

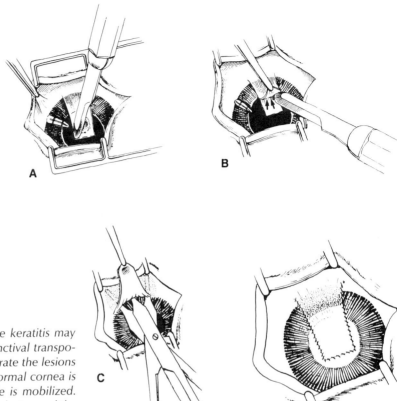

Figure 5-7. *Deep stromal ulcerative keratitis may be treated by corneal, scleral, conjunctival transposition.* **A,** *Divergent incisions incorporate the lesions and extend toward the limbus.* **B,** *Normal cornea is dissected midstromally.* **C,** *A pedicle is mobilized.* **D,** *The pedicle is transposed over the lesion and the wound is closed with simple continuous sutures.*

Two simple interrupted sutures are placed in the corners of the pedicle and a continuous suture pattern is added to satisfactorily close the lesion (see Fig. 5-7D). Biodegradable 7-0 material is used with a spatula Atraloc needle. Even though the material is biodegradable, the sutures should be removed in 14 days.

Postoperative care should be directed toward the manifest ocular disease. If severe anterior segment disease is present, systemic antibiotics and steroids may be indicated. Topical drugs should include antibiotics (specific if sensitivities are available) t.i.d. to q.i.d., mydriatic/cycloplegics (atropine sulfate 1% b.i.d. to q.i.d), anticollagenase (acetylcysteine 10% q.i.d.) and artificial tears, the frequency depending on the severity of the corneal or anterior segment disease. The sutures are removed in 7 to 10 days. Ocular therapy is adjusted depending on clinical signs.

The results of this surgery provide a relatively clear central cornea in lieu of the dense scar that would result from a conjunctival flap. Cosmetically and functionally, this transposition procedure is more effective than a flap and can be performed with a little practice. Because of the predisposing lagophthalmos, a permanent lateral or medial tarsorrhaphy may be indicated either at the time of surgery or after the transposition heals. The exciting predisposition must be corrected or the lesion can recur.

Instruments
Beaver handle and #64 blade
Castroviejo suture forceps
Castroviejo needle holder

Colibri iris forceps
Wire lid speculum
Tenotomy scissors
Desmares corneal dissector (optional)
7-0 biodegradable suture
Weckcell sponges

Keratectomy

Superficial keratectomy is the partial or entire removal of the superficial cornea, including the epithelium and/or superficial stroma. A keratectomy is indicated when the cornea has a superficial opacity that interferes with vision or predisposes the eye to further ocular damage; examples are focal neoplasms, epithelial inclusion cysts, and focal granulomas. The most frequent lesions corrected by keratectomy are the corneal dermoid (choriostoma) seen in most species and recurrent erosion or "Boxer" ulceration. The dermoid is located at the limbus and may involve the cornea and conjunctiva. It is composed of hair follicles, sebaceous glands, fibrous tissue and fat; in other words, a dermoid is an ectopic island of skin. Because of their obvious presence, these lesions are diagnosed while affected animals are quite young.

Other conditions warranting a keratectomy are dense, superficial corneal dystrophies that interfere with vision. Most dystrophies do not interfere noticeably with vision, and surgery is at the discretion of the clinician or owner. Corneal dystrophy is a noninfectious avascular lesion of the superficial corneal stroma. It may be inherited; however, many dystrophic-like lesions are idiopathic. They may contain lipids (cholesterol) or calcium salts. Some lipid dystrophies have been attributed to hypothyroidism. This is manifested by a central white crystalline opacity underlying an intact epithelium and is a degenerative lesion that often contains blood vessels. Dystrophies can appear at any age and in any breed. There is no known medical treatment and usually the lesion persists. The lesion can ap-

pear with or without other ocular disease. Evidence suggests an hereditary predisposition in some breeds.

Conditions for which keratectomy is not recommended are degenerative pannus (common in German shepherds) and full-depth leukomas or staphylomas. Degenerative pannus can best be treated medically, and a keratectomy only temporarily relieves the corneal pannus and promotes permanent scarring. Full-depth leukomas cannot be removed sufficiently for the animal to see without the danger of corneal perforation. Healed staphylomas not only have the same inherent dangers as leukomas, but additionally, the corneal stroma is usually thinner than normal.

Technique

After appropriate preoperative preparation and adequate draping and irrigation of the conjunctival cul-de-sac with sterile saline or eye wash, the globe is stabilized with suture forceps. These forceps are used on the sclera nearest the corneal lesion. A #64 Beaver blade is used to incise the cornea. The incision is perpendicular to the surface of the cornea and is made in the form of a triangle with the apex of the triangle at the center of the eye and the base at the limbus. The incision is carried beyond the lesion until it crosses the adjacent incision, making an X (Fig. 5-8A). The depth of the incision should be sufficient to be just beneath the lesion. The apex of the incision is grasped with a pair of iris forceps or small conjunctival forceps, and the stromal lamellae are separated by using a #64 Beaver blade or a Desmares corneal dissector (Fig. 5-8B). Care should be taken when using a blade since it is easy to go from one stromal plane to the other; the corneal dissector tends to remain in one plane of the stroma during dissection. If the lesion is a dermoid and involves the perilimbal sclera, the dissection must be carried through the limbus and affected sclera. Hemorrhage will occur at this point. Covering the wound or cautery are unnecessary.

The animal is sent home on topical antibi-

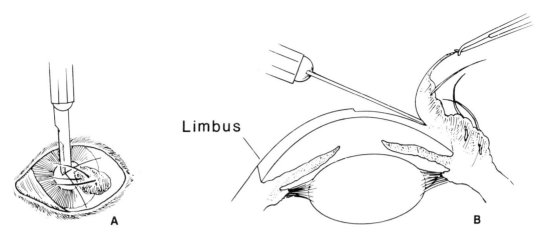

Figure 5-8. *Superficial keratectomy is used for superficial to midstromal disease of the cornea.* **A,** *The lesion is outlined by intersecting incisions made with a No. 64 Beaver blade.* **B,** *A cross-section shows the correct position of the blade and the proper depth of the incision for lamellar separation.*

otics because of the vulnerability of the iatrogenic corneal ulcer to infection. Atropine sulfate 1% solution may be indicated if anterior segmental disease is present. The wound should epithelialize in a few days. Excessively deep wounds will not regenerate a full thickness of stroma. Scarring of the cornea as a result of surgery is minimal when secondary infection is prevented.

Instruments
Beaver handle and #64 blade
Castroviejo suturing forceps
Desmares corneal dissector
Colibri iris forceps
Lid speculum

Corneal Epithelial Abrasion

Conditions under which the corneal epithelium is scarified or scraped off the underlying stroma are superficial, chronic, nonresolving corneal ulcers with redundant borders.

Indolent corneal ulceration, common in the boxer dog, is the most common syndrome requiring epithelial abrasion. The disease manifests itself as a persistent, nonhealing, superficial corneal ulceration. Characteristically, it is differentiated from other longstanding corneal ulcers by the absence of corneal vascularization in and around the ulcerated area. An overlapping border is best demonstrated by fluorescein dye. The fluorescein will stain only the portion of the eye that has no epithelial covering or is attached to the stroma. Consequently, the examiner will see the edge of the ulcer as a green stain and then notice that the stroma is stained, usually a lighter green, a few millimeters beyond the apparent border of the ulcer. There is a defect in the basement membrane of the corneal epithelium that predisposes to erosion of epithelial cells as well as to separation of one epithelial cell from another. Subsequently, these cells "fall" out of position without exciting the fifth nerve endings in the cornea. The resultant minimal irritation of the ulcer and lack of inflammatory response does not elicit vascularization. Some dogs, however, demonstrate severe signs of irritation as seen by marked blepharospasm, conjunctival erythema, mucopurulent exudate, and even corneal vascularization. This represents complications, probably due to secondary bacterial infection rather than a primary healing response to the ulcer.

The cornea is anesthetized with a topical anesthetic, and the redundant borders of the ulcer are rubbed with a dry sterile cotton-tipped swab (Fig. 5-9A). The perilesional epithelium is removed by applying gentle pressure toward the limbus and away from the ulcer (Fig. 5-9B). This results in removing the redundant tissue that is not firmly adherent to the underlying stroma. Because of the ulcer, prophylactic antibiotics are given in an attempt to control the bacterial flora within the palpebral surfaces. The lesion should be restained and reevaluated in 72 hours; it should be at least half the original size at that time. The epithelium will still be loose, since firm adherence will take at least 6 weeks. This must be considered when reevaluating the eye and should be uppermost in your mind when irrigating the eye after staining. Overzealous manipulation may result in iatrogenic injury.

Other conditions in which this technique may be used in conjunction with other modes of therapy include precipitates of calcium salts in the cornea, fungal keratitis, and deep infectious keratitis. Scraping removes debris and infected tissue, increasing the effectiveness of treatment with antibiotics and other topical drugs as well as providing a cytologic or culture specimen for diagnostic purposes.

Instruments
Proparacaine HCl topical anesthetic
Castroviejo suturing forceps
Sterile cotton applicators

Transposition of the Parotid Duct

This procedure is used to replace lacrimal secretion in the treatment of absolute keratoconjunctivitis sicca. It is used when all hopes of return of lacrimal gland function have been exhausted. Surgery should be considered when the Schirmer tear test is 0 mm per minute and medical therapy has not been satisfactory to patient or owner.

The surgeon first should review the anatomy of the area (Fig. 5-10). The proximity of the dorsal and ventral buccal nerves and the facial vein is important to consider when invading this area surgically.

Treatment with broad-spectrum antibiotics for 24 to 48 hours is optional to control the microbial population in the cul-de-sac and mouth. Dental prophylaxis is also advisable 1 to 2 weeks before surgery if feasible and indicated. The parotid duct empties into the mouth adjacent to the third and fourth upper cheek teeth. A visible papilla can be distinguished in this area. Parotid gland function should be determined before attempting surgery. This may be accomplished by placing a drop of 1% atropine solution on your finger and rubbing it on the dog's gum. The bitter taste will stimulate profuse salivation in the normal animal; saliva should visibly flow from the papillas. The absence of flow negates this surgery.

The eye should be thoroughly irrigated with sterile eye wash. The parotid duct is identified by cannulating it with a 0 monofilament suture. The lateral aspect of the jaw, including the commissures of the lips and ex-

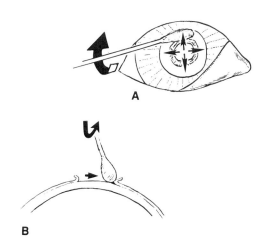

Figure 5-9. *Treatment of indolent corneal ulceration. A, The lesion is rubbed with a dry sterile swab. B, Gentle rotating pressure on the limbus removes redundant tissue.*

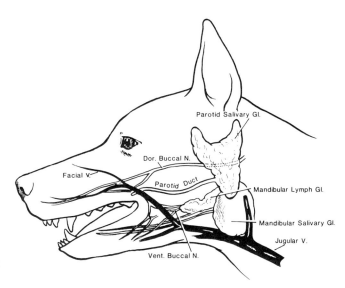

Parotid Salivary Gl.

Dor. Buccal N.

Facial V.

Parotid Duct

Mandibular Lymph Gl.

Mandibular Salivary Gl.

Jugular V.

Vent. Buccal N.

Figure 5-10. *The anatomy of the parotid duct and adjacent structures.*

tending 2 to 3 cm caudal to the lateral canthus, is clipped and surgically prepared.

A triangular circumpapillary incision is made 4 to 5 mm from the cannulated papilla (Fig. 5-11*A*). The incision can be made with a #15 Bard-Parker blade. It should be meticulously performed so as to ensure sufficient buccal mucosa around the papilla for adequate suture placement without occluding the duct. By carefully dissecting caudally from the papilla through the circumpapillary incision, the surgeon can free the duct along its buccal course. In many dogs, the duct can be completely freed in this manner without making a facial skin incision.

A skin incision may be made between the parotid gland and the lateral canthus to facilitate isolation of the parotid duct and papilla in some animals (see Fig. 5-11*B*). This may be either an elliptical or straight incision, depending on the surgeon's preference and the patient's skull type. The subcutis and platysma muscle are dissected bluntly to expose the masseter muscle and the cannulated parotid duct. By blunt dissection, the duct may be freed and a piece of sterile moistened umbilical tape placed around it to manipulate the duct more safely. Meticulous care must be exercised while manipulating the duct to prevent

trauma and tears, which may lead to adhesions predisposing failure. Identification of the buccal nerves (dorsal and ventral branches) is necessary to avoid neurectomies, and the facial vein must also be avoided.

The duct must be mobilized along its course to the parotid gland regardless of whether the closed method through the buccal incision or the open method through the skin incision is used. The freed duct and papilla are moved toward the lateral canthus and should reach it with little or no tension on the duct per se. If tension is demonstrated, further dissection is indicated.

A lateral canthotomy, which allows better exposure for suture placement, may be used. Mosquito forceps are placed in the lateral ventral cul-de-sac and gently pushed into the operative field. A small nick incision is made between the arms of the forceps and they are forced through, producing a track through which the cannulated duct is drawn (see Fig. 5-11*B*). The papilla is placed between the third eyelid and the lateral lower lid. Suture placement must ensure good apposition between the epithelial edges of the transplanted papilla and conjunctiva. The conjunctiva is sutured to the papilla with three or four 6-0 or 7-0 biodegradable sutures using an everting mattress

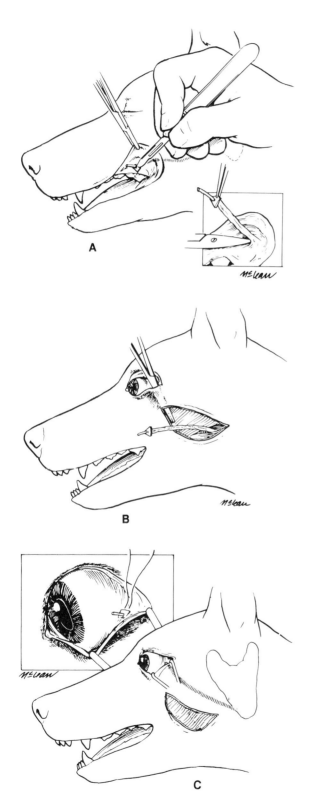

suture pattern (Fig. 5-11*C*). This suture pattern causes the papilla to protrude well into the cul-de-sac, decreasing the chance of scar retraction and postoperative constriction.

The canthotomy and facial skin incisions are closed with 6-0 simple interrupted nonabsorbable sutures. The skin sutures are removed in 7 to 10 days.

Postoperative care should include systemic antibiotics, warm compresses over the jaw, and frequent stimulation of salivation. Stimulation can be produced following surgery by placing a drop of atropine on your finger and rubbing it on the gums. This should not be overdone, lest atropinization occur. The bitter taste produces copious saliva. When the animal is fully recovered from anesthesia, or 12 to 24 hours postoperatively, salivation may be stimulated by offering the animal food or a treat. Some owners can train their pets to respond to the telephone bell by offering a treat when the owner rings a bell; subsequently, if the client is away from home for several hours, a telephone call can provide the sound that stimulates the pet to salivate, thus moistening the eye.

The pH of the new "tears" should be tested. Some animals whose saliva is alkaline (pH 7 to 8) may have a predisposition to forming calcium precipitates. Although this may not be completely eliminated, it may be reduced by acidifying the animals's diet as for urolithiasis.

A successful result of this surgery does not eliminate ocular therapy but changes the frequency of therapy, which can benefit the owner and patient. The surgery provides saliva, not tears, and the surgeon must be aware of this limitation. Dogs that salivate profusely will often develop moist facial dermatitis as a

Figure 5-11. *Transposition of the parotid duct.* **A,** *The duct is cannulated and an incision frees the duct around the papilla to permit dissection within the cheek (inset).* **B,** *Forceps are used to form a track through which the duct is drawn.* **C,** *The papilla is sutured to the conjunctiva.*

complication. Failure to secrete may be due to scar formation or inspissation of saliva within the duct. It is important to instruct the owners to be certain the dog salivates when stimulated and that "saliva tears" are seen within the palpebral fissure.

Instruments

Castroviejo needle holders
Castroviejo suture forceps
0 monofilament sutures
Blunt tenotomy scissors
Bard-Parker handle and #15 blade
Four straight mosquito forceps
1/4" umbilical tape, 6 to 8" long
6-0 biodegradable suture
6-0 nonabsorbable suture

Enucleation

There are three forms of removing all or part of the orbital contents. Exenteration is the removal of all the orbital contents. This is reserved for neoplastic disease that has extended beyond the globe itself. Evisceration is the removal of all the contents of the globe, retaining the fibrous tunic (cornea and sclera). This is used for intraocular prosthetics. Enucleation, by definition, is removing only the globe and retaining all adnexal tissue. Most surgical procedures requiring removal of the globe in animals also include portions of the adnexal tissues that have secretory function, such as the tarsal glands, intraepithelial goblet cells, and gland of the third eyelid.

Enucleation is indicated when the eye is painful, such as in severe glaucoma or severe traumatic injury not amenable to medical therapy. Primary intraocular neoplasia without metastasis and phthisis bulbi also may require enucleation. There are other indications, all of which are last resorts; the decision for enucleation should be carefully evaluated.

The objectives for the surgery are to alleviate pain, resolve an untreatable medical disease, prevent further or additional complications, and provide the most aesthetic appearance possible. Many methods have been advocated. The transpalpebral technique results in minimal tissue injury and preserves orbital tissue while removing all potential secretory tissues.

The animal is routinely anesthetized and the periocular region is preoperatively prepared as previously described. An incision is made in the medial canthal region as close to the free lid margin as possible extending it dorsally and ventrally, parallel to the upper and lower lids respectively (Fig. 5-12A). This preserves the integrity of the medial canthal ligament while avoiding the large angularis oculi vein in the medial canthal region. The incisions through the lid should be through skin and orbicularis, but not through the conjunctiva. This results in retaining the free lid margin and tarsal glands on the conjunctival pedicle.

Dissection should be continued at the medial canthal region. Tension with Adson tissue forceps on the lid margins containing the tarsal glands facilitates dissection. The #15 Bard-Parker blade is directed toward the conjunctiva and the dissection is continued until the globe itself is reached. This essentially means that the conjunctiva is freed from the underlying tissue and results in "straightening out" the conjunctiva. The third eyelid and gland is excised in this method; as the dissection continues in the medial aspect of the globe, the gland protrudes and is easily identified. A pair of mosquito forceps are inserted between the gland and globe and closed to facilitate hemostasis and ligation of the third eyelid stump, including the basilar artery to the gland (see Fig. 5-12B). The membrane, including its gland, is excised as close as possible to the posterior pole. As dissection continues and the surgeon reaches the globe, Tenon's capsule is incised at the limbus, a muscle hook is used to engage each of the extrinsic muscles, and myectomies are performed as close as possible to the sclera. This is continued to include the retractor oculi muscle bundles, which attach posterior to the equator. The muscle hook can be used to determine if any residual muscle

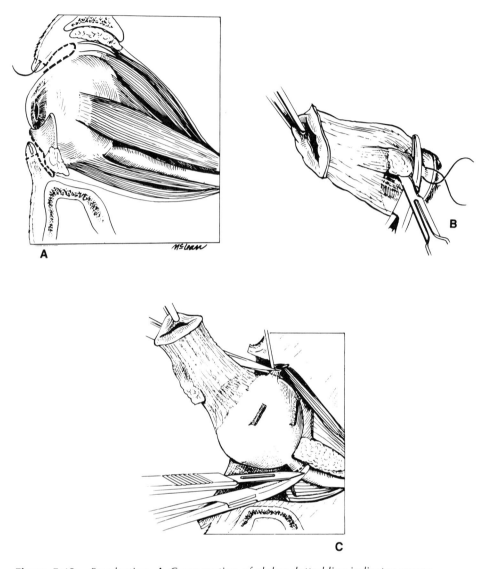

Figure 5-12. *Enucleation.* ***A,*** *Cross-section of globe; dotted line indicates course of dissection through the skin and represents the conjunctiva, which is straightened by dissection.* ***B,*** *Forceps retracting the base of the third eyelid, and ligation and excision of the entire third eyelid structure, including the gland.* ***C,*** *Cross-section showing myectomy, forceps attached to the nerve, and method of neurectomy to deliver the globe.*

attachment is present. If there is none, a curved mosquito forceps is placed medially to clasp the optic nerve and vessels surrounding it (see Fig. 5-12C). A #15 Bard-Parker blade on a handle is placed on the forceps handle that is used as a guide to sever the optic nerve. The globe, third eyelid, conjunctiva, and free lid margins containing the tarsal glands are all removed (see Fig. 5-12C). A 3-0 biodegradable suture is placed around the nerve and vessels and ligated. The forcep is removed.

To minimize premature tissue shrinkage,

the periorbit is closed by beginning either medially or laterally at the orbital rim with a simple continuous suture pattern of 3-0 biodegradable suture. The skin is then closed with a simple continuous suture of 5-0 nonabsorbable sutures. To decrease dead tissue space, a large mattress suture is placed behind the lid closure and allowed to remain for 3 days. This technique forms a large lid scar to aid in slowing orbital sinking. Eventually, the absence of tissue pressure will result in atrophy and orbital sinking; however, this technique allows owner conditioning and is, initially, aesthetically more acceptable. The prognosis is excellent, particularly when all secretory tissues have been removed.

Instruments
Castroviejo needle holders
Castroviejo suture forceps
Castroviejo standard 6″ needle holders
Blunt-blunt tenotomy scissors
Muscle hook
2 straight mosquito forceps
2 curved mosquito forceps
Adson tissue forceps
Bard-Parker handle and #15 blades
3-0 biodegradable suture
5-0 nonabsorbable suture
4-0 nonabsorbable suture

Intrascleral Prosthesis

Artificial eyes as used in human ophthalmology are not as effective in dogs and cats. An alternative in veterinary ophthalmology is a nonreacting intrascleral implant such as a silicone sphere. Ocular conditions that lend themselves to this option include nonresponsive painful glaucoma; post-traumatic noninfectious endophthalmitis such as scleral lacerations and shotgun injuries; postinfectious endophthalmitis with a predisposition to phthisis bulbi; and others. Conditions that do not lend themselves to this procedure are primary and secondary intraocular neoplasms

involving the fibrous tunic or orbital content. Acute infectious endophthalmitis is also a contraindication. The eviscerated tissue in all procedures should be thoroughly examined grossly and histologically to exclude the possibility of neoplastic or infectious disease.

The animal's periorbital region is prepared routinely and the conjunctival cul-de-sacs irrigated thoroughly. The anesthetized animal is placed in a dorsal recumbency with the head position adjusted so the cornea is parallel to the table top. A lid speculum is placed in the interpalpebral space and the globe is fixed with Castroviejo suture forceps so that the 12 o'clock position is exposed. A fornix-based conjunctival flap is fashioned about 3 mm posterior to the limbus to expose the sclera. This extends approximately 160° in the dorsal aspect of the globe (Fig. 5-13A). An incision is made in the exposed sclera with a #64 Beaver blade approximately 4 mm posterior to the limbus (see Fig. 5-13B). The incision should be a "scratch" incision through the sclera, to the choroid but not into it. The incision may be 5 to 6 mm long parallel to the limbus. A cyclodialysis spatula is inserted between the fibrous and vascular tunics and the two layers are separated (cyclodialysis) (see Fig. 5-13C). This is easily accomplished everywhere except at the iridocorneal angle and the vortex vein emissaries. Bleeding may be profuse when these vessels are torn, but it is transient.

The initial scleral incision is enlarged medially and laterally using straight blunt-blunt tenotomy scissors. Place one blade of the scissors between the sclera and underlying choroid. Care must be exercised so as not to penetrate the vascular tunic (choroid). When the scleral incision is elongated, further cyclodialysis is performed until the fibrous and vascular tunics are separated completely to the optic nerve. The optic nerve is separated and the entire contents of the globe are removed (see Fig. 5-13D). It is important to list the tissues that must be removed, including the vitreous, retina, lens, choroid, ciliary body, and iris. These tissues should be inspected grossly and histologically, depending on the reason for

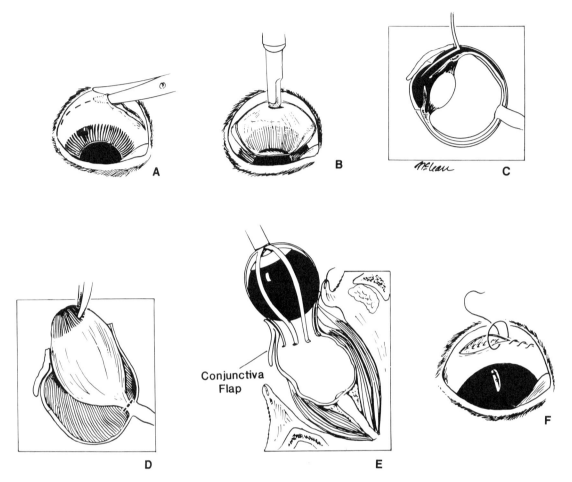

Figure 5-13. *Intrascleral prosthesis.* ***A,*** *Enlarging the conjunctival flap to 160 degrees.* ***B,*** *"Scratch" incision through sclera to cornea.* ***C,*** *Cross-section demonstrating separation of the cornea from sclera by the cyclodialysis spatula.* ***D,*** *Delivering the uvea; dotted line indicates where optic nerve is severed.* ***E,*** *Placement of the silastic prosthesis.* ***F,*** *Closure of sclera and conjunctiva.*

the surgery, to provide an accurate prognosis more effectively.

A small brain aspirator is helpful in inspecting the inner surface of the fibrous tunic. The surgeon must protect the cornea during the entire procedure. Unnecessary endothelial injury will result in postoperative complications and poor aesthetic result.

A sphere introducer is used to insert the proper-sized sphere (14 to 18 mm for the average globe). The ends of the introducer with the

sphere inside are inserted through the 160° scleral incision and the sphere is placed within the fibrous tunic (see Fig. 5-13*E*). The scleral incision is closed with 6-0 biodegradable simple continuous sutures. Tenon's capsule and conjunctiva are closed with 6-0 or 7-0 biodegradable simple continuous sutures (see Fig. 5-13*F*).

Because of the predisposition of microbial contamination in a closed system, postoperative therapy is recommended (Amoxicillin, 10 mg/kg p.o. b.i.d. for 7 days). Due to the severe postoperative inflammation that often accompanies this surgery, antiprostaglandins are recommended. Aspirin is effective at 15 mg/kg p.o. b.i.d. for 7 days. Swelling and discomfort is not uncommon for the first 3 days after surgery, and it may be prudent to hospitalize the patient during this period. The patient often exhibits discomfort, which dictates keeping the animal under observation and allowing for analgesic management. Corneal vascularization is a common response to an intrascleral prosthesis but regresses and becomes cosmetically acceptable when healing occurs. Many clients are more amenable to this option than to enucleation, which is an alternative.

Instruments

Eyelid speculum
Castroviejo suturing forceps
Castroviejo needle holders
Colibri forceps
Cyclodialysis spatula
Cyclodialysis cannula
Small brain aspirator
Intraocular sphere introducer
Beaver handle and #64 Beaver blade
Blunt-blunt straight tenotomy scissors
6-0 and 7-0 biodegradable sutures

Jordan's Implant (Jordon Plastic Research Corp., Southfield, MI)

Surgical exploration of the orbit and related structures is described under "Zygomatic Salivary Gland" in Chapter 6.

Several intraocular surgical procedures, such as cyclodialysis and lendectomy, may be indicated in veterinary patients. Because of the specialized diagnostic and surgical instrumentation necessary, and the need for specific training in these procedures, they are beyond the scope of this book. A veterinary ophthalmologist should be consulted.

Suggested Readings

Bistner SI, Aquirre G, Batik G. Atlas of veterinary ophthalmic surgery. Philadelphia: WB Saunders, 1977.
Gelatt KN. Treatment of canine keratoconjunctivitis sicca by parotid duct transposition. J Am Anim Hosp Assoc 1970;6:1.
Paton, Smith, Katzin, Stilwell. Atlas of eye surgery. 2nd ed. New York: McGraw-Hill, 1962.
Roper-Hall MJ. Stallard's eye surgery. 6th ed. Philadelphia: JB Lippincott, 1980.
Slatter DH. Fundamentals of veterinary ophthalmology. 1st ed. Philadelphia: WB Saunders, 1981.

6

Colin E. Harvey

Oral and Dental Diseases and Procedures

The oral cavity often is the site of surgical procedures in dogs and cats. In fact, teeth cleaning is one of the most common surgical procedures in small animal practice.

Significant anatomic features are the teeth, which are covered by an inert enamel substance on the exposed crown; the jaws, with alveolar spaces that contain the roots of the teeth; and the muscular system, which permits food and fluid to be prehended and swallowed. Salivary gland secretions lubricate the passage of food to the stomach. The oral environment is always grossly contaminated; however, the oral tissues are very well supplied with blood vessels because of the need to replace abraded oral epithelium and handle the constant contamination. As a result, the squamous epithelium of the oral cavity heals more rapidly than does that of skin: the inflammatory response develops more rapidly, and epithelial replication and collagen formation occur earlier.

Until recently, dental procedures in small animals, other than teeth cleaning, have been considered rather exotic, to be performed only occasionally and by a collaborating dentist. This need not be the case; many veterinary dental procedures can be performed by veterinarians.

Equipment and Supplies

Some specialized instruments are necessary for the more common veterinary dental procedures. The most important is a dental engine and handpiece. A dental handpiece is held like a pencil, using the other fingers as stabilizers pressed against adjacent teeth or jaw to support the hand as close as possible to the instrument's working tip. An air-driven unit is ideal because of its high speed (350,000 to 400,000 rpm); at this speed, tooth structure and bone can be resected with maximum control and minimum heat production. A second advantage of a turbine handpiece is its built-in cooling spray, which further reduces the likelihood of tooth or bone damage from heat build-up.

An ultrasonic scaler speeds teeth cleaning, but hand scalers are essential. The Roto-Pro bur (Henry Schein, Port Washington, NY), used in an air-driven handpiece, can perform the same function as an ultrasonic scaler. An electroscalpel with a variety of tips is useful for gingival surgery.

Dental radiographs are essential for many veterinary dental procedures. When examining teeth radiographically, use parallel technique when possible (the x-ray film is parallel to the long axis of the tooth, and the x-ray beam is perpendicular to both). If true parallel position is not possible, use bisecting angle technique to minimize foreshortening. Other materials and supplies needed are described with the specific procedures.

Periodontal Disease

Periodontal disease is the most common disease in dogs and cats. It is caused by accumulation of plaque, the bacteria-rich layer that adheres to the tooth surface. Two types of periodontal disease are gingivitis and periodontitis (the more severe form, in which bone supporting the tooth is gradually lost, leading eventually to loss of the tooth).

When treating periodontal disease, the major goal is to prevent plaque build-up, lest it mature into the gram-negative anaerobic flora that destroys tissue. Professional treatment, such as teeth cleaning and other procedures requiring general anesthesia, is of long-term value only if followed by frequent, effective home care. The deposition of calculus (minerals from salivary secretions that precipitate onto the plaque-covered crown or exposed root surfaces) exacerbates plaque deposition and development of periodontal disease.

Though it is not an essential cause of periodontal disease, calculus should be removed because it forms a rough, plaque-retentive surface.

The extent of periodontal disease is evaluated by inspecting the mouth, using a periodontal probe gently inserted between the gingiva and tooth to measure the pocket depth (normally 1 to 2 mm in a dog and 0 to 1 mm in a cat). The periodontal probe causes bleeding when inserted gently into an acutely inflamed periodontal pocket. The extent of plaque accumulation can be measured by applying disclosing solution, which stains bacteria and other organic material, onto the tooth surfaces.

Treatment of Periodontal Disease

First, assess the owner and patient. Is compliance with brushing instructions likely? If not, more radical treatment such as extraction should be considered for severely affected teeth. Companion animal dogs and cats manage very well without teeth. If it is unclear from a preliminary discussion whether the owner is likely to comply with instructions for follow-up care (daily brushing), have him or her try brushing for a week or two to evaluate the extent of compliance before anesthetizing the animal.

Very mobile teeth that can be moved back and forth with gentle pressure are not salvageable and should be extracted. In an animal where long-term compliance with brushing is not expected to be good, somewhat mobile molar and premolar teeth with deep pockets (>4 mm) should be extracted, leaving the more accessible and more aesthetically important incisor and canine teeth to be cleaned and subsequently brushed by the owner.

Teeth-cleaning procedures require general anesthesia because of the discomfort associated with subgingival manipulation and need for careful inspection. The procedure starts by removing grossly obvious supragingival calculus and plaque; this can be performed rapidly with an ultrasonic unit. Do not keep the tip pressed firmly against the tooth surface or keep it in contact with the same area for several seconds, and be sure the water spray works correctly. If these precautions are not taken, the tooth surface may be severely gouged and the pulp tissue may be injured and undergo necrosis. Move the instrument continuously, keeping as much of the tip surface in contact with the tooth as possible.

A similar ultrasonic calculus dislodgement effect can be achieved with the Roto-Pro bur in an air-driven high-speed handpiece. However, this unit should be used carefully, because if applied at an incorrect angle the shape of the tip of the straight-sided bur in most common use can damage the tooth surface and attachment tissues. Units generating ultrasonic frequencies contaminate the immediate environment with bacteria-laden water droplets; masks should be worn by all personnel in the immediate vicinity when this equipment is in use, and sterile surgical procedures should not be scheduled in the same work area immediately afterward.

It is impossible to perform teeth scaling adequately using ultrasonic equipment only, and such equipment is not necessary for the procedure. Ultrasonic units produce clean white crowns rapidly and easily and, if used with care, can start the subgingival cleaning process very efficiently, but an animal with established periodontitis needs hand scaling.

The basic set of hand instruments consists of a periodontal scaler, curette, hoe, and chisel. The scaler, hoe, and chisel are used to remove supragingival calculus concretions (Fig. 6-1) and are not essential if ultrasonic equipment is available. The scaler and hoe are used with a pull stroke: they are inserted below the calculus mass, then pulled forcefully toward the tip of the crown (coronally). The chisel is used with a push stroke toward the tip of the root (apically). Because of the direction a chisel is applied, it can cause a great deal of damage to soft tissue and bone if not used under close control.

The most important hand instrument is the curette. A double-ended curved blade is

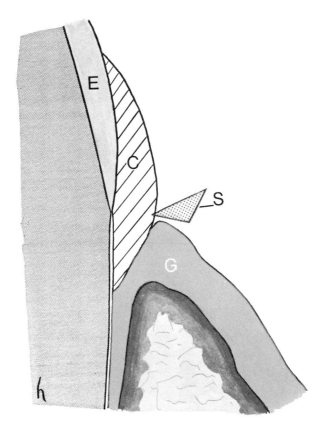

Figure 6-1. *Placement of a scaler for removal of supragingival calculus. E = enamel; C = calculus; G = gingiva; S = scaler. (Harvey CE, ed. Veterinary dentistry. Philadelphia: WB Saunders, 1985)*

best for veterinary use. It is inserted gently into the pocket along the side of the root until resistance is felt (Fig. 6-2), then pressed forcefully against the root surface as it is pulled out. One such stroke will clean about 10 to 20 percent of the circumference of the root, so several strokes are necessary to clean the entire circumference. The purpose of forcefully applying a curette against the root ("root planing") is to remove all subgingival calculus and a thin layer of the superficial cementum, which is loaded with bacterial toxins that will inhibit healing if left in place. To determine if a crown or root is thoroughly clean, gently run a curette or periodontal probe over the surface; it will "skip" if deposits or rough areas are still

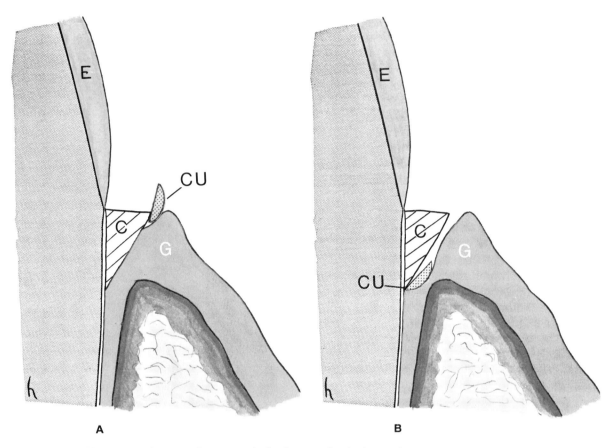

Figure 6-2. *Placement of a curet for removal of subgingival calculus and root-planing.* ***A,*** *The curet is inserted at the gingival margin.* ***B,*** *It is advanced to the attachment point, then the cutting edge is engaged against the root. E = enamel; C = calculus; G = gingiva; CU = curet. (Harvey CE, ed. Veterinary dentistry. Philadelphia: WB Saunders, 1985)*

present. In deep pockets with abscessation, necrotic soft tissue debris, and irregular bone loss, the curette is used by directing it forcefully against the soft tissue and bone to create a fresh wound that may go on to heal.

Because curettes, scalers, chisels, and hoes need a sharp edge, they require weekly or more frequent use of a sharpening stone and oil.

The final step in conservative treatment of periodontal disease is polishing the teeth to smooth any rough surfaces caused by the scaling procedure. A mildly abrasive paste is applied to the surface of the teeth with a pro-phylaxis cup mounted in a prophylaxis angle in a slow-speed (<5,000 rpm) handpiece. The cup is moved over the surface, flaring out the edges to dip below the gingival margin.

Thorough teeth-cleaning procedures are time consuming; they can be performed very efficiently by veterinary technicians, provided that supervised hands-on instruction is given and that a veterinarian examines the dog's mouth before and after the procedure to determine if additional procedures, such as gingival surgery or extraction, are indicated.

For deep periodontal pockets (> about 4 mm), additional treatment is needed, because the bristles of even a conscientiously applied toothbrush cannot reach the bottom of the pocket. The general principle is to uncover the area of unattached root that is covered with gingival tissue so that subsequent home care can prevent plaque from building up in the pocket. Either gingivectomy or gingivoplasty (flap surgery) is used, and the specific technique depends on the depth of the pocket relative to the mucogingival junction. At least 2 mm of normal full-thickness gingiva should be saved whenever possible.

The incision line for gingivectomy is determined by measuring the pocket depth. Bleeding points can be created with the periodontal probe or a pocket depth marker to form a visible line, though the incision should be beveled away from the tooth so that a pocket is not reformed following healing (Fig. 6-3). When using the electroscalpel for gingival surgery, make only one pass of the instru-

ment. The densely fibrous gingival tissue will not separate, and further passes of the instrument will cause periodontal bone destruction. Use a sharp scalpel or dental scaler to complete the resection. A loop tip can be used very effectively to sculpt the gingival margin for gingivectomy, particularly between the incisor teeth.

When the remaining gingiva must be saved because so little is left, an apically based flap is used to permit repositioning of the gingival margin. Two incisions through the gingiva and subgingival connective tissue are made with a scalpel parallel to the long axis of the tooth at either end of the tooth or teeth; these initial incisions are connected by an incision at the gingival margin. If the flap extends along several teeth, the gingival margin incision is not a straight line: it extends between the teeth to include the interdental papilla. The gingival tissue is elevated and re-

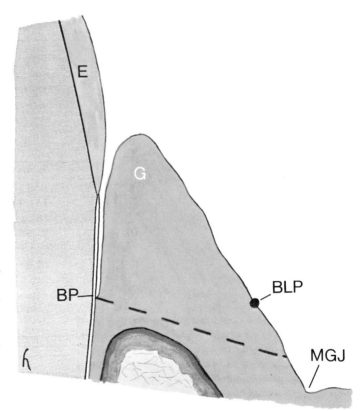

Figure 6-3. *Gingivectomy for treatment of gingival hyperplasia or excessive pocket depth with sufficient attached gingiva. The dashed line represents the line of resection to achieve a beveled incision. G = gingiva; BP = bottom of pocket; BLP = bleeding point created by pushing probe into gingiva at a distance equivalent to pocket depth; MGJ = mucogingival junction. (Harvey CE, ed. Veterinary dentistry. Philadelphia: WB Saunders, 1985)*

flected, the exposed roots are cleaned thoroughly and polished, and the flap is sutured at each end so the gingival margin is level with the attachment point (Fig. 6-4), then sutured between teeth to conform the new gingival margin to the attachment line around individual teeth. Absorbable suture material is used to avoid the need for suture removal.

Postpone brushing for about a week after gingival surgery.

Two additional procedures that can be used to treat periodontitis are splinting and contouring. These procedures are time consuming and should only be used in animals whose owners are willing and able to perform daily home care conscientiously.

Splinting is used to stabilize mobile incisor teeth. The crowns and roots are thoroughly scaled and polished with a non-fluoride dental polish. A groove is cut in the enamel of the teeth at the level of the lateral cusp tips, the teeth are acid-etched, and a length of transpar-

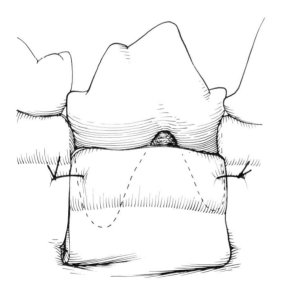

Figure 6-4. *Apically positioned gingival flap surgery for treatment of excessive pocket depth with insufficient attached gingiva for gingivectomy. The gingiva and alveolar mucosa have been incised and the flap dissected to permit the gingival margin to be relocated at the level of the existing attachment and held in place with two sutures.*

ent nylon or fiberglass material is glued into the groove with composite resin. Additional composite resin is placed as necessary and finishing discs and burs are used to shape and smooth the surface of the teeth. The bonding technique is described in more detail below.

Contouring is a somewhat controversial technique because part of the tooth is deliberately removed. The enamel bulge of the tooth is burred away just above the neck of the root to provide a smooth straight surface for subsequent brushing of the exposed root. The burred surface must be smoothed with a sanding disc and polished; otherwise, this area will retain plaque.

Home Care

To improve the owner's compliance, give specific instructions and gradually introduce the animal to brushing. Daily brushing is best: powders or sprays that do not require brushing suppress the halitosis odor but mask the continuing disease in the periodontal pocket. Chlorhexidine has been proved effective in many trials and is available as a palatable oral solution (Novaldent, Fort Dodge Laboratories, Fort Dodge, Iowa). Other preparations palatable to dogs and cats are available, for example CET dentifrice (St. JON Laboratories, Harbor City, CA).

The following sequence works well for many owners. With the finger and thumb of one hand placed gently around the muzzle to keep the mouth closed, start by brushing only the external surface of the canine and incisor teeth. After a few days, extend the brush into the cheek pouch to reach the lateral surfaces of the premolar and molar teeth. When the animal is comfortable with the taste of the material and the sensation of brushing, open the mouth by holding the head back as far as possible with one hand, then brush the palatal and lingual surfaces of the teeth.

Routine antibiotic treatment is not necessary when cleaning the teeth of dogs and cats, as the inevitable bacteremia is cleared within about 30 minutes by the reticuloendothelial filtering system. Exceptions to this rule are animals with immune-suppressive diseases or those under treatment with immune-suppressive medications, and those with clinical evidence of cardiac disease where there may be a risk that bacterial endocarditis will develop. In these animals, a single intravenous dose of ampicillin, 20 mg/kg, given when anesthesia is induced, is sufficient. Antibiotic treatment should begin before surgery and should continue for 4 to 5 days afterward in animals in which teeth cleaning is combined with a sterile surgical procedure elsewhere in the body.

Periodontal Disease in Cats

The general cause and effects of periodontal disease in cats are similar to those in dogs. Cats' teeth are smaller and more difficult to clean. A dry-food diet results in better gingival health than does a soft-food one.

The two specific abnormalities associated with periodontal disease in cats make the disease in this species more difficult and frustrating to treat. Both result in oral pain and thus loss of appetite. The first is neck lesions (external odontoclastic cavitation, seen most commonly in the cemento-enamel junction area). The cavitations are diagnosed by running a sharp-pointed dental explorer over the surface of the tooth at the gingival margin. The lesions are sometimes visible grossly as areas of red granulation tissue emerging from the gingival margin. They are treated by extraction (see "Teeth Extraction" below) or, if the owner desires that the tooth be retained and the cavitation has not penetrated the pulp canal, by cavity preparation and filling. A glass-ionomer/silver restorative material is simple to use and effective, because it leaches fluoride to retard plaque and desensitize dentin on a long-term basis (see under "Dental Restorative Procedures" below).

The second species-specific periodontal abnormality in cats is plasmacytic-lymphocytic gingivitis-stomatitis. Protuberant ulcerated soft tissue lesions that often spread beyond the mucogingival junction, these lesions often cannot be controlled by conservative periodontal therapy. Corticosteroids combined with antibiotic administration often provides temporary relief. In severe cases, extraction of all the premolar and molar teeth is required to control the symptoms. Because of the neck lesions, fractured root segments are common and may cause continuing disease after removal of all externally visible tooth structure. An intraoral radiograph is needed to demonstrate retained root segments.

Conditions Affecting Teeth

Endodontics

Endodontic treatment is indicated when disease (external trauma, heat damage, caries exposure, and vascular damage at or close to the apex) has caused the pulp tissues to become inflamed or avascular, with little chance of recovery. Swelling caused by hemorrhage or inflammation within the pulp canal system causes necrosis of the pulp canal contents because they are contained in a rigid tube and there is no room for the pressure to be relieved by expansion.

The purpose of endodontic (root canal) therapy is to prevent the pulp canal from becoming, or continuing to be, a source of contamination that will result in leakage of cellular debris, bacteria, and other toxic products through the apex of the root, because these materials can destroy the bone surrounding the root. Eventually, the periapical pathology resulting from endodontic disease will cause an apical abscess, fistula, or loss of the tooth.

The steps in the basic endodontic technique (nonsurgical endodontic treatment) (Fig. 6-5) are as follows. Radiographs are taken periodically during the procedure to ensure that the entire pulp canal is cleaned and filled.

Access: Often the access opening into the pulp chamber already exists because of fracture of the crown. In a long-crowned tooth with a curved root, such as a canine tooth of a large

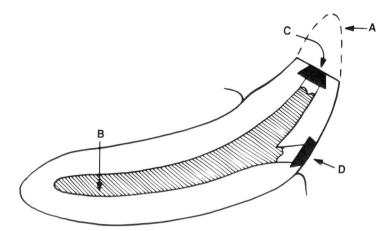

Figure 6-5. A completed conservative endodontic procedure in the canine tooth of a dog. A = fractured crown; B = root canal packed with, e.g., gutta percha/zinc oxide-eugenol; C = coronal access site; D = gingival margin access site. Both access sites are closed with a restorative material (dark shaded undercut area), and an intermediate base (white area) if the root canal filling material and restorative material are not compatible.

dog, it is often necessary to make a second access opening with a round or pear-shaped diamond- or carbide-tipped bur at the gingival margin. Access openings must be made carefully so that the pulp cavity is entered without destroying excessive crown structure. The surgeon must allow for the angle of divergence of the canine tooth from the midline when making the gingival access opening, particularly for mandibular canine teeth.

Cleaning and Shaping: In a large-pulped tooth, a barbed broach is useful but not essential for extracting the soft tissue mass. Endodontic files are used to file away remaining pulpal soft tissue or debris and the innermost dentinal layer. Early in the filing process, insert a file as far as possible and take a radiograph to assess the canal length. Particularly for canine teeth, a full set (#15 to #80) of the 55 mm or 60 mm length veterinary Hedstrom files must be available. Failure to adequately clean all the dentinal surface will leave necrotic soft tissue or debris that will cause problems later. The files are used by inserting them until meeting resistance, then pulling forcefully on the out stroke only. By curving the instrument before insertion, and deflecting its long axis while it is inserted, the cutting edges of the file may be directed against the whole circumference of the canal. Use files only in a moist canal.

Sterilization: Strict sterile technique during access and filing is not essential; it is more important to remove all the tissue and debris in the canal. Using a sterilizing agent such as bleach periodically during filing keeps the canal moist and removes gross contamination. Hydrogen peroxide is usually used sequentially with bleach to help froth out debris. Repeat the bleach and H_2O_2 flushes several times once filing is complete so that the canal is sterile before drying and filling. A final rinse with sterile saline is used to wash out the bleach and hydrogen peroxide.

Drying and Filling: There are many filling materials, almost all of which require a dry canal. Dry the canal with a filtered air jet (if available) and sterile paper points; again, the 55-mm veterinary length will be necessary for many canine teeth. The standard human filling material is gutta percha (rolled latex rubber that is radiopaque, nonabsorbable and nonsoluble, and shaped for placement in the canal). In humans, the gutta percha point is placed and then condensed mechanically; however, this is often impractical in veterinary patients, as the gutta percha is not yet available in a full range of lengths and widths.

In veterinary patients, gutta percha is often used to augment a paste filler. Paste fillers usually consist of a mixture of zinc oxide and eugenol. The materials are mixed with a spatula on a glass slab and inserted to fill the canal, using a pressure injection syringe or a lentulo spiral filler; 60-mm lentulo spirals for veterinary use are available. After filling, another radiograph should be made to check that the filling is acceptable (*i.e.*, that there are no obvious areas of radiolucency).

Sealing: The sealer is often also the restorative material that will be used. When a paste material has been used to fill the canal, a cement may be needed as a base or stiffening layer between the filling material and the restorative material, particularly when amalgam is used because of the need for mechanical compression.

Endodontic Treatment of Multi-Rooted teeth

Treatment of carnassial abscess endodontically has been described, with good long-term results. The three-root pulp canals of the upper carnassial tooth all connect with the single crown pulp chamber. Either all three canals are treated, or the small medial root is sectioned and extracted, the two large lateral roots are treated, and the opening to the medial root is filled (see "Apicoectomy" below). The pulp chamber's shape requires a very large access site, which means some of the crown is lost and restoration to full crown height and shape is impractical.

Endodontic Complications

Hemorrhage during cleansing or filing of the canal can sometimes be difficult to control. Epinephrine soaked into a paper point that is inserted to the bottom of the canal and left in place may be satisfactory, although often pressure from a dry paper point is enough. Patience is the most important consideration: 3 to 5 minutes of continuous pressure is more likely to be successful than many rapid insertions and removals.

Open apex is a developmental stage. Until about 24 to 30 months of age in the dog the root is still developing and the apex is open to allow access for larger blood vessels. Once the root is fully formed, the apex radiographically appears to be complete, but it is pierced by small neurovascular channels forming an apical delta. In a young dog, the pulp should be retained if possible to allow for subsequent normal development. For a fresh crown fracture, this can be done by performing a pulpotomy rather than full endodontic treatment if viable (red or bleeding) pulp is visible at the fracture site.

Pulpotomy: Ideally, this procedure is performed within a few hours of injury. About 3 mm of the pulp and immediately adjacent dentin is removed with a sterile bur, calcium hydroxide is placed over the pulp either as a powder or as a cement if an amalgam restoration is to be used, and the crown is restored. Systemic antibiotic treatment is given. The disadvantage of pulpotomy is that its long-term results are much less predictable than with full endodontic treatment. Periodic radiographic examination to assess progress after pulpotomy is often impractical because of the need for anesthesia in veterinary patients.

Root apex damage or obstructed canal require a second opening to clean the canal thoroughly from the root apex (apicoectomy). The presence of an externally obvious abscess or fistula, or of extensive radiographically obvious resorption of apical bone, are not necessarily indications for apicoectomy. Abnormality in the shape of the root, combined with local bone radiolucency (absence of lamina dura), suggests apical root resorption and the need for apicoectomy.

Apicoectomy is performed by incising the mucosa and burring away bone lying over the root tip. The root canal is entered laterally with a bur, the canal is cleaned, the root apex is bevelled to allow better access for the apical restoration, and the apex is sealed before the rest of the canal is filled. Amalgam is used for the restoration. The mucosal wound is sutured closed.

Dental Restorative Procedures

Restorative procedures can be divided into those requiring endodontic treatment before restoration (most commonly, treatment of a fractured tooth) and those in which the pulp chamber or root canal has not been penetrated (such as for teeth with enamel hypoplasia, caries, or superficial neck lesions in cats). A sharp-pointed dental explorer is used to determine if there is penetration into the pulp system.

For large flat surfaces requiring restoration (e.g., enamel hypoplasia), a composite resin system is used. This material is simple to use, bonds well to enamel, and is enamel-colored, but does not bond to dentin and does not tolerate high occlusal pressures well. Commercial bonding kits contain all the materials needed. For dogs and cats, the lightest shade ("universal") is used.

Bonding Procedure

1. Thoroughly clean and polish the surface with a non-fluoride paste (the usual human prophylaxis pastes containing fluoride are not suitable because the fluoride interferes with normal setting of the resin material).
2. Etch the enamel surface to be covered with phosphoric acid (etching gel or solution). Leave it in place for 60 seconds, then rinse it off thoroughly with water and dry it with an air jet. Do not rub the surface to dry it, because this will crush the etched enamel surface.
3. Mix the bonding agent (unfilled resin) and catalyst and apply it with a brush tip.
4. Mix equal amounts of the two parts of the composite resin on a paper mixing plate to form a uniform paste (use different spatulas for the two materials), then spread it on to the area to be covered and press it into place with a plastic spatula or mylar strip.
5. After the composite material has fully set (about 5 to 7 minutes), remove the excess material with burs and then sanding discs to provide a smooth surface.
6. If desired, add a finishing layer of bonding agent for a final smooth glossy appearance.

For very wide surfaces, furrows should be burred in the enamel before etching to improve mechanical retention. A light-activated composite is more convenient but much more expensive for the limited use likely in a veterinary practice.

Where aesthetics are of less concern but occlusal stress is more severe, other systems are used. The standard is dental amalgam (a mixture of silver and mercury plus trace metals), which requires several specialized instruments (amalgam mixer, carrier, condenser, burnisher) for correct use. Because there is no chemical bond between amalgam and tooth substance, the tooth structure must be undercut with an inverted cone bur (the cavity is made larger at the bottom than at the surface) so that the amalgam plug will not fall out once it has set. Other materials with satisfactory occlusal-resistance properties are now becoming available. These are much more practical for veterinary use because there is no need for additional specialized equipment.

Glass-ionomer cements sintered with silver bond directly to enamel, dentin, and metals and can be used in a wet field without the need for undercutting. Thus, they are ideal for restoring neck lesion preparations in cats and can be used wherever amalgam would otherwise be used. Diseased tooth substance (e.g., caries lesion or neck lesion in a cat) is removed with a bur. Avoid penetrating the pulp chamber; if the pulp is exposed or almost exposed, a pulp-capping procedure (applying a layer of $Ca(OH)_2$ to the exposed pulp) is necessary before commencing the restorative procedure. Fluid in the area to be filled is removed by wiping any obvious puddles, but the area is not air-dried. The material is mixed, applied, pressed into place, and shaped, and excess is removed. Then it is allowed to set, with a layer of varnish or petroleum jelly on the surface to retard drying. Finally, the surface is polished with sanding discs or burs.

Reinforced Restorations

When crown height has been lost and restoration is desired, the major considerations are occlusal stress and cost. For a working dog (*e.g.*, a military or police dog) with a fractured canine tooth, any restorative procedure short of a custom cast post and crown is very likely to fail, but this procedure requires at least two anesthetic episodes and the services of a dental laboratory. In the first procedure, the tooth is treated endodontically, part of the pulp chamber filling material is removed to provide space for a tapered post extending well down into the root, and a layer of enamel is burred away to provide a shoulder for the metal crown. An accurate impression of the post preparation is made using a high-quality rubber- or plastic-based impression material. A second impression, using alginate material, is made of the affected and opposing jaw so the dental laboratory knows how much space is available for the crown to be fabricated. Models made from the impressions are sent to the dental laboratory, where they are used to shape and cast a metal tooth (post and crown sections separately). The post and crown should include channels to permit excess cement to escape and prevent rotation and subsequent dislodgement of the crown. Stainless steel is the cheapest and strongest material available. At a second anesthetic episode, the post and crown are trial-fitted, trimmed if necessary after checking occlusion, and cemented in place. A porcelain veneer can be incorporated onto the surface of the crown, but it is expensive and subject to surface fracture from occlusal stress.

A less expensive option that can be used to restore incisor tooth height, or to restore partial height to a canine tooth in a small or medium-sized dog, is a standard post or pin-reinforced glass-ionomer or composite restoration. The post is a metal stem inserted into the pulp canal after endodontic treatment. The pin is a very small threaded metal pin inserted into dentin. Dentinal pins are very adaptable, as several can be used to prevent rotational disruption and can be used in conjunction with a standard preformed post. The steps in dentinal pin placement are as follows.

1. Identify the border between the outer enamel and inner dentin areas. The enamel is too hard to permit placement, so if a pin must pass through enamel (as when the pins are used to anchor a composite bridge for fracture fixation), a small round-head bur is used to penetrate the enamel and then the pin drill is applied to the exposed dentin.

2. Use the custom-sized drill bit supplied with the dentinal pin kit (*e.g.*, Whaledent Minim) in a low-speed handpiece. Drill directly into the dentin to the full depth of the bit. Avoid wobble, as this will increase the diameter of the hole and decrease the strength of the retention. Additional holes well separated from each other are made as necessary for the planned restoration. Locate the tip of the pin in the opening of the hole, then at very low speed allow the handpiece to twist the pin into the hole. The pin is designed to break off when it has reached its correct depth. The pins are supplied either premounted on a plastic latch-grip contra-angle shaft or with a shaped end to fit into a pin driver, and are available either in single or multiple-stack pin sets. Bend the pins to form the core of the desired shape using a pin bender or wire twister. If the pin is not stable after placement because the hole is too large and there is no space for another hole, coat the pin with glass-ionomer cement and re-seat it.

3. If using a glass-ionomer-silver cement for the base of the restoration, mix it, apply it to coat the pins, and press it to the correct shape. If using a composite resin as a surface layer for aesthetic reasons, once the

glass-ionomer cement has set, acid-etch the surface of the glass-ionomer material and the surrounding enamel for attachment of the final composite layer (see above). A combination silver glass-ionomer/composite restoration is stronger than a restoration made of composite resin only.

If a composite material is to be used alone, apply a layer of dentinal adhesive to the area of exposed dentin and allow it to dry, then proceed with etching and bonding as described above to build up the crown.

Carnassial Abscess

Carnassial abscess (facial abscess, dental fistula) is seen as a swelling or draining tract below the medial canthus of the eye, typically in older dogs. The cause is unknown. Affected teeth often are fractured, or periodontal disease is obvious, but in some cases the tooth is normal externally. Root abscessation may be visible on a radiograph as an area of radiolucency. Carnassial abscess is treated by extracting the upper carnassial tooth and draining the swelling. A similar condition occurs occasionally, affecting the upper first molar tooth or lower carnassial tooth. Carnassial abscess can also be treated endodontically, but this requires removing a large part of the crown of the tooth to fully expose and prepare the pulp chamber and root canals.

Avulsion of Teeth

Teeth are occasionally avulsed from the alveoli as a result of trauma. If the root is fractured, the situation is essentially hopeless. For incisor teeth, which are most commonly avulsed in dogs, a missing tooth can be created from composite resin (or the original crown, if intact and available) and included in a transparent bridge attached to adjacent teeth.

If the trauma is recent, the avulsed tooth is intact, and the jaw appears clinically and radiographically intact, an attempt can be made to reseat the tooth. This is best done within 24 hours. The tooth is replaced in the alveolus (without any attempt to clean the root, as this will only damage any remaining viable periodontal cells) and will probably need to be splinted to hold it in place for 10 to 14 days. Endodontic treatment is then performed. The prognosis depends on the viability of the periodontal cells: if there are areas of nonviable periodontal surface, there will eventually (a year or more later) be external resorption and ankylosis, and the tooth will eventually be exfoliated or will shatter.

Teeth Extraction

The most common indication for extraction in dogs and cats is periodontal disease, particularly in animals that are difficult for the owner to manage because follow-up oral hygiene is likely to be ineffective. Judicious extraction of crowded or rotated teeth can reduce the likelihood that periodontal disease will lead to loss of the remaining teeth. Other indications for extraction are fractured teeth that cause the animal pain or have resulted in an apical abscess, teeth that prevent normal occlusion, dental caries, carnassial abscess, and neck lesions in cats. For many of these conditions, alternatives to extraction are available, such as endodontic, restorative, or orthodontic procedures, if the owner wants the tooth or teeth saved.

Techniques

Generally, the tooth is loosened with a root elevator, and wedge leverage is applied. The fingers and palm of the hand are used to support the jaw and to limit the force applied to any one point on the jaw. Only rarely do the dental extraction forceps fit the neck of a canine or feline tooth accurately, and use of forceps alone often will fracture the tooth.

For wedge leverage to be successful, the root elevator or other wedging instrument must be applied by twisting or levering between teeth (or sections of the same tooth, if extracting a multi-root tooth) until resistance to further distraction is felt. It is then held in that position for several seconds so that the periodontal fibers are stretched and torn. For a single-root tooth, the root elevator is inserted between the gingival margin and the crown or exposed root. Pressure is applied while rotating the elevator through a small arc, keeping the instrument at a 30° to 45° angle to the long axis of the root to avoid slipping and injuring the gingiva. A finger extended along the blade of the elevator acts as a stop should the instrument slip.

The root elevator is used against all available surfaces of the root until the tooth begins to loosen. Elevators with offset jaws are useful for reaching caudal teeth.

Canine Teeth

These teeth have massive roots. In large dogs, it is best to incise and reflect the mucoperiosteum on the lateral surface of the tooth, then resect the alveolar bone overlying the root with a dental bur or orthopedic chisel. The mucosal incision is best made caudal to the root so that sutured tissues are not directly over the resulting void. The gingival and subgingival tissue is reflected with a periosteal elevator. If a bur is used, a channel is cut full-thickness through the lateral alveolar plate in a U or V shape along the rostral and caudal margins to meet at the palpable root apex. The rostral, medial, and caudal surfaces of the root are loosened with a root elevator. Once the tooth moves slightly, the tooth is grasped with extraction forceps and twisted until resistance is felt, then held for a few seconds. This movement is alternated in both directions until the tooth can be lifted out. The gingival flaps are sutured with simple interrupted absorbable sutures.

In narrow-nosed dogs with extensive periodontal disease, where the risk of creating an oronasal fistula after canine tooth extraction is greatest, take particular care to avoid damaging the bone medial to the root. When using forceps, do not lever the crown of the tooth laterally, as this pushes the root medially into the nasal cavity. If penetration into the nasal cavity is obvious during the extraction procedure (from observing hemorrhage or emergence of flushing solution from the nostril), try to prevent a fistula from forming by placing one or two absorbable sutures through the lateral and medial gingivae, pulling the two edges together to collapse the soft tissues. The alveolus can be packed loosely with a shaped cube or granules of polylactic acid; this will retain a blood clot within the alveolus and encourage granulation tissue to form. If an oronasal fistula does form and causes nasal discharge or difficulties during eating, treatment is closure of the fistula by creating a flap of buccal epithelium (see "Oronasal Fistula" below).

Multi-Rooted Teeth

Multi-rooted teeth can be removed as one unit by loosening the roots with a root elevator before applying extraction forceps. However, it is much easier to extract the tooth if it is first separated into single root sections, because the sections can be levered against each other (Fig. 6-6) and then forcefully rotated individually. The best implement for this purpose is a taper cross-cut fissure bur (#701, 702, or 703), as this creates a channel of the right width for starting the wedging process. A diamond disc or even a hacksaw blade can be used, but the risk of damaging adjacent bone and soft tissue is higher. Each piece is then taken out as a separate one-root tooth.

Two-Rooted Teeth

In the dog, two-rooted teeth are the upper second and third premolar teeth, and all of the lower premolar and molar teeth except PM1; in the cat, all of the premolar and molar teeth except the upper PM1 and PM3 are two-rooted.

Starting from the furcation (the area where the roots join to form the crown), separate the tooth into rostral and caudal sections. Insert the root elevator into the channel be-

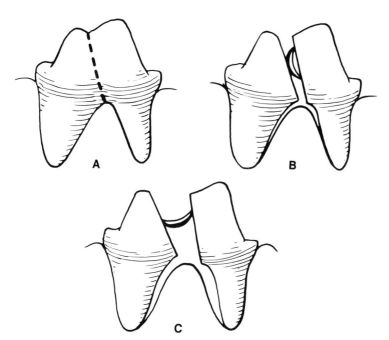

Figure 6-6. *Extraction of a two-rooted tooth.* ***A,*** *The tooth is sectioned from the furcation to the crown (dashed line).* ***B,*** *A root elevator is inserted between the crown sections perpendicular to the long axis of the roots.* ***C,*** *The root elevator is twisted and held to separate the crown sections and stretch and tear the periodontal fibers.*

tween the sections and twist until resistance is felt, then hold under tension for several seconds. Then twist the other way and hold under tension. The leverage effect is greater if the elevator is applied horizontally (with the blade perpendicular to the long axis of the roots). Continue with this back-and-forth twisting-and-holding action until one of the root sections loosens, then apply the extraction forceps and continue the twist-and-hold sequence until that section can be lifted out. Often, the second tooth section is still rather firmly attached. Apply the root elevator between the tooth and bone adjacent to the next tooth and lever towards the previously removed section. Then apply the extraction forceps and use the same twist-and-hold action until it can be lifted out.

Three-Rooted Teeth

Three-rooted teeth are the upper 4PM, M1,2 in the dog and the upper 3PM in the cat. The upper carnassial tooth is the largest of the three-rooted teeth and the one that is most often removed, because of carnassial abscess. It can be removed as easily as a two-rooted tooth by separating the small medial root from

the main part of the tooth, then levering the medial root against the rest of the tooth. Once the medial root is extracted, the two lateral roots are dealt with as for the lower carnassial tooth.

An alternative technique for multi-rooted teeth is to make a passage through the furcation area between the roots with the tip of a root elevator. The root elevator is then passed through the channel between the roots and rotated, forcing the angled handle of the instrument into the furcation as a wedge and forcing the intact tooth from its sockets.

Deciduous Teeth

When the developing bud of the permanent tooth is not in direct alignment with the root of the deciduous tooth, the deciduous root resorption process does not proceed normally as the permanent tooth develops. The permanent tooth may develop in abnormal position, and correction may require extraction of the deciduous tooth. Deciduous and permanent versions of the same tooth should not be in erupted position in the mouth at the same time. Deciduous teeth usually are easier to extract than permanent teeth. The danger is that the developing permanent tooth may be damaged if the extraction instruments penetrate too deeply; thus, extraction of deciduous teeth requires particular care and patience.

Extraction of Teeth in Cats

Tooth extractions in cats are performed in similar fashion as for dogs, although the surgeon must remember that the skull of the cat is much smaller and more fragile than that of the dog. The tooth sectioning and leverage technique can be used, but the crown sections are more likely to fracture unless the force is applied very gradually. The typical veterinary root elevators are often too large for convenient use in cats; a #11 straight-edge scalpel blade mounted on a scalpel handle makes a convenient root elevator to start the process; a small root elevator is inserted once the scalpel blade has formed an initial channel between root and bone. An alternative technique is to use a dental bur in a dental handpiece to cut away all the root tissue; with a high-speed handpiece the process is very quick, and the cooling water jet keeps the field clear of blood and root fragments.

Complications of Extraction

Bleeding often continues for a day or two after extraction. Packing the empty alveolus with gauze is sufficient to prevent further bleeding. Packing the alveolus with polylactic acid granules will speed granulation and prevent dry-socket formation, although this is rare in dogs and cats.

A fractured root, with retention of the tip in the alveolus, is common, particularly if excessive force is applied before the periodontal fibers have been loosened sufficiently. A snapping sound may be obvious, or a sharp edge will be palpated at the end of the coronal segment. Root tips that contain necrotic pulp or deep periodontal pockets will cause bone lysis and subsequent fistula or abscess formation. Fractured root tips are removed by one of

two methods: either a root-tip pick or a narrow-bladed root elevator is inserted into the alveolus and levered between the root and alveolar bone until the tip is loose and extracted, or a dental bur in a handpiece is used to cut away the remaining tooth root structure.

Fracture of the mandible should be prevented by careful extraction technique. Small dogs with extensive periodontitis have the highest risk of fracture of the jaw during tooth extraction and are also those with the least desirable conditions for fracture healing.

Postoperative infection in the soft tissues immediately surrounding the extraction site is very uncommon. Infections in the deeper soft tissues, such as the orbital or intermandibular areas, are seen occasionally as a result of contamination from inadvertent penetration of the elevator into these areas. Treatment is drainage of the abscess that results.

Necrosis of bone around the extraction site occurs occasionally, particularly if the bone was severely infected before extraction or if the extraction procedure was excessively traumatic or caused loss of vascular supply to a segment of alveolar bone. Conservative treatment is unlikely to be effective. Surgical treatment is removal of the affected bone with a curette or rongeur until healthy bleeding bone is reached. The surgical site is left uncovered.

Jaw and Occlusion Abnormalities

Jaw Fractures

Because the jaws do not bear weight, healing by formation of a fibrous union is usually satisfactory. If the fracture causes malocclusion, normal or near-normal occlusion must be restored and maintained during the healing process. Many fractures of the mandible and maxilla do not need surgical fixation, particularly those in which the fracture lines are contained within the areas of attachment of the masticatory muscles, as these muscles effectively splint the fracture during healing. Even for horizontal ramus fractures, the most common location in dogs, a bandage around the muzzle for 3 to 4 weeks is often sufficient if the jaws are in normal occlusion. The bandage can be made by placing a loop of surgical tape, adhesive side facing out, around the muzzle, then placing a second layer, adhesive side facing in, over the first loop. The loop should be adjusted so that the tips of the canine teeth interlock to maintain normal occlusion, but it should be loose enough to allow the incisor teeth to open and the tongue to protrude, permitting intake of fluid and slurried food.

Mandibular Fractures

Even in cats and small dogs, the mandible is thick enough to accommodate pins, plates, and screws. Use of these standard orthopedic techniques requires a surgical approach through the oral mucosa or ventrolaterally through a skin incision. The ventrolateral approach can be extended caudally by reflecting the digastricus muscle medially when necessary.

However, performing these orthopedic techniques is more involved and time consuming than using a simple muzzle or alternative techniques that use teeth as fixation points. The screws attaching a plate to the horizontal ramus are likely to penetrate through or interfere with the blood supply to the roots of the mandibular teeth, with resulting endodontic disease (see above). The mandible has a medullary canal that will accept small Steinmann pins or Kirschner wires; however, the canal is curved, and the pin or wire must exit through the ventral cortex in the caudal part of the horizontal ramus to prevent dorsal spreading of the fracture line. Orthopedic wire, used in a simple loop or in a figure-8 pattern, can be placed through holes made in the mandible with a dental bur or Kirschner wire; two or more wires can be used to prevent overriding.

Cross-pinning to the other mandible can be used successfully, either by itself or combined with tension wires. Tension wires can be used alone. If a cross-pinning and external fixation technique is used, the weight of the external fixation device can be reduced by using an acrylic sidebar. Biphase external splints used in humans are not necessary and are not practical for any but the largest dogs because of their weight. The principles of use of orthopedic techniques are described in Chapter 20.

An alternative external fixation device is wiring of teeth. It is lightweight and quick (no surgical approach or closure is needed), it avoids surgical exposure of the mandible (and thus avoids further disruption of the mandibular blood supply and contamination of the fracture site), it does not involve placing foreign material in the fracture site, and it permits the surgeon to align the fracture fragments as necessary during manufacture of the device to achieve normal occlusion. This technique is suitable only when two or more uninjured teeth are on either side of the fracture site; the device can be made to span missing jaw or tooth segments but does require anchoring at both ends. Thus, its practical limitations for use are fractures rostral to the fourth premolar tooth.

Wires are attached around or to the teeth, then immersed in a quick-setting acrylic plate made directly in the mouth. Once it has set, the plate will hold the wires in place to maintain occlusion in the desired position. If there is existing periodontitis, the wire will fit around the neck of the tooth below the enamel bulge. If it slips off the crown, as often happens, a groove is cut in the enamel just above the gingival margin to retain the wire. The wire loop is tightened and the ends are cut, leaving a 2- to 3-cm tail facing onto the lingual surface.

Because the upper premolar and molar teeth occlude on the lateral aspect of the lower teeth, the plate must be made on the lingual (medial) aspect of the jaw, or on the lateral aspect ventral to the mucogingival junction (in the latter case, the wires are bent ventrally). Acrylic powder and liquid are mixed together. When a dough-like consistency is obtained, the acrylic material is pressed into position and the mandible is aligned, with the wire ends pressed into the plastic until the plate has hardened. More powder and/or liquid is added as necessary to thicken and position the plate and cover the ends of the wires. Cold-curing acrylic should be used for fabricating plates directly in the mouth as described here. The teeth should be brushed and the device rinsed with dilute chlorhexidine solution daily. The device is removed about 3 to 4 weeks later by cutting the wires. If grooves were required to retain the wires, the grooves are filled with composite resin, sanded, and polished.

For severe mandibular fractures that have caused malocclusion but no loss of teeth, an alternative technique using dentinal pins seated in each canine tooth can be used. Pins are placed in the crown of the canine teeth on one or both sides perpendicular to the long axis of the tooth. Aim the miniature drill used to seat the pins so that the pins will not penetrate the pulp canal. Bend the pins so they will lie close together when the jaws are held in normal occlusion, then etch the surrounding enamel and cover the pins with composite resin to stabilize the teeth and jaws. This technique is particularly suitable for use in cats.

Fractures of the vertical ramus that are not splinted in satisfactory occlusion by the masticatory muscles can be held in fixation by wiring the mandibular teeth to the maxillary teeth in normal occlusion. The jaws are wired by placing and twisting 24- to 28-gauge wire subgingivally around several incisor and premolar teeth, placing the jaws in occlusion, and twisting the wires together, leaving 1 to 2 mm of movement available.

In the latter techniques, the upper and lower jaws must be held in a partially closed position. Alimentation by injection through the cheek pouch or through a gastrostomy tube is necessary for about 4 weeks, until the jaw has healed.

Complications of mandibular fracture fixation include malocclusion, bone resorption and subsequent nonunion, periodontal disease and tooth loss, and mandibular osteomyelitis. When a healed mandibular fracture has resulted in locking of teeth to the point that the animal cannot close its jaws completely, extraction of one or more teeth is often sufficient to restore normal ability to eat. If nonunion or delayed union causes malocclusion, a rigid fixation device is required. Transfixation splints with acrylic bridges, or biphase external fixation splints are tolerated by dogs for several months if necessary. When greater bone loss has occurred, grafts of rib or ilium can be used; the likelihood of acceptance is good on the mandible or maxilla. Up to 2 cm of mandibular length can be replaced if a bridging bone plate is left in place for up to 4 months.

In cats, mandibular symphyseal separation is the most common fracture site. Sufficient fixation to achieve fibrous union can be obtained by wiring the two sides together caudal to the canine teeth, using a hypodermic needle or suture passer to feed the wire subcutaneously. If the fracture is comminuted, there may be symphyseal collapse and distortion of the angle of the canine teeth; additional stabilization with interdental wiring and an acrylic splint or a cross-pin or Kirschner wire is indicated. The fixation device can usually be removed in 2 to 3 weeks.

Maxillary Fractures

Although many maxillar fractures require only conservative treatment, others are more complex to manage. The maxilla is a relatively thin bone supporting the teeth and framing the nasal cavity. Rigid fixation of these thin plates of bone is rarely possible. An additional complication is that the nasal cavity may be exposed as a result of the fracture, and there is often damage to intranasal structures that may reduce or prevent air movement through the nose for a period of time after the injury.

Maxillary fractures often are left untreated. If the nasal cavity is exposed, the palate must be repaired to close off the airway to prevent aspiration during eating or drinking. In some animals, sutures in the mucoperiosteum are sufficient to achieve this; in other cases, the fracture must be held in fixation or the oronasal defect must await later reconstructive surgery if the maxilla is extensively damaged. Closure of palate defects is described below.

Primary fixation of large fragments of the premaxilla and maxilla is achieved with sutures or tension wires. A severely deformed maxilla may be returned to normal occlusion and held in fixation by placing Kirschner wires or small Steinmann pins through the fractured segments and adjacent normal bone, and attaching them to an external fixation frame.

An alternative and simpler technique is the use of circumdental wires held in an acrylic plate; the technique is described above (see "Mandibular Fractures," above). During the setting of the acrylic plate, the canine teeth can be held apart and at the correct angle of divergence.

Jaw fractures predispose the animal to more rapid development of periodontal disease because of the soft-food diet required during the healing phase or permanently if occlusion is no longer normal.

Maxillary or Mandibular Osteomyelitis

Severe osteomyelitis or sequestrum formation occurs occasionally secondary to inappropriate extraction technique, severe periodontal disease, or occlusive trauma. There may be considerable necrosis and new bone formation. Following biopsy to rule out neoplasia as a cause of the swelling, conservative treatment is attempted first: any remaining teeth in that jaw segment are removed, necrotic bone is thoroughly curetted, and clindamycin (20 mg/kg orally for 10 to 14 days) or tetracycline (20 mg/kg orally t.i.d. for 4 to 6 weeks) is given. If no improvement results, radical maxillectomy or mandibulectomy is indicated.

Occlusal Abnormalities

Orthodontic procedures are infrequently indicated in dogs and cats because of the ethical implications of correcting congenital or inherited disease. According to AVMA guidelines, it is unethical to alter the natural dental arcade, and American Kennel Club rules state that correcting a defect so that a dog conforms to a breed standard makes that animal ineligible for showing. It is ethical to correct a congenital abnormality if the defect interferes with the health of the animal; these dogs should be neutered. When the abnormality results from an acquired condition, such as a fracture, correction is not unethical.

The abnormality may be due to abnormal jaw length or to abnormal position of the teeth within the jaw. Extraction is a simple, effective but aesthetically displeasing alternative.

Because there is a differential rate of growth during jaw development, an abnormality that is obvious at 5 or 6 months of age may have corrected itself by 10 or 12 months of age. Unless the teeth are interlocked in an abnormal pattern (e.g., the lower canine is caudal to the upper canine), an orthodontic device should not be placed until growth has ceased.

The most common orthodontic abnormality causing secondary soft tissue or bone disease is abnormal position of the lower canine teeth so that the crown tips are medial to the upper canine teeth crowns; pressure from the lower teeth crowns causes ulceration of the palate. The problem can be corrected by extracting the malpositioned lower teeth and the upper canine tooth, producing a natural hollow to accommodate the lower canine tooth. This leaves the aesthetically and functionally more important lower canine teeth in place. An alternative is to move the lower teeth orthodontically.

Principles of Orthodontic Movement

To ensure that the abnormality is fully understood, and to facilitate creation of an appliance if needed, an alginate impression is made; from the impression, a model of both the upper and lower jaws is made from dental stone. In a dental laboratory, the stone models are mounted on an articulator to ensure the device fits accurately.

Orthodontic devices must have a firm base: the force directed against the tooth to be moved will be directed with equal but opposite force against the anchor, which may cause movement of the anchoring teeth unless they are more firmly anchored in the jaw than the target tooth. Usually multiple teeth, or at least a multi-rooted tooth, are used as anchors. Two or more teeth can be anchored together by wires placed around or bonded to the teeth and incorporated into a single metal or acrylic anchor. Depending on its design, the device must be attached to the target tooth or placed so that the target tooth is pressed against it when the jaws are closed. Attachment brackets for wires or elastic bands can be bonded directly to the tooth surface (see acid-etch composite technique as described above under "Bonding Procedure," p. 148). If possible, the device should be designed to avoid contact with the tongue or cheek, or it should be covered with a smooth layer of composite to protect adjacent mucosa.

After movement to the desired position has been achieved, maintain the device in place in neutral tension for several more weeks to ensure that the new position is retained; some devices must be removed and replaced with a separate neutral retainer for this period.

Orthodontic devices work by creating pressure: the compression effect on one side of the tooth causes resorption of periodontal bone, and the tension on the other side stimulates periodontal bone production. These tissue pressures cause periodontal disease by interfering with the normal blood supply of the gingiva and subgingival tissues. The effect is exacerbated by the direct pressure that some devices place on the gingival soft tissues. The owner of an animal with an orthodontic device in place should be instructed to irrigate the animal's mouth daily with an oral antiseptic such as Novaldent chlorhexidine oral rinse, and should expect obvious gingival inflammation when the device is removed.

Detailed descriptions of orthodontic techniques are beyond the scope of this text (see Suggested Readings).

Severe Jaw Length Abnormalities

To shorten the mandible in an animal with a major occlusal abnormality, remove a section of mandible by osteotomy caudal to the root of the canine tooth. One or more premolar teeth may have to be removed. Hold the fractured ends in apposition with small bone plates. The neurovascular bundle within the mandible can be preserved by enlarging the medullary canal at the osteotomy site. To lengthen the mandible, perform a step osteotomy and plate fixation. Similar procedures can be performed on the maxilla, but are complicated by the nasal cavity and contents.

Temporomandibular Joint (TMJ) Abnormalities

Congenital Abnormalities

TMJ Dysplasia

In some Irish setters and bassets and occasionally in other breeds, the dorsal tip of the coronoid process of the mandible becomes locked outside the zygomatic arch, and the dog is unable to close its mouth. The locking episode may correct spontaneously or the jaw may need to be manipulated back into place. If the problem recurs, remove part of the ventral aspect of the zygoma, forming a notch to prevent locking, or perform a condylectomy on that side (see "TMJ Condylectomy" below).

Acquired Abnormalities

Trauma

Fractures of the TMJ are most common in cats but are difficult to differentiate from luxation without a radiograph of excellent quality. Surgical fixation of fractures is rarely possible. Chronic abnormality is treated by condylectomy (see below). Luxation, which also is more common in cats, can result from trauma such as falls from a height. Luxation usually is rostral, so the luxated mandible is deviated medially. The luxation can be reduced by placing a wood dowel or plastic rod (such as a ball-point pen) between the carnassial teeth on the luxated side, closing the jaws firmly, and forcefully pushing the jaw caudally to reseat the condyle. If the luxation cannot be reduced and malocclusion continues, condylectomy (see below) eventually may be necessary.

Degenerative TMJ Disease

Treatment of chronic TMJ diseases (such as fracture or arthritis that limits ability to open the mouth, or TMJ dysplasia that results in jaws that persistently lock in the open position) that are not manageable conservatively is condylectomy.

TMJ Condylectomy

One or both condyles can be removed in the dog and cat with little or no clinically evident abnormality in prehension. The approach is made through the masseter muscle, avoiding the buccal nerves and parotid duct, transecting the lateral ligament and exposing the meniscotemporal and meniscomandibular joints. The condylar process and meniscus are removed with a bur, rongeurs, or a wire saw, leaving the edges as smooth as possible. The masseter muscle aponeurosis incised edges are apposed with sutures. There is usually slight malocclusion immediately after the operation, but dogs and cats eat well and the malocclusion corrects itself over the next several weeks.

Palate Defects

Defects of palatal structures that separate the oral and nasal cavities may be inherited or may result from an insult during the critical stage of fetal development when the two palatine shelves fuse, or from trauma, surgery, or radiation. Affected animals usually are presented because of nasal discharge. The prognosis without surgical repair is guarded because of the risk of airway aspiration.

Surgical correction of congenital cleft palate usually is possible if the animal can survive and grow to a size suitable for anesthesia and surgery. Tube-feeding several times daily is necessary in most dogs and cats to avoid recurrent aspiration pneumonia. The larger the animal is at the time of surgery the better, as more tissue and surgical working space are available and the anesthetic risk is lower; most procedures of this sort are performed on animals 3 to 4 months of age.

Congenital cleft hard palate is almost always midline and is associated with midline soft palate abnormality. Soft palate defects without hard palate defects may be midline or unilateral. Harelip (defect of the primary palate) sometimes occurs in association with midline cleft palate. Repair of harelip is described in Chapter 7, under "Diseases of the External Nares and Lips."

Repair of Palate Defects

The principles of surgical treatment of palate defects are:

1. The covering flaps should be large compared to the size of the defect. This minimizes tension on the suture line and may permit overlapping of tissues to provide support for the suture line.
2. Locate and avoid or retract the major blood supply, usually the palatine artery, which emerges onto the ventral surface of the palatine bone about 0.5 to 1 cm medial to the carnassial tooth.
3. Make incisions, create flaps, and suture tissues so as to appose cleanly incised epithelial edges. A flap sutured to an intact epithelial surface will not heal.
4. Where possible, arrange suture lines so they lie over connective tissue rather than over the defect. This will prevent drying and contamination of the connective tissue side of the flap, decreasing the likelihood of dehiscence.
5. Suture the tissues gently and carefully to avoid tearing the epithelium, using large

bites of tissue to minimize tension and interference with blood supply at the wound edges.

The surgical working space is limited by the presence of the mandible and tongue, particularly for repair of soft palate defects. Mandibular symphysiotomy provides additional exposure, although it is very rarely necessary. Use of pharyngostomy tubes postoperatively has been recommended, but is unnecessary; using such devices to avoid swallowing movements will not prevent dehiscence of a surgical wound resulting from an inadequately planned or performed procedure.

Midline Palate Defects

The above principles are best met for midline congenital defects by using the overlapping flap technique. Incisions are made in the palate mucosa down to bone, and a periosteal elevator is used to separate the mucoperiosteum from the bone. Two flaps are formed; one flap is

hinged at the edge of the cleft, and the other is attached at the lateral aspect of the palate (Fig. 6-7A). Hemorrhage, which is usually brisk, is controlled by pressure. The incisions extend to the junction of the hard and soft palate. The flap hinged at the defect margin is turned under the other flap, and the connective tissue surfaces of the two flaps are kept in apposition by preplaced horizontal mattress sutures of synthetic absorbable material (Fig. 6-7B). This technique does not result in apposition of epithelial cut edges, but does provide a wide area of connective tissue contact without tension. The epithelial defect fills in by epithelialization. Breakdown of repair following use of this technique is rare if the flaps formed retain sufficient vascularity. Identifying the palatine artery is particularly important on the side with the overturned flap, as the artery will be stretched.

The alternative technique, forming two symmetrical flaps by making incisions at the edges of the defect, then suturing the flaps over

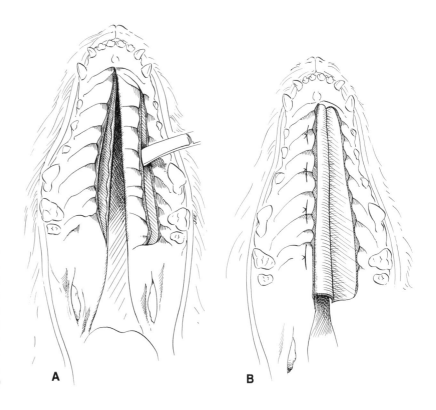

Figure 6-7. *Closure of a midline hard palate defect. A, Two incisions are made, one on the edge of the defect, the other close to the dental arch, to form two flaps. B, The flap hinged at the mid-line is turned under and sutured to the opposite flap. (Harvey CE, ed. Veterinary dentistry. Philadelphia: WB Saunders, 1985)*

A B

the defect, is no longer recommended because dehiscence is frequent. This technique results in tension at the suture line, which is located directly over the defect.

Closure of the soft palate defect, performed at the same time, is described under "Pharynx," below.

Acquired Palate Defects

The most common cause of acquired defects between the nasal and oral cavities is severe periodontal disease or extraction of the upper canine tooth (oronasal fistula). Trauma (dog bites, electric-cord injury), severe chronic infections, and surgery and radiation therapy of palatal tumors are other causes.

Oronasal Fistula

An established fistula is repaired by creating a buccal flap that extends well onto the lateral surface of the maxilla, advancing it over the defect, and suturing it to a cleanly incised epithelial edge on the palatal margin (Fig. 6-8). Results are excellent with this technique if the flap is large enough and includes some connective tissue to retain vascularity. The plane of dissection must extend through the fibrous connective tissue layer that attaches the lip to the maxilla just dorsal to the mucogingival margin. Closure of a defect caused by tooth extraction is described above, under "Teeth Extraction—Canine Teeth."

Acquired Defects of the Hard Palate

Many defects in the hard palate can be closed by some form of mucoperiosteal flap. Because the hard palate mucoperiosteum has little elasticity, it cannot be stretched to cover a large area. Therefore, planning of the flap position is essential to obtain a large enough area of tissue that will retain its vascularity. Rotation and advancement flaps can be created; in general, use the technique that will provide the largest flap. For small circular defects, rotation flaps usually are best. For long midline or para-

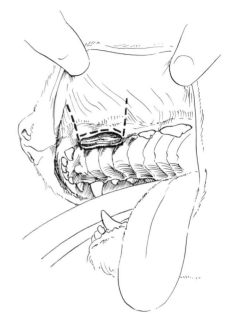

Figure 6-8. *Closure of an oronasal fistula. The dashed lines are the incisions to form a flap that extends well onto the buccal mucosa and that is carried down to the bone of the maxilla. The dotted lines are the incision to form a freshly incised edge to which to suture the flap.*

midline defects (such as those resulting from midline palatal separation in cats), the overlapping technique described above for congenital defects can be used if the epithelium at the defect has matured, or relieving incisions can be made to allow two lateral flaps to be apposed if the bony defect is very narrow. The donor site area of hard palate that is left devoid of mucosa heals by epithelialization.

Fresh midline lacerations in the palate of cats may not need surgical repair if there is no bubbling through the defect from the nose, as the stump of the vomer bone or nasal septum plugs the defect until a blood clot forms and healing commences. Fresh defects with obvious communication into the nasal cavity can be closed successfully by placing sutures to join the tissue edges, as for a clean skin wound.

Large defects that cross the midline can be closed with an advancement flap; this requires elevating the mucoperiosteum caudally to include part of the soft palate so that sufficient tissue can be pulled forward to prevent tension on the suture line. With flaps of any shape, the epithelium around the defect must be removed to provide an epithelial cut edge to which to suture the flap. For very large defects (covering more than half the width of the palate), a buccal-based flap can be formed and sutured across the defect, although the teeth and remaining palatal mucosa adjacent to the defect first must be removed. An alternative method is to create a permanent or removable acrylic or metal obturator, which may require the services of a dental laboratory.

Oral Neoplasia

Most oral masses are benign. The most common are generalized gingival hyperplasia and fibromatous epulis lesions. If these firm, nonulcerated masses interfere with the function of the teeth or are abraded and bleed, they can be removed surgically. Electrosurgery is very useful in reducing hemorrhage. The lesion is removed down to the underlying bone, which is left bare of epithelium. Recurrent lesions are treated by more radical excision or radiotherapy.

Malignant neoplasms are common and often difficult to treat. The major tumor types are malignant melanoma (of the palate, mandible, or tongue, typically in an older pigmented dog, although the lesion may be amelanotic), fibrosarcoma (usually of the palate or mandible, occurring at a younger age in larger dogs), and squamous-cell carcinoma (of the gingiva). Lymph node and lung metastasis is frequent with malignant melanoma, less so with gingival squamous cell carcinoma, and infrequent with fibrosarcoma. In cats, the most common malignancy is squamous-cell carcinoma of the gingiva or tongue.

Thoracic radiographs should be made in all animals with suspected oral malignancies, as the oral lesions often cannot be diagnosed on gross examination alone. Biopsy is essential for prognosis and treatment decisions. Chemotherapy is of little or no value as the primary treatment of oral malignancies. Bone invasion is usual, so conservative surgery is not beneficial. Cryo- and electrosurgery are of no particular benefit; they destroy tissue effectively though without accurate delimitation and do not permit primary reconstruction. Radiation therapy generally produces poor long-term results, although recently a combination therapy and hyperthermia has been shown to be as effective as radical surgery.

Surgery for Oral Mass Lesions

Radical (en-bloc) surgical resection of maxillary and mandibular lesions may allow complete removal of some malignant lesions, including the zone of microscopic invasion that results in recurrence after less radical procedures. Aesthetically, maxillectomy causes minor facial abnormality; after mandibulectomy in dogs, the tongue often hangs out on one side, although this can be partially corrected by narrowing the commissure of the lips and forming a sling to contain the tongue. Osteomyelitis, cystic disease, and benign neoplasms are other possible indications for resection of major oral segments.

Temporary occlusion of one or both carotid arteries through an incision in the neck should be considered if extensive surgery is likely.

Maxillectomy

The procedure begins with an incision in the palatal, gingival, and buccal mucosa outlining the extent of resection, staying at least 1 cm away from the gross margins of the lesion (Fig. 6-9A). The epithelium is reflected to expose the underlying bone. Hemorrhage is controlled by pressure until the resected tissue is lifted out, when the vessels themselves can be located and ligated or electrocoagulated. The maxilla and palate are fractured along the incision lines with a diamond wheel, dental bur, or osteotome. The tissue to be resected is le-

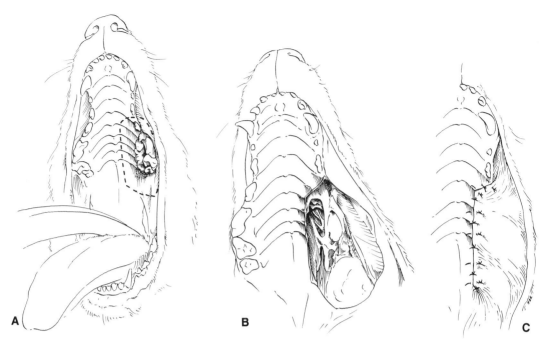

Figure 6-9. *Maxillectomy.* **A,** *The incisions in normal tissue surrounding the lesion are shown as dashed lines.* **B,** *The resected tissue exposes the nasal cavity and periorbital area.* **C,** *The oronasal defect is closed with a buccal-based flap sutured to the palatine incision. (Harvey CE, ed. Veterinary dentistry. Philadelphia: WB Saunders, 1985)*

vered up, remaining attachments are separated, and the section, usually including several teeth in situ, is removed en-bloc. If the tissue is levered gradually, vessels are stretched and exposed and can be identified and ligated. Full-thickness maxilla and palate are removed, exposing the nasal passages (Fig. 6-9B). Hemorrhage is controlled, blood clots are removed, and the remaining tissues are examined. If areas of nasal conchae were partially severed or traumatized during the resection, they are cut with scissors to leave a clean edge. Hemorrhage that cannot be controlled by ligation or pressure may respond to surface application of 5% cocaine solution. Use of dilute epinephrine solution (1:100,000) is more problematic because of the risk of cardiac arrythmias in an anesthetized dog.

The defect between the nose and mouth is covered with a buccal flap created by incising the buccal mucosa and undermining it until enough tissue is formed to cover the defect without tension (Fig. 6-9C). Most of the connective tissue layer is left attached to the buccal mucosa to ensure viability of the flap in its new position. Closure is made with simple interrupted or vertical mattress synthetic absorbable sutures. Wound disruption is more common if the incision is made with an electroscalpel. Drains are unnecessary. The connective tissue surface of the flap that faces the nasal cavity heals by granulation and epithelialization of the nasal mucosa.

The most common complication is breakdown of the sutures holding the flap in place 2 to 3 days after surgery. This occurs in about 20% of dogs and is more common with caudal maxillectomy than rostral resection. The flap is resutured. Feeding the animal through a pharyngostomy or gastrostomy tube is of doubtful value in preventing dehiscence. Antibiotics are unnecessary. The animal should be fed a soft diet and prohibited from chewing hard objects for the next several weeks to protect the flap while it heals.

The extent of tissue that can be resected by adapting this basic technique is remarkable. Resecting the entire premaxilla will cause the tip of the muzzle to droop slightly. The entire secondary palate (all of the teeth bilaterally from the canine teeth caudally) can be removed en-bloc, with closure of the huge oronasal defect by bilateral buccal-based flaps.

Mandibulectomy

In general, for malignant lesions, resect the entire affected hemimandible. Because there is a medullary cavity, vascular invasion leads to recurrence on the remaining mandibular segment if partial mandibulectomy is performed. For acanthomatous epulis lesions, a block of bone containing at least one tooth on either side of the visible lesion is resected; this technique permits retention of the symphysis and thus the normal length of the mandible. If the symphysis is disrupted by removal of all or a significant part of the mandible, the opposite mandible will shift toward the midline. This does not create problems for the dog, and will not be very evident to the owner unless the dog's tongue hangs from the mouth. If less than the entire hemimandible is resected but the symphysis is disrupted, attempts to stabilize the mandibles with cross-wires or screws are unnecessary and may result in migrating wires that cause complications.

Hemimandibulectomy incisions are made well away from the lesional tissue in the free gingiva (Fig. 6-10A), and the mandible is undermined by blunt dissection. The symphysis is separated by bone cutters or scissors and the lateral attachments of the tongue are separated, leaving the mandibular and sublingual gland ducts intact if they can be identified. The mandible is rotated to facilitate dissection of the masseter and pterygoid muscles from their attachments (Fig. 6-10B). Exposed or incised vessels are ligated, including the mandibular artery that enters the mandible medially at the angle of the jaw. The thick lateral temporo-mandibular ligament is exposed by rotating the mandible medially, then incised; remaining attachments are transected and the mandible is lifted out. A drain can be placed in the cavity beneath the suture line, exiting through the skin. The incision is closed by absorbable sutures apposing the incised oral mucosal edges (Fig. 6-10C).

The opposite mandible will swing over toward the midline; because of this movement and the absence of the mandible and canine tooth on the operated side, the tongue tends to hang out from that side in a dog. The lip commissure on the operated side can be shortened to lessen or prevent this constant extrusion of the tongue. About 1 cm of the mucocutaneous junction tissue is resected all the way around the upper and lower lips to the level of the new commissure, which is generally located level with the first premolar tooth. The mucosal edges of the upper and lower lips are sutured together with absorbable sutures, and the skin edges are sutured as a separate layer.

A soft-food diet probably will be necessary for the rest of the animal's life, although the animal will be able to eat and swallow by itself. Regular daily tooth-brushing and periodic professional periodontal care are recommended, as normal dietary abrasion is no longer available.

For lesions such as multilobulated osteochondroma that can occur on the coronoid process, resection of the coronoid process is possible. The surgical approach is made by resecting the zygomatic arch and separating the masseter muscle aponeurosis, then dissecting between the exposed temporal and pterygoid muscles. Surgery of the temporomandibular joint area is described above, under "Temporomandibular Joint (TMJ) Abnormalities."

Neoplasms of the Tongue and Lips

Surgical resection of the tongue is limited to the rostral half if swallowing function is to be retained. For lesions in rostrodorsal position, resection is simple, but hemorrhage must be controlled. A wedge of tissue is resected and the epithelial edges are apposed. A change of

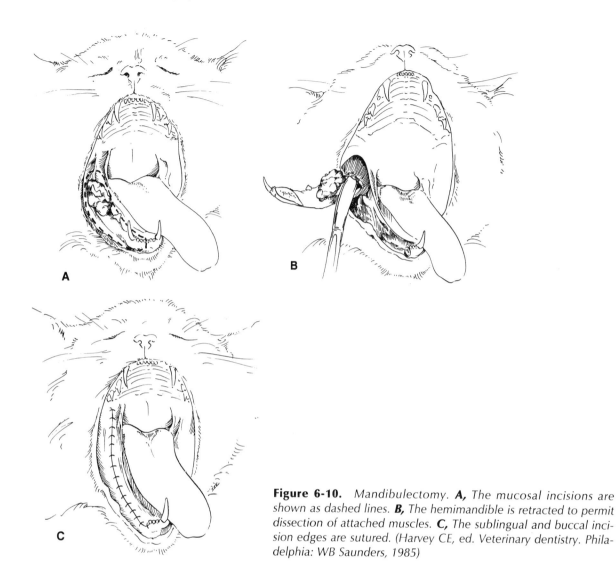

Figure 6-10. *Mandibulectomy. **A,** The mucosal incisions are shown as dashed lines. **B,** The hemimandible is retracted to permit dissection of attached muscles. **C,** The sublingual and buccal incision edges are sutured. (Harvey CE, ed. Veterinary dentistry. Philadelphia: WB Saunders, 1985)*

diet may be necessary, and some animals may be unable to groom themselves. Resection of the base of tongue area is impractical; unfortunately, this area is a typical site for squamous-cell carcinoma in cats.

Lip lesion surgery is described in Chapter 7, under "Surgery of the Lips."

Pharynx

The most common indications for pharyngeal surgery are overlong soft palate due to brachycephalic head shape, defects of the soft palate, and tonsillar lesions. Pharyngeal salivary mucocele and nasopharyngeal inflammatory polyps in cats are other indications.

Dogs with airway obstruction conditions severe enough to consider surgical treatment must be treated very gently to prevent exacerbating the obstruction and possible asphyxiation. Physical examination findings often are vital in making clinical decisions, because many of these dogs will not tolerate physical restraint for radiographic or other examinations without struggling and exacerbating respiratory distress. Careful auscultation usually is sufficient to localize the point of maximum loudness of respiratory noise, thus differentiating pharyngeal, laryngeal, and tracheal abnormalities.

Recovery from anesthesia for an animal with uncorrected airway obstruction often is difficult. For this reason, these animals should be anesthetized only if the expertise and facilities to correct the cause of obstruction are available, or at the least if equipment is available for tracheotomy to bypass upper airway obstruction. In some dogs, a primary or obvious upper airway problem may be combined with a tracheal abnormality, such as tracheal stenosis (hypoplasia) in bulldogs with brachycephalic upper airway disease.

Pharyngeal surgery may cause postoperative edema that can result in airway obstruction. An emergency tracheotomy may be indicated in an animal that is breathing with great effort and is collapsed or cyanotic after pharyngeal surgery.

Tonsils

Tonsillitis

Tonsillitis may cause vomiting, coughing, retching, salivation, and fever. The tonsils are deep red bilaterally and enlarged and stand out of their crypts. Tonsillitis often is secondary to other conditions causing vomiting or coughing. Primary recurrent tonsillitis is most often seen in young miniature or toy poodles and usually disappears when the dog matures. Antibiotics and nursing care are sufficient treatment for acute episodes; tonsillectomy is reserved for severe recurrent cases.

Neoplasia

Squamous-cell carcinoma is the most common tonsillar neoplasm, most often seen as a small ulcerated lesion on a tonsil, but with massive and very hard retropharyngeal node metastasis. Lung metastasis is frequent. These lesions are not radiosensitive and usually metastasis has occurred by the time of diagnosis, so the prognosis is very poor. Tonsillectomy

can be combined with mandibular or retropharyngeal lymph node resection as a palliative procedure. If the lesion has invaded the lateral pharyngeal wall, surgical treatment is impractical.

Lymphosarcoma usually is bilateral. The tonsils are enlarged, smooth, and cream colored. Lymphosarcoma lesions are often obvious in other lymph nodes. Tonsillectomy can be used only as a palliative treatment or in conjunction with chemotherapy for generalized lymphosarcoma.

Tonsillectomy

An endotracheal tube is essential. Pull the tonsil out of the crypt and cut the pedicle with scissors or an electroscalpel. Pick up and ligate bleeders, then place absorbable sutures in the epithelial edges. An alternate technique is tonsillar snare excision, although this is less accurate than scissors or electroscalpel excision. Watch for respiratory distress as a result of pharyngeal swelling for 24 hours, and feed soft food for a few days.

Soft Palate Lesions and Surgery

Overlong Soft Palate

Overlong soft palate is a major part of the brachycephalic airway syndrome. Soft palate resection is effective in relieving respiratory distress, particularly when combined with stenotic nares resection in dogs without severe laryngeal abnormality. After pharyngoscopy/laryngoscopy, an endotracheal tube is placed (or a tracheotomy tube if laryngeal surgery is also to be performed). Prednisolone (1 mg/kg) is given. There is no obvious difference in long-term results between the scissors resection/suturing technique and the electroscalpel technique when prednisolone is used. The extent of resection is to the midpoint of the tonsil. Resection of too much tissue is unlikely in a brachycephalic dog; it is somewhat more likely in the less common semibrachycephalic dog with an overlong soft palate, such as a St. Bernard or a cocker spaniel.

The soft palate and pharyngeal tissues distort when retracted for incision; remember the three-dimensional relationships of the pharyngeal structures when resecting the palate. Avoid pulling the lateral edge medially, as this will tent the lateral pharyngeal wall. Resect a rectangular or U-shaped area of tissue; trim off pharyngeal tags or flaps. Control arterial bleeding by ligating the clamped vessel, incorporating the bleeding point into a suture, or touching the hemostat clamping the vessel with the electroscalpel. To be of any benefit, sutures must appose the nasal and oral epithelial edges to facilitate first-intention healing. After resection, the nasal epithelial cut edge retracts dorsally; use the point of a curved needle to pull it back into view. If the lateral pharyngeal wall cut edges gape in the area where the palate tissue was resected, appose these edges with sutures also.

After soft palate resection, most dogs gag or vomit occasionally for several days. Because surgical manipulation may cause hemorrhage into tissue planes, or inflammation and edema, airway obstruction may be just as severe immediately after surgery as it was before, even when prednisolone is used. Equipment and personnel should always be available to perform tracheotomy if needed.

Resection of mucosal folds rostral and ventral to the epiglottis is used in dogs when the folds are full enough to be sucked over the epiglottis during inspiration. The mucosa is trimmed with scissors conservatively.

Other aspects of surgical treatment of the brachycephalic airway syndrome are described elsewhere (see "Stenotic Nares," Chap. 7, and "Laryngeal Abnormalities," Chap. 8).

Closure of Soft Palate Defects

Closure of Midline Soft Palate Defects

Closure is performed by making incisions at the junction of the oral and nasal epitheliums to the level of the middle of the tonsils (Fig. 6-11A). These incisions are deepened by gentle blunt dissection with scissors to form a dorsal and ventral flap on each side. The dorsal flaps are sutured with absorbable material to appose the nasal epithelial edges, placing the suture knots on the epithelial surface to minimize scar tissue formation within the muscle tissue of the palate (Fig. 6-11B). The ventral flaps are then sutured together to appose the oral epithelium. Closure of soft palate defects in cats is similar; the tissues are thinner and must be handled gently.

Unilateral Soft Palate Defects

These are less common than midline cleft of the hard and soft palate. Unilateral hypoplasia or failure of fusion of the soft palate on one side occurs sporadically. The simple flap technique described above for closure of midline soft palate defects often is not successful on unilateral soft palate flaps, perhaps because the tension produced by muscle activity during swallowing is more disruptive when the repair is not symmetrical. More elaborate flap techniques are necessary. The tonsil on the affected side can be removed, providing tissue for a dorsal and ventral flap that can be sutured to flaps made by incising the palatal edge on the normal side. If this repair breaks down, the entire lateral pharyngeal wall is available for creating mucomuscular flaps.

Inflammatory Nasopharyngeal Polyps in Cats

Nasopharyngeal polyps are resected by reflecting the soft palate forward, then grasping the polyp with a hemostat. If the polyp recurs, ventral bulla osteotomy offers a greater likelihood that the site of origin of the polyp will be resected (see Chap. 7, The Ear and Nose).

Salivary Glands

Salivary Mucocele

The most common indication for salivary gland surgery in small animal practice is salivary mucocele, a mucus-filled swelling caused by

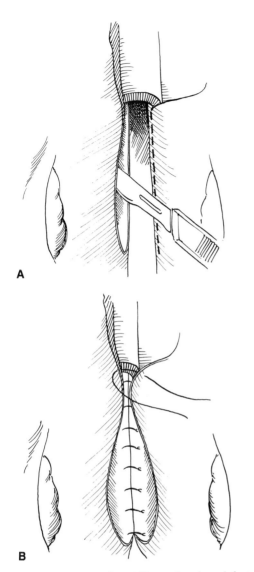

Figure 6-11. *Closure of a midline soft palate defect. **A,** Incisions are made along the edges of the defect. **B,** The nasal edges are sutured, followed by the oral edges. (Harvey CE, ed. Veterinary dentistry. Philadelphia: WB Saunders, 1985)*

disruption of a salivary gland or duct seen in the intermandibular-cranial cervical area (cervical mucocele), in the mouth under the tongue (ranula), or occasionally in the pharynx. The swelling is soft and not painful. Diagnosis is confirmed by aspirating a mucoid material that may be blood-stained. Treatment is either conservative (draining the mucocele as

needed, especially in a dog that is a poor surgical risk) or by mandibular-sublingual gland resection.

The gland affected is almost always the sublingual, although because of the close approximation of the mandibular and sublingual glands, both are removed during surgical treatment. Often the side affected is obvious from the history or physical examination results. If not, either the glands are removed on both sides, or an incision is made into the mucocele and a finger is inserted to palpate for the track or channel connecting the gland to the mucocele. The glands are approached through an incision in the neck over the palpable mandibular gland (Fig. 6-12A). The firm mandibular gland capsule is incised (Fig. 6-12B) and the mandibular gland is followed cranially to find the sublingual gland. The sublingual gland is long and requires digital dissection to get sufficient length to prevent recurrence. The sublingual branch of the lingual artery lies on the surface of the sublingual gland and should be identified and avoided.

As dissection proceeds, the gland and ducts are grasped with a hemostat and retracted caudally; this brings further glandular tissue into view, which is also grasped with a hemostat (Fig. 6-12C). This blunt dissection process is continued until the gland and duct separate by forceful retraction. The gland or duct stump does not require ligation. The mandibular capsule tissue, subcutaneous tissue, and skin are sutured. The mucocele itself is drained, but no attempt is made to resect the lining tissue, as it does not contain secretory cells. The mucocele recurrence rate after mandibular and sublingual gland resection is less than 5%.

A pharyngeal mucocele may present because of airway obstruction. For emergency relief of respiratory distress, lance the pharyngeal swelling.

Other salivary gland problems seen occasionally are neoplasia, mandibular gland necrosis, and fistula secondary to trauma. Mandibular gland necrosis results from acute enlargement of the gland that is held in a tight, strong capsule. The cause of the glandular swelling is unknown; the effect is very severe

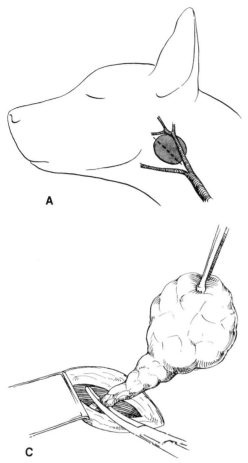

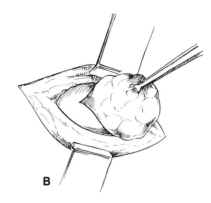

Figure 6-12. *Sublingual-mandibular gland resection.* **A,** *The incision is made over the gland where it lies between the lingual-facial and maxillary veins.* **B,** *The mandibular gland capsule is incised and the gland is retracted.* **C,** *The sublingual gland is dissected. (Harvey CE, ed. Veterinary dentistry. Philadelphia: WB Saunders, 1985)*

pain in the dog's neck. Treatment by mandibular gland resection is usually not successful. Mandibular and sublingual resection technique is used to resect mandibular gland tumors.

Parotid Gland and Duct

Parotid fistula, parotid sialocele, and congenital enlargement of the parotid gland can be effectively treated by parotid duct ligation. For a fistula or sialocele, the duct must be ligated proximal to the lesion. The duct is ligated using two or three ligatures, with the most distal (oral) ligature pulled the tightest and the more proximal ligatures slightly less tight. Anastomosis of the duct, or transposing the duct into the mouth, is also possible but unnecessary.

Parotectomy may be required for treatment of parotid masses. This is a difficult, tedious procedure because of the diffuse nature of the gland and the many neurovascular structures that run in and under the gland. It is rarely successful as treatment of an infiltrating tumor.

Zygomatic Gland

Diseases of the zygomatic gland are rare, although mucoceles and tumors arising from this gland are occasionally seen, usually causing exophthalmos. The gland can be biopsied or removed by orbital exploration. An incision is made along the dorsal rim of the zygomatic arch, the periosteum is reflected, and part or all of the zygoma is removed. The zygomatic gland is found in the orbital fat ventrolateral to the globe. It is gently dissected free, vessels and ducts are ligated, and the gland is removed. A soft rubber drain is placed, and the incision is closed by suturing the periosteum, subcutaneous tissues, and skin.

Drooling

Drooling is very rarely due to excessive salivation. Oral pain or swallowing dysfunction are much more common causes and should be investigated before salivary gland surgery is considered. In some giant breed dogs, such as St. Bernards and Newfoundlands, the shape and size of the lower lip predisposes to accumulation of saliva in mucoid ropes hanging from the lower jaw. Treatment by cheiloplasty (resection of part of the lip and commissure to tighten the lower lip) is possible. A simpler alternative is to ligate the mandibular and sublingual ducts bilaterally through incisions in the sublingual tissue. The ducts can be identified by threading black monofilament nylon into the duct openings. As in parotid duct ligation, two or three ligatures are placed with the most distal (oral) ligature pulled tightest.

Suggested Readings

Eisenmenger E, Zetner K. Veterinary dentistry. Philadelphia: Lea & Febiger, 1985.

Glen JB. Canine salivary mucoceles: results of surgical treatment in 50 cases. J Small Anim Pract 1972;13:515.

Harvey CE. Soft palate resection in brachycephalic dogs. J Am Anim Hosp Assoc 1982;18:538.

Harvey CE. Oral surgery: radical resection of maxillary and mandibular lesions. Vet Clin Nor Am 16;983, 1986.

Harvey CE, ed. Veterinary dentistry. Philadelphia: WB Saunders, 1985.

Hedlund CS, Tangner CH, Elkins AD, Hobson HP. Temporary bilateral carotid artery occlusion during surgical exploration of the nasal cavity of the dog. Vet Surg 1983:12;83.

Howard DR, Davis DG, Merkley DF, Krahwinkel DJ, Schirmer RG, Brinker WO. Mucoperiosteal flap technique for cleft palate repair in dogs. J Am Vet Med Assoc 1974:165;352.

Lantz GC, Cantwell HD, VanVleet JF, Cechner PE. Unilateral mandibular condylectomy: experimental and clinical results. J Am Anim Hosp Ass 1982:18;883.

Ross DL. Canine endodontic therapy. J Am Vet Med Assoc 1981:180;356.

Sumner-Smith G, Dingwall JG. The plating of mandibular fractures in the dog. Vet Rec 1971: 88;595.

Withrow SJ, Holmberg DL. Mandibulectomy in the treatment of oral cancer. J Am Anim Hosp Assoc 1983;19;273.

Zetner K. Results following repair of mandibular fractures in dogs and cats using parapulpar pins and composite bridges. Personal communication, 1987.

7

Colin E. Harvey

The Ear and Nose

The Ear

Anatomically and functionally, the ear can be divided into four sections; the pinna, the external ear canal, the middle ear, and the inner ear. The most externally obvious, but least important functionally and clinically, is the pinna, which is either erect or pendulous in dogs, and short and erect in cats. The pinna is attached to the cartilages forming the external ear canal. The auricular and annular cartilages of the external ear canal form a cartilaginous tube lined by stratified squamous epithelium and a rich layer of sebaceous (ceruminous) glands. The canal ends medially at the tympanic membrane. Medial to the tympanic membrane is the middle ear cavity (osseous bulla), an air-filled bony shell lined by ciliated columnar epithelium. The middle ear cavity has a large lateral opening covered by the tympanic membrane, a medial opening (the au-

ditory tube) leading to the pharynx, and, dorsally in the epitympanic recess, the round and oval windows leading to inner ear structures. The tympanic membrane and oval window are connected by the ear ossicles, which transmit and amplify sound waves. In the cat, a prominent bony shelf divides the middle ear cavity into dorsal and ventral compartments. The middle ear cavity is traversed by the bone-encased chorda tympani nerve, which carries parasympathetic nerve fibers to the glands of the head via the trigeminal nerve. The inner ear consists of fluid-filled tubes and neural structures that transmit sound and perceptions of equilibrium to the brain.

Ear Canal Disease

In dogs, ear canal disease is very common and often severe. Causes include infection (bacterial, fungal, and mite infestation), skin disease (atopy, seborrhea, hypothyroidism), trauma, foreign bodies, conformation, and neoplasia. Most other species, including cats, suffer much less often from external ear canal disease. This difference is due to the anatomy of the dog's ear canal; because it is long, narrow, and tortuous, it is easily damaged and discharge is eliminated only with difficulty. The normal defense mechanisms that protect skin—the thickening of the squamous epithelium and the increased secretion of sebaceous fluid onto the surface—compound the problem in many dogs, because they result in further narrowing of the ear canal lumen. This causes the epithelial surface to become warmer and more moist, promotes bacterial activity, and makes resolution of common skin lesions more difficult. Unlike the gastrointestinal and urinary tracts, the ear canal cannot be cleared of debris by peristalsis. The ear canal of wild canidae is wider and more conical than that of most developed breeds. Understanding these anatomical and associated factors is a prerequisite for the correct use of surgical procedures in the treatment of external ear canal disease.

External ear canal disease in the dog traditionally has been treated as an infection by using various chemicals; first caustics, later antiseptics, and now various combinations of antibiotics and antimycotics have been used. We probably make things worse in many dogs by eliminating the normal skin surface flora, thus encouraging the growth of resistant organisms, such as Proteus and Pseudomonas, that often are impossible to control. A second element of treatment that may worsen the disease is ear cleaning. In some dogs this leads to rupture of the eardrum, which often goes unrecognized at the time and allows infection to become established in the bony middle ear cavity, where it is safe from contact with ear medications and can continue to feed discharge into the ear canal.

Except in the most severe cases, there is rarely an absolute indication for surgical treatment. The general principles for managing ear canal disease in the dog are as follows:

- Examine and treat skin disease if present.
- Consider whether conservative (medical or local cleansing) treatment is likely to be effective.
- Is the ear canal lumen visible at the external ear canal opening? If not, medical treatment is very unlikely to be successful.
- Are the owner and dog amenable to home medical treatment? All too often, a medication or cleansing regime that may be effective if used correctly cannot be applied as directed.

If both answers are "yes," medical treatment is appropriate. However, warn the owner that ear canal disease often recurs, and that each recurrence contributes to the gradual thickening of the ear canal lumen. Select the simplest medication likely to be effective. Use a miticidal agent if there is any suspicion that mites may be present (even if they cannot be seen on a smear of discharge from the ear canal). Antibiotics should be reserved for the occasional situation when acute control of all flora is essential. Baby oil helps loosen clumped seborrheic secretions. Rubbing alcohol dries and cleanses the ear canal. Dilute vinegar prevents growth of most bacteria, but lowers the ear canal surface pH for only an hour or less. Potentially irritating medications such as alcohol or vinegar should not be used when the ear canal epithelium is acutely ulcerated. Squeezing a drop or two of medication into the ear canal is of little value if the ear is full of discharge. Mildly antiseptic and soothing ear cleansing solutions (malic-salicylic acid and propylene glycol) have the advantage that they can be used in large volume (several ml rather than one or two drops each time).

A gentle massaging and flushing action after instilling an ear cleansing solution (and allowing the dog to shake its head afterwards) is very useful in cleansing the ear canal, but the canal should not be cleaned mechanically without adequate restraint. Suction is needed to remove all debris from the ear canal and prevent damage to the eardrum, and dogs will not tolerate it without general anesthesia. Therefore, ear cleaning should be reserved for dogs that have not responded to more conservative treatment. In many dogs, a point will be reached when the ear canal will no longer be amenable to conservative treatment. Simply put, the longer the decision to perform an ear canal wall resection is put off, the less likely the animal will obtain significant long-term relief from pain as a result of the procedure. When conservative treatment is not effective in a young dog or recurrence is frequent, and systemic disease has been ruled out, surgical treatment should be recommended early, before chronic changes occur in the horizontal ear canal.

- Consider the age and medical condition of the dog as a candidate for anesthesia. A chronic condition that will worsen is a clear indication for surgical treatment in a young or middle-aged healthy dog, but may be less appropriate in an aged, sick animal.
- Consider the risk of deafness. Many dogs with severe external ear canal disease are clinically deaf before surgery, in which case it is irrelevant to consider whether the procedure will cause deafness. In most dogs, clinical deafness results from ear canal ablation and lateral bulla osteotomy. If preserving current hearing is a major consideration, a less radical procedure (*e.g.*, lateral ear canal resection combined with ventral bulla osteotomy) may be indicated, with ablation and lateral bulla osteotomy as a standby procedure should the conservative surgical treatment fail to provide sufficient relief.

Ear Canal Surgery

Examine the horizontal ear canal and eardrum before surgery to attempt to give the owner a more accurate prognosis.

Ear Canal Resection

Lateral wall resection (Zepp procedure), the procedure of choice in most cases, has become the standard procedure. It is indicated only if a lumen is visible at the horizontal canal level. Otoscopic examination, therefore, is indicated in all dogs before performing ear canal resection surgery. In some dogs, the vertical ear canal epithelium is too hyperplastic to permit otoscopic examination of the horizontal ear canal level, although the hyperplasia may be less severe at the horizontal ear canal level. In this circumstance, the most practical approach is to incise the tissues as though a lateral ear canal resection procedure is to be performed, thus allowing examination of the horizontal canal area. If the horizontal canal has even a minimal lumen, the lateral ear canal resection procedure can be completed. If the horizontal canal is occluded, ablation and lateral bulla osteotomy can be performed through the ear canal resection incisions. If the horizontal canal is severely hyperplastic, it is advisable to contact the owner after determining the state of the horizontal canal, particularly if bilateral surgery is to be performed, because of the potential for hearing loss associated with lateral bulla osteotomy.

The lateral ear canal resection procedure seems simple to perform, but is made more demanding by the canal's irregular surface and shape. When making the incisions in the cartilages, keep in mind the desired end result: to bypass the vertical ear canal and maximally enlarge the opening of the horizontal canal.

Clean the ear as thoroughly as possible before surgery. Clip hair from around the ear, and pluck hair from within the ear canal. Flush the canal gently but copiously with a surgical scrub solution. Two parallel incisions are made, starting at the indentations on either side of the tragus, the cartilaginous prominence that forms the lateral edge of the vertical ear canal opening. The incisions are directed ventrally and slightly rostrally, parallel to the ear canal itself, and extend about 1 cm ventral to the palpable ear canal (Fig. 7-1A). Inserting a probe or closed hemostat into the ear canal has been recommended as a means of marking

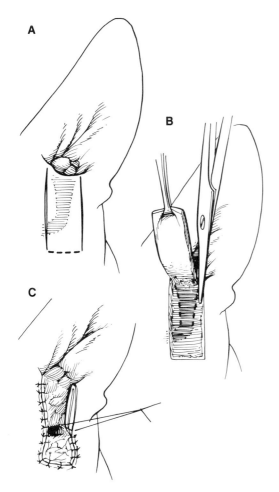

Figure 7-1. *Zepp lateral ear canal wall resection.* **A,** *Skin incisions.* **B,** *Scissors are inserted to incise the cartilage.* **C,** *The edges of the cartilaginous and skin incisions are sutured to maximally expose the horizontal ear canal.*

the direction and length of the canal, but this may cause ulceration of epithelium if held in place as the ear is manipulated and is not necessary, as the canal can be palpated to determine its limits.

The two incisions are joined ventrally by a third incision, and the rectangle of skin thus outlined is dissected free and reflected dorsally. It is either excised at the ear canal opening or used as a handle during the initial stages of dissection of the cartilage. The extent of soft tissue covering the ear canal cartilage depends

on the breed and obesity of the dog. If the cartilage cannot be palpated accurately, soft tissue covering it is dissected and reflected, avoiding or reflecting ventrally the parotid salivary gland tissue and the great auricular artery. The lateral wall of the ear canal is separated by making two ventrally directed incisions through the cartilage. Although the use of an initial marking incision with a scalpel has been recommended, it is easier to correctly incise this thick tissue with scissors, one blade inserted into the lumen of the canal and one blade outside (see Fig. 7-1*B*). The rostral incision is made directly ventral from the notch at the rostral end of the external canal opening (the tragohelicine incisure). The caudal incision is made from the caudal notch of the ear canal opening (intertragic incisure), but with the scissors initially directed caudoventrally. This is because the intertragic incisure notch is not located at the caudal end of the canal opening, but rather about one third of the circumference of the ear canal opening from the tragohelicine incisure notch, so that incisions made directly ventral parallel from these notches will lead to formation of a narrow ventral flap and wide retained medial ear canal wall, with less-than-optimal exposure of the horizontal canal.

The cartilaginous incisions are extended, usually by 1-cm lengths on alternating edges so the direction of the canal and incisions can be checked constantly and minor adjustments to direction made. The direction of the incisions is made more difficult by the presence of cartilaginous folds in the wall of the canal: the folds tend to lead spirally and if followed will result in a small or nonexistent ventral flap. As the vertical canal merges with the horizontal canal, the incisions must be turned from ventral to ventromedial and then directly medial if the ventral flap is to be maintained. The entire auricular cartilage must be split, as the shape and stiffness of the cartilage will cause the ventral flap to deflect dorsally if incompletely incised. Except in dogs with an extreme amount of calcified cartilage, the ventral flap will remain in its deflected position with minimal pressure once the auricular cartilage has been completely incised. The incisions in the cartilage at the opening of the horizontal ear canal should split the canal to form two equal surfaces, thus maximizing the opening. Bleeding vessels are clamped, avoiding inclusion of cartilage in the clamp if possible, and ligated. Some surgeons prefer to bluntly dissect the epithelium and connective tissue from the cartilage of the ventral flap and to resect the cartilage, again in an attempt to maximize the horizontal canal opening.

If the tissues gape considerably, subcuticular/subchondral absorbable sutures can be used to appose the epithelial edges. Sutures are used to appose the cut edges of the skin and ear canal epithelium (see Fig. 7-1C). Because the ear is a contaminated structure and contains cartilage (which has a poor blood supply), some discharge is very common for 1 to 2 weeks after surgery. Disturbed healing of the apposed edges also is common: sometimes the edges fail to remain apposed, with exposure and drying of an incised cartilaginous edge and wound breakdown. For this reason, protruding cartilaginous corners or edges should be excised at the time of surgery, and sutures placed so as to avoid or bury the cartilage. In other cases the epithelium overgrows the suture knots, making suture removal difficult for the veterinarian and painful for the animal. For these reasons, use of an absorbable material such as monofilament PDS is suggested.

The first sutures are placed with the flap reflected ventrally to maximally expose the horizontal canal. The tissues apposed are of very different stiffnesses, and the ear is subject to considerable tension if the dog shakes its head; again, the result may be dehiscence of the wound. This can be avoided in most animals by careful suture technique, such as including full-thickness cartilage and epithelium in each suture if the ventral flap cartilage is left in place and taking a much larger bite (1.5 to 2 cm) on the skin side of the incision to spread the tissue tension over a larger area.

Bandages that cover the incision closely will permit contaminated wound fluids to accumulate and are unnecessary. If the dog attempts to scratch at the surgical site, an Elizabethan collar is helpful. The detrimental effect of head-shaking can be reduced in a dog with pendulous ears by wrapping the ears on top of the head under a tubular bandage, although the surgical site should be left exposed by cutting a window in the bandage. Antibiotic treatment is not indicated. If part of the wound dehisces, repair is not necessary provided the ventral flap stays in position. The most common area of dehiscence is the medial ear canal wall at or just above the horizontal canal. If discharge accumulates around the surgical site, gently rinse the area with dilute chlorhexidine solution once or twice daily, or leave the surgical site alone if the dog is not willing to cooperate with rinsing.

Several studies of the long-term effects of ear canal resection surgery have concluded that only 30 to 50 percent of dogs having ear canal resection surgery (Zepp procedure) benefit greatly from the procedure. The problem is not the surgical healing (though it is possible to perform the surgery poorly by not extending the incisions sufficiently far ventromedially). In most of the 50 to 70 percent of dogs that do not respond well, the procedure was performed too late to be curative or, even had it been performed earlier, was never likely to be effective (*e.g.*, in cocker spaniels with congenital proliferative-seborrheic otitis externa).

An alternative to the Zepp ventral flap procedure for lateral ear canal resection (and, in fact, its predecessor) is the procedure commonly known as the Lacroix procedure in the United States and the Hinz procedure in Europe. Two incisions in the shape of a V are made in the skin, subcutaneous tissues, and cartilage, with the bottom of the V at the level of the horizontal ear canal. The ear canal epithelium and skin are then sutured together to leave the medial wall of the vertical ear canal exposed. This procedure is slightly quicker and simpler to perform than the Zepp procedure, but produces a less-than-optimal horizontal ear canal opening. Because the two incisions join at the acute angle formed by the V, accurate epithelial apposition at this location is very difficult to achieve, and granulation tissue can lead to occlusion of the horizontal ear canal opening.

Vertical Ear Canal Ablation

Vertical ear canal ablation with retention of the horizontal ear canal is indicated in animals with severe hyperplastic, seborrheic disease of the vertical canal wall, where the horizontal canal has a visible lumen. The purpose is to remove as much as possible of the hyperplastic skin, which often has a foul-smelling deep *Pseudomonas* or *Proteus spp.* pyoderma. The major consideration is to retain the horizontal canal opening, as resection of too much tissue will result in stenosis of the horizontal ear canal opening and development of more severe clinical signs.

The procedure begins with an incision around the external ear canal opening, with a ventral extension over the palpable ear canal. Scissors are used to dissect the ear canal free; the dissection plane should stay very close to the cartilage to avoid damaging the parotid salivary gland and nearby major vessels and facial and trigeminal nerve branches. The vertical ear canal is transected where it starts to turn medially, then two 1-cm incisions are made through the horizontal canal wall at its most rostral and caudal limits to form dorsal and ventral flaps. These are sutured in place as for the Zepp procedure. The remaining exposed tissues dorsal to the reformed horizontal canal opening are closed by apposing the skin edges with subcutaneous and skin sutures. The most awkward area to suture is the junction of the skin and the transected cartilage and epithelium of the pinna, as they do not conform readily.

Another variation on the basic ear canal resection procedure is designed to minimize the surgical wound and remove most of the vertical ear canal. The vertical canal is dissected free through a circumferential incision at the external ear canal opening. Then a separate incision is made at the horizontal canal level, the dissected canal is pulled through, the vertical canal is resected, and dorsal and ventral flaps are created to form the new horizontal canal opening. The initial dorsal incision is closed separately.

For dogs with erect ears where any risk of the ear no longer standing normally is not acceptable to the owner, a variation on lateral ear canal resection/ablation is performed. A complete cartilaginous and epithelial ring 1 cm long is retained at the external ear canal opening, then the rest of the vertical canal is ablated. The procedure begins with a horizontal skin incision 1.5 cm below the external ear canal opening, extending to and transecting through the vertical ear canal cartilage, then proceeding as for vertical ear canal ablation. The incised ventral edge of the skin covering the retained ear canal dorsal ring is sutured to the incised ventral epithelial edge attached to the lateral wall of the ring. The horizontal canal opening is reformed with a dorsal and ventral flap as described above.

All the techniques described above are of value only if the horizontal canal is at least partially patent. If the canal is completely occluded, or if a previous procedure designed to permit medical treatment of a partially occluded horizontal canal has failed to relieve ongoing or recurring discomfort, a more radical procedure is necessary.

The radical alternative surgical techniques are ear canal ablation, either by itself or with ventral or lateral bulla osteotomy. These procedures leave no external opening from the middle ear cavity. Thus, if there is residual or recurrent disease in the middle ear cavity or if pockets of horizontal canal epithelium are left in place, discharge with no natural drainage route will build up and cause an abscess or fistula on the side of the face. Often there will be considerable extension of this infected tissue in other directions also, making treatment very difficult and the prognosis for preventing further spread of infection very poor. Insufficiently radical surgery, such as ablation without bulla osteotomy, often results in recurrence. Ventral bulla osteotomy is a way to clean the middle ear cavity very thoroughly; combined with ear canal ablation, it allows a moderately thorough removal of the medial horizontal canal lining. Lateral bulla osteotomy combined with ear canal ablation permits a much more thorough resection of the horizontal canal epithelium, but causes hearing loss.

There is little risk to the function of the animal from vertical ear canal resection procedures. Procedures such as ventral and lateral bulla osteotomy carry a much greater risk of permanent functional neurological impairment, but are necessary in dogs with ongoing or recurrent painful ear disease involving the horizontal canal.

Ear Canal Ablation and Lateral Bulla Osteotomy

Ear canal ablation is indicated for severe hyperplastic otitis extending into the horizontal ear canal. Usually a T-shaped incision is used. The top bar of the T consists of two incisions, one made in the skin on the lateral edge of the ear canal opening, the other extending medially to transect the cartilage and inner hairless epithelium of the pinna. The medial incision is the most awkward, because of the undulating shape and varying thickness of the cartilage and the risk of penetrating through to and lacerating underlying auricular arteries and veins. The vertical incision is made over the palpable ear canal cartilage. The soft tissues over the cartilages are reflected, and the cartilaginous ear canal tube is dissected free (Fig. 7-2). The plane of dissection must be on the cartilage itself to avoid extension into potentially dangerous areas. The dissection continues to spiral down the cone ventrally. At the level of the junction of the auricular and annular cartilages, the facial nerve is identified as it courses around the ventral half of the horizontal canal. In animals such as cocker spaniels with extensive calcification of adjacent connective tissue, the facial nerve may be incorporated into the connective tissue mass.

A second difficult area is the membranous part of the canal where the cartilagi-

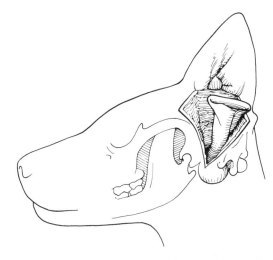

Figure 7-2. *Ear canal ablation. The auricular cartilage is dissected free.*

nous canal and bony canal join. In a dog with a normal canal, this area is not readily distinguishable from the rest of the canal, but in a severely affected dog the membranous portion often bulges because of epithelial and subepithelial tissue proliferation within the canal. This is a convenient area to cut and remove the canal. Because of the angle of the scissors when inserted to excise the ear canal, often some cartilage is left adhered to the skull bone; this is removed by further dissection with scissors. The epithelium and subepithelial glandular tissue in the remaining bony horizontal ear canal must be removed by curettage; this tissue often is pigmented and thus can readily be identified. The curette is inserted through the tympanic membrane into the bulla cavity. This inevitably damages the tympanic membrane, although usually it is already ruptured. The muscular attachments on the ventrolateral aspect of the bony horizontal canal and lateral external surface of the bulla are reflected with a periosteal elevator; this must be done with care because the facial nerve is contained in the tissue that is reflected ventrally to permit the dissection.

When the bony rim of the canal is fully exposed, one blade of a narrow-beaked rongeur is inserted into the canal opening with the other ventral to the canal, and the ventral rim is resected. This tissue is very hard and is much more dense than normal bone ("petra" as in "petrous temporal bone" means "rock"), so a heavy-duty rongeur is used. If the rongeur blade will not fit into the canal, the opening is enlarged by inserting a curette slightly larger than the opening and forcibly rotating it. Once the bulla is exposed, the middle ear cavity is curetted and flushed until all visible soft tissue is removed. The oval and round windows to inner ear structures are somewhat protected in the epitympanic recess, so acute vestibular damage is rare immediately postoperatively. A drain is placed in the incision and the soft tissues and skin are closed, leaving no external ear canal opening. The drain is removed once wound fluid flow slows, usually in 2 to 3 days. Antibiotic treatment is not necessary.

The major complication of ear canal ablation performed without lateral or ventral bulla osteotomy is continuing middle ear disease, as infection now has no natural way of discharging. Fistulas form on the side of the face from this deep-seated infection, which is essentially impossible to treat. For this reason, ear canal ablation is not recommended when middle ear disease or rupture of the eardrum is present or suspected, unless a middle ear drainage procedure such as lateral bulla osteotomy is performed at the same time. Other possible complications are facial paralysis and hemorrhage, and sloughing of areas of exposed pinna cartilage following dehiscence of the wound. On prick-eared dogs, the initial incision is made as far ventral as possible, to form a base for the pinna. In dogs with severe seborrheic otitis, the opposite is done: the incision is made high on the pinna to remove as much of the seborrheic tissue mass as possible. Ear canal ablation with lateral bulla osteotomy gives excellent long-term results in dogs with end-stage otitis externa.

The ear canal of the cat is shorter and cone-shaped rather than tubular as in the dog. Otitis externa is much less common, with the exception of ear-mite infestation. Polyps presenting as horizontal canal masses in fact originate from the middle ear cavity. Lateral ear canal resection is occasionally indicated to obtain surgical access to middle ear polyps in the horizontal canal.

Atresia of the ear canal or occlusion of the ear canal external opening occurs occasionally. It usually is possible to open the remaining ear canal lumen by performing a variation on the vertical ear canal surgical procedure described above. If the canal is completely atretic, ablation and lateral bulla osteotomy are performed.

Surgical Treatment of Otitis Media

In dogs, bacterial infection of the middle ear most often results from otitis externa, or overzealous ear cleaning. Otitis media is much more common than clinical signs would suggest, as many dogs with external ear canal disease and extension of that disease through a ruptured tympanum do not show the classical vestibular signs. In cats, otitis media is more commonly associated with upper respiratory infections or middle ear polyps.

The need for treatment is based on viewing a ruptured (or, less commonly, bulging) eardrum on otoscopic examination, or neurological vestibular disturbance or radiographic evidence. If the connection of the middle ear cavity with a facial fistula or abscess is not clear due to a blocked or ablated ear canal, a radiographic contrast agent may be injected into the fistula or though a narrow plastic catheter worked into the ear canal opening and a radiograph is made.

The treatment selected depends on whether external ear canal disease is present also. If there are neurological signs without severe horizontal ear canal disease, conservative treatment is appropriate initially: systemic administration of an antibiotic (ampicillin or Tribrissen) and treatment of coexisting otitis externa. If neurological signs are very acute, oral or injectable prednisolone (1 mg/kg) is given. If the response to conservative treatment is poor or if clinical signs recur, the bulla is flushed with saline under anesthesia via the external ear canal, followed by systemic administration of an antibiotic. Myringotomy (incision through the tympanum into the middle ear cavity) is necessary if the tympanum is intact; this is done by advancing a metal suction catheter through the horizontal ear canal until the bony medial wall of the bulla is encountered. Using aminoglycoside antibiotics, chlorhexidine, and full-strength povidone-iodine in the middle ear cavity should be avoided; they are ototoxic. Resecting the lateral ear canal allows better access for flushing and helps in treatment of coexisting otitis externa. This semiconservative treatment is successful in about half the established cases of otitis media. Some advocate using the auditory tube to insufflate and drain the middle ear cavity, but this procedure has not been widely accepted.

If conservative treatment is unsuccessful, surgical drainage of the bulla cavity is indicated. Bulla osteotomy can be performed either laterally or ventrally. The lateral approach is useful in conjunction with ear canal ablation but results in considerable hearing loss, as the eardrum is partially removed to allow access to the bulla. The procedure is described above, under "Ear Canal Ablation and Lateral Bulla Osteotomy."

The ventral approach is indicated if the horizontal ear canal is not totally occluded and the owner wishes to make every effort to retain some of the animal's hearing. A ventral incision is made medial to the mandibular salivary gland, and dorsal dissection between the mandibular salivary gland and digastric muscle reveals the hypoglossal nerve, carotid artery, and lingual artery (Fig. 7-3A). The bulla lies under a thin layer of muscle in the triangle formed by these structures. It is penetrated with a Steinmann pin (Fig. 7-3B), and the opening is enlarged with rongeurs until about a 1-cm hole is made. Debris in the bulla is removed with suction and curettage, the bulla is flushed, and a soft rubber drain is placed, exiting ventrally. The drain can be placed by inserting a small hemostat through the horizon-

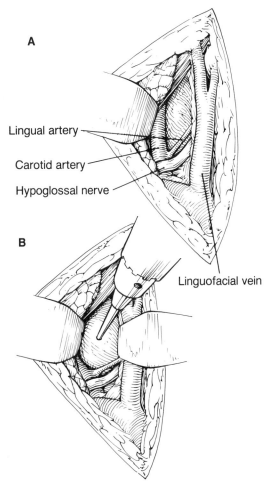

Figure 7-3. *Ventral bulla osteotomy.* **A,** *The mandibular salivary gland is reflected to expose the hypoglossal nerve, carotid artery and lingual artery (beneath the hypoglossal nerve).* **B,** *A hole is drilled in the ventral aspect of the bulla with a Steinmann pin.*

tal ear canal into the bulla, and then feeding the drain into the jaws of the hemostat and pulling it through and out the surgical opening. It can be tied in a loop on the side of the face. It is usually left in place for 7 to 10 days.

Bulla osteotomy in cats is complicated by the almost complete division of the bulla into dorsal and ventral compartments by a bony shelf; this shelf must be penetrated and removed by curettage for satisfactory completion of the procedure.

Complications of bulla osteotomy include

tongue paralysis; chorda tympani damage, causing interference with parasympathetic supply to the lacrimal, nasal, and salivary glands; hemorrhage; and recurrence or failure of clinical signs to improve. Generally, the more severe vestibular signs (stumbling, circling, nystagmus) improve within a few days; however, the head tilt often takes much longer to correct or may never return completely to normal.

The Pinna

Aural Hematoma

Aural hematoma is caused by head-shaking or scratching at the ear, usually as a result of otitis externa. A blood vessel ruptures as it passes through the ear cartilage, forming a cartilaginous inner lining on both inner surfaces of the hematoma. Treatment is directed at the two following areas:

1. To prevent further damage, by taping the ear over the top of the head and looking for and treating the cause (otitis externa).
2. To aspirate or drain to speed resolution of the hematoma. Many methods have been described, but the simplest is probably the best (inserting a Penrose drain through incisions at the extreme ends of the hematoma). Leave the drainage system in place for at least 2 weeks (or longer in dogs such as Weimaraners with wide, long, thin pinnas). The hematoma will resorb without surgery; in fact, the only reason for surgery is to prevent scar tissue cicatrization resulting in crinkling of the ear, particularly in erect-eared dogs. Several techniques designed to maintain the two sides of the hematoma in apposition have been described, such as through-and-through sutures or sutures clamping plastic tubing or radiographic film to both sides of the ear. These latter techniques have the disadvantage of encouraging loculation of hematoma fluid away from the drainage incision. More recently, treatment with

corticosteroid medications at anti-inflammatory dosages without surgery has been shown to speed resolution of the hematoma; it is not yet clear whether this effect is due to suppression of ear canal inflammation or to a specific immunologic effect in the hematoma wall.

Trauma

Frostbite damage usually requires no treatment. If the result is a jagged edge to an erect ear, additional pinna tissue can be resected to smooth the edge. Bite-wound trauma may be more severe; cartilaginous edges are apposed by suturing the epithelium on both sides, and the pinna is placed on top of the head within a tubular stockinette bandage to prevent disruption as a result of head-shaking. Cosmetic repair using a flap of skin from the neck is possible.

Tumors of the Ear

The Pinna

Squamous-cell carcinoma due to solar sensitization is seen on the ear tips of white cats; there may be multicentric lesions on the eyelids or lips. Local resection or radiotherapy is effective treatment. Mast-cell sarcoma is seen on the pinna in dogs; wide excision (partial or complete pinna excision) is necessary because of the likelihood of local invasion. The entire pinna can be removed without functional impairment, but with a potential aesthetic problem; when making the excision, retain enough of the ventral aspect of the vertical ear canal to permit formation of dorsal and ventral Zepp flaps.

The External Ear Canal

Ceruminous adenocarcinoma usually is seen in the vertical ear canal as a raised, sometimes ulcerated lesion. Vertical ear canal resection is performed to expose the lesion, which is then surgically excised, by ablating the entire ear

canal if necessary. Ear canal ablation is very practical because this will be a unilateral procedure, and hearing loss associated with lateral bulla osteotomy will have little clinical relevance.

The Middle Ear Cavity

Inflammatory polyps of the middle ear of the cat arise from the middle ear epithelium or underlying connective tissue and present because of chronic discharge (usually seborrheic or purulent) from the external ear canal, or as a nasopharyngeal mass. Treatment of a mass in the middle ear extruding through the horizontal canal is by resecting the lateral ear canal, then grasping the polyp with a hemostat; usually part of the stalk is left, but hemorrhage prevents further tissue removal through this approach. Complications are otitis media and a 50% chance of recurrence. A ventral bulla osteotomy is performed to permit more radical resection of recurrent lesions. Inflammatory polyps extending into the nasopharynx are treated by reflecting the soft palate with a spay hook or hemostat, then grasping the polyp with a hemostat and pulling out the polyp. Polyps usually are firm, and a long stalk can be removed if the pulling is gradual.

Nasal Cavity, Nares, and Lip Surgery

The nose is a complex bony box that filters, humidifies, and warms inspired air, adjusts body temperature, optimizes airway resistance, and exposes the olfactory sensory nerve endings.

The external nares are mounted on a cartilaginous framework. Within the fibrocartilage surrounding the external nares are arterial circles, branches of the lateral nasal arteries. The rest of the nasal structures also are richly supplied with blood vessels.

The interior of the nasal cavity is filled with bony projections (conchae and ethmoturbinates). The nasal mucosa covering the conchae is well equipped with cellular and humoral antimicrobial defenses.

Most dogs have well-defined frontal sinuses dorsocaudally and less obvious sphenoidal sinuses ventrocaudally. Cats generally have a small frontal sinus and a well-defined sphenoidal sinus beneath the ethmoturbinates and cribriform plate. The nasofrontal opening is large, but mostly occupied by the fingerlike ectoturbinates that extend into the sinus. There is no true maxillary sinus in the dog or cat, only a slight outpouching of the nasal cavity covered by a fold of the ventral conchae.

Superficial structures and the structures framing the external nares are supplied by the lateral and dorsal nasal arteries that run between the skin and the bones forming the nose. These can be avoided by keeping incisions to the midline, although there are two large veins that join in the midline just rostral to the junction of the two nasal bones with the nasal cartilages. Most of the contents of the nose, except the ethmoid area, are supplied by the sphenopalatine and major palatine arteries, both of which penetrate into the nose ventrally.

Stenotic nares contributing to upper airway obstruction occur as a congenital condition in some brachycephalic dogs. Treatment of this condition is described below, under "Brachycephalic Airway Obstruction—Stenotic Nares."

Management of Nasal Trauma

Control of Epistaxis

Nasal hemorrhage, whether caused by external trauma, neoplasia, fungal disease, surgery, or coagulopathy, can be very severe because of the rich blood supply; the volume of blood lost based on external pooling may be underestimated because of swallowed blood. The most effective way to control severe nasal hemorrhage is by occluding one or both carotid arteries through an incision in the neck.

The occlusion can be temporary (by umbilical tape loops encased in plastic tubing) if the source of bleeding is known and will be handled subsequently, or permanent (by ligation). Packing the external nares is very ineffective because the blood loss can continue, exiting from the nose through the pharynx at a rate unknown to the observer. Packing both internal and external nares requires general anesthesia. A probe is passed through the nasal cavity to allow a pack to be pulled up into the nasopharynx, but this is uncomfortable for the animal while it is in place and eliminates nasal air flow. Dogs are semiobligate nasal breathers and will become hypoxic if forced to breathe through their mouths acutely. Flushing with vasoconstrictive agents such as epinephrine is unlikely to control hemorrhage.

Relief of Obstruction

Blood clots and debris resulting from nasal trauma are cleared by the mucociliary system within a few days of trauma in an otherwise healthy animal. A decision to resort to radical surgical exploration is best delayed, although during this period the hypoxia-inducing effect of nasal obstruction must be appreciated and the animal closely observed. If the animal has a combination of acute blood loss and cranial trauma that may suppress the respiratory center, tracheotomy (and controlled or assisted ventilation) may be indicated; at the same time, the nasal cavity can be flushed gently to remove the larger clots hindering the major airways.

If nasal airflow obstruction is obvious several days after trauma, or if there is an area of obvious compressive injury, surgery is indicated. The nasal passages are flushed firmly to dislodge debris. Areas of severe compression can be reformed by gently inserting a curved blunt-ended bone elevator into the external naris on that side and forcing the compressed maxillary and nasal bone fragments back into normal alignment. This will damage the conchae, possibly leading to conchal necrosis and chronic nasal discharge, and the reformed area

may collapse again as a result of minor trauma (such as may result from violent sneezing caused by the irritation of the procedure).

A better but more involved technique is to incise the skin over the compressed area, remove any very small fragments, and knit together larger fragments. This is done with sutures of absorbable material placed in holes drilled with a dental bur or Kirshchner wire. As the area is not weight bearing and some of the bones are thin, fracture fixation by standard orthopedic techniques is neither necessary nor possible.

Diagnosis and Management of Chronic Nasal Discharge

For anatomical reasons, effective nasal surgical exploration requires removing all the contents of the nasal cavity. This may be necessary for management of some diseases causing chronic nasal discharge, such as nasal neoplasia, or may be indicated if more conservative diagnostic techniques have not provided a clinical diagnosis. The surgeon must differentiate between the most common causes of chronic nasal discharge, which in dogs are neoplasia, fungal disease (aspergillosis/penicilliosis), and chronic inflammatory or traumatic nonspecific rhinitis. The differential list in cats is somewhat different (see "Nasal Disease and Surgery in Cats," below). Alternatives to radical nasal exploration in dogs follow.

Endoscopic Examination

To progress beyond the nasal vestibule, this requires a small-diameter (4 to 6 mm) flexible endoscope or an arthroscope.

Radiographic Examination

This is particularly useful in distinguishing between neoplastic and fungal disease. The two radiographic signs of diagnostic importance

are destruction of bone, particularly the major bones forming the shape of the nose, and areas of increased lucency seen within the conchal area on the occlusal radiograph, particularly if they coalesce to form lucent pools 2 cm or more in diameter. Bone destruction is present in about half the dogs with nasal cancer, but in less than 5% of dogs with fungal infections. Lucent areas are present in about half the dogs with fungal infections, and rare in dogs with neoplasia. Foreign bodies generally are rare, but when present usually are obvious. Grass awns are common nasal foreign bodies in some areas and are not radiodense.

Biopsy

Samples of nasal tissues can be obtained by blind biopsy using long-handled biopsy forceps (or laryngeal cup forceps). The latter are available with smaller cup sizes and are therefore more useful in the nose than the typical uterine biopsy forceps. A sharp-pointed stiff plastic cannula also can be used and works well when combined with flushing. Both techniques necessarily destroy some nasal structures and do not permit the tissue to be selected by direct observation. The general area to biopsy can be determined from radiographs.

An alternative technique is to flush the nasal cavity with saline under high pressure, using an ear-flushing syringe pushed firmly into the external naris. The syringe is squeezed firmly and rapidly, with flow through the nasal cavity exiting from the mouth via the nasopharynx. Gently flushing for collection of samples for cytological examination is very unlikely to provide diagnostic information.

Bacterial Culture

This very rarely provides useful diagnostic information in dogs with chronic nasal disease; the organisms and their frequency of isolation from normal dogs are almost identical to those from dogs with chronic nasal discharge. Fungal culture also is of questionable value, as 40%

of normal dogs are positive. The most frequent growth is *Aspergillus*. Fungal culture of nasal discharge from dogs with proven fungal disease is not always positive, and contamination by nonpathogens is common. Serological diagnosis of aspergillosis is more reliable.

Dogs with a diagnosis of chronic active rhinitis from biopsy, or when no specific diagnosis is made from any of the tests described above, can be treated by turbinectomy, both as a diagnostic measure and as a way of clearing the nasal cavities of areas of turbinate trauma or necrosis that may be obstructing normal nasal function and allowing areas of secondary infection to reside.

Nasal Surgery

Turbinectomy

Surgical exploration (turbinectomy) is performed through a dorsal flap incision, either unilaterally or bilaterally. Skin and periosteum are incised on the midline, and the periosteum is stripped from the maxillary and nasal bones dorsolaterally. The bones are incised along parallel lines with a diamond cutting wheel or bone saw (Fig. 7-4*A*), or a hole is made with a Steinmann pin and bone is removed with a rongeur. If the bone flap approach is used, the flap is discarded, as it may become a sequestrum or contain neoplastic or fungal tissue. The flap is not needed to provide support for the dorsal aspect of the nasal cavity.

The exposed turbinates are removed with curettes and hemostats. Hemorrhage, which usually is brisk, can be controlled by temporarily occluding or ligating the carotid arteries, or by intranasal pressure, packing one end of the surgically exposed area while working on the other end (see Fig. 7-4*B*). The maxilloturbinates are removed completely. The ethmoturbinates, identified by the green-brown color of the mucosa, are removed more gently, curetting dorsoventrally rather than craniocaudally to avoid penetrating the cribriform plate. During nasal surgery in dogs, the position of

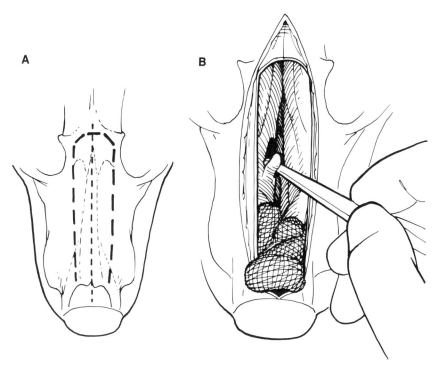

Figure 7-4. *Nasal exploration.* ***A,*** *Incisions for bone flaps to expose the nasal cavity (short dashed line is the skin incision).* ***B,*** *The nasal conchae are removed with a curet from the caudal half of the incision while sponges are packed into the rostral half of the incision.*

the cribriform plate can be estimated by dividing the dorsal-ventral nasal height on a line between the medial canthi into thirds: the dorsal third is the nasofrontal opening, the middle third is the cribriform plate, and the ventral third is the sphenoidal sinus recess and nasal meatus. The cribriform plates are protected by a substantial midline bony septum extending from the frontal bone ventrally. At the end of surgery, the dorsal surface of the palate and the lining of the frontal sinuses should be clean, and the caudal nasal opening should be free of bone splinters that may occlude the airway. The sphenopalatine arteries and accompanying nerves that enter the nasal cavity caudoventrally are ligated or cauterized. Packing is continued until hemorrhage is controlled. If possible, no packing material is left in the nasal cavity during the postoperative period. Although packing controls nasal hemorrhage, it also induces hypoxia in dogs.

Neoplastic tissue is grossly different from the usual gray-purple crunchy nasal conchae or green-brown ethmoturbinates. It is curetted until normal firm bone is reached. Particular care is needed when the tumor extends caudally into the cribriform plate area or caudolaterally through the thin medial wall of the orbit, because excessively vigorous curettage can result in penetration into the cranial vault or eyeball.

To prevent subcutaneous emphysema after surgery, a short length of plastic tubing (a blow-off tube) is placed into the frontal sinus through a skin incision and a hole in the frontal bone made with a Steinmann pin. The tube is attached to the skin of the skull immediately adjacent to the incision with a butterfly tape and sutures. The periosteum, which has little elastic tissue, is closed by suturing the connective tissue adjacent to it. Subcutaneous tissue and skin are closed routinely.

The prognosis after nasal surgery depends on the disease treated. Dogs tolerate the procedure well and complications due to the surgery itself are rare, except for hemorrhage and complications due to weakness of bone as a result of malignant invasion. Hematocrit and pulse strength and rate should be monitored closely for 24 hours after surgery. There is usually intermittent hemorrhagic discharge for several days, followed by a serosanguinous and sometimes purulent discharge for up to a month. In the long term, there is some serous or mucoid discharge periodically as a result of the disrupted mucociliary system. Occasionally, a repositioned bone flap may fail to reattach and form a sequestrum.

The prognosis for dogs with intranasal malignancy is grave unless radical treatment is performed. Surgery by itself is of little or no value. With a combination of turbinectomy and orthovoltage radiation therapy, a mean period free from clinical signs of tumor of about 16 months can be obtained. Results are better following treatment of the occasional benign nasal tumor and with chondrosarcoma.

Frontal Sinus Surgery

Occasionally, radiographic evidence of disease is limited to the frontal sinuses. The sinuses can be cleaned surgically by making a more limited dorsal flap directly over the sinus. Debris in the sinus is removed, and the sinus is flushed. The ectoturbinates that extend into the nasofrontal opening are resected to enlarge the opening and prevent subsequent obstruction of drainage into the nose. The incision is closed as for nasal flap surgery. A blow-off tube is placed if surgery is performed bilaterally, as blood clots may obstruct the nasal passages temporarily.

The procedure is similar for local treatment of nasal aspergillosis with enilconazole. After entering the frontal sinuses and clearing out debris and the ectoturbinate projections, two tubes are placed, one leading into each nasal cavity. The tubes are fenestrated liberally and attached by butterfly tapes to the skin of the skull. Short sections of secondary intra-venous tubing sets are convenient to use because they end in a syringe adaptor, which makes subsequent injection of enilconazole easier. The incision is closed, and the dog is permitted to recover from surgery. The next day, when swallowing reflexes are fully returned, the first injections (20 mg/kg) into the frontal sinuses and nasal cavities is given. Injections are continued daily for 14 days. The tubes are removed; closure of the opening is not necessary. Long-term improvement or cessation of nasal discharge is seen in 90% of dogs treated by this method.

Nasal Disease and Surgery in Cats

The differential diagnosis list for cats with chronic nasal discharge is different from that of dogs. The most common cause is chronic inflammatory disease secondary to conchal damage caused by acute feline viral rhinotracheitis or feline calicivirus infection. This condition has been referred to incorrectly as "chronic sinusitis." The frontal sinuses are involved, but the major problem is chronic disease of the conchae and ethmoturbinates, which causes retention of secretions and secondary bacterial activity in protected pockets. Nasal tumors are less common than in dogs but usually more malignant, with extensive erosion of facial structures. Nasal fungal disease occurs, but most commonly is the result of *Cryptococcus neoformans* infection. Cryptococcosis rarely requires surgical attention because it usually can be diagnosed from microscopic examination of a smear of nasal exudate and is amenable to treatment with ketaconazole (except when the disease has extended beyond the cribriform plate into the cranial vault). A diagnosis unique to cats is inflammatory polyps that arise from the middle ear cavity or auditory tube. These polyps block the nasopharynx, producing snorting respiration and nasal discharge; they are obvious on pharyngoscopic examination under anesthesia if the soft palate is retracted. Treatment is described under "Pharynx" in Chapter 6, Oral and Dental Diseases and Procedures.

Cats with chronic rhinitis-sinusitis usually are treated conservatively (periodic antibiotics) until the frequency of recurrence or need for nursing care to maintain nutrition dictate more radical treatment. Treatment by trephining and flushing the frontal sinuses has a very short-term effect; it is of no more benefit than simple but vigorous flushing of the nasal cavities. Treatment by radical nasal exploration provides long-term relief, and the cat is usually considerably improved once healing is complete. Nasal surgery in cats must be performed with considerable care; compared to dogs, the nasal cavity is much smaller, and the bones that form the external structure of the nose (including the cribriform plate) are much thinner and more liable to be damaged if treated in the same rather forceful way required for nasal exploration in dogs. The large sphenoidal sinus directly ventral to the cribriform plate contains ectoturbinates that must be curetted to remove tight spaces that can continue to promote virus replication and chronic rhinitis.

Frontal sinus mucosal ablation and replacement with a pad of fat has been described; ectoturbinates projecting into the frontal sinuses must also be resected for the procedure to be successful. Overall, the procedure is more involved than standard turbinectomy and no more successful.

Resection of nasopharyngeal polyps arising from the middle ear is described under "Pharynx" in Chapter 6, Oral and Dental Diseases and Procedures.

Diseases of the External Nares and Lips

Harelip

Congenital abnormalities of formation of the primary palate (incisive bone) appear as harelip. They may be associated with abnormalities of the secondary palate (hard and soft palate), but rarely result in clinical signs in and of themselves. Repair is made for aesthetic reasons. The defect may be unilateral or bilateral, and is often difficult to correct aesthetically; without detailed planning of the incisions, dehiscence is common. The floor of the nasal vestibule and roof of the mouth must each be reformed with separate flaps. Often one or more incisor teeth are located in the defect; these must be extracted.

Brachycephalic Airway Obstruction—Stenotic Nares

Stenotic nares are an externally obvious part of the brachycephalic airway obstruction syndrome; however, not all obstructed brachycephalic dogs have stenotic nares. Bulldogs are often affected, the small-breed brachycephalic dogs less so. Clinical signs are noisy breathing, dyspnea, and collapse. In many cases, considerable relief from respiratory distress can be provided by correcting stenotic nares and overlong soft palate. However, there is considerable danger of immediate postoperative airway obstruction if other airway abnormalities (such as everted laryngeal ventricles, laryngeal collapse, or tracheal hypoplasia) are not recognized. Thus, the entire respiratory tract should be examined (pharyngoscopy, laryngoscopy, tracheal palpation, thoracic radiographs) in any dog with airway obstruction.

Stenotic nares are simple to correct: symmetrical wedges of the lateral nasal folds are removed by making connecting dorsolateral and ventromedial incisions (Fig. 7-5). The fibrocartilage and thick epithelium prevent vessel retraction and simple apposition of tissue, so hemorrhage often is brisk from the transected lateral nasal artery branches. Suture the epithelial edges to control hemorrhage; use a large cutting-edge needle, take deep bites, and pull the tissues snugly together to control bleeding. Using absorbable material avoids the need for suture removal, with the risk of iatrogenic ocular proptosis in an uncooperative brachycephalic dog. Not all brachycephalic dogs with airway obstruction have stenotic nares, but long-term results show that if stenotic nares are present, correction improves

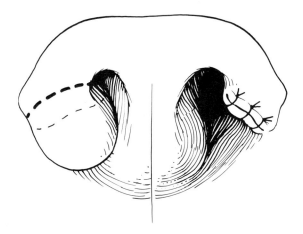

Figure 7-5. *Incisions and sutures for correction of stenotic nares.*

the overall results of airway surgery. Therefore, it is not justifiable to avoid correcting stenotic nares when treating palatine and laryngeal abnormalities just because the owner wants to avoid an external indication of airway surgery. Correction of this congenital abnormality rules the dog ineligible for showing, and these dogs should be neutered.

Other External Nares Lesions

Occasionally, squamous-cell carcinoma arises from the epithelium of the planum nasale, or nasal vestibule. The extent of the lesion can be determined by rhinoscopy or by making an incision on the lateral aspect of the nasal vestibule. Adequate surgical excision requires resecting the planum nasale, which is practical but disfiguring. Larger tumors may require resecting the planum nasale and premaxilla, with reconstruction of the rostral nasal opening.

Surgery of the Lips

Trauma

The lips often are injured in falls or in automobile trauma. The principle of treatment is to salvage or reform the mucocutaneous junction as rapidly as possible, as this is an area subject to considerable ongoing trauma and contamination during feeding. If the lower lip is intact but avulsed, it should be restored to its normal position as soon as possible and retained in position with sutures around the incisor or canine teeth if necessary. Rotation or advancement flaps from the cheek can be used to reform the upper lip; the parotid duct must be identified and avoided or ligated during these procedures.

Lip-Fold Dermatitis

The deep pyoderma of the lower-lip furrow commonly seen in cocker spaniels often can be managed conservatively. Surgical treatment is very satisfactory and is more permanent. A full-thickness wedge of lip tissue is resected; it should be centered on the furrow and should include the lateral frenulum of the lower lip. Hemorrhage is brisk; individual vessels are located and ligated. The wound is closed in two layers, commencing with absorbable sutures in the buccal mucosa. If the connective tissue between the mucosal and skin epitheliums is thick, some subcutaneous sutures are placed, then the skin is closed with polydioxanone or nonabsorbable suture material.

Lip Tumors

Several types of malignant and benign tumors occur on the mucosa and skin of the lip. Squamous-cell carcinoma of the buccal mucosa can be removed successfully by local resection if diagnosed early. Tumors arising from either epithelial surface that have invaded the connective tissue of the lip should be treated by resection of a full-thickness wedge of lip, as described for lip-fold dermatitis above.

Suggested Readings

Denny HR. Results of surgical treatment of otitis media and interna in the dog. J Sm Anim Pract 1973;14:585.

Evans SM, Goldschmidt MH, McKee LJ, Harvey

CE. Radiation therapy for intranasal neoplasms in dogs: long-term results and prognostic factors. J Am Vet Med Assoc 1989;194:1460.

Fraser G, Withers AR, Spreull JSA. Canine ear disease. J Sm An Pract 1970;10;725.

Gregory CR, Vasseur PB. Clinical results of lateral ear canal resection in dogs. J Am Vet Med Assoc 1983;182:1087.

Harvey CE. Stenotic nares surgery in brachycephalic dogs. J Am Anim Hosp Ass 1982;18:535.

Harvey CE, Goldschmidt MH. Inflammatory polypoid growths in the ear canal of cats. J Sm Anim Pract 1978;19:669.

Hedlund CS, Tangner CH, Elkins AD, Hobson HP. Temporary bilateral carotid artery occlusion during surgical exploration of the nasal cavity of the dog. Vet Surg 1983;12:83.

Howard DR, Merkley DF, Lammerding JJ, et al. Primary cleft palate (harelip) closure in puppies. J Am Anim Hosp Assoc 1976;12:636.

Mason KA, Harvey CE, Orsher R. Results of treatment of end-stage otitis externa in dogs with total ear canal ablation and lateral bulla osteotomy. Vet Surg 1988;17:263.

Sharp NJH, Sullivan M, Harvey CE, Richardson D. Aspergillosis in dogs; treatment with enilconazole. [Abstr]. Int Vet Ear Nose Throat Assoc, 1989.

Siemering GH. Resection of the vertical ear canal for treatment of chronic otitis externa. J Am Anim Hosp Assoc 1980;16:753.

Thrall D, Harvey CE. Radiation therapy for nasal neoplasia; results in 21 dogs. J Am Vet Med Assoc 1983;183:663.

8

Dennis D. Caywood

The Larynx, Trachea, and Thyroid and Parathyroid Glands

The Larynx

The larynx, a musculocartilaginous structure lined with mucous membrane, is located in the cranioventral aspect of the neck, between the base of the tongue and the trachea. The muscles of the larynx are responsible for both the sphincter action that closes off the lower airway during swallowing and the process of vocalization.

The laryngeal cavity is divided into three segments: the vestibule, which extends from the laryngeal opening to the ventricular folds; the glottis, which consists of the paired arytenoid cartilages dorsally and the paired vocal folds ventrally; and the infraglottic cavity, which extends caudally from the glottis to the trachea.

The blood supply to the larynx comes from the cranial laryngeal artery and laryngeal branch of the cranial thyroid artery. The nerve supply to the larynx is derived from the cranial and caudal laryngeal nerves, medial laryngeal nerve, and pharyngeal ramus of the vagus.

The larynx may be examined by external palpation; it normally is a firm but movable structure. Pressure may elicit a cough. Internal examination requires general anesthesia or heavy sedation and topical anesthesia.

Eversion of the Laryngeal Ventricles and Collapse of the Arytenoid Cartilages

Brachycephalic dogs with stenotic nares and elongation of the soft palate produce abnormally high negative air pressures in the larynx during inspiration. The inspiratory negative pressure often results in structural changes of the larynx, causing respiratory dysfunction. The laryngeal ventricles, which have the least resistance of any structure in the larynx, become everted into the laryngeal lumen. This obstruction leads to further increase in negative inspiratory pressure, which may be sufficient to displace initially the cuneiform and later the corniculate cartilages. The situation may become severe enough to cause total laryngeal collapse.

Clinical findings include stenotic nares, overlong soft palate, and inspiratory dyspnea. An upper respiratory stridor, cyanosis of mucous membranes, and exercise intolerance are also often seen.

General anesthesia is required to examine the larynx. Ultra-short-acting intravenous barbiturate anesthesia is usually adequate for examination. The everted laryngeal ventricles are seen as mucous-membrane-covered balloonlike structures in the ventral aspect of the laryngeal lumen. Laryngeal collapse is seen as a narrowed laryngeal lumen resulting from medial displacement of the cuneiform and corniculate cartilages.

Treatment depends on the severity of the condition. It is important to first correct the stenotic nares and overlong soft palate. Everted laryngeal ventricles are easily amputated with scissors through an oral approach. Partial laryngectomy or permanent tracheostomy may be necessary with severe laryngeal collapse.

These patients are extremely poor anesthesia risks and should be monitored closely until they have recovered completely from anesthesia. Tracheal intubation should be performed immediately after laryngoscopy and surgical procedures, and the tube should be maintained in place until recovery. Oxygen administration may be necessary.

Laryngeal Ventriculectomy (Fig. 1)

Hold the patient's mouth wide open with an oral speculum. Pull the tongue rostrally and direct the epiglottis rostroventrally to expose the laryngeal lumen. Grasp the lateral laryn-

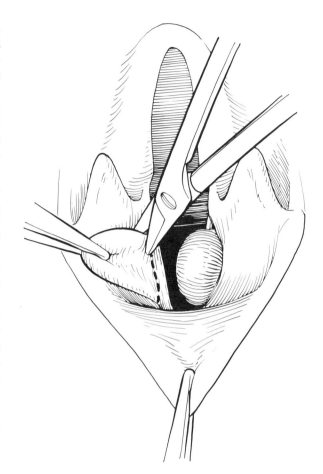

Figure 8-1. *The exposed everted ventricles are excised with Metzenbaum scissors.*

geal ventricles with a forceps and excise them with Metzenbaum scissors or an electrosurgical snare. Immediately intubate the animal and allow it to recover from anesthesia. Although hemorrhage is usually minimal, it should be carefully assessed as the patient recovers.

Laryngeal Paralysis

Laryngeal paralysis is an upper respiratory disturbance caused by dysfunction of the laryngeal abductor (dorsal cricoarytenoid) muscles. Neurogenic muscle atrophy follows Wallerian degeneration of the recurrent laryngeal nerves. There may be unilateral or bilateral nerve and muscle involvement. The disease is often slow in onset and the underlying cause is unknown. External trauma, chronic stretching due to cervical or thoracic lymphadenopathy, and cardiopulmonary disease have been suggested as possible causes of the nerve damage, but most animals have no demonstrable underlying cause. The problem may be observed in any breed and at any age in the dog and cat. However, inherited spontaneous laryngeal paralysis has been observed in a large group of young Bouviers. Other breeds known to show congenital laryngeal paralysis are bull terriers, malamutes, and huskies. Laryngeal paralysis is rare in cats.

Clinical signs include decreasing exercise tolerance, increasing laryngeal stridor, increasing dyspnea, cyanosis, and vomiting. The bark decreases in volume and changes in character.

Laryngeal function may be evaluated by laryngoscopy under light general anesthesia with the animal in sternal recumbency. An ultra-short-acting barbiturate is administered intravenously until there is a loss of resistance to opening the mouth. Laryngeal movements are observed as the animal recovers from anesthesia. The vocal folds and arytenoid cartilage remain motionless and more to the midline on the affected side. The function of the larynx cannot be evaluated under deep anesthesia.

Partial laryngectomy (vocal fold resection and partial arytenoidectomy), bilateral arytenoid cartilage lateralization, and castellated laryngofissure are three separate surgical procedures recommended for managing laryngeal paralysis in the dog and cat. Vocal fold resection is also combined with castellated laryngofissure. Each procedure increases the glottic diameter to improve airflow. Evaluation of a study in normal canine cadavers revealed a mean increase in the glottic cross-sectional area of 182.5% after bilateral arytenoid cartilage lateralization and 84.8% after partial laryngectomy. Castellated laryngofissure was not compared. Results of functional studies (tidal breathing flow volume loops) of a modified castellated laryngofissure in 12 dogs did not correlate with clinical results. Clinical results have been similar for partial laryngectomy, bilateral arytenoid cartilage lateralization, and castellated laryngofissure. Resolution or improvement of clinical signs of upper airway obstruction is reported for each procedure.

Although results with the other techniques are similar, I prefer partial laryngectomy because it is faster and easier to perform than the other procedures.

Vocal Fold Resection

This technique is commonly used to decrease noise produced from the barking dog. The intensity and character of a loud bark is usually reduced to a coughlike sound. The bark may return with time, as vocal folds tend to regrow through scarring after incomplete resection. Vocal fold resection is routinely performed on dogs in research colonies and occasionally on canine companions when their barking becomes a nuisance.

Therapeutically, vocal fold resection is an ancillary procedure to increase the size of the laryngeal lumen in cases when it has been reduced in size by various obstructive laryngeal diseases. It may be particularly beneficial in the surgical management of paralysis or collapse of the larynx.

The oral approach is rapid and more easily performed than laryngotomy. An intravenous ultra-short-acting barbiturate will give the appropriate depth of anesthesia and allow enough time to perform a vocal fold resection through an oral approach. Place the animal in sternal recumbency with the mouth held open with an oral speculum. Grasp the epiglottis with a forceps and pull it rostroventrally to reveal the laryngeal lumen and vocal folds. Grasp a vocal fold with a long forceps and excise it using a Metzenbaum scissors. Cut the vocal folds 1 to 2 mm dorsal to the ventral commissure of the glottis, leaving a small stump of vocal fold separated by epithelium ventrally to avoid webbing. An electrocautery wire loop or an alligator biopsy forceps may also be used. Hemorrhage is usually minimal. Place an endotracheal tube to prevent aspiration of blood and to maintain a patent airway until the animal recovers.

Partial Laryngectomy (Vocal Fold Resection and Partial Arytenoidectomy) (Fig. 2)

Partial laryngectomy is used to correct laryngeal air passage obstruction encountered with laryngeal paralysis or laryngeal collapse. The procedure is easily performed through an oral approach. Intravenous ultra-short-acting barbiturates may be used for anesthesia. An endotracheal tube should be available for intubation immediately after the procedure.

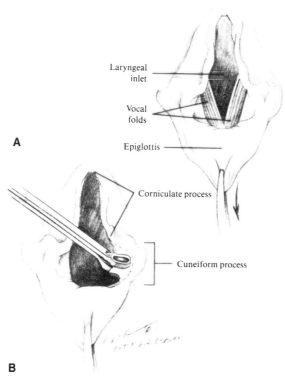

A

Laryngeal inlet

Vocal folds

Epiglottis

Corniculate process

Cuneiform process

B

Figure 8-2. **A,** *The epiglottis is grasped with a forceps, pulling it rostroventrally.* **B,** *The vocal folds are excised and the cuneiform process is removed piecemeal in bites using a laryngeal cup forceps. (Caywood DD, Lipowitz AJ. Atlas of general small animal surgery. St. Louis: CV Mosby, 1989:61)*

Place the animal in dorsal recumbency with the mouth held open with an oral speculum. Grasp the epiglottis with a forceps and pull it forward to expose the surgical field. The extent of the laryngectomy should have been previously determined by laryngoscopy. The object of the surgery is to create a functional air passage without severely compromising the larynx's ability to close. Overzealous laryngectomy may result in chronic aspiration.

Remove the vocal folds as described for vocal fold resection. Beginning at the aryepiglottic fold ventrally, remove the cuneiform process piecemeal in bites using a laryngeal cup forceps. Take care to avoid extending dorsally into the corniculate process. The procedure is usually confined to the most severely affected side, if possible, even with bilateral paralysis. Alternatively, curved scissors may be used. In older dogs the laryngeal cartilages become calcified and may be more difficult to resect.

Hemorrhage is usually minimal. An endotracheal tube should be inserted on completion of surgery to prevent aspiration. After intubation, hemorrhage may be controlled with pressure using gauze sponges held in a long-handled forceps.

No attempt should be made to suture the wound. Corticosteroid therapy may be beneficial in preventing excessive postoperative swelling and edema. Healing is usually rapid.

One potential complication involves the formation of granulation tissue or mucosal webs across the resected site, causing chronic air passage obstruction. These are more likely with extensive or bilateral resections. Anti-inflammatory doses of corticosteroids given for 30 to 60 days after surgery may reduce laryngeal web formation.

Bilateral Arytenoid Cartilage Lateralization to Correct Laryngeal Paralysis (Fig. 3)

Anesthetize the dog with inhalant anesthetic, using an endotracheal tube, and position it in dorsal recumbency. Make a paramedian inci-

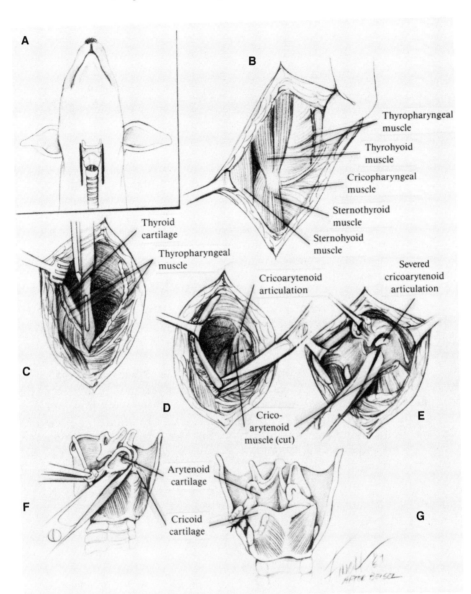

Figure 8-3. *A,* Arytenoid cartilage lateralization is performed with the animal positioned in dorsal recumbency. A paramedian incision is made lateral to the larynx in the jugular forrow. *B,* The sternohyoideus, sternothyroideus, thyrohyoideus, cricopharyngeal, and thyropharyngeal muscles are exposed, and the edge of the thyroid cartilage is grasped through the thyropharyngeus muscle and rotated laterally. *C,* The thyropharyngeus muscle is transected along the dorsocaudal edge of the thyroid cartilage. *D,* The rim of the thyroid cartilage is elevated, and the articulation of the thyroid and cricoid cartilages is incised, exposing the intrinsic laryngeal muscles. *E,* The cricoarytenoideus muscle is transected just caudal to its insertion on the arytenoid cartilage and retracted, exposing the articulation of the arytenoid and cricoid cartilages. The articulation is cut with scissors. *F,* The arytenoid cartilage is retracted rostrally and the arytenoid articulation is cut with scissors without incising the laryngeal mucosa. *G,* A single interrupted 2-0 nonabsorbable monofilament suture is passed through the cricoid articulation of the arytenoid cartilage and the caudodorsal border of the thyroid cartilage, bringing the cartilages into apposition. The thyroropharyngeus muscle is apposed. (Caywood DD, Lipowitz AJ. Atlas of general small animal surgery. St. Louis: CV Mosby, 1989:63)

sion alongside the larynx, approximately in the jugular furrow. Continue the incision through superficial muscle and subcutaneous fat to expose the sternothyroideus, thyrohyoideus, cricopharyngeus, and thyropharyngeal muscles. A portion of the sternohyoideus muscle will be visible through the incision. Grasp the edge of the thyroid cartilage of the larynx through the thyropharyngeus muscle and rotate it dorsolaterally. Transect the thryopharyngeus muscle along the dorsocaudal edge of the thyroid cartilage. Elevate the exposed rim of the thyroid cartilage and incise the articulation of the thyroid and cricoid cartilages, exposing the intrinsic muscles of the larynx. Transect the dorsal cricoarytenoideus muscle just caudal to its insertion on the arytenoid cartilage and retract it rostrally to expose the articulation of the arytenoid and cricoid cartilages. Cut this articulation with scissors. Retract the arytenoid cartilage rostrally, and insert scissors between the arytenoid and cricoid cartilages to transect the arytenoid-arytenoid articulation on the dorsal midline of the larynx without incising the mucosa of the larynx. With a single simple interrupted stitch of 2-0 nonabsorbable monofilament suture material, appose the cricoid

articulation of the arytenoid cartilage to the caudodorsal border of the thyroid cartilage. The exact placement of this stitch to produce maximal abduction of the arytenoid cartilage is determined with the help of an assistant who, after temporarily removing the endotracheal tube, can see the increase in the size of the air passage.

Reunite the thyropharyngeus muscle with a simple continuous suture pattern of 3-0 synthetic absorbable material. Repeat the identical procedure on the other side of the larynx, and close the neck incisions in standard fashion.

Castellated Laryngofissure and Vocal Fold Resection for the Correction of Laryngeal Paralysis (Fig. 4)

Place the animal in dorsal recumbency with the neck arched to better expose its ventral aspect. Make a midline incision directly over the larynx to about the level of the fourth tracheal ring. Incise the fascia overlying the sternohyoideus muscle on the midline and by blunt dissection separate the muscle on the

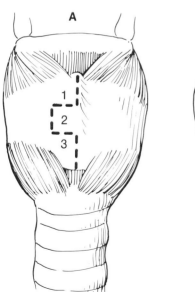 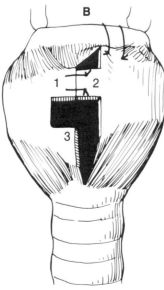

Figure 8-4. *Castellated laryngofissure. **A,** The distance between the cranial and caudal aspects of the thyroid cartilage on the central midline is divided into three equal portions (1, 2, and 3) and the thyroid cartilage and cricothyroid ligament are incised, exposing the laryngeal lumen as illustrated. **B,** The central cartilaginous flap 2 is aligned with the opposite edge of the laryngeal incision (flap 1). The flap is fixed in position using two or three 3-0 interrupted monofilament nonabsorbable sutures through the flap and around the basihyoid bone. Two 3-0 interrupted monofilament nonabsorbable sutures are used to appose flaps 1 and 2.*

midline to expose the ventral aspect of the larynx and cranial aspect of the trachea. Insert a tracheotomy tube through a vertical incision in the second and third tracheal rings.

Measure the distance between the cranial and caudal aspects of the thyroid cartilage on the ventral midline and divide it into three equal portions (1, 2, and 3). Incise the larynx and cricothyroid ligament as illustrated. Remove the vocal folds.

Align the central cartilaginous flap (2) with the opposite edge of the laryngeal incision (1). This widens the thyroid cartilage by the length of the central flap and creates a reversed L-shaped defect in the larynx.

Fix the flap in position by inserting two or three 3-0 monofilament nonabsorbable sutures through the cartilage flap and around the basihyoid bone. Insert one or two sutures through the flap to appose it to the opposite cranial thyroid segment. Additional sutures may be inserted through the middle and caudal aspects of the flap and into the soft tissues cranial to the hyoid bone to prevent the caudal end of the flap from obstructing the laryngeal lumen.

Cover the defect created in the larynx by close approximation of the overlying sternohyoideus and sternothyroideus muscles. Skin closure is routine. The tracheotomy tube can be removed in 3 or 4 days.

Laryngeal Spasms

Spasms of the larynx are seen more commonly in cats than in dogs because cats have a much more developed laryngeal sensory nerve supply. The condition results from reflex closure of the vocal folds after irritation of the respiratory mucosa along the upper or lower respiratory tract. Laryngeal spasms result in an inspiratory stridor and varying degrees of cyanosis.

Spasms occur more often in lightly anesthetized animals, particularly after intubation attempts or inhalation of concentrated anesthetic gases. Barbiturates tend to increase sensitivity to irritating stimuli.

The main complication of laryngospasm is associated with tracheal intubation during anesthetic induction. Forcible intubation through a closed glottis can cause trauma and subsequent edema. Atropine has no therapeutic value in the management of laryngeal spasms. Spasms may be prevented or controlled by topical application of 4% lidocaine spray to the larynx; intubation should be attempted only after the loss of the reflex.

Trauma and Foreign Bodies

Laryngeal trauma may result from external fracturing of the laryngeal cartilages or from foreign bodies that damage laryngeal soft tissues and cause obstruction. It may also be iatrogenically induced after endotracheal intubation or laryngeal surgery. Clinical signs include dyspnea, cyanosis, respiratory stridor, and laryngeal edema. Subcutaneous emphysema and hemorrhage are seen in more severe cases. Severe deformity of the larynx and stenosis may be associated with fracture of the cartilage.

It is often difficult to determine the extent of a traumatic laryngeal lesion. Diagnosis must be based on palpation, laryngoscopy, and radiographic evaluation.

Hemorrhage into the laryngeal lumen or stenosis of the larynx generally requires intubation or tracheostomy to ensure adequate ventilation. Severe hemorrhage necessitates laryngotomy to allow access to large bleeding vessels for ligation. Corticosteroids and diuretics may relieve laryngeal edema when present. Tracheostomy is often necessary for 24 to 48 hours in severe cases to allow the resolution of laryngeal swelling and the resulting obstruction of the upper air passages.

Fortunately, laryngeal foreign bodies are uncommon. When present, they are usually aspirated food particles. Stomach contents may enter the larynx after vomiting, especially during anesthesia. Most foreign bodies can be removed under anesthesia using a combination of instrument manipulation, lavage, and aspiration. Rarely, laryngotomy may be necessary to remove a foreign body.

Laryngeal Cysts and Neoplasms

Aspiration of the occasional laryngeal cyst is ineffective; surgical excision or stripping of the cyst wall is necessary, with good results.

Neoplasms arising from the larynx are uncommon. However, many types of tumors may be encountered, originating from epithelial tissue, connective tissue, or cartilaginous structures. Lymphosarcoma is the most common laryngeal tumor in the cat.

Clinical signs depend on the location and characteristics of the neoplasm. Dyspnea is observed with a luminal mass or when displacement or compression of the larynx occurs. Epiglottal hyperplasia and laryngeal cysts may produce clinical signs and appear similar to laryngeal neoplasms. Inflammatory proliferation should be considered in differential diagnosis. Diagnosis must be based on histologic evaluation of biopsy specimens.

Treatment involves surgical excision of the neoplasm. Tumors protruding into the laryngeal cavity often require laryngotomy to give adequate surgical exposure. Invasive malignant neoplasms have a poor prognosis. Total laryngectomy and permanent tracheostomy may be used as a salvage procedure in selected cases.

Laryngotomy

Laryngotomy is used to explore internal laryngeal structures and the lumen of the larynx. It may also be used to remove laryngeal foreign bodies, cysts, or neoplasms or to excise the vocal folds more completely.

After induction of general anesthesia, place the animal in dorsal recumbency and make a 3- to 5-cm incision on the ventral mid-line over the larynx. Bluntly separate the sternohyoid muscles and retract them to expose the thyroid cartilages and the cricothyroid membrane. Incise the thyroid cartilage on the midline from its cranial extent caudally to the cricothyroid membrane. Retract the edges of the incision to reveal the laryngeal lumen and the vocal folds.

To close the larynx, reappose the incised thyroid cartilage with interrupted 3-0 absorbable sutures. Then suture the sternohyoideus muscles, subcutaneous tissue, and skin. A ventral incision in the larynx is often associated with epithelial webbing; anti-inflammatory doses of corticosteroids given for 30 to 60 days after surgery may reduce laryngeal web formation.

The Trachea

The trachea is a ciliated columnar epithelial tube supported by a series of incomplete hyaline rings extending caudally from the cricotracheal membrane to the tracheal bifurcation at the base of the heart. The coordinated cranial movement of the cilia allows the elimination of secretions and particulate matter.

Blood supply is segmented and arises from a number of major vessels in the cervical region and mediastinum. When mobilizing the cervical region, care must be exercised to avoid damaging the recurrent laryngeal nerves that lie on the right and left dorsolateral aspect of the trachea.

The trachea may be compressed or deviated by surrounding masses, such as tumors, abscesses, or foreign objects. Such masses may be palpated or demonstrated by radiographic examination. By using a bronchoscope to examine the lumen of the trachea, acute or chronic inflammation, injuries, foreign objects, tumors, parasites, and congenital and acquired constrictions can be detected. A portion of a tumor can be removed with a long biopsy punch for diagnosis; parasitic nodules of *Filaroides spp* can be removed in the same way.

Transtracheal Aspiration

Transtracheal aspiration is valuable if the culture and sensitivity of organisms in tracheal secretions or cytological examination of cellular elements would be useful in the diagnosis of respiratory disease.

Sedation is usually unnecessary. After the hair is clipped and the skin prepared over the ventral aspect of laryngeal and cranial tracheal areas of the neck, infiltrate with lidocaine the area between the caudal larynx and the first tracheal cartilage, or between two of the first three or four tracheal cartilages.

Grasp the trachea with the thumb and fingers, with the skin held taut over the site at which the needle is to be inserted. Insert a 16- to 20-gauge needle into the trachea at a 90° angle and direct it caudally. Pass an intravenous catheter of suitable diameter through the needle to the tracheal bifurcation, approximately 4 cm beyond the thoracic inlet.

Rapidly inject 10 ml (less for small dogs or cats) of physiological saline solution through the catheter into the trachea. As soon as the animal coughs, immediately aspirate the injected solution by withdrawing the plunger of the syringe. Usually only 1 to 2 ml of fluid and secretions can be recovered after the injection of 10 ml of solution.

After the tracheal secretions are aspirated, remove the needle before withdrawing the plastic catheter. If the catheter is withdrawn first, it might be severed by the sharp edge of the needle and a portion left in the trachea.

Tracheotomy and Tracheostomy

These procedures are performed to provide a temporary or permanent opening into the cervical trachea. They allow inspection of the tracheal lumen, facilitate the removal of a foreign body, aid in the aspiration of tracheal secretions, or, more commonly, relieve upper airway obstruction.

A tracheostomy results in reduced closed glottic pressure, which may be beneficial in the postoperative management of the suture lines placed above or below the tracheostomy. In addition, anesthetic gases can be administered through a tracheostomy tube.

Tracheostomy tubes are available in a variety of materials and designs (Fig. 5). They may be of metal, plastic, or rubber and can be cannulated or cuffed. Cannulated tubes facilitate the frequent cleaning and removal of secretions that must be done, while maintaining a patent air passage. Cuffed tubes are useful for providing mechanical ventilation. Caution must be exercised when using cuffed tubes, as excessive inflation of the cuff can result in necrosis of the tracheal mucosa and subsequent stenosis.

When possible, the procedure should be performed in an aseptic manner. It is rarely necessary to perform an emergency tracheostomy because an endotracheal tube can be used to bypass the obstruction, allowing aseptic preparation of the cervical area. The patient is placed in dorsal recumbency and a ventral midline approach is made midway between the manubrium and the larynx. The sternohyoid muscles are bluntly separated laterally to expose the trachea.

To perform a tracheotomy, use either a horizontal incision through the annular ligament between tracheal rings or a vertical (longitudinal) incision through one or more rings. The horizontal (transverse) incision is recommended for short-term tracheostomies, as healing is rapid and postoperative stenosis minimal.

A tracheotomy performed by incising the ventral aspect of an annular ligament parallel to the tracheal rings should not involve more than one third the diameter of the trachea. This approach gives limited exposure to the trachea, allowing the passage of a small tracheal tube distally, the removal of small tracheal foreign bodies, or the aspiration of tracheal se-

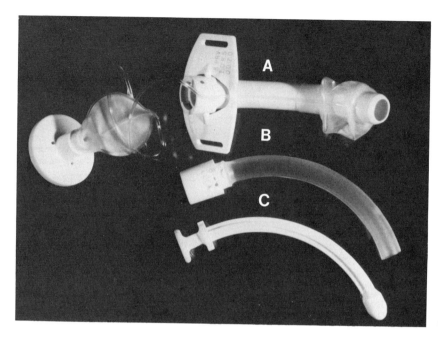

Figure 8-5. **A,** A cuffed tracheostomy tube; **B,** cannula; and **C,** obturator. The cannula (inner tube) is removed and cleaned periodically.

cretions. A more extensive tracheotomy is often necessary, especially when placing a tracheostomy tube.

Make a longitudinal incision through the first three tracheal cartilages at right angles to their long axis. A tracheostomy tube may be inserted and anchored to the neck by umbilical tape tied around the neck. The tube may also be sutured to the skin. After tube placement, appose the soft tissues with absorbable suture and close the skin with interrupted nonabsorbable monofilament sutures.

Constant care and observation is important in management of tracheostomy tubes. Because tubes quickly occlude with mucus and other secretions, possibly resulting in asphyxia, the tube must be cleaned and aspirated frequently. Allow the wound to heal by second intention following removal of the tube to prevent complications resulting from infection and subcutaneous emphysema.

Permanent Tracheostomy (Fig. 6)

Permanent tracheostomy is indicated in patients requiring long-term tracheostomy maintenance after laryngeal-tracheal reconstructive procedures and radiation therapy of the oropharynx and upper respiratory tract. Permanent tracheostomy may also be used as a salvage procedure to manage laryngeal paralysis, laryngeal collapse, and neoplasms of the upper respiratory system.

After the animal is prepared for surgery and under general anesthesia, position it in dorsal recumbency. Incise the skin and subcutaneous tissues on the ventral midline of the neck. Separate the sternohyoid muscles on the midline by blunt dissection and retract them laterally to expose the trachea. Bluntly dissect the tissues surrounding the trachea (including the carotid sheaths) from it to permit its elevation to the level of the skin incision.

Preplace one or two mattress sutures beneath the dorsal aspect of the trachea; insert them in the sternohyoid muscles and tie them. This brings the muscles into apposition on the dorsal aspect of the trachea and elevates it to the level of the skin. Excise a rectangular section of the trachea approximately encompassing four cartilage rings and one third the circumference of the ventral trachea, but take care not to excise the mucosa underlying the cartilages. Excise a section of skin about the

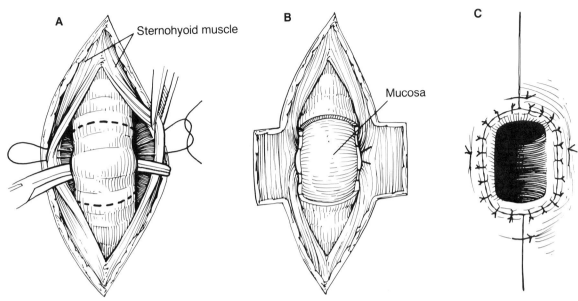

Figure 8-6.   *Permanent tracheostomy. **A,** The proximal trachea is isolated and two absorbable mattress sutures are placed through the sternohyoid muscles, tying them beneath the trachea and elevating the trachea to the level of the skin. **B,** A rectangular section of trachea encompassing three or four tracheal rings is cut from the ventral third of the trachea. **C,** A section of the skin the size of the stoma is excised, the edges of the skin incision are sutured to the trachea proximal and distal to the stoma, and the tracheal mucosa is incised and sutured to the skin, creating a stoma.*

size of the proposed tracheal stoma. Using simple interrupted absorbable sutures, suture the edges of the skin incision to the external fascia on the lateral aspect of the trachea and to the annular ligaments proximal and distal to the stoma. Incise the tracheal mucosa on the midline and suture its edges to the edges of the skin with a series of simple interrupted absorbable sutures inserted approximately 2 mm apart. Close the remainder of the skin incision routinely.

Alternatively, make a full-thickness H incision on the ventral third of the trachea, creating cranial and caudal tracheal flaps. Excise a section of skin about the size of the stoma and flaps. Suture the skin to the flaps and the margins of the tracheal wound using simple interrupted sutures.

Management of permanent tracheostomies is less demanding than tube tracheostomies. The stoma should be cleaned three or four times a day the first week and once or twice a day as secretions diminish. The hair must be clipped around the stoma to prevent matting and obstruction.

Tracheal Collapse

Collapse of the trachea is observed in toy and miniature breeds of dogs, particularly the toy poodle, Yorkshire terrier, Chihuahua, and Pomeranian. The disease is generally encountered in older obese animals. The cause is unknown. The major pathological feature is a weakened, flaccid tracheal muscle and weakening and stretching of the annular ligaments. This allows flattening of the trachea and narrowing of the tracheal lumen in a dorsoventral direction due to the elastic nature of the tracheal rings.

Diagnosis is based on history, physical, and radiographic findings. Differential diagnosis should include other types of obstructive diseases of the air passages such as laryngeal collapse, eversion of the laryngeal ventricles, and hypoplastic trachea.

The history includes a chronic cough and respiratory distress exacerbated by stress. Animals with tracheal collapse are prone to paroxysmal coughing that has a characteristic "honking" sound. Physical examination reveals an animal with respiratory embarrassment. Palpation of the trachea tends to initiate coughing.

The most important diagnostic tool is radiography. Plain lateral cervical and thoracic radiographs often are diagnostic. The most frequent sites of collapse are the caudal cervical and cranial thoracic areas of the trachea. Fluoroscopy is often beneficial in evaluating the condition. Although a number of surgical techniques have been devised to manage tracheal collapse, the main goal is to restore a functional tracheal diameter without disrupting normal ciliary function.

Patients with less severe disease and collapse of minimal anatomic extent may be managed by a combination of tracheal ring chondrotomy and plication of the tracheal muscle. More severe cases with more extensive lesions are best managed using a extraluminal prosthetic device. Severely obese animals, those with concomitant cardiopulmonary disease, and those with extensive lesions have a poor prognosis.

Postoperative care should include steroid and antitussive agents to decrease inflammation and prevent damage of the suture line.

Tracheal Ring Chondrotomy

This technique may be combined with plication of the tracheal muscle to manage less severe cases of collapsed trachea. Repair by chondrotomy involves exposing the trachea through a ventral midline approach. Alternate tracheal cartilages in the affected area are incised at the midline in a craniocaudal direction. Care should be taken to avoid cutting the underlying mucous membrane and entering the tracheal lumen.

Plication of the Tracheal Muscle

Approach the cervical trachea through a ventral midline incision and identify the collapsed area. Free the trachea from surrounding loose fascia and rotate it to expose its dorsal aspect in the collapsed area. If the collapsed segment of the trachea is located within the thoracic inlet, it can usually be retracted cranially, thus avoiding a thoracotomy approach. A 2- to 4-cm segment of thoracic trachea can be reached in this manner. Place interrupted monofilament synthetic horizontal mattress sutures approximately 0.5 cm apart through the dorsal tracheal muscle. Place the sutures in the muscle at the medial edges of the cartilage at right angles to the long axis of the trachea. Direct the sutures so that the plicated area is everted from the tracheal lumen. Allow the trachea to return to its normal position and close the surgical wound routinely.

Extraluminal Spiral Tracheal Ring Prosthesis (Fig. 7)

External support of the collapsed trachea using an extraluminal spiral ring prosthesis is a salvage procedure used to treat patients with clinical signs associated with severe collapse of the cervical and thoracic trachea. The procedure provides uniform support of the collapsed trachea while maintaining tracheal flexibility. It is preferred to internal supports because extraluminal devices do not interfere with ciliary dynamics or cause irritation that may perpetuate infection or result in granuloma formation.

The prosthesis is made from a 3-cc syringe case. Using a rigid- edge razor blade, remove the top and bottom of the case, leaving a hollow cylinder. Beginning at either end, make a spiral cut at a 15° angle, continuing down the

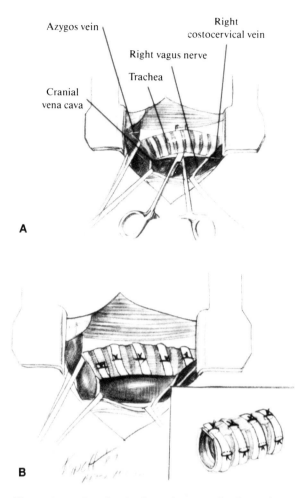

Figure 8-7. *Extraluminal spiral ring tracheal prosthesis. A, The trachea is isolated from the azygus vein, cranial vena cava, and right vagus nerve. B, Simple interrupted 4-0 polypropylene sutures are placed to incorporate each turn of the prosthesis and individual cartilage rings. The sutures enter the lumen. (Caywood DD, Lipowitz AJ. Atlas of general small animal surgery. St. Louis: CV Mosby, 1989:81)*

length of the cylinder, leaving 9 mm between each cut. Remove the tapered ends of the cylinder. Make a second cut 3 mm from the first, following the same angle. The second cut divides the cylinder into a spiral with 3-mm turns and a spiral with 6-mm turns. Remove the 3-mm spiral and cut the 6-mm ring in half. The resulting three (3 mm × 5.5 cm) polypro-

pylene spiral ring prostheses should be autoclaved or gas-sterilized before implantation.

Approach the cervical trachea by a ventral midline incision and identify the lesion. Mobilize the trachea, taking care to identify the recurrent laryngeal nerves to avoid incorporating them between the trachea and the prosthesis. Approach the thoracic trachea through a right third intercostal thoracotomy. Retract the right cranial lung lobe caudally and pack it off using moistened laparotomy sponges to expose the thoracic trachea. Carefully isolate the trachea from the azygos vein, cranial vena cava, right costocervical vein, and right vagus nerve.

Direct the end of the spiral ring prosthesis around the trachea and rotate it onto the trachea by turning the free end of the spiral. Position the caudal end of the prosthesis as close to the tracheal bifurcation as possible. Place simple interrupted 4-0 polypropylene sutures to incorporate each turn and individual cartilage rings. All sutures should enter the tracheal lumen. The trachea is supported from the bifurcation to the thoracic inlet.

Place a thoracostomy tube, approximate the ribs with 0 or 00 absorbable sutures, and close the chest routinely. The thoracostomy tube may be removed when negative intrathoracic pressure is established.

Immediate postoperative edema may be minimized by administering a preoperative or intraoperative dose of dexamethasone (1 to 2 mg/kg). Observe the patient closely for immediate postoperative respiratory distress. Cough suppressants, bronchodilators, glucocorticoids, antibiotics, and sedatives can be used as needed. The animal should be placed in a quiet environment for 5 to 7 days after surgery.

Foreign Bodies

Tracheal foreign bodies, rare in the dog and cat, are usually aspirated while the animal is playing or running. Clinical signs are those associated with dyspnea and upper airway obstruction, but can vary depending on whether the object is movable or embedded. Clinical signs include choking, coughing, retching, and vomiting. Cyanosis occurs; the degree of obstruction determines its severity.

Diagnosis may require radiography and endoscopy. Often, foreign bodies can be removed by endoscopy and long retrieval forceps. Care should be taken when removing sharp irregular objects, because considerable damage to the trachea can occur. Embedded foreign bodies and those not retrievable by endoscopy should be removed by tracheotomy. Cervical foreign bodies are best approached through the ventral midline, while thoracic tracheal foreign bodies are best approached through a right lateral thoracotomy with the incision placed at the appropriate interspace. Right cranial lung lobectomy has been described as a means of obtaining exposure to the carina.

Stricture

Stricture of the trachea is rare. When encountered, it is usually the result of scarring occurring after tracheal intubation, tracheostomy, endoscopy, or trauma. Common signs include respiratory stridor and dyspnea. Tracheal strictures are best managed by resection of the stenotic area and tracheal anastomosis.

Trauma

Cervical bite wounds are the most common cause of trauma to the trachea; lacerations or avulsions of the trachea may also result from blunt trauma or penetrating injuries. External injuries may result in subcutaneous emphysema, sometimes so extensive that the entire body is affected. Rubber bands placed around the necks of puppies and kittens can constrict and eventually penetrate the trachea.

Cervical lacerations may produce a nonproductive cough, hemoptysis, dyspnea, and cyanosis. Subcutaneous and mediastinal emphysema are often seen with larger tears. Rupture of the mediastinal pleura from trauma or from the increased pressure from air leakage produces tension pneumothorax. Rupture of the thoracic trachea or bronchi causes progressive tension pneumothorax, resulting in severe dyspnea and cyanosis.

Diagnosis is based on history, clinical signs, and physical examination. Plain and positive-contrast cervical and thoracic radiographic evaluation can often localize the wound, but endoscopy may be necessary to delineate and determine the severity of the lesion.

Emergency therapy includes administration of oxygen and treatment for shock, when present. If dyspnea and cyanosis are severe, it is necessary to perform conventional tracheal intubation or intubation through either pharyngostomy or tracheostomy to ensure a patent airway. Tension pneumothorax is managed by inserting a chest tube and using a system for continuous evacuation of air (Heimlich valve or a continuous suction system).

Small lacerations and puncture wounds are best treated conservatively. Intubation through pharyngostomy or tracheostomy is beneficial in reducing intraluminal pressure, allowing small leaks to seal. Larger lacerations and smaller wounds that persist in leaking over a 3- to 4-day period should be corrected surgically.

Neoplasia

Primary tracheal neoplasms are rare. Reported cases have included osteochondroma, chondrosarcoma, and osteosarcoma. These neoplasms appear to arise from the hyaline cartilage of the tracheal rings. Physical signs include dyspnea, cough, and hemoptysis. Diagnosis is based on radiography, endoscopy, and biopsy results.

Surgical treatment is tracheal resection and anastomosis when possible. Permanent tracheostomy may be an alternative when neoplasms are confined to the cranial cervical trachea. When extensive resection is necessary, prosthetic materials and grafts may be used. These alternatives should be avoided whenever possible because of the extremely high frequency of complications associated with grafts and prostheses in the trachea.

Repair of Tracheal Wounds and Defects

Small wounds of the cervical part of the trachea can be repaired by making a ventral midline incision and suturing with synthetic absorbable material. The use of a tissue cement has also been described. Any necrotic or infected tissue present must be debrided and local and systemic antibiotic therapy instituted. Emphysema usually is rapidly resolved after the tracheal defect is closed.

Larger wounds must be adequately exposed, then debrided and closed with a series of interrupted mattress sutures.

Mucosal wounds of the trachea heal by migration, mitosis, and differentiation. Within 48 hours, the wound becomes covered with transitional epithelium; by 96 hours, it differentiates into ciliated and goblet cells.

Injuries affecting the submucosa heal by granulation. A reduction in the diameter of the tracheal lumen is to be expected following second-intention healing.

Primary healing of full-thickness wounds follows precise anatomic reconstruction provided that only minimal tension is placed upon the sutures. Excessive tension on the suture line can lead to disruption and increases the likelihood of stenosis. Following meticulous anastomosis, the epithelium becomes ciliated within 6 months and stenosis is minimal.

Reconstruction of the trachea must be meticulous to avoid postoperative stenosis or leakage of air with subsequent subcutaneous emphysema. Nonabsorbable sutures and intraluminal tubes should be avoided, as they may cause ulceration of the mucosa and a granulomatous reaction that will interfere with mucociliary transport. Postoperative complications are more common following the use of grafts or prosthetic devices.

Primary end-to-end anastomosis is the preferred method of tracheal reconstruction. Excessive tension on the suture line must be avoided, as this can result in separation of the anastomosis, scar tissue formation, and stenosis of the tracheal lumen.

Tracheal Resection and Anastomosis

Resection and anastomosis is indicated in the management of tracheal stricture, severe traumatic lesions with necrosis, and neoplastic lesions involving the tracheal wall. Success depends on adequately mobilizing the trachea, avoiding excessive tension at the anastomotic site, avoiding excessive granulation at the anastomosis, and preserving normal ciliary and tracheal luminal dynamics.

The most important consideration in avoiding complications in tracheal anastomosis is the degree of tension at the anastomotic site resulting from the number of excised cartilages. Predictable primary healing will occur if tension is kept less than 1,000 g (3 to 10 cartilages removed) in the young animal and 1,700 g (8 to 23 cartilages removed) in the adult animal.

Approach the cervical portion of the trachea through a ventral midline incision in the neck. Separate and retract the sternohyoideus muscles. Approach the thoracic portion through a right lateral thoracotomy at the level of the defect. When the trachea has been exposed, the surgical techniques used for repair are similar. Three techniques for tracheal reconstruction are commonly used; in all three, the preliminary steps in approaching the trachea are identical.

Bluntly dissect the peritracheal fascia from the affected portion and adjacent trachea to permit mobilization of the operative area. Before transecting the trachea, insert one stay suture around one tracheal ring cranial to and one caudal to the area to be resected. These sutures permit manipulation and prevent retraction of the severed ends. Immediately after transection, it is important to insert an endotracheal tube into the distal segment of the trachea to maintain ventilation and anesthesia. If the lesion is in the most distal part of the trachea, a sterile tube can be passed through the surgical wound into the distal segment temporarily. Remove secretions and blood clots from the tracheal lumen and bring the severed ends into apposition by tying three or four preplaced simple interrupted synthetic absorbable sutures through the dorsal tracheal membrane. This maneuver is common to both the following procedures. Although the annular ligament technique may be necessary in small dogs and cats, the split cartilage tech-

nique is preferred because it results in more precise anatomic alignment with less luminal stenosis.

Split Cartilage Technique (Fig. 8)

In transecting the trachea, split in half circumferentially one tracheal ring at each end of the area to be resected and continue the incision through the dorsal membrane and mucosa. After resecting the affected area, bring the severed ends into apposition with three simple interrupted monofilament synthetic absorbable sutures placed through the dorsal membrane. Anastomose the cartilaginous portions with a series of simple interrupted sutures inserted circumferentially 2 mm apart around the trachea. The sutures should be inserted through

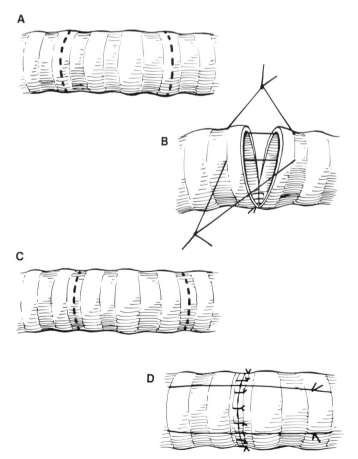

Figure 8-8. *Split cartilage technique of tracheal resection and anastomosis. **A,** One tracheal ring at each end of the area to be resected is split in half circumferentially. The incision is carried through the dorsal membrane and mucosa. **B,** The severed ends are brought into apposition using interrupted nonabsorbable monofilament sutures in the dorsal tracheal membrane. The cartilaginous portions are apposed with interrupted nonabsorbable monofilament sutures inserted circumferentially 2 to 3 mm apart.*

*Annular technique of tracheal resection and anastomosis. **C,** The annular ligaments and mucosa are incised just cranial and caudal to the lesion and the trachea is resected. **D,** The trachea is anastomosed by inserting interrupted nonabsorbable monofilament sutures through annular ligaments and mucosa cranial and caudal to the anastomotic site, encircling tracheal rings. Retention sutures may be placed around tracheal rings two cartilages cranial and caudal to the anastomosis to relieve tension on the suture line.*

the annular ligaments and mucosa so as to include the split cartilage rings. Tie the knots extraluminally.

Annular Ligament Technique (Fig. 8)

In this technique, resect the trachea by incising through the annular ligament and dorsal ligament at each end of the affected area. After resection, suture the dorsal membrane to achieve apposition. The remainder of the anastomosis is completed by inserting a series of simple interrupted sutures through the annular ligaments and mucosa cranial and caudal to the anastomotic site, encircling the tracheal rings.

With each technique, retention sutures may be placed around the tracheal rings two cartilages cranial and caudal to the anastomosis to relieve tension on the suture line.

Immediate postoperative edema may be minimized by administering a preoperative or intraoperative dose of dexamethasone (1 to 2 mg/kg). Observe the patient closely for immediate postoperative respiratory distress. Cough suppressants, bronchodilators, glucocorticoids, antibiotics, and sedatives may be used as needed. Extension of the neck is discouraged, especially if large tracheal segments have been excised. The animal should be placed in a quiet environment for 5 to 7 days after surgery.

Thyroid and Parathyroid Glands

The thyroid glands of the dog and cat consist of paired structures referred to as lobes. Each lobe is positioned ventrolaterally on the trachea. Between the glands is a poorly developed to nonexistent isthmus. In the dog, the right lobe of the thyroid is located slightly cra-nial to the left lobe, with the cranial pole of the right beginning at the caudal aspect of the cricoid cartilage extending caudally to the level of the fifth tracheal ring. The left lobe runs from the third tracheal ring caudal to the eighth tracheal ring. Each gland is embedded in deep cervical fascia and closely adheres to the trachea.

The thyroid lobes are covered laterally by the sternocephalicus and sternohyoideus muscles and ventrally by the sternothyroideus muscle. Ectopic thyroid tissue is not unusual in dogs and cats and may be located anywhere in the cervical area from the hyoid apparatus caudally along the trachea to the level of the heart. Two branches of the common carotid artery, the cranial and caudal thyroid arteries, supply blood to the thyroid gland. The glands are drained by the cranial and caudal thyroid veins.

The thyroids produce the thyroid hormones thyroxine (T_4) and triiodothyronine (T_3), which exert major control on metabolic processes in the body. The thyroid glands also produce thyrocalcitonin, which lowers the blood calcium concentration.

The parathyroid glands are intimately related structurally to the thyroid glands. The location and number of parathyroids varies in the dog and cat, but there are usually four, two associated with each thyroid lobe. The cranial parathyroid is usually external to the thyroid, especially in the cat, where it is usually located near the thyroid's cranial pole. The caudal parathyroid is located on the surface or buried within the parenchyma of the caudal portion of the thyroid gland. Accessory parathyroid tissue is common in dogs and cats and may be located in a number of areas in the neck and thorax, similar to ectopic thyroid tissue. The parathyroid glands share blood supply with the thyroid glands. The parathyroids produce parathormone, which mobilizes body stores of calcium.

The thyroid gland can be examined directly by palpation if enlarged or by surgical exposure and inspection. By pushing the larynx to one side, each lobe can be palpated, but this enables the surgeon to determine only whether the gland is enlarged.

Laboratory evaluations of thyroid function include measuring plasma T_3 and T_4 concentrations, thyroid radioiodine uptake, and thyroid-stimulating hormone (TSH) stimulation.

Examining the gland after exposing it surgically is unlikely to reveal a purely functional disorder. In such cases, the microscopic appearance of a resected specimen may not be a reliable indication of function. Microscopic examination will reveal atrophy, inflammation, or neoplasia.

Radiologic examination helps to disclose hepatic and cardiac enlargements, which accompany severe hypothyroidism, or demineralization of bone associated with hyperparathyroidism. The cardiac enlargement results from fatty infiltration of the myocardium. Therefore, anesthesia should be administered carefully and, if possible, only after the animal has been treated with exogenous thyroxine.

Determining blood calcium and phosphorus concentrations can be informative when hyperparathyroidism is suspected.

Feline Hyperthyroidism

In the cat, hyperthyroidism is commonly a result of functional thyroid adenomas or adenocarcinomas producing thyrotoxicosis. The disease is usually observed in cats older than 10 years of age. There is no breed or sex predilection. Clinical signs commonly include weight loss, hyperexcitability, polyphagia, vomiting, tachycardia, cardiac murmur, polyuria, polydipsia, a matted, greasy hair coat, and bulky stools. An enlarged palpable mass in the area of one or both thyroid lobes is often found on physical examination.

Evaluation of thoracic radiographs may reveal mild to severe cardiomegaly. Pleural effusion and pulmonary edema may be present in long-standing disease, resulting in congestive heart failure. Feline cardiomyopathy must

be ruled out as a diagnosis. Tachycardia (heart rate above 240 beats/minute), tall R waves, shortened QT intervals and paroxysmal arrhythmias can be observed on electrocardiographic evaluation. Premature atrial contractions, and atrial and ventricular bigeminy are less common findings. The cardiac abnormalities often resolve following resolution of the thyrotoxicosis.

Treatment of cardiac abnormalities is necessary before correction of thyrotoxicosis, particularly if surgery is to be the therapeutic approach. Propranolol should be given for 5 to 7 days before surgery to stabilize cardiac function and reduce the heart rate. Beta-adrenergic blockers counter the effect of excessive thyroid hormones on the heart. It appears that cardiac beta-adrenergic receptor sites are increased or amplified in thyrotoxicosis.

Antithyroid drugs, thyroidectomy, and ^{131}I can be used to manage feline hyperthyroidism. Propylthiouracil and methimazole are antithyroid drugs that can be used on a short-term basis before surgery or for long-term control of hyperthyroidism. Propylthiouracil results in some major adverse reactions in cats, including anemia, thrombocytopenia, and a positive antiglobulin test. Side effects are less common with methimazole, but pruritus, anorexia, vomiting, lethargy, thrombocytopenia, and agranulocytosis have been observed in treated cats. ^{131}I therapy is an effective and safe way to selectively obliterate functional thyroid tissue (normal and abnormal) in the cat. Unfortunately, it has limited use because of government regulations, unavailability of facilities, and required quarantine periods.

Thyroidectomy is commonly used to treat feline hyperthyroidism. Only the grossly enlarged thyroid lobe is removed, but bilateral thyroidectomy is necessary when both glands are involved. In some instances, it may be difficult to remove both thyroid glands without sacrificing a significant amount of parathyroid tissue. Staged bilateral thyroidectomy may be considered. The cranial external parathyroid gland or ectopic parathyroid tissue often remain to provide a functional parathormone concentration.

Serum calcium concentrations should be monitored closely for 48 to 72 hours after thyroidectomy. Signs of acute hypothyroidism including depression, anorexia, diarrhea, and hypothermia require thyroxine therapy. Most cats with unilateral thyroid involvement and those with ectopic thyroid tissue resolve most or all of their clinical signs of hypothyroidism. Total thyroidectomy may also cause hypoparathyroidism and resulting hypocalcemia. If hypocalcemia develops, calcium and vitamin D therapy is indicated.

Functional accessory parathyroid tissue often exists and may allow discontinuation of therapy within a few weeks. Thyroid replacement therapy is necessary with bilateral thyroidectomy.

Postoperatively, thyroid hormone concentrations should be monitored every 3 to 4 months, as adenomatous changes may occur in the remaining lobe and adenocarcinomas commonly metastasize to regional lymph nodes and lungs.

Thyroidectomy (Fig. 9)

An intracapsular dissection is recommended for thyroidectomy in cats with hyperthyroidism. With the animal positioned in dorsal recumbency, incise the skin and subcutaneous tissues on the midline, starting cranial to the larynx and extending caudally almost to the thoracic inlet.

Bluntly separate and retract laterally the sternohyoideus and sternothyroideus muscles to expose the thyroid and parathyroid glands. Identify and isolate the recurrent laryngeal nerves, which lie dorsomedial to the glands. The external parathyroid lies at the cranial pole of the thyroid, while the internal parathy-

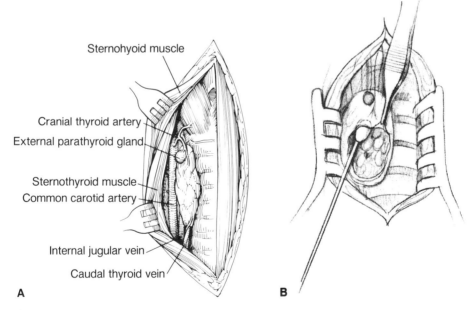

Sternohyoid muscle

Cranial thyroid artery
External parathyroid gland

Sternothyroid muscle
Common carotid artery

Internal jugular vein

Caudal thyroid vein

A   B

Figure 8-9. ***A,*** *The sternohyoideus and thyrohyoideus muscles are separated, exposing the thyroid and parathyroid glands. The caudal thyroid vein is ligated and the capsule is incised.* ***B,*** *The capsule is separated from the gland using a sterile cotton-tipped swab, leaving the external parathyroid gland, the thyroid capsule and cranial vessels intact. (Caywood DD, Lipowitz AJ. Atlas of general small animal surgery. St. Louis: CV Mosby, 1989:91)*

roid lies within the thyroid parenchyma. The parathyroid glands are lighter in color than the thyroid glands.

Ligate and transect the caudal thyroid vein as it exits the thyroid gland. Carefully incise an avascular area on the caudal aspect of the thyroid capsule and separate the capsule from the gland using a sterile cotton-tipped swab. Strict hemostasis is essential. Remove the thyroid gland, leaving the external parathyroid gland, the thyroid capsule, and the cranial thyroid vessels intact. For bilateral disease, the procedure may be repeated on the opposite lobe.

Unlike those in cats, thyroid neoplasms in dogs are generally locally invasive and seldom managed by intracapsular dissection. Canine thyroid adenocarcinomas often require extensive cervical dissection, ligation of the cranial and caudal thyroid arteries, and, when possible, removal of an extensive margin of normal tissue.

Primary Hyperparathyroidism

Primary hyperparathyroidism is the result of either a functional parathyroid adenoma, adenocarcinoma, or glandular hyperplasia. The condition is rare and is seen primarily in adult dogs. Clinical signs are invariably a result of increased calcium mobilization and hypercalcemia. Signs may include anorexia, vomiting, constipation, muscular weakness, severe skeletal demineralization, polyuria, and polydipsia.

Laboratory evaluation reveals hypercalcemia and hypophosphatemia. Differential diagnosis must include pseudohyperparathyroidism, renal secondary hyperparathyroidism, neoplasms with bony metastasis, and hypervitaminosis D. Primary hyperparathyroidism is the least likely disease among those producing hypercalcemia. Pseudohyperparathyroidism secondary to lymphoma or other neoplasms is the most common cause of elevated calcium concentration.

Diagnosis is usually made by excluding the more likely causes of hypercalcemia. Radiographs may be beneficial in ruling out direct osteolytic effects of bony metastasis, while analysis of serum parathormone levels may help differentiate pseudohypoparathyroidism from primary hyperparathyroidism. Definitive diagnosis of primary hyperparathyroidism is made by microscopic identification of parathyroid neoplasia or hyperplasia associated with appropriate clinical signs and laboratory data.

Initial treatment should involve lowering serum calcium levels and rehydrating the patient. Hypercalcemia causes nephrocalcinosis and renal damage. Fluids not only restore fluid volume, but also increase renal excretion of calcium. Furosemide also enhances calcium diuresis. When the animal has been rehydrated and serum calcium levels approach normal levels, surgical exploration of the parathyroid glands is recommended. Neoplasms are usually associated with parathyroid glands, but ectopic parathyroid tissue involvement is also possible. Adenomas and glandular hyperplasia are more common than adenocarcinomas.

Following surgery, if all abnormal tissue has been excised, serum calcium levels should fall to normal or subnormal levels within the first 12 hours. Postoperative management requires frequent monitoring for hypocalcemia. Clinical signs of hypocalcemia include tetany, muscular fasciculations, and hyperexcitability. If signs of hypocalcemia appear, calcium should be administered to control tetany. If hypocalcemia persists, serum calcium levels are maintained by oral administration of calcium and vitamin D.

Parathyroidectomy

The surgical approach to the parathyroid glands is the same as that to the thyroid glands (see "Thyroidectomy" above). The cranial parathyroid glands may be external to the thyroids, especially in the cat, where they are near the cranial pole of the thyroids. In the dog, the cranial parathyroid is often embedded in the cranial pole of the thyroid lobe. In both the dog and cat, the caudal parathyroid gland is embedded within the parenchyma of the caudal portion of the thyroid lobe.

The main indication for parathyroidectomy is a functional adenoma of the parathyroid gland. Fortunately, parathyroid carcinomas are extremely rare in dogs and cats. If the cranial parathyroid gland is abnormal, then parathyroidectomy is possible. Generally, parathyroid adenomas are managed by unilateral thyroparathyroidectomy.

Thyroid Neoplasms

Thyroid neoplasms occur in adult or aged dogs and cats. Carcinomas are observed more frequently than adenomas in the dog; in cats; adenomas predominate. About 90% of all clinically diagnosed canine thyroid tumors are carcinomas. The beagle, boxer, and golden retriever have a significantly greater risk for thyroid carcinoma than do other breeds of dogs. No breed predilection has been observed for thyroid neoplasms in the cat. Unlike humans, in which females are more often affected, dogs and cats have no sex predilection.

Clinical signs associated with thyroid neoplasms differ significantly in the dog and cat (see "Feline Hyperthyroidism" above). Hyperthyroidism is rarely associated with thyroid neoplasia in the dog. The main clinical sign in the dog is dyspnea. Clinically, canine thyroid carcinomas are rapidly growing, locally invasive neoplasms with metastasis occurring in 60 to 80% of the cases. The tumors commonly metastasize to the lungs, regional lymph nodes, and jugular veins. Larger tumors have a greater tendency to metastasize. Pulmonary metastasis occurs early and is often present before local involvement is apparent. Although most cases (64%) of canine thyroid carcinoma are unilateral, bilateral involvement indicates a more extensive neoplastic process.

Presumptive diagnosis of canine thyroid adenocarcinoma is initially based on the identification of a painful cervical mass in the laryngeal area. It must be differentiated from a cervical abscess, cervical foreign body, and granuloma or carcinoma of the tonsil with retropharyngeal lymph node metastasis. Plain radiography may reveal ventral displacement of the trachea, with a soft tissue mass between the trachea and vertebrae. The larynx or cervical vertebrae may show evidence of lysis due to tumor invasion. Thoracic radiography is necessary to rule out pulmonary metastasis. Radionuclide imaging using $^{99m}TcO_4$ and ^{123}I can greatly aid in the diagnosis of canine thyroid carcinoma. Scintigraphic evaluation not only reveals abnormal uptake of nuclide by the primary thyroid tumor, but also may demonstrate uptake at sites of neoplastic metastasis. Scintiscans appear to be more accurate than plain radiography in confirming pulmonary metastasis of canine thyroid carcinomas.

Excision is the primary therapy for thyroid carcinoma, but surgery is often limited to biopsy. Complete excision is often difficult because of extensive local invasion and vascularity of thyroid carcinoma in the dog. In addition, widespread pulmonary metastasis is common. In cases in which complete tumor excision is impossible, adjuvant therapy is indicated. Therapy with ^{131}I produces tissue destruction by beta radiation following uptake of the nuclide by the neoplasm. The combination of surgery and radiotherapy offers the best chance of controlling the spread of thyroid carcinoma.

Hypothyroidism and hypoparathyroidism are both possible complications after tumor excision. Neoplasms are highly vascular and invasive and anatomic relationships are difficult to maintain. Postoperative monitoring of T_3 and T_4 levels should be done and serum calcium concentrations should be monitored. The appearance of clinical signs of thyroid and parathyroid deficiency indicates the need for thyroxine or calcium and vitamin D therapy.

Suggested Readings

Berger B, Feldman EC. Primary hyperparathyroidism in dogs: 21 cases (1976–1986). J Am Vet Med Assoc 1987;181:350.

Birchard SJ, Peterson ME, Jacobson A. Surgical treatment of feline hyperthyroidism: Results of 85 cases. J Am Anim Hosp Assoc 1984;20:705.

Fingland RB, Dehoff WD, Birchard SJ. Surgical management of cervical and thoracic tracheal collapse in dogs using extraluminal spiral prostheses: Results in seven dogs. J Am Anim Hosp Assoc 1987;23:173.

Gourley IM, Paul H, Gregory C. Castellated laryngofissure and vocal fold resection for the treatment of laryngeal paralysis in the dog. J Am Vet Med Assoc 1983;182:1084.

Harari J, Patterson JS, Rosenthal RC. Clinical and pathologic features of thyroid tumors in 26 dogs. J Am Vet Med Assoc 1986;188:1160.

Harvey CE. Review of results of airway obstruction surgery. J Small Anim Pract 1983;24:555.

Hedlund CS. Tracheal anastomosis in the dog: Comparison of two end-to-end techniques. Vet Surg 1984;18:135.

Hedlund CS, Tangner CH. Tracheal surgery in the dog, Part I. Compen Contin Ed Pract Vet 1983; 5:599.

Hedlund CS, Tangner CH. Tracheal surgery in the dog, Part II. Compen Contin Ed Pract Vet 1983; 5:738.

Lumb WV, Jones EW. Anesthetic emergencies. In: Lumb WV, Jones EW eds. Veterinary anesthesia. Philadelphia: Lea & Febiger, 1973;579.

Mitchell M, Hurov LI, Troy GC. Canine thyroid carcinomas: Clinical occurrence, staging by means of scintiscans and therapy of 15 cases. Vet Surg 1979;8:112.

Rosin E, Greenwood K. Bilateral arytenoid cartilage lateralization for laryngeal paralysis in the dog. J Am Vet Med Assoc 1982;180:515.

Rubin GJ, Neal TM, Bojrab MJ. Surgical reconstruction for collapsed tracheal rings. J Small Anim Pract 1973;14:607.

Venker-Van Haagen A, Goedegebure SA, Hartman W. Spontaneous laryngeal paralysis in young Bouviers. J Am Anim Hosp Assoc 1978;14:714.

9

Anthony Schwartz
Cheryl J. Mehlhaff Schunk

The Thorax

Surgical Principles and Instrumentation

Surgical exposure of thoracic structures interferes with respiratory and cardiovascular function. This chapter first describes the particular consequences of thoracic surgery and the techniques used to avoid or minimize them, and then describes surgical abnormalities of the following thoracic structures: chest wall, pleural space, diaphragm, mediastinum, and bronchi and lungs. Cardiovascular surgery is described in Chapter 10.

The contents of the thoracic cavity, particularly the lungs, are intolerant of crushing, puncturing, or clamping. To minimize pleural irritation, which may lead to postoperative adhesions, pleural surfaces should be kept moist with warm sterile isotonic solution, and potentially irritating glove powder should be removed with a moistened gauze sponge before surgery.

Following incision into the thorax, a self-retaining retractor is placed to widen the incision and give proper exposure. We suggest the Finochietto retractor, which is available in various styles and in pediatric and adult sizes. To avoid tissue trauma or pressure necrosis, moistened gauze pads should be placed beneath the retractor blades, and the retractor should be repositioned about every 30 minutes. Hand-held retractors also are useful for exposing otherwise inaccessible areas. One type, the "malleable" (ribbon) retractor, which can be purchased in several widths, is bent to the desired shape for use.

Careful hemostasis and evacuation of blood clots prevent excessive blood loss and provide for better visibility and, therefore, faster and more accurate surgery. A cutting and coagulating electrosurgical unit is indispensable. A bipolar cautery pinpoints coagulation, thereby helping to prevent nonspecific tissue damage. A suction device can be lifesaving by facilitating the rapid localization and control of sites of major intraoperative hemorrhage. The Poole sump-type suction tube consists of an inner suction tip surrounded by a multifenestrated outer sleeve. It is useful for removing large volumes of fluids because it does not tend to become plugged or to cause suction-induced tissue damage, compared to tubes with a single opening. Single-hole fine tips are more useful for localizing points of hemorrhage; the outer sleeve of the Poole suction tube may be removed in order to use it in this way.

To avoid tissue trauma, hemostatic gauze sponges should be used with a blotting rather than a wiping technique. Sponges should be counted before both incision and closure to avoid leaving one in the chest. Because small sponges are easily misplaced in the thoracic cavity, only larger laparotomy sponges should be used. These have long ends that can be "tagged" outside the chest with an instrument. In addition, all sponges used in a body cavity should have radiopaque markers, so they may be detected easily postoperatively, if necessary.

Vascular forceps are best for manipulating delicate structures, because although they do not have penetrating teeth, they grasp securely with minimal trauma. Cardiovascular instruments are discussed in Chapter 10. Curved Metzenbaum scissors are very useful for dissection. Isolation and mobilization of tubular structures in the chest often depend on a combination of blunt and sharp dissection. Sharp dissection usually causes the least tissue trauma; blunt dissection of fascial planes is more traumatic but often is safer. Blunt dissection may be performed by opening the jaws of blunt-nosed instruments (such as Metzenbaum scissors or right-angle hemostats) in the desired tissue plane or by wiping apart delicate tissues with miniature ("peanut") sponges held with forceps.

Anesthesia for Thoracic Surgery

Manually or mechanically controlled intermittent positive pressure ventilation in a closed or semiclosed system is required if the chest is opened or if a condition exists that limits lung expansion or effective chest wall movement (*e.g.*, pneumothorax, pleural effusion, diaphragmatic hernia, pulmonary tumor, flail chest, etc.).

Induction of anesthesia should progress rapidly, particularly if one of the above conditions that reduces tidal volume exists. If possible, air or fluid should be removed from the pleural space before induction of anesthesia in animals with pneumothorax or pleural effusion. Removing hair from the surgical field before induction of anesthesia reduces the total anesthesia time. Surrounding the patient with circulating warm-water blankets or warm-water bottles (changed hourly) decreases the significant tendency toward hypothermia that accompanies an open thoracic cavity. Any pre-anesthetic sedatives or tranquilizers used should have minimal respiratory depressant effects (*e.g.*, butorphanol tartrate, 0.2 to 0.4 mg/kg SQ [Torbugesic, Bristol-Myers, Syracuse, NY]). Less excitable patients may be allowed to breathe 100% oxygen by face mask for several minutes before anesthesia induction.

Due to its ease of control, gas anesthesia is suggested for maintenance. Induction with a gas anesthetic by face mask eliminates problems due to barbiturates, but it may cause excitement in some irritable or frightened patients. This may lead to anoxia, particularly when there is marginal pulmonary function and/or tidal volume. Therefore, rapid induction with a thiobarbiturate anesthetic, intubation, and subsequent application of a gas anesthetic in 100% oxygen may be more appropriate for the early phase of anesthesia. Thereafter, the concentration of oxygen in the anesthetic mixture may be lowered, as long as good oxygenation of the blood persists. In many cases it is important to assess blood gas values periodically pre-, intra-, and postsurgically.

Nitrous oxide tends to diffuse from the blood and accumulate in gas-filled spaces. Therefore, its use in cases of pneumothorax is worrisome, as it may result in an increase in intrathoracic pressure, *i.e.,* diffusion hypoxia, even to the point of tension pneumothorax (see "Pneumothorax," p. 230). Because of this, nitrous oxide should not be used as an adjunct to inhalation anesthesia before entering the chest when pneumothorax exists. It may be used after the chest has been opened, during the main part of the surgical procedure, but it should be turned off at least 5 minutes before chest closure to reduce its concentration in the blood. Some anesthesiologists advise against using nitrous oxide at all in thoracic surgery because 50% nitrous oxide in combination with "packing off" the lungs may result in a dangerous degree of hypoxia.

Surgical Approaches to the Thoracic Cavity

A thoracotomy is a surgical incision into the thoracic cavity, entering the pleural space. It may be performed by one of several techniques: left or right lateral thoracotomy, in which part of one half of the thoracic cavity is exposed; or the longitudinal, sternum-splitting, median sternotomy or transsternal bilateral intercostal approaches, both of which expose both sides of the chest. Occasionally, limited thoracic exposure is provided during a celiotomy by incising the diaphragm (see "Diaphragm," p. 243).

Lateral Thoracotomy With or Without Rib Resection

Lateral thoracotomy without rib resection is the most common method of entering the chest, because it usually provides satisfactory,

although limited, exposure and it is associated with minimal morbidity. Because of limited exposure, the selection of the interspace for incision is important. Table 9-1 lists approximate locations for lateral thoracotomy to approach specific organs or to perform specific procedures. Because of anatomical variations, or displacement or enlargement of the underlying thoracic viscera, thoracic radiographs should be examined to determine the exact interspace to choose for the specific patient. An error of one interspace may necessitate rib resection or may tempt the surgeon to continue with an improper and potentially dangerous exposure. A two-interspace error could require closure and a new thoracotomy.

The patient is placed in lateral recumbency and the entire lateral chest wall, to just beyond the dorsal and ventral midlines and from the scapulohumeral joint to the caudal edge of the rib cage, is prepared for surgery. A small rolled towel placed beneath the chest, opposite the intercostal space to be opened, helps spread the ribs after incision. The forelimb on the side to be operated is secured cranially in a comfortable position. The skin at the appropriate intercostal space is marked with a scalpel nick or a sterile marking pen, and the incision site is draped. The skin is incised midway between two ribs, and parallel to the curve of the ribs, from near the head of the rib to just beyond the costochondral junction. The subcutaneous tissues and cutaneous trunci muscle then are incised and hemostasis is effected. The ribs are counted again to confirm the desired intercostal space. In cranial incisions, the latissimus dorsi muscle is undermined and transected over the intercostal space. In a more caudal approach, it may be retracted dorsally without cutting. The muscular bundles of the serratus ventralis and external abdominal oblique muscles then are separated bluntly (not cut) in the direction of their fibers, exposing the intercostal muscles (Fig. 9-1). In a cranial thoracotomy, the ventrally located scalenus muscle must be transected.

The intercostal muscles are incised midway between the ribs, exposing the normally transparent parietal pleura. Care should be taken to avoid the intercostal artery, vein, and nerve, which lie just caudal to the rib. The pleura is opened during the patient's expiratory phase, and the incision is extended dorsally to the paravertebral region and ventrally to within 3 to 4 cm of the sternum, taking care not to transect the internal thoracic artery or vein, on the dorsal surface of the sternum. Occasionally, in long-standing inflammatory conditions of the pleural space, the lung adheres to the parietal pleura. Thus, the pleural incision should be made with caution.

Before the thoracotomy is closed, the lungs should be inflated fully to expand atelectatic areas. To avoid pulmonary injury, a maximum of 20 cm H_2O of pressure should be applied to the ventilator bag. Gently massaging the lung tissue, while applying pressure, will help with lung inflation. Full inflation should be avoided, however, in acutely damaged lung tissue, or if long-term atelectasis exists (e.g., in association with chronic diaphragmatic hernia or pleural effusion), as reperfusion pulmonary edema might result.

A thoracostomy tube generally is placed for evacuation of the chest (see "Chest Drainage," p. 218), and the wound is closed. Alternatively, residual air may be aspirated via a needle inserted through an intercostal space after the incision is closed, or through a cannula placed temporarily between sutures of the thoracotomy closure. This cannula is removed after the closure is deemed airtight and when the lungs have been inflated maximally. Aspiration may be via a suction apparatus or a syringe attached to a three-way stopcock.

The rolled towel beneath the patient is removed to facilitate the placement of sutures. A series of five or six interrupted (pericostal) sutures is placed around adjacent ribs (during the patient's expiratory phase, to avoid puncture of a lung) but not tied (Fig. 9-2). Absorbable (e.g., surgical gut or polydioxanone) or monofilament nonabsorbable (e.g., nylon or polypropylene) suture material may be used. Wire should be avoided, as it may cut through the ribs or break at a later date, possibly causing damage to the lung. Before tying the sutures, the ribs are brought together in a natural degree of separation with rib approximators or

Table 9–1. Location of Lateral Thoracotomy Incisions in the Dog and Cat

Thoracic Structure and/or Surgical Problem	Intercostal Space (left side)	Intercostal Space (right side)
Thoracic trachea for collapsing trachea		3
Cranial mediastinum, esophagus (cranial to heart)	3–4	3–4
Patent ductus arteriosus, persistent right aortic arch, pulmonic stenosis	4	
Esophagus (at heart base), cardiopulmonary bypass		4–5
Cranial lung lobe, pericardium	5	5
Middle lung lobe		6
Caudal lung lobe, accessory lung lobe	5–6	5–6
Esophagus (caudal to heart base), diaphragm	7–10	7–10
Thoracic duct, dog		8–10
Thoracic duct, cat	8–10	
Intervertebral disc fenestration T_{10} through L_2	11	11

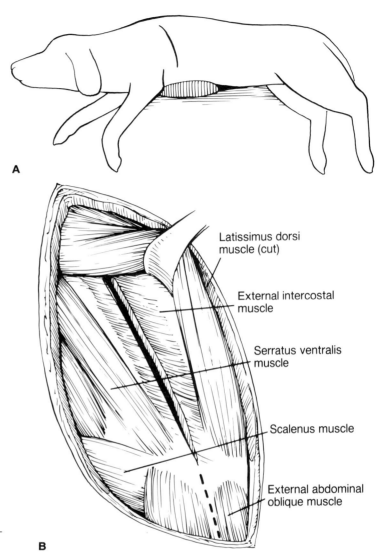

Figure 9-1. *Skin **(A)** and muscular **(B)** incisions for cranial lateral thoracotomy.*

towel clamps or by having the assistant cross the ends of an adjacent suture and apply tension. Excessive closure causes overlap of the caudal over the cranial rib and is unnecessary. To avoid hemorrhage from the intercostal vessels, the blunt rather than the sharp end of the swaged-on needle may be pushed through the intercostal space.

The above closure generally does not create an airtight seal. The more superficial layers of continuous or interrupted sutures generally accomplish that goal when placed (1) in the serratus ventralis and external abdominal oblique muscles, (2) in the latissimus dorsi muscle, and (3) in the cutaneous trunci muscle and subcutaneous tissues. Occasionally, however, it may be possible (but not necessary) to seal the pleural space by closing the parietal pleura and intercostal muscles as a separate layer of simple continuous sutures. In the smallest patients, this may be done without prior pericostal sutures.

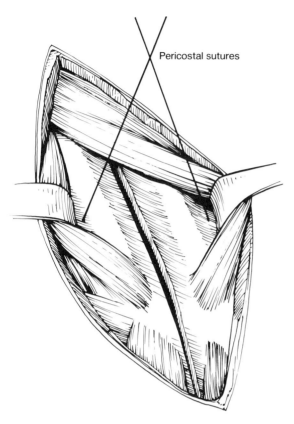

Figure 9-2. *Closure of lateral thoracotomy by pericostal sutures.*

Lateral Thoracotomy With Rib Resection

The approach is as described for intercostal thoracotomy, but once the intercostal muscles and ribs are exposed, a longitudinal incision is made in the periosteum of the rib to be resected, which then is elevated ("stripped") from the bony surface of the rib. The rib is transected with rib cutters at the dorsal and ventral ends of the stripped portions. The former medial portion of the periosteal "hose" then is incised longitudinally, opening the thoracic cavity. Closure is accomplished by a continuous suture placed in the periosteum. Other layers are closed as described above.

Further modifications of the lateral thoracotomy technique include the cranial wall flap, which gives greater exposure.

Median Sternotomy

The sternal-splitting technique is a ventral midline approach to the chest (Figs. 9-3, 9-4) that gives access to both pleural spaces as well as the lungs, mediastinum, and heart. This approach sometimes is combined with a ventral

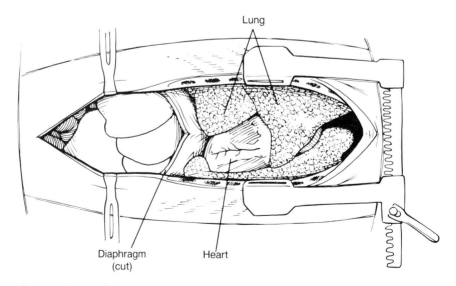

Figure 9-3. *Median sternotomy to approach the thorax; dog's head to the right.*

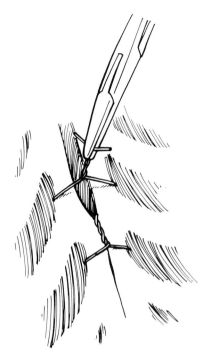

Figure 9-4. *Closure of median sternotomy with wire sutures.*

midline abdominal incision to expose the diaphragm for hernia repair.

With the patient in dorsal recumbency, the ventral and lateral neck, thorax, and abdomen, from the larynx to the umbilicus, are prepared for surgery. A midline skin incision is made over the sternum from cranial to the manubrium to caudal to the xyphoid. The median raphe of the sternum is incised and the pectoral muscles are elevated slightly and retracted laterally. The exposed sternum then is split, using a power-driven oscillating saw, beginning at the fifth sternebra, where the sternum is widest. Thereafter, the incision is extended cranially and caudally through the manubrium and xyphoid, respectively. It may be desirable, however, not to separate the two halves of the sternum completely in large dogs, if exposure of the entire chest is not needed. This reduces sliding of the two sides on each other and postoperative pain. The sternum also may be split, although probably less accu-

rately (especially in cats and small dogs), with an osteotome and mallet or with rib cutters. The ventral part of the diaphragm also may be incised slightly to increase exposure. The internal thoracic arteries and veins are located dorsal and lateral to the sternum. If severed, they bleed profusely and require ligation.

The sternal halves are reapposed with orthopedic wire. Holes for the wire are drilled with a Kirschner wire using a Jacobs chuck, or a large suture needle. The wires are tightened only when all are in place. The cut ends are bent back toward the sternum so they do not protrude into overlying soft tissues. Accurate apposition of the two halves of the sternum is important to prevent immediate postoperative discomfort and to ensure proper healing. Before closure, one or more chest drains are placed in the pleural space, exiting through the lateral chest wall. Subcutaneous tissues and skin over the sternum are closed routinely.

Transsternal Thoracotomy

This rarely used approach essentially is a bilateral intercostal incision that is carried across the ventral midline of the sternum. It has been advocated for cardiac surgery and for repair of diaphragmatic hernia.

Postoperative Management

As surgery nears completion, the vaporizer setting is decreased and finally turned off, allowing recovery from anesthesia. Weaning the patient from oxygen to an oxygen/air mixture is begun. Following skin apposition, residual air in the pleural space is removed by thoracocentesis. The endotracheal tube is disconnected and the rate and depth of spontaneous breathing are evaluated. If tidal and minute volumes are adequate, the patient is allowed to breathe room air and is placed in sternal recumbency, the most physiologic position for matching ventilation and perfusion. Extubation is delayed as long as possible.

If minute volume is inadequate, it may be necessary to aspirate fluids that have collected in the endotracheal tube and tracheobronchial tree, using a sterile catheter. The patient then is turned and positive-pressure respiration is given; these techniques help prevent atelectasis. Overfilling of the lungs or excessive frequency of positive-pressure ventilation should be avoided. Hypocarbia, which can result from hyperventilation, eliminates the most effective stimulus to breathing. During recovery, a laterally recumbent patient must be turned frequently to decrease atelectasis and hypostatic congestion. Respiratory stimulants rarely are needed.

Chest Drainage (Thoracostomy) Tubes

Chest drainage tubes often are indicated for withdrawal of fluid and air from the pleural space after thoracic surgery. Inserting them before closure allows accurate placement. Adequate evacuation helps maintain the integrity of the pleural space, allows the lung lobes to expand fully, and maintains an intrathoracic negative pressure. Chest tubes are indicated following surgery for pneumothorax, pleural effusion, or hemothorax or if there is concern that one of these conditions may develop. The tubes allow monitoring of the rate of accumulation (production/removal) of air or liquid from the chest. Further, they assist in removing infectious exudates, such as empyema, or exudates created when an intrathoracic abscess or mediastinal infection has been drained into the pleural space.

For thoracic drainage (or lavage), a large-bore silastic or polyethylene pediatric pleural catheter with a radiopaque marker (and with a trocar, for closed chest placement) can be used. The marker identifies the location of the tube and the last hole on postoperative radiographs. Tube sizes used for cats and small dogs usually are 10 to 16 French; for large dogs, up to size 32 to 38 French. Several additional side holes may be placed in the tube. Care should be taken not to make the fenestrations too close together or too large, because this may result in weakening of the tube wall, with subsequent kinking or collapse when suction is applied, or tearing on removal, with retention of a tube tip in the chest.

The chest tube is introduced through the mid-thoracic wall, usually one or two interspaces caudal to the incised one (in cranial and mid-thoracic incisions). If needed, drains may be placed bilaterally. A stab skin incision is made, and the skin is moved forward a distance of 1 or 2 interspaces. The tip of a closed curved Kelly forceps is pushed through the intercostal space and out through the stab incision (from within) and used to pull the tip of the catheter into the thoracic cavity. The skin is released, creating a sealing subcutaneous tunnel as it moves back into position. The tube is advanced through the chest until its distal end is in the thoracic inlet area. It is securely fastened to the skin with a purse-string suture (which seals the skin around the tube) affixed to the skin with a butterfly tape or a "Chinese finger trap" friction suture (Fig. 9-5). At this point, if the chest is closed, the external portion of the tube is aspirated and clamped; alternatively, it may be attached to a suction device. If the tube is clamped while bronchopulmonary air leaks continue, particularly with continuing positive-pressure ventilation, tension pneumothorax might develop.

The chest is bandaged so that all tubular connections are accessible for inspection but are covered to prevent trauma to the tubing by the patient. Chest tubes may remain in place for several days; in special cases, a week or more. They require careful ongoing monitoring for patency and protection against leakage at connections.

Intrathoracic negative pressure is maintained by using a one-way Heimlich (flutter) valve (Heimlich Chest Drain Valve, Bard Parker, a division of Becton Dickinson, Rutherford, NJ) (Fig. 9-6), by gravity drainage into a chest bottle with an underwater seal, or by intermittent or continuous aspiration.

Advantages of the Heimlich valve are its small size and simplicity. Air is expelled

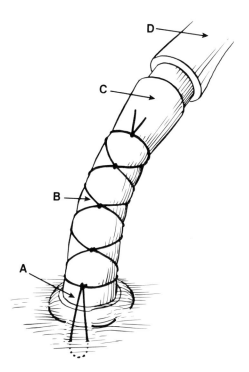

Figure 9-5. *The "Chinese finger trap" friction suture for retention of a thoracostomy tube. The suture first is tied without tension to prevent irritation of the skin* **(A).** *Thereafter, in a criss-cross fashion, multiple surgeon's knots are tied around the tube* **(B)**; *chest catheter* **(C)**; *extension tubing to drainage bottle or to a suction system* **(D).**

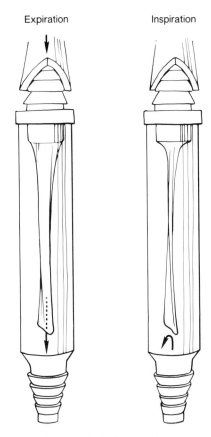

Expiration   Inspiration

Figure 9-6. *The Heimlich flutter valve. During expiration, as intrapleural pressure increases, air is forced out of the pleural space through the tube and the one-way valve. During inspiration, this valve collapses and remains closed so no air can enter the thoracic cavity.*

through the valve during expiration, when intrathoracic pressure increases to above atmospheric level. Dead space in the system is minimal. However, the valve is dangerous if misused; for example, proteinaceous fluid may clot or otherwise adhere to the sides of the valve, preventing drainage. Therefore, fluid production is a contraindication for the Heimlich valve. Careful monitoring of the valve is required, and changing the valve at least every 24 hours is advisable. Some clinicians believe that Heimlich valves should be used only in dogs heavier than 15 kg because smaller animals may have an insufficient tidal volume or intrapleural pressure to allow the drains to work properly. These valves have been very effective, however, in treating pneumothorax,

not only in larger dogs, but in small dogs and even in cats, as long as their use is carefully managed.

Simple gravity drainage can occur via a catheter line inserted into a single drainage bottle, which serves as a water seal, a one-way valve, a manometric control, and a collection reservoir in one bottle. The end of the catheter is attached to a rigid tube submerged in 3 to 5 cm of water in a water seal (air-trap) bottle (equivalent to the center bottle in Fig. 9-7, had the right tube been attached to the chest catheter, with the left tube open to the air). Thus, excess pleural air or liquid will enter the bottle at expiratory pressures greater than 3 to 5 cm

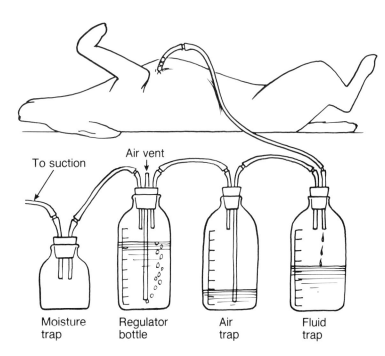

To suction

Air vent

Moisture trap

Regulator bottle

Air trap

Fluid trap

Figure 9-7. *A conventional three-bottle system for drainage. The regulator bottle is known also as the manometer bottle, the air trap as the water seal, and the fluid trap as the collection bottle.*

of water. As the bottle fills, the positive pressure must increase further in the chest before air bubbles through the fluid in the bottle. Reflux from the bottle into the pleural space is avoided by keeping the bottle 20 cm or more below the patient's chest. Managing a catheter line that runs to an underwater seal involves "stripping" to draw thick fluids down the tube, thereby preventing them from accumulating within and blocking the lumen.

In a two-bottle continuous suction system, the second bottle acts as a manometer or regulator. When suction is applied to the system, the negative pressure to the patient equals the depth of the manometer tube in cm H_2O minus the depth of the water seal tube in cm H_2O, with a recommended negative pressure of 10 to 20 cm H_2O. Excessive suction can increase the intrathoracic negative pressure to a point that the lungs may be partially prevented from deflating; according to some clinicians, more than 25 cm of vacuum may cause lung injury or persistence of a pneumopleural fistula.

Negative pressure to the patient de-

creases as fluids accumulate in the water seal bottle of a two-bottle system. This can be avoided by adding a third, fluid trap or collection bottle (right bottle, Fig. 9-7), converting this to a three-bottle system. Several three-bottle systems are on the market; in some, the "bottles" are combined in a single partitioned plastic unit. The latter avoids many of the potentially dangerous tube connections and is easier to use than conventional systems, but it is expensive if used as a disposable unit as recommended by the manufacturer.

An alternative to continuous suction is intermittent suction, in which the chest tubing is attached to a three-way valve and fluid or air is periodically aspirated using a syringe. While this precludes constant elimination of unwanted thoracic contents, it allows accurate estimation of fluid or air production (with continuous suction, air production cannot be estimated). It may also decrease the need for constant patient monitoring, because the tubing is kept under bandages except during aspiration.

The most dangerous complication of chest tube placement is pneumothorax and even death from air leakage. This may occur if segments of the catheter line become disconnected, if the patient bites the tube, if air leaks around the tube because an inadequate subcutaneous tunnel has been created, or if the last hole of the catheter backs out of the thorax. Because of the threat of ascending infection, asepsis is required in placing and managing the tubes. Antibiotic administration has not been proven effective in preventing infection associated with tube placement.

Chest drain tubes should be removed as soon as possible. They are foreign bodies that cause local pleuritis, with the associated production of as much as 100 ml of effusion per day. Most surgeons prefer to remove the tube before the end of the day of surgery, if possible. The tube may be removed if liquid production is less than 5 to 10 ml per hour on several successive aspirations in a medium-sized (15- to 20-kg) dog and if air production is less than 10 ml over a 12-hour period.

Alleviating Post-Thoracotomy Pain

Some patients suffer severe pain after a thoracotomy. Pain may be relieved with potent centrally acting agents such as oxymorphone, 0.05 to 0.1 mg/kg, (Numorphan, Endo Laboratories, Garden City, NY) or butorphanol tartrate, 0.2 to 0.4 mg/kg (Torbugesic, Bristol-Myers, Syracuse, NY). Perineural injections of bupivicaine hydrochloride (Marcaine Hydrochloride with Epinephrine, 1:2,000,000, Breonn Laboratories, Inc., New York, NY), a long-acting local anesthetic, give up to 6 hours of pain relief. If given intraoperatively, 0.25 ml is infiltrated adjacent to the intercostal nerve root in the intercostal space in which the incision was made, and two spaces to each side, cranially and caudally. If given pre- or postoperatively, a subcutaneous wheal of the anesthetic is injected over the rib. The needle is then "walked off" the caudal margin of the rib. Injection accuracy is more difficult, so up to 2 ml per site may be required, depending on the dog's size. Bupivicaine is available in 0.25 and 0.5% concentrations; 0.5% may give longer pain relief.

Complications of Thoracotomy

Most complications of thoracotomy are not associated with entry or closure of the chest, but rather result from procedures carried out within the thorax. These are discussed in other sections. Occasionally, however, an unexplained postoperative lung lobe torsion or chylothorax may occur. Further, subcutaneous edema for 2 to 5 days after surgery may result from trauma or partial disruption of lymphatic drainage after lateral thoracotomy. Subcutaneous seroma formation also occurs occasionally after cranial lateral thoracotomy, often due to inadequate closure of subcutaneous dead space and/or excessive postoperative exercise. Surgical or needle drainage of the seroma may be necessary. Dehiscence of one of the deeper layers, such as the latissimus dorsi muscle, may occur due to improper closure technique, inappropriate choice of suture material, and/or excessive postoperative exercise. Wound infection and partial superficial dehiscence may occur after contaminated surgery (*e.g.,* of the esophagus, of a lung abscess). Chest tubes can become kinked and nonfunctional, allowing fluid or air to accumulate; the tube connections also can leak, the tube may back out of the thorax, or a hole may be chewed, resulting in pneumothorax and death (see "Chest Drainage (Thoracostomy) Tubes," p. 218).

Chest Wall

The thoracic wall includes the thorax (thoracic vertebrae, ribs, and sternum) and its associated skin, fascia, and muscles.

Congenital Defects

Pectus excavatum is a rare congenital deformity of the thorax of dogs and cats. It is characterized by a dorsal depression of the caudal portion of the sternum and the attached costal cartilages, resulting in a ventral concavity of the caudal thoracic wall. Although many animals with this condition are asymptomatic, severely affected kittens and pups may have retarded growth. The deformed sternebrae may interfere with cardiopulmonary function, which can result in exercise intolerance and respiratory distress. Chronic respiratory infection also may be present. In severe cases, excision of the caudal sternum and costal cartilages may be attempted. Alternatively, costal cartilages may be sutured to an external support formed from thermoplastic material that will prevent collapse during further development and calcification of the chest wall structures.

Other abnormalities of the bony thorax include malformed (fused, misshapen, etc.), missing, or extra ribs. Generally, no treatment is required. Repair of spinal column abnormalities, including kyphosis and/or scoliosis, is not suggested. Orchiectomy or ovariohysterectomy is suggested for any animal with congenital deformities because of the possibility of heritability.

Infection

Infection of the ribs and soft tissues of the chest wall can result from direct extension of a pulmonary or pleural infection or, more commonly, from penetrating foreign bodies, bite wounds or other lacerations, or postsurgical wound infection. Once pleuritis is excluded, workup and treatment are as for any soft tissue infection or osteomyelitis. Fungal and/or bacterial culture and bacterial antibiotic sensitivity testing should be performed, followed by appropriate antibacterial or antifungal therapy, and debridement and Penrose tube drain-

age of the infected area. At times, excision of a rib affected with osteomyelitis is necessary. Occasionally, extensive subcutaneous sinus formation necessitates massive skin and subcutaneous soft tissue excision. When costal and intercostal tissues are infected, excising part of the thoracic wall may be necessary to control the infection, to remove a foreign body, or both. Reconstructive procedures and plastic surgical techniques may be needed to repair the resulting defect (see "Reconstructive Surgery," p. 227). A positive contrast fistulogram may help determine the full extent of the infection and its source, such as a foreign body.

Neoplasia

Soft Tissue Tumors

Although a wide variety of soft tissue tumors affect the thoracic wall, lipomas deserve special mention. Occasionally these tumors are large, dissecting between muscular and fascial planes, so their complete removal is difficult without resecting surrounding tissues. A small subcutaneous lipoma may have a larger intrathoracic component. Therefore, before removing a lipoma on the rib cage, thoracic radiography is indicated to define its extent.

Benign Rib Tumors

Osteochondromas are benign, cartilage-capped tumors of dogs and cats that protrude from the cortical surface of the ribs, vertebrae, or other bones, where they may occur singly or in the form of osteochondromatosis. The tumors usually stop growing at the time of skeletal maturation in dogs, and they often are asymptomatic, unless they interfere with adjacent structures. In some cases, most notably in cats, growth may continue, or even accelerate, in mature animals. Rarely, they may transform to osteogenic sarcomas or chondrosarcomas. Local excision of these benign neoplasms should be wide enough to ensure their complete removal.

Malignant Rib Tumors

Most primary and secondary malignant chest wall tumors of dogs and cats arise from the ribs. Although they are rare, osteosarcomas are the most common primary malignant canine rib tumors (infrequently, they are metastatic to the ribs), followed by chondrosarcomas. Other, more unusual primary and secondary tumors of the rib include fibrosarcomas, mast cell sarcomas, multiple myelomas, hemangiosarcomas, and squamous cell carcinomas. Osteosarcomas of the ribs occur in younger dogs (mean 4 to 5 years of age) than do those of the appendicular skeleton (mean 7 to 8 years of age). Rib osteosarcomas and chondrosarcomas are very rare in cats.

Osteosarcomas and chondrosarcomas are hard, painless swellings of the thoracic wall, often at the costochondral junction, usually at or caudal to the fifth rib. Sometimes a small mass on the rib may be attached to a much larger intrathoracic mass—the "iceberg" effect. Although they often are asymptomatic, the presence of large tumors may be associated with weight loss, and dyspnea may result from pulmonary atelectasis due to extensive intrathoracic growth, secondary pleural effusion, and/or pulmonary metastasis. Hypertrophic osteopathy also has been associated with these tumors. Although both types of tumor metastasize, osteosarcomas tend to do so earlier in their course. The lung is the most common site of metastasis, but it also occurs to the pleura, skeletal muscle, heart valves, kidney, liver, and other areas.

Radiography can confirm the presence of a rib tumor and help estimate the extent of intrathoracic and chest wall involvement, pulmonary metastasis, and pleural effusion. It cannot distinguish between osteosarcoma and chondrosarcoma. A fine needle biopsy or pleural fluid cytology may help differentiate an infectious from a neoplastic process, but only histological examination of a biopsy specimen provides a definitive diagnosis.

Treatment of rib tumors is by full-thickness en bloc excision. Large lesions may re-quire resection of multiple ribs and excision of adhesions to underlying structures such as the pericardium, lung, or diaphragm. This is followed by reconstructive chest wall surgery (see "Reconstructive Surgery," p. 227). The margins of the excised tissues should be examined histologically for evidence of tumor. Due to early metastasis, the prognosis for osteosarcomas is poor (less than 10% one-year survival). The prognosis for chondrosarcoma is guarded because affected animals tend to survive longer (approximately 50% three-year survival) and there are some long-term cures. The presence of metastasis or pleural effusion is a poor prognostic sign.

Trauma

Trauma to the chest is common in both dogs and cats. Because the thoracic wall is resilient, particularly in young animals, there may be significant intrathoracic injury without any apparent thoracic wall damage. If there is thoracic wall damage, internal injuries often are very severe. A scheme for assessing patients with acute chest trauma is presented in Figure 9-8.

Penetrating Wounds

Penetrating wounds of the thoracic wall may be caused by weapons (such as bullets, knives, or arrows), bites, or impalement. Even minimal superficial damage, other than a small-diameter hole, may result in open pneumothorax and internal damage that can be quite severe. Concurrent injuries include lacerations of the great vessels causing fatal hemorrhage, cardiac puncture leading to hemopericardium and cardiac tamponade, hemothorax, pneumothorax, pulmonary contusion, and esophageal perforation.

Diagnosis of a penetrating wound is easy if a sucking chest wound or a large foreign body exists, but smaller wounds in long-haired dogs may be more difficult to detect. Visual

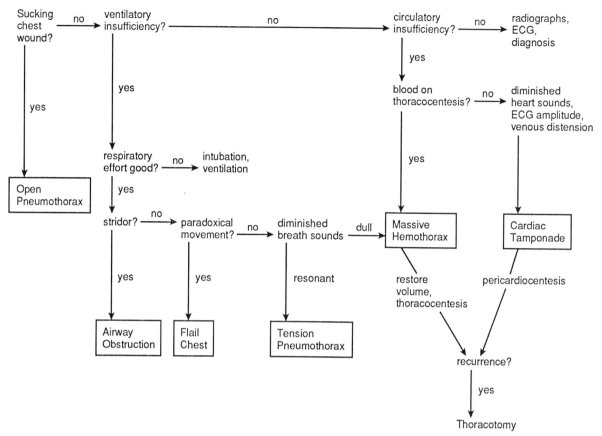

Figure 9-8. *Assessment of acute thoracic injury. (Spackman CJA, Caywood DD. Management of thoracic trauma and chest wall construction. Vet Clin North Am 1987;17:431.)*

examination, palpation, and auscultation help confirm signs of trauma, such as wounds, subcutaneous emphysema, pneumothorax, and hemothorax. Radiography helps confirm pleural space penetration by demonstrating pneumothorax, pleural fluid (hemothorax), and pulmonary hemorrhage.

The first step in treating an open chest wound is to occlude it to prevent further entry of air into the chest. A sterile petrolatum gauze pack or other dressing should be placed over the wound to temporarily close it, converting an open to a closed pneumothorax. The pack should extend 5 cm wider than the wound on all sides and should be taped to the skin. Air is aspirated from the chest via a tube at this time.

The patient should be stabilized medically and then should be prepared for surgical exploration of the wound. Care must be taken when probing a chest wall wound because this may complete a partial penetration, resulting in pneumothorax that had not previously existed. The surgeon should be prepared for positive-pressure ventilation of the patient should entry of the pleural space occur. The skin of the entire side of the thorax should be prepared aseptically because a full-length lateral thoracotomy is needed to explore the pleural space thoroughly and ventral drainage may be needed. If an object lodges in the thoracic wall, the hole may be plugged, preventing pneumothorax. The protruding foreign body should not be removed until radiographs are obtained (depending on the animal's condition) and the thorax is surgically opened. Pneumothorax is discussed in more detail below.

Complications of penetrating chest wounds include infection, with breakdown of the repair, local infection, and/or empyema. Infection is not likely if the source of contamination is eliminated, drainage is established, air or blood is removed, and the lungs are reinflated. Other complications are related to specific internal organ damage.

Bite wounds and sometimes even blunt trauma may result in stripping of intercostal muscles from one or more ribs. This may be associated with herniation of a lung lobe into the subcutaneous space and/or with paradoxical movements of the skin of the chest wall, which must be differentiated from flail chest (see "Flail Chest," below). Subcutaneous muscle may be crushed as well as torn and ribs may be fractured, sometimes resulting in flail chest. In addition, particularly when a cat or a small dog is attacked by a large dog, pulmonary parenchyma and vasculature or other major intrathoracic structures may be damaged. Pulmonary lacerations should be repaired, obviously devitalized muscle should be excised, and contaminated soft tissues debrided. Ribs stripped of intercostal muscle then may be approximated with monofilament synthetic nonabsorbable pericostal sutures. The chest wall must be sealed by suturing any residual intercostal and more superficial muscles. In some animals, extensive chest wall defects require reconstructive surgery (see "Reconstructive Surgery," p. 227).

Initially, a broad-spectrum antibiotic, such as cephalothin (22 mg/kg, IV or SQ, every 6 hours) or trimethoprim—sulfadiazine (Tribrissen, Cooper Animal Health, Kansas City, MO) (15 mg/kg [combined] every 12 hours, SQ) should be administered as for any contaminated wound, later selecting specific therapy based on bacterial culture and antibiotic sensitivity testing. In general, postoperative bandaging of the chest should be avoided. When needed to cover drains, the bandage should be loose to avoid restricting chest excursions and causing hypoxemia.

Blunt Trauma

Blunt trauma to the bony thorax is the most common cause of rib fractures. Most often, simple fractures result. Breaks may occur in several adjacent ribs. Overlying soft tissue damage may be so severe that necrosis occurs and there is not enough healthy tissue to hold sutures. Fractured rib segments may penetrate the skin, but more commonly they cause deeper injury, including pulmonary contusion or laceration of an intercostal artery (hemothorax), lung parenchyma, or, less commonly, the heart, diaphragm, liver, stomach, or gall bladder.

On physical examination, crepitus may be found. The patient with one or more rib fractures is in pain, causing a decreased tidal volume and an increased rate of ventilation. This may result in increased physiologic dead space, retention of secretions, and atelectasis. Radiography allows evaluation of the thoracic contents and the chest wall and usually but not always demonstrates an existing rib fracture (some fractured ribs spring back into position after causing damage).

For patients with nondisplaced rib fractures and no pneumothorax, cage rest is indicated. If the animal is ambulatory, it should be walked to encourage lung expansion. If other orthopedic injuries exist, frequent turning and rolling are essential to prevent hypostatic congestion. Binding the chest with a light bandage provides some pain relief, but further compromises ventilation. Narcotic analgesics may be considered, but because they depress ventilation they should be used with caution. If an analgesic is necessary, butorphanol tartrate, 0.2 to 0.4 mg/kg (Torbugesic, Bristol-Myers, Syracuse, NY), only minimally depresses ventilation. Intercostal nerve blocks may be considered (see "Alleviating Post-Thoracotomy Pain," p. 221).

Cases in which rib fragments are grossly displaced into the pleural cavity are treated surgically to remove the threat of further internal damage. An incision is made over the affected site, parallel to the normal rib bed. By the time muscle separation and fracture reduction are accomplished, the chest is open and controlled ventilation is required. The fracture ends may be fixed internally with an intramedullary Kirschner wire, wire sutures (Fig. 9-9), etc. Alternatively, the rib may be resected. Closure of the pleura and overlying muscle is done in layers and must be airtight.

Flail Chest

Flail chest is a very serious chest wall injury, often associated with dog-bite wounds. It is caused by the fracture of several adjacent ribs, dorsally and ventrally, in two or more places, resulting in a grossly unstable, freely floating region of the chest wall (the flail segment). Paradoxical respiration results: when the patient inspires, the flail segment moves inward (as it would in normal expiration). Conversely, the segment moves outward during expiration. This instability prevents adequate tidal volume and precludes effective coughing. Pleural effusions, damage to the pulmonary parenchyma and other organs, and poor cardiac function may further compromise respiratory function. Respiratory embarrassment is compounded by the accumulation of secretions in the airways, atelectasis, decreased compliance, and patient fatigue. The eventual outcome may be hypoxia, hypercapnia, respiratory acidosis, and cardiac arrhythmias.

Applying a soft compression bandage or temporary traction to the flail segment with a towel clamp will limit inappropriate excursion until the patient can be stabilized, which should occur before definitive therapy. In minor cases, the above treatment may be all that is required. Tracheal intubation through the oropharynx or via tracheostomy with intermittent positive-pressure ventilation may be indicated. With the latter, muscle-blocking agents may allow better ventilation. As surgery begins, the patient must be watched closely for signs of pneumothorax. Pain control may be very important to optimize respiratory effort.

The flail segment may be stabilized by wiring the affected ribs to adjacent normal ribs. Any rib fragments that cannot be repaired probably should be removed. An external aluminum or plastic (Orthoplast, Johnson & Johnson, New Brunswick, NJ) frame apparatus also may be used (Fig. 9-10). In the latter case, under local anesthesia, sutures of heavy monofilament nonabsorbable material, such as nylon, polypropylene, or stainless steel, are

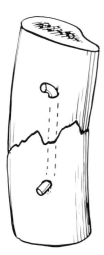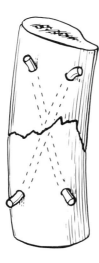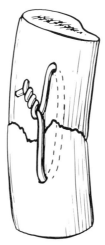

Figure 9-9. *Fractured ribs may be pinned or sutured with surgical wire.*

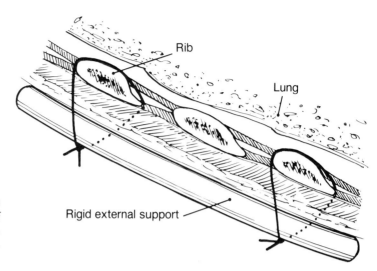

Figure 9-10. *In cases of flail chest, the affected ribs may be secured to a frame of aluminum rod, which prevents medial displacement and reduces paradoxical motion.*

passed around the ribs of the flail segment and tied without tension to the apparatus. Two sutures are placed around each rib to prevent pivoting of the segment around a single row. The splint and sutures are left in place for 2 to 4 weeks; by that time, although the fracture will not have healed, callus formation and soft tissue healing should be adequate to prevent paradoxical movement. Fracture fixation also may be accomplished using wires or pins. Soft tissues often are severely traumatized, but the pleural cavity must be closed at all cost. The primary closure usually can be reinforced by mobilizing and sliding a viable portion of the latissimus dorsi or external abdominal oblique muscles, or both. For extensive avulsion, en bloc excision with reconstructive surgery is necessary (see below).

Pleural drainage is required in pneumothorax or hemothorax. Postoperatively, flail chest patients may be shocky and unstable and may require respiratory assistance or oxygen therapy for several hours. Use of broad-spectrum antibiotics, analgesics, fluids, steroids, warmth, and humidified oxygen may be necessary as well. If treated quickly, many such patients will survive and return to normal. The prospects for recovery are poor with a late or conservative effort.

Reconstructive Surgery

Reconstruction of the thoracic wall usually is required when en bloc resection of three or more ribs is necessary, because the defect created is too large to be closed by apposing remaining soft tissues. Closure may be performed using polypropylene mesh (Marlex mesh, Davol Rubber Co., Providence, RI) with or without an omental pedicle flap, or repositioning the latissimus dorsi or the abdominal muscles. Polypropylene mesh is resistant to infection but generally should not be implanted in an infected wound. It has high tensile strength, can be autoclaved, causes little tissue reaction, and serves as a framework for fibroblastic ingrowth. But if the tissues surrounding the mesh do become infected, draining tracts often result, requiring its removal. This is difficult to do because of tissue ingrowth. A thoracic drain always must be inserted before placing the mesh. The mesh is positioned intrapleurally (Fig. 9-11), and monofilament nylon or polypropylene pericostal sutures are used to attach it to the adjacent ribs. If possible, the latissimus dorsi muscle then is undermined and it is sutured over the graft. A subcutaneous Penrose drain is placed and the wound is closed.

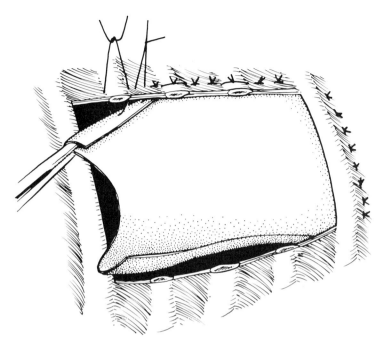

Figure 9-11. *Suture placement to affix polypropylene mesh in chest wall reconstruction. The suture technique shown ensures intrapleural placement of the mesh and a good bond between the mesh and the tissues. A slight lateral pull of the mesh toward the free edge, when placing the sutures under the ribs and to the interosseous musculature, ensures the proper degree of tension on the mesh. Suture placement on the dorsal and right borders is repeated on the ventral and left borders, respectively. The cut edge of the mesh is turned outward as a hem to prevent laceration of the lung during respiratory movement.*

If the overlying musculature had to be removed during the procedure, an omental pedicle flap may be used to cover the mesh, filling the gap and providing additional blood supply. This aids healing and helps prevent infection. A paracostal approach to the abdomen is made, and the omental pedicle is prepared on the greater curvature of the stomach. A subcutaneous tunnel is created between the two skin incisions, through which the pedicle is drawn. One or more layers of the flap are sutured over the mesh to the soft tissues at the edge of the defect, using 2-0 or 3-0 nylon or polypropylene. Using similar sutures, the paracostal incision is partially closed (leaving a gap of approximately 5 cm to prevent strangulation of the pedicle), and the omentum is tacked to the abdominal musculature, just cranial to the paracostal incision. If the deeper thoracic wall is airtight, subcutaneous Penrose drains may be placed both at the abdominal and thoracic surgical sites before skin closure. Both incision sites are bandaged until the drains are removed, usually after 3 to 5 days.

Mesh may not be able to prevent paradoxical movement in large thoracic wall defects. In such cases, plastic spinal fixation plates (Lubra plate, Lubra Co., Fort Collins, CO) are affixed to the cut edge of the rib with orthopedic wire, and the polypropylene mesh is placed superficial to the plates.

Large defects of the most caudal and the most rostral parts of the lateral thoracic wall often can be closed without mesh or rib prostheses. A defect in the chest wall, from the 9th to the 13th rib, may be closed by moving the diaphragmatic edge cranial to the defect and suturing it to the epaxial and intercostal muscles with nylon or polypropylene sutures. This converts a thoracic to an abdominal defect. Closure involves a transpositional flap from the transversus abdominus muscle, if necessary. The size of the thoracic cavity is reduced by this procedure, but not enough to cause respiratory compromise. Similar muscle-movement closure can be achieved for extensive defects of the cranial chest wall—ribs 1 to 5 can be replaced by sewing together the latissimus dorsi, scalenus, and external abdominal muscles, without the need to implant a prosthesis.

Pleural Space

Anatomy and Physiology

The pleura is a serous membrane lining the thoracic cavity. It is composed of a mesothelial cell layer and a subjacent layer of elastic connective tissue, rich in lymphatic and blood vascular channels. The parietal pleura includes costal, mediastinal, and diaphragmatic components. The visceral pleura invests the lungs. The mediastinum is functionally incomplete in dogs and cats, so pleural fluids and air tend to distribute bilaterally. Sporadic reports of unilateral effusions and pneumothorax probably are due in part to mediastinal thickening from inflammation, fibrosis, etc. Diaphragmatic pores and lymphatics also allow some communication between the pleural and peritoneal cavities.

Normally, the visceral and parietal pleurae slide readily on each other due to a small amount of lubricating fluid (2 to 3 ml in a 10-kg dog) in the pleural space. According to some investigators, the fluid is formed primarily by the parietal pleura and absorbed by the visceral pleura, based on differences between systemic and pulmonary capillary hydrostatic pressures (Fig. 9-12). Other investigators say the systemic bronchial vessels are the source of visceral pleural capillaries, so production and absorption occur from both surfaces. Pleural fluid turnover is a very active process (about 5 L/day in a large dog). Protein and cells are removed primarily by subserosal lymphatics; electrolytes and water are absorbed mainly by visceral blood capillaries. When excess fluid is present, lymphatics also drain fluid and electrolytes. In cats, the mediastinal lymphatics are most involved in resorption. Respiratory movements enhance lymphatic flow. Colloids pass between mesothelial and endothelial cells; the ability to pass depends on molecular size. For example, albumin and small globular proteins pass easily but larger globulins, lipids, and lipoproteins remain in the blood. Cells pass between endothelial and mesothelial cells. Normal fluid has less than 500 cells/μl and less than 1.5 gm of protein/dl.

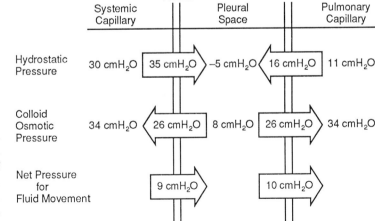

Figure 9-12. *Hydrostatic, colloid osmotic, and net Starling pressures that influence the movement of fluid into and out of the pleural space. (Orton EC. Pleura and pleural space. In: Slatter DH, ed. Textbook of small animal surgery. Philadelphia: WB Saunders, 1985:547.)*

Thoracocentesis

Needle Thoracocentesis

In thoracocentesis, fluid or air is aspirated from the pleural space for diagnostic and/or therapeutic purposes. Needle thoracocentesis usually is performed in the 6th to the 9th intercostal space and on the right side, because the presence of the cardiac notch on that side decreases the chance of inadvertently injuring the lung. Hair is removed from an area 7.5 to 10 cm in diameter around the aspiration site, and the area is prepared for surgery aseptically to avoid iatrogenic contamination. Normally, neither local anesthesia nor tranquilizers is necessary. To avoid lung damage, in cases of pneumothorax the needle should be inserted two thirds up the chest wall from the sternum while the patient is in a standing or sternal recumbent position, because the partially collapsed lungs tend to drop ventrad, out of the way of the needle. It also may be inserted at a point midway between the sternum and the spinal column, with the patient in a lateral recumbent position, because the lung falls away from the chest wall. For pleural effusion, the needle is inserted in the lower third of the intercostal space while the patient is standing, because the lungs tend to float above the site of needle insertion and this position is most comfortable for the patient. An 18- or 20-gauge needle is inserted into the pleural cavity midway between the ribs, to avoid the intercostal vessels. It is then attached to a sterile extension tube, a three-way valve, and a syringe. To decrease the likelihood of lacerating the lung, needle movement should be minimized, and after passing through the pleura the needle tip should be angled so the point is against the parietal pleura, with the bevel facing the pleural space. To further decrease the possibility of iatrogenic lung damage, a blunt-tipped teat cannula (the insertion of which first requires a small skin incision) or

an over-the-needle intravenous catheter may replace the needle.

Tube Thoracostomy

Tube thoracostomy is indicated if frequent or more thorough evacuation of the pleural space is required than is possible with needle thoracocentesis, if pleural lavage is indicated, or if the effusion is viscous. A tube also is less likely to lacerate the lung than is repeated needle aspiration. Hair is removed from an area 10 to 15 cm in diameter, and the skin is prepared and draped as if for sterile surgery. The site of incision is moved cranially two intercostal spaces so it overlies the site of penetration into the thoracic cavity (same location as for needle thoracocentesis, above). A local anesthetic is injected from skin to pleura over the region of tube insertion, and a small skin incision is made. The catheter tip then is placed into the incision and is thrust through the intercostal space. Either a commercially available catheter with a trocar-pointed stylet is used, or the tube may be inserted while its end is held between the tips of the jaws of a Carmalt or Kelly forceps. The stylet or the forceps then is removed and the skin is allowed to slide back into its normal position, creating a two-intercostal space sealing tunnel that prevents entry of air along the tube and into the chest. The tube then is clamped rapidly, attached to suction or a three-way valve and managed as discussed earlier in "Chest Drainage (Thoracostomy) Tubes."

Pneumothorax

Pneumothorax is the accumulation of air or gas in the pleural space. It may be classified by etiology (i.e., spontaneous, traumatic, or iatrogenic) and pathophysiology (i.e., open or closed). In open pneumothorax, there is free communication between the pleural space and the external environment; in closed pneumothorax, there is not.

Pathophysiology

The severity of the effects of pneumothorax is directly related to the volume of air in the pleural space. Tachypnea, often the first response to a small amount of pleural air, progresses to hyperventilation (with increased rate and depth of respiration) as the volume increases. When air enters the pleural space, although the lungs collapse due to their elastic recoil, the elastic thoracic wall expands. Therefore, the net decrease in functional lung volume may be only half that of the air entering the pleural space. The intercostal, caudal cervical, and cranial abdominal muscles and the diaphragm become involved in forced respiration. As pneumothorax increases, compensatory mechanisms fail, hypoxemia and respiratory acidemia become severe, and death can result. The loss of intrapleural negative pressure decreases venous return to the heart and, therefore, cardiac output and systemic arterial pressure. Mediastinal and cardiac position shifts may cause the conus venosus to kink, further decreasing venous return.

Tension pneumothorax exists when intrapleural pressure becomes equal to or greater than atmospheric pressure. It results from a one-way valve effect, usually in closed pneumothorax, in which air enters the pleural space but cannot escape. The patient shows progressive respiratory distress and less effective respiration until the chest becomes barrel-shaped and fixed in maximal expansion. The combination of underventilation and decreased cardiac output leads to total cardiopulmonary failure, shock, and death, unless emergency evacuation of the chest is performed. Administering oxygen therapy and inserting a needle into the chest to relieve intrapleural positive pressure can be lifesaving first steps.

Traumatic Pneumothorax

Trauma is the most frequent cause of pneumothorax in dogs and cats. Pneumothorax occurs in nearly half of canine chest injury patients and in about 20% of cats and dogs suffering automobile trauma. Penetrating chest wounds are termed "sucking" wounds when the influx of air into the chest during inspiration is accompanied by a characteristic sound. If the wound is large, intrapleural and extrapleural pressures are equal; if it is smaller than the opening of the glottis, some negative intrapleural pressure is maintained. Rarely, a flap-like effect results in open tension pneumothorax.

Direct blunt trauma to the chest or indirect trauma to the abdomen or limbs can cause bronchial or pulmonary damage and closed pneumothorax. The transfer of pressure into the chest may increase bronchopulmonary pressure in the presence of a closed glottis, causing a blow-out, causing shearing forces to develop between organs of different inertias, or causing pulmonary tissue to tear because of fractured ribs. Occasionally, closed pneumothorax results from rupture of the esophagus or trachea, even in the cervical region, because air will migrate down tissue planes and, with rupture of the mediastinum, into the pleural space. Such cases often are associated with subcutaneous emphysema and pneumomediastinum.

Often, the injury results from a fall from a height, a dog fight, a gun-shot or knife wound, a motor vehicle accident, or similar trauma. Clinical signs include varying degrees of dyspnea, associated with tachypnea and anxiety, and frothy blood may exude from the nose and mouth. In severe cases, cyanosis, pale mucous membranes, open-mouth breathing, and signs of tension pneumothorax may develop (see "Pathophysiology," above). Cutaneous hemorrhage, subcutaneous emphysema, a penetrating foreign body, or a sucking or gaping chest wound may be detected, associated with fractured ribs, flail chest, and abdominal breathing. Auscultation of the chest may reveal an absence of normal pulmonary sounds dorsally and muffled cardiac sounds ventrally. The chest may be hyperresonant on percussion or even tympanic if tension pneumothorax exists.

The diagnosis often may be made on the basis of the history, clinical signs, and physical examination. If the diagnosis is obvious and the patient is extremely dyspneic, immediate thoracocentesis is indicated. Further workup should be done after the patient is stabilized. Radiography confirms the presence of pneumothorax and provides a baseline for evaluation of progress. Classically, the air-filled pleural space is wider than normal and the lung margins are retracted from the chest wall, particularly in a horizontal beam recumbent or standing lateral view. In a vertical beam recumbent lateral view, the heart appears to have moved dorsal to the sternum. This is due to a pendulum effect in which the apex of the heart shifts toward the lower lung, which is no longer expanded adequately to support the heart in its normal position. In some instances, pneumothorax may be observed primarily or (rarely) wholly on one side, accompanied by mediastinal shift. Traumatic pneumatocysts occasionally may be observed radiographically. Bronchoscopy may allow tears of the tracheobronchial tree to be located.

Spontaneous Pneumothorax

This condition, which tends to recur, results from pulmonary leakage occurring without known trauma. Although sometimes called "idiopathic," it is secondary to pulmonary lesions, such as congenital cysts, bullae, blebs, bullous emphysema, chronic obstructive pulmonary disease, granulomas, pneumonia, abscesses, or neoplasia, which may not be readily identifiable without surgery. In more than 80% of cases in dogs, the right lung is affected. Deep-chested breeds of dogs (average

age of 6 years) are affected, though there is no specific breed or sex predilection. Cats are affected infrequently. Presurgical localization of the leak to one lung may not be possible, although radiographic evidence of an underlying lesion or greater collapse of one lung may suggest the affected side. Expanding the lungs by evacuating air from the chest increases the likelihood of identifying a primary pulmonary lesion. Pleural effusion may accompany pneumothorax. If so, bubbles, a fluid line, or both may be visible on radiographs.

Laboratory studies should include a complete blood count and a serum chemistry profile and electrolyte assay, for evidence of underlying infection or systemic disease. Arterial blood gas evaluation often is important. Tachypnea may result in respiratory alkalemia. As tissue hypoxia progresses, metabolic acidemia with respiratory compensation occur, and with respiratory failure hypoxemia and respiratory acidemia develop.

Iatrogenic Pneumothorax

Iatrogenic pneumothorax may occur at the time of chest tube placement or removal or may be due to dehiscence of thoracotomy incisions, thoracic disc fenestration, celiotomy for diaphragmatic hernia, rupture of the trachea due to overinflation of an endotracheal tube, etc. Closed pneumothorax may result from percutaneous lung biopsy, or barotrauma from overinflation of the lungs. The latter can lead to tension pneumothorax.

Treatment of Pneumothorax

Treatment varies with the cause, magnitude, and clinical signs. Open chest wounds require emergency treatment (see "Penetrating Wounds," p. 223). If the diagnosis of closed pneumothorax is obvious and the patient is extremely dyspneic, immediate thoracocentesis is indicated. Minor lacerations of the pulmonary parenchyma often heal spontaneously, so if the degree of closed pneumothorax and clinical signs are not severe, careful monitoring and cage rest for 48 hours may be all that is needed. Cage rest decreases pulmonary movement and pleural friction, which promotes fibrin sealing of minor bronchial and pulmonary tears. Excitement or restraint should be minimal to avoid respiratory arrest.

The pleura is permeable to gases. Normally, pleural pressure is approximately -5 cm H_2O in relation to atmospheric pressure. Because the total pressure of gases in the systemic venous blood is -73 cm H_2O, gases tend to be pulled from the pleural space into the capillaries, at a rate of absorption of about 1.25% of the air volume per day. Inhalation of oxygen increases the rate of resorption to about 4.2% per day.

Thoracocentesis should be performed if the magnitude of pneumothorax is sufficient to cause clinical signs of dyspnea. Needle thoracocentesis is adequate for treating small leaks (see p. 230). If, following aspiration, radiography and clinical signs show slow recurrence of pneumothorax, a second aspiration should be performed. If more than two thoracocenteses are needed within 24 hours or if tension pneumothorax exists, tube thoracostomy is indicated (see "Tube Thoracostomy," p. 230).

Should pneumothorax continue to develop after tube placement, without evidence of decreasing formation, if there are more than two recurrent episodes of spontaneous pneumothorax, or if a source of leakage (a radiographic lesion) is identified, thoracotomy is indicated. If the affected side is known, lateral thoracotomy is performed; if it is not, median sternotomy is suggested. Bilateral lesions are commonly encountered. The recurrence rate after surgical intervention for spontaneous pneumothorax in the dog is nearly 25%. When diffuse disease is found, or if it is recurrent, pleurodesis should be considered (see "Pleurodesis," p. 242).

Pleural Effusion

Etiology

A pleural effusion is an abnormal accumulation of fluid within the pleural space. The causes of various types of effusions are presented in Table 9-2. Pleural effusion results from interference with pleural fluid reabsorption or, more often, from excess fluid production. The rapid turnover of pleural fluid (as much as 75% each hour) determines and alters its composition.

Diagnosis

History and Clinical Signs

Often, there is no relevant history except for recent or past trauma in some cases. Minor effusions generally cause few or no signs. Larger effusions decrease lung expansion and increase abnormalities in gas exchange, resulting in dyspnea and rapid, shallow breathing. Patients prefer standing or recumbent sternal positions to recumbent lateral positions. Lethargy, decreased exercise tolerance, open-mouth breathing with extension of the head and neck, and cyanosis may be seen. Coughing usually is due to underlying pulmonary disease rather than to the effusion. Nonspecific signs, such as anorexia, malaise, and weight loss may be present, depending on the underlying etiology. A barrel-chest appearance may exist in animals with chronic effusion, due to prolonged respiratory effort. Animals with significant signs should not be restrained, manipulated, or excited excessively lest respiratory arrest result.

Auscultation allows detection of ventrally muffled respiratory and cardiac sounds. Normal sounds may be heard dorsal to the horizontal level of fluid accumulation. Percussion of the chest reveals ventral dullness. Infrequently, these changes are unilateral. Animals with inflammatory effusion also may have fever and show painful respiration.

Radiography

Radiography confirms the presence of pleural fluid, estimates its volume, and helps determine a suitable site for thoracocentesis. In order to show up on radiographs, about 50 ml must be present in the pleural space of a cat or a small dog and about 100 ml in a larger dog. Small amounts of fluid may be detected more readily by using the erect position with an horizontal beam. Although ventrodorsal and lateral recumbent views are best for detecting pleural effusion, dorsoventral and horizontal beam standing views usually are adequate for diagnosis and avoid excessive and dangerous restraint during radiography. A series of horizontal beam projections help discriminate free fluid from solid masses or trapped or encapsulated fluid. Positive contrast pleurograms also may be helpful for this.

Table 9–2. Causes of Pleural Effusion

Pure Transudate
Hypoalbuminemia

Modified Transudate
Congestive heart failure
  Cardiomyopathy
  Cardiac anomalies
  Pericardial effusion
  Feline hyperthyroidism
Ascites
Nephrotic syndrome
Pulmonary atelectasis
Lung-lobe torsion
Diaphragmatic hernia
Thromboemboli
Mediastinal tumors
Other tumors

Chylous Effusion
True chylous effusion
  Congenital
  Trauma
  Neoplasia
  Lymphangiectasia
  Cardiac failure
    Cardiomyopathy
  Fungal granuloma
  Obstructed cranial vena cava
  Diaphragmatic hernia
  Dirofilariasis
  Sepsis
  Idiopathic

Pseudochylous Effusion
  Cardiomyopathy
  Chronic pleural effusion
  Idiopathic

Inflammatory Exudates
Nonseptic Inflammatory Exudate
  Feline infectious peritonitis
  Post-thoracic surgery
  Sterile foreign bodies
  Chest drains
  Chronic pleural effusion
  Diaphragmatic hernia
  Esophageal or pulmonary parasites
  Viral infections
  Steatitis
  Idiopathic

Septic Inflammatory Exudate
  Extension from thoracic structures
  Hematogenous
  Foreign body
  Penetrating wounds

Neoplastic Effusion
Primary
  Mesothelioma

Secondary
  Adenocarcinoma (bronchogenic, bronchoalveolar)
  Lymphoma (mediastinal)
  Mast cell sarcoma
  Metastatic neoplasia

Hemorrhagic Effusion
  Trauma
  Pulmonary infarction
  Lung lobe torsion
  Neoplasia
  Thoracic surgery
  Coagulopathies
  Idiopathic

(Modified from Christopher MM. Pleural effusion. Vet Clin North Am 1987;17:255.)

Common radiographic signs of pleural effusion include a homogeneous, water density within the thorax, interlobar pulmonary fissure lines, rounded lung margins at the costophrenic angles, separation of the borders of the lungs from the thoracic wall, scalloping of the lung border dorsal to the sternum, masking of the cardiac and diaphragmatic silhouettes, and fluid lines (in the presence of hydropneumothorax when horizontal beam radiography is used). The pleura itself usually cannot be detected unless there is fibrin deposition or fibrosis or calcification in association with chronic disease. The cause may not be detectable until fluid is removed from the chest, which may require bilateral drainage.

Fluid Evaluation

Usually, analysis of 5 ml or more of fluid is required for diagnosis. Therapeutic thoracocentesis should occur simultaneously, if necessary. Cytologic evaluation is most important for diagnosis. A sample for cytology should be collected in EDTA to avoid clotting, and direct smears should be prepared before performing other procedures, because cell morphology may change rapidly. Depending on the total cell count, it may be necessary to concentrate the cells by centrifugation and prepare smears from the sediment. Occasionally, a specific etiologic diagnosis may be made by examining the smear (*e.g.*, finding a fungus or identifying tumor cells). Samples collected in sterile tubes should undergo aerobic and anaerobic bacterial and/or fungal culture and antibiotic sensitivity testing. These samples may be discarded if other analyses suggest that culture is unnecessary. Three or four milliliters are placed in a tube for physicochemical evaluation, which along with cytologic examination aids in classifying the fluid (see Table 9-3). The sample also is tested for odor, the presence of chylomicrons, and cholesterol and triglyceride concentrations.

Table 9–3.   Characteristics of Transudates and Exudates

	Pure Transudate	Modified Transudate	Exudate
Turbidity	Clear	Variable	Turbid
Viscosity	Low	Variable	High
Color	Pale-straw	Variable	Variable[c]
Protein	<1.0 gm/dl	1.5–3.0 gm/dl[a]	>3.0 gm/dl
Specific Gravity	<1.005	1.012–1.018	>1.018
Nucleated Cell Count	<500/μl	1,000–5,000/μl	>5,000/μl[d]
Cell Types	Mesothelial cells and occasional lymphocytes and monocytes	Variable[b]	Variable[e,f]

[a] May reach 5 to 7 gm/dl, especially when lymph is present, and/or due to obstruction.

[b] Variably present are reactive mesothelial cells, neutrophils, eosinophils, plasma cells, lymphocytes, mast cells, and erythrocytes. An inflammatory component may develop in obstructive effusions if organ or tumor necrosis occurs, so increased neutrophils and macrophages may be present. In chronic transudates, long-lived cells such as lymphocytes may predominate, and plasma cells may increase in numbers.

[c] Septic inflammatory exudates may be sanguineous, brown, or tan, or may be typical of green or white pus.

[d] The neutrophil count, especially in acute septic inflammatory exudates, may reach 100,000/μl.

[e] Nonseptic inflammatory exudates contain, predominantly, nondegenerate hypersegmented neutrophils, plus variable number of macrophages, lymphocytes, and erythrocytes.

[f] The neutrophils of acute septic inflammatory exudates usually are degenerate, indicating the effect of bacterial toxins. The degeneracy is correlated with the severity of infection. In chronic septic inflammatory exudates, up to 30% of the cells are actively phagocytizing. Lymphocytes and plasma cells also are present in increased numbers.

(Modified from Christopher MM. Pleural effusions. Vet Clin North Am 1987;17:255.)

Treatment

Pleural drainage is indicated to treat respiratory distress. Specific therapy varies with the type and cause of the effusion (see below).

Transudates—Hydrothorax

Hydrothorax is the presence of a pleural transudate. The various causes of transudates are presented in Table 9-2, and their physical and cellular characteristics in Table 9-3. Pure, modified, and chronic transudates occur.

Pure Transudates

Hypoalbuminemia, which decreases plasma osmotic pressure, is the sole cause of a pure pleural transudate. Abdominal effusion and pitting edema of the extremities may be concurrent. The causes of hypoalbuminemia (*e.g.*, malnutrition, portosystemic shunt, hepatic cirrhosis, protein-losing enteropathy, and glomerulonephropathy) must be treated to prevent continued fluid formation.

Modified Transudates

Long-standing pure transudates become modified transudates as exfoliating mesothelial cells, erythrocytes, and/or inflammatory cells increase in number. Modified transudates are subclassified as obstructive effusions, neoplastic effusions, or chronic transudates. Only neoplastic effusions (discussed separately, below) present specific cytologic appearances.

Obstructive effusions result from passive congestion. The most frequent cause is cardiac failure; other causes are lung-lobe torsion or incarceration of a liver lobe in a diaphragmatic hernia. In such cases, transudation of fluid occurs due to elevated hydrostatic pressure, secondary to obstruction of venous and lymphatic drainage. Chronic transudates from any cause appear similar (see Table 9-3).

Inflammatory Exudates

The presence of an exudate is a sign of an inflammatory disease involving the pleural surface. Fluid accumulates because of increased capillary permeability due to inflammation or endotoxemia. Inflammatory exudates may be nonseptic or septic.

Nonseptic Inflammatory Exudate

A nonseptic inflammatory exudate may have some characteristics of both transudates and exudates (see Table 9-3). It usually arises by continued modification of a transudate, but there are other causes (see Table 9-2). After thoracic surgery, a nonseptic effusion may develop as a response to surgical trauma or to the continued presence of a thoracic drain. Treatment usually involves removing the inciting cause, followed by chest drainage (unless it is caused by a drain). Feline infectious peritonitis virus causes a viscous, yellow, turbid nonseptic effusion.

Septic Inflammatory Exudates

Purulent pleuritis, also known as pyothorax, or empyema, results from bacterial or fungal infection. Infection arises due to penetrating thoracic wounds, particularly the following: animal bites; extension from pneumonia; migrating foreign bodies, such as grass awns; esophageal perforation; and extension of cervical, lumbar, or mediastinal infections.

Presentation often is delayed due to an insidious course. The diagnosis is based on typical signs, radiographic evidence of pleural fluid, and fluid analysis. Clinical signs include respiratory distress and evidence of systemic infection, such as fever and malaise.

Bacteria usually cause acute septic inflammatory exudates, but fungal infections commonly cause chronic exudates. Typical characteristics of septic exudates are presented in Table 9-3. Centrifugation of septic exudates yields a clear supernatant, distinguishing them from chylous or pseudochylous effusions.

Culture always should be performed before starting antibiotic therapy. Bacteria may be seen in the cytoplasm of neutrophils, or extracellularly in overwhelming infections, in new methylene blue or Wright-stained cytologic smears. Gram stains may give early partial identification of the causative agent(s). Organisms isolated from canine cases commonly are the anaerobic filamentous rod *Nocardia asteroides* and the anaerobe *Fusobacterium*; from feline cases, *Pasteurella multocida* and anaerobes. Other causative obligate anaerobes include *Bacteroides, Fusarium,* and *Peptostreptococcus,* often mixed with facultative anaerobes. Filamentous bacteria, including *Actinomyces* spp. and *Nocardia asteroides* may be associated with the presence of sulfur granules. Culturing these organisms is difficult. *Streptococcus, Escherichia coli,* and *Corynebacterium* are commonly isolated aerobic bacteria. Many other causative agents have been reported, including *Proteus, Enterobacter, Pseudomonas,* spirochetes, *Aspergillus,* and *Cryptococcus.*

Treatment must be aggressive to succeed. Emergency treatment includes relieving respiratory embarrassment by tube thoracocentesis. If the patient is in acute distress, in which case tube thoracocentesis would be dangerous, needle thoracocentesis should be performed. Intravenous fluids should be given to correct dehydration and acid-base and electrolyte disturbances. After collecting fluid for aerobic and anaerobic culture and antibiotic sensitivity testing, systemic antibiotic therapy should be started. An initial combination of sodium penicillin G (40,000 units/kg every 6 hours) and gentamycin (2.2 mg/kg every 8 hours) has been useful; the treatment should be modified as indicated by the culture results.

Medical treatment includes pleural drainage and lavage, via a thoracostomy tube placed on one or both sides as necessary, once the patient is stable. After fluid evacuation, the pleural space is lavaged by injecting 20 ml/kg of warm lactated Ringer's solution twice daily, then draining the fluid 1 hour later. Proteolytic enzymes, such as chymotrypsin (50,000 units/100 ml of lavage), added to the lavage fluid may help digest exudative debris, although not all clinicians consider this effective. About 25% of the fluid is absorbed during the 1-hour wait. Although the intrathoracic administration of antibiotics after lavage has not been proven effective, some clinicians advocate injecting half the systemic antibiotic dose by this route.

Surgical exploration is indicated if improvement does not occur within 72 hours, if encapsulated fluid cannot be drained, or if radiography shows nonresolving lung consolidation (indicating a possible pulmonary abscess) or an intrathoracic foreign body. Exploration is by median sternotomy if the condition appears to be bilateral. Lateral thoracotomy is adequate for the occasional unilateral empyema. The goals of surgery are:

1. Detecting the source of infection;
2. Disrupting adhesions and freeing loculated fluid, to encourage uniform drainage;
3. Excising infected tissue, including the ventral mediastinum (which may consist of a large soft granulomatous mass that is distinctly different from normal mediastinal pleura; removal of the ventral mediastinum also allows bilateral drainage and lavage from a single chest tube);
4. Removing consolidated lung tissue, which may already be or may become a source of infection;
5. Decorticating the lung, to help prevent or treat constrictive pleuritis (see below); and
6. Providing thorough lavage with warm isotonic fluid and proper placement of chest drains.

Postoperative lavage is continued for 2 or 3 days. The prognosis for successful treatment of septic pleuritis is guarded to poor, but not hopeless. Many animals respond well to early appropriate therapy.

Constrictive Pleuritis

Constrictive pleuritis is a serious sequela of septic pleuritis or trauma to the chest. Pleural adhesions and a fibroelastic pleural peel form due to fibrin deposition, resulting in an inability to fully inflate the lungs. Pleural thickening is seen radiographically. If the condition is diffuse, surgical dissection (decortication) of the visceral pleural peel may be necessary. This is easiest to perform within 5 weeks of the pleural insult, before fibrous infiltration of the visceral pleura. Thereafter, decortication becomes difficult and dangerous because it is easy to lacerate the lungs. The pleural peel is torn and undermined initially at the hilus or mediastinum, then the edge facing the lung is worked free by digital and blunt instrument dissection. Referral is suggested.

Chylous Effusions

Chylous effusions are milky, white or pink, opaque modified transudates or exudates. There are two kinds of chylous effusions: true chylous and pseudochylous.

True Chylous Effusions

True chylous effusions result from the accumulation of chyle in the pleural space, causing chylothorax. True chylous effusions contain 0.2 to 0.8 μm lipid droplets called chylomicrons that move by Brownian motion on wet-mounted slides, stain with lipophilic dyes (such as the orange dye Sudan III), and form a chylomicron band on lipoprotein electrophoresis. They separate into an opaque upper fatty "cream" layer and a lower aqueous layer on standing or after centrifugation. Their opacity often clears after adding ether and shaking, but sometimes only if the fluid is alkalinized with sodium bicarbonate. In chronic chylous effusions, however, the concomitant inflammatory response may prevent complete clearing of the fluid (see below). The specific gravity of chylous effusions generally is greater than 1.012, often over 1.020, with protein concentrations of 2.0 to 6.0 gm/dl.

A true chylous effusion is much higher in its triglyceride concentration than is the serum, and the cholesterol is low (the cholesterol:triglyceride ratio is less than 1.0). This is the most reliable means of distinguishing between true chylous and pseudochylous effusions, although effusions with intermediate characteristics do arise. Especially in early chylothorax, the cells in the effusion are predominantly small lymphocytes with some larger lymphocytes, 1 to 2% blast cells, and other inflammatory cells and mesothelial cells. The underlying cause may be masked by con-

tamination with hemorrhage, iatrogenic infection due to contaminated thoracocentesis, or a nonseptic inflammatory response, particularly in long-term chylous effusions (perhaps due to the irritative nature of the chyle). Because of inflammation, in many (perhaps most) true chylous effusions the predominant cells are neutrophils (13 of 19 in one series) and less often macrophages (4 of 19 in the same series).

Pseudochylous Effusions

The milky, opalescent appearance of pseudochylous effusions is caused by the presence of lecithin-globulin complexes or cholesterol granules. Often, these effusions arise from the products of degeneration of exfoliated mesothelial, inflammatory, or tumor cells; the specific gravity of these fluids usually is less than 1.016. They do not contain chylomicrons, they generally do not separate into creamy and aqueous layers on standing or after centrifugation, they do not clear with ether, their cholesterol concentrations are higher than that of the serum, and their triglyceride concentrations are low.

Chylothorax

Although in most cases the etiology of chylothorax is idiopathic, in many and perhaps most instances it appears to result from inhibition to drainage of the thoracic duct into the great veins. This may be caused by obstruction of the duct or the cranial vena cava, or from right-sided heart failure (which also causes increased hepatic lymph production). The obstruction leads to lymphatic hypertension, lymphangiectasia, and increased thoracic duct permeability and the formation of a true chylous effusion (see "Chylous Effusions," above). In some cases, this is associated with intestinal lymphangiectasia. Other causes of thoracic duct obstruction (and invasion or rupture) include thoracic neoplasia (5 of 34 dogs with chylothorax in one series), cranial mediastinal neoplasia (particularly lymphoma in the cat), and fungal infection. Trauma (5 of 34 in one series), including blunt external trauma and trauma secondary to thoracic surgery, is another possible cause of chylothorax. Although laceration of the thoracic duct has been implicated as a cause, this has not been documented in dogs or cats. Afghan dogs are at greater risk of developing idiopathic chylothorax than other breeds (8 of 24 cases in one series), perhaps associated with congenital thoracic duct anomalies (one has been reported). Lung-lobe torsion has been associated with chylothorax. It is more likely that chylothorax precedes, rather than follows, the development of lung-lobe torsion, but this has not been confirmed. Feline chylothorax has been associated with cardiomyopathy, diaphragmatic hernia, dirofilariasis, and lymphangiectasia.

Diagnosis

Fluid evaluation is necessary to distinguish chylothorax from other pleural effusions (see "Fluid Evaluation," p. 235). Ultrasonography can help identify a cranial mediastinal mass; positive contrast angiography may reveal an intravenacaval mass or thrombus; a thorough cardiac workup may demonstrate the existence of underlying heart disease; and antifungal antibody titers can help identify a fungal infection.

Treatment

Treatment is directed at the primary cause, if one can be discovered. If not (*i.e.*, in idiopathic chylothorax), medical therapy for 2 to 4 weeks usually is the first approach, because it is successful in some animals and does not require a major surgical procedure, which is not always successful. The irritating effusion is removed at least once daily or, preferably, continuously via a thoracostomy tube; the volume, color, and character of the fluid are recorded daily.

The metabolic effects of chylous effusion usually are more serious than the respiratory effects. This is due to a loss of proteins (which may result in hypoalbuminemia and peripheral edema), fats, fat-soluble vitamins, water,

and electrolytes into the pleural space, which is compounded by their repeated aspiration from the thorax. T-cell lymphopenia may result as well. Because of these substantial losses, aggressive supportive management usually is necessary. Parenteral fluid therapy is required, including administration of plasma if hypoproteinemia occurs. A diet low in long-chain triglycerides is indicated because they significantly increase chyle formation and because they are absorbed via the lymphatics and deposited in the pleural cavity, where they appear to irritate the pleura. The prescription diet R/D (Hill's Pet Products, Inc., Topeka, KS) may serve as a basis of the patient's diet. Calories are replaced by starchy foods (depending on weight loss) and 1 to 2 ml/kg per day of medium-chain triglycerides (*e.g.*, MCT Oil, Mead Johnson and Co., Evansville, IN), which are absorbed directly by the portal circulation. Fat-soluble vitamins should also be added to the diet.

Theoretically, intravenous hyperalimentation is an alternative to the above, but it is expensive, the intravenous catheter is difficult to maintain, and thrombophlebitis may result. The effectiveness of giving diuretics to reduce pleural fluid formation is unproven.

The other choices for therapy include surgery (ligation of the thoracic duct caudal to the site of leakage) or, more recently, pleurodesis. Due to the serious systemic effects of chronic removal of the chylous effusion, this may be necessary before the end of the suggested 2- to 4-week attempt at medical management. Ligation is warranted only if no underlying cause (*e.g.*, malignant neoplasm, fungal disease, heart disease) can be identified; in such cases, ligation is of no long-term benefit for the patient, and management of the underlying cause would be more successful.

In the dog, the thoracic duct collects lymph from the entire body, except the right forelimb and the right side of the head and neck (which is collected by the right lymphatic duct). Intestinal and other abdominal lymphatics drain to the cisterna chyli, the source of the thoracic duct. In the dog, the duct usually branches into multiple vessels in the mediastinum, on the right dorsolateral aspect of the aorta, ventral to the azygous vein. The duct then crosses from right to left at the level of the 5th or 6th thoracic vertebra and empties into the venous system at the junction of the left jugular vein and the cranial vena cava, or the left brachiocephalic, left subclavian, azygous, or other vein. Valves prevent venous-lymphatic regurgitation and lymphatic backflow. The thoracic duct is similar in the cat, but is located completely on the left side.

Lymphangiography can improve the chance of successful ligation by providing intraoperative, preligation evaluation of the degree of arborization and postligation confirmation of the completeness of ligation of thoracic duct radicles. Via a right paracostal incision, a 20- to 22-gauge intravenous catheter is inserted into one of the large lymphatics in the ileocecocolic region. Lateral and ventrodorsal radiographs are obtained immediately after injecting 1 ml/kg of an aqueous iodinated contrast agent (e.g., Renovist, Squibb, Princeton, NJ), which is warmed and diluted by one third with saline to decrease its viscosity. Intraoperative identification of the mesenteric lymphatics and the thoracic duct branches may be facilitated by feeding 10 to 30 ml of cream or corn oil 3, 2, and 1 hours preoperatively, which outlines the lymphatics in white. Adding a dye such as Sudan black to the cream aids visualization of the duct. Another method is to inject 2 to 4 ml of 1% methylene blue solution (Elkins-Sinn, Cherry Hill, NJ) into the mesenteric lymphatic catheter or mesenteric lymph nodes. Dyes may actually decrease visualization, however, by staining the tissues; this is aggravated if a duct is inadvertently ruptured during surgery.

The thoracic duct is approached via a 10th intercostal thoracotomy, on the right in the dog and on the left in the cat. Ligation is performed as far caudad in the thorax as possible and/or at the site at which ligation is deemed easiest (fewest branches) by lymphangiography. The pleura is incised on the dorso-lateral aspect of the aorta, and all branches of the duct are bluntly isolated and then ligated with a nonabsorbable material that holds knots well, such as 3-0 silk. Metallic clips may be used for ligation, to facilitate orientation for finding and ligating any additional branches of the duct that appear on the immediate postligation lymphangiogram. Ligating all branches of the duct visible in at least two inter-intercostal artery spaces may improve success. To facilitate bilateral postoperative drainage of the chest, the ventral portion of the caudal mediastinum is fenestrated widely. Before closing the paracostal incision (used for lymphangiography), a full-thickness small intestine biopsy should be obtained to examine for lymphangiectasia.

A thoracostomy tube is left in place until pleural effusion decreases adequately. In some animals, chylous effusion may be detected for 3 to 5 days postoperatively. A low-fat diet should be fed for 2 to 3 weeks postoperatively, to allow time for alternate lymphatic and/or lymphaticovenous channels to develop. Animals with intestinal lymphangiectasia should remain on low-fat diets indefinitely.

The poorest results have occurred in Afghans, about half of which continue to produce chylous effusions even after complete thoracic duct ligation, as confirmed by lymphangiography. A non-chylous serosanguinous effusion develops and persists postoperatively for several weeks or even longer in about one third of non-Afghan dogs. This may be due to low-grade pleuritis or extraductal lymphatic dysfunction. Diuretic therapy may be attempted if the amount of fluid remains stable. In some cases, the production of such fluid is substantial and intractable (sometimes in even greater quantity than the original chylous effusion), requiring pleurodesis or a pleuroperitoneal shunt (see "Pleuroperitoneal Shunt," below).

Pleurodesis also has been used for primary management of chylothorax. In one study, there were very promising results in 8 of 10 dogs and in the 1 cat tested.

Hemorrhagic Effusions— Hemothorax

Hemothorax results from bleeding into the pleural space. Secondary transudation of fluid lowers the packed cell volume; hemoglobin levels rarely are more than 1 gm/dl. Nearly all pleural effusions contain some erythrocytes, and only 5,000 to 6,000 cells/μl give a red tint. Erythrocyte concentrations greater than 100,000/μl generally indicate pleural hemorrhage or contamination with blood during thoracocentesis. Platelets commonly are present in recent hemorrhage. Erythrophagocytosis with release of hemoglobin occurs within a few hours after hemorrhage, resulting in a xanthochromic supernatant. Even relatively fresh hemorrhagic pleural effusions generally do not clot after their removal from the chest, due to mechanical defibrination and activation of fibrinolytic mechanisms. Coagulation of the fluid is impaired further by consumption of platelets within 8 hours. Therefore, clotting of a sample implies very recent hemorrhage or traumatic thoracocentesis. If clotting occurs, as in severe trauma associated with tissue thromboplastin release, lysis of the clot usually is complete by 7 to 10 days. Diffuse clots may organize and mature into a fibrous layer (see "Constrictive Pleuritis," p. 237).

The most common cause of hemothorax is trauma, especially that associated with fractured ribs. Inadvertent laceration of an intercostal or other vessel during thoracotomy should be considered as a cause if bleeding follows thoracic surgery. Hemorrhage may also be caused by coagulation disorders or infiltrating neoplasms; rare causes include *Spirocerca lupi*—induced bleeding from the aorta, or *Dirofilaria immitis*—induced changes in the pulmonary artery. Hemorrhage may be idiopathic.

Bleeding from the comparatively low-pressure pulmonary vasculature, particularly from small vessels, generally is self-limiting. Clotting is enhanced by the tamponade-like effect of the relatively fixed size of the pleural space and any free air from concomitant pneumothorax. Bleeding from the diaphragm, chest wall, or cardiac vessels is at a higher pressure, so bleeding may continue.

Clinical signs depend on the rapidity and amount of hemorrhage. A small amount of hemorrhage may go unrecognized. In rapid, major hemorrhage, respiration is impaired and right to left shunting occurs, leading to dyspnea, restlessness, decreased heart and lung sounds, dullness on percussion, cyanosis, and signs of shock. In animals with a history of trauma, no overt bleeding, and signs of hypovolemic shock, the possibility of thoracic hemorrhage should be considered.

Hemothorax does not necessarily require thoracocentesis, unless respiration is compromised. Otherwise, the bleeding may be self-limiting, and about 70% or more of the erythrocytes are absorbed intact (autotransfusion). Hypovolemia should be treated first by fluid volume expansion with crystalloids, followed by blood transfusion if indicated (see "Surgical Principles and Instrumentation," above).

Autogenous transfusion of blood removed by thoracocentesis or during surgery may be considered. The blood should be mixed with an anticoagulant and passed through a micropore filter to remove platelet aggregates and microthrombi. Complications of autotransfusion include microembolization, hemolysis, coagulopathies, hypofibrinogenemia, and disseminated intravascular coagulation, but the technique is practical and lifesaving and should be considered, particularly when blood from another canine or feline source is not available.

Serial radiographs help evaluate the progression or cessation of hemorrhage. Massive hemorrhage, or deteriorating clinical signs with evidence of continuing hemorrhage, calls for surgical exploration and ligation of bleeding vessels. Often, the treatment of massive hemothorax is not successful. While intercostal vessels lacerated by rib fractures sometimes can be ligated without thoracotomy (*e.g.*, by placing a suture-ligature around the rib above and below the bleeding point), entry into the chest usually is necessary to deal with a major thoracic vessel. Lateral thoracotomy or median sternotomy may be used, depending on whether there are signs of lateralization of the hemorrhage. Postoperative tube thoracostomy is indicated, with the tube removed when hemorrhage has ceased.

Neoplastic Effusions

Neoplastic effusions are exudates, chylous effusions, or modified transudates that often are hemorrhagic and frequently but not always contain neoplastic cells. Many primary and metastatic pleural neoplasms, including lymphoma, mesothelioma, and pulmonary carcinoma are commonly associated with effusions.

Cytology may prove an effusion to be of neoplastic origin, but specific cell identification often is difficult. Sarcomas generally do not readily exfoliate cells into body fluids. Mesothelioma cells and blast-transformed nonmalignant mesothelial cells are difficult to differentiate from carcinoma cells. The presence of mast cells in large numbers or in the absence of an inflammatory response suggests neoplasia. Increased numbers of lymphoblasts suggest lymphoma. A pleural punch biopsy, performed after a small skin incision, or exploratory thoracotomy is indicated if parietal pleural neoplasia is suspected. Management of specific neoplasms is discussed in the appropriate section.

Treatment of Intractable Pleural Effusion or Repeated Pneumothorax

Pleurodesis

Pleurodesis is the obliteration of the pleural space by fusing the parietal to the visceral pleura. It is considered when two properly managed episodes of pneumothorax are followed by a third episode, when pleural effusion is refractory to conventional medical or surgical therapy, or more recently as primary therapy for idiopathic chylothorax. Dry-sponge abrasion of the visceral pleura, and several intrathoracically placed sclerosing agents, such as sterile talc or tetracycline, have been used to attempt pleurodesis in dogs and cats. Although tetracycline is the most popular of these agents, there are only anecdotal published reports of its successful use. This might be due to poor application of the technique, although further studies are necessary to develop an optimal protocol. In addition, success has been measured by a decrease in clinical signs, and/or by lessened fluid or air accumulation in the chest. There has been no published evidence for the formation of widespread adhesions of the lung to the chest wall, although localized adhesions have been discovered after intrapleural tetracycline administration. Therefore, the term "pleurodesis" may be a misnomer; a more appropriate description is "sclerotherapy," as all the techniques cause pleural surface sclerosis, which may decrease the production of gas or fluid by lessening its ease of crossing the pleura, without adhesion formation.

One technique involves thorough drainage of the pleural space via bilateral thoracostomy tubes placed under general anesthesia. A total of 1 gm of tetracycline hydrochloride, diluted in 40 to 100 ml of saline, is infused divided between the two chest tubes. The tubes then are clamped and the animal is placed in dorsal, right lateral, left lateral, and sternal recumbencies for 10 minutes each to distribute the fluid. Thereafter, under careful monitoring, constant suction is required to empty the pleural space of the irritant and to bring the lungs against the chest wall, facilitating adhesion. Post-treatment pain might require analgesia, although this appears to be unusual. Constant suction is continued until air stops forming (in cases of pneumothorax), or fluid formation decreases to 1 or 2 ml/kg of body weight. This requires about 10 to 14 days. Some fluid may form after treatment is completed, but after 6 months, as shown by radiography, this has been less than that present when the chest tubes were removed. Routine radiographic follow-up occurs periodically for 1 year after treatment in cases of chylothorax. This is accompanied by dietary and supportive management as described under "Treatment," p. 239.

Pleuroperitoneal Shunt

Intractable effusion has been treated with a Denver peritoneal-venous shunt (Denver Biomedicals, Evergreen, CO). The pump is installed subcutaneously on the lateral aspect of the chest wall. Percutaneous compression of the pump by the owner several times each day moves fluid from the thoracic to the peritoneal cavity, from which it is absorbed.

Diaphragm

The diaphragm is a musculotendinous organ that separates the abdominal and thoracic cavities, thus keeping the abdominal organs in place. As it contracts, negative intrathoracic pressure is increased, resulting in inspiration. Contraction also provides the abdominal press, which is important for excretion and parturition. Surgery of the diaphragm in dogs and cats is confined almost exclusively to the repair of defects (hernias) caused by congenital malformation or trauma.

Congenital Diaphragmatic Hernias

The diaphragm develops from six embryonic segments, the largest of which is the septum transversum. Congenital hernias develop when the embryonic segments fail to fuse and vary from a small defect to complete absence of the diaphragm. Fewer than 10% of diaphragmatic hernias in small animals are congenital.

Congenital Pleuroperitoneal Hernias

Pleuroperitoneal hernias are very rare and may have an hereditary origin. The diaphragmatic central tendon and crural attachments are absent, and only traces of lateral attachments are present. Affected animals generally die early in life, probably because of concomitant pulmonary hypoplasia, cardiovascular defects, renal agenesis, and other anomalies.

Congenital Peritoneopericardial Hernias

Peritoneopericardial hernias are the most common of the congenital diaphragmatic hernias of small animals. They are more common in dogs than in cats, with a possible breed predisposition in Weimaraners and German shepherds. The hernia occurs through a ventral midline defect in the diaphragm, which exists because of faulty development of the septum transversum. Rather than closing normally, this structure fuses with the mediastinum and the pericardium, allowing herniation of the abdominal organs into the pericardial sac. Associated anomalies are common, including a cranial ventral abdominal wall defect (omphalocele, found in about half of these patients), umbilical hernia, and/or cardiac or sternebral malformations.

Often, clinical signs of peritoneopericardial hernia are absent and its presence is an incidental finding in an adult animal. Clinical signs may be caused by malpositioning, entrapment, or dysfunction of herniated organs. For example, if the stomach and intestines are in the pericardial sac, postprandial dyspnea, vomiting, or diarrhea may occur. Entrapment of the liver or spleen may lead to pericardial effusion, resulting in cardiac tamponade. Distention of the pericardial sac with herniated organs may cause compression of the heart, lungs, and major veins of the chest. This leads to respiratory and cardiovascular signs, ranging from tachypnea and tachycardia to cyanosis, respiratory distress, and right-sided cardiac failure.

Physical findings include absent or muffled heart sounds; occasionally, borborygmi are heard on chest auscultation. The point of maximal intensity of cardiac contraction may not be palpable in its normal position at the left sternal border, from the 4th to the 6th intercostal space. Deep palpation of the cranial abdomen may allow detection of the diaphragmatic defect and the apex of the heart, particularly if an omphalocele exists.

Typically, thoracic radiographs show a large, globoid cardiac silhouette that must be differentiated from cardiomegaly or pericardial effusion. Echocardiography, electrocardiography, and/or the radiographic presence of barium or gas-filled bowel loops within the pericardial sac help to differentiate these conditions. Occasionally, contrast peritoneography is needed to confirm the defect.

Surgical treatment involves reducing the herniated organs and repairing the diaphragmatic defect and is best performed via a cranial ventral midline celiotomy. Although entry into the pleural space rarely occurs, respiratory support with intermittent positive-pressure ventilation is recommended to counter the effects of surgical manipulation and compression of the lungs by the dilated pericardial sac. Adhesions occur only rarely, so hernial contents generally are reduced easily by gentle traction.

The most frequent contents of the hernia include the liver, with or without the gall bladder, small intestines, and omentum. Spleen, pancreas, falciform ligament, and mesentery also may be involved. Chronic passive congestion of the spleen or liver can make them difficult to reduce. If so, the hernial opening should be enlarged (thus entering the pleural space) to ease reduction. The margins of the hernial sac usually include a dense fibrous ring that supports sutures very well. Debriding the edges is unnecessary. Suture material and patterns are as described under "Treatment," p. 246.

Closure of the abdomen usually is routine, but the presence of an omphalocele adds several problems. The rectus fascia must be apposed over a significantly greater volume of abdominal viscera than was present before herniorrhaphy. Therefore, significant tension may be placed on the incision line, so retention sutures may be required. Further, cardiovascular collapse may occur during closure if the increased intra-abdominal pressure obstructs venous return to the heart. Negative intrathoracic pressure should be re-established, either by thoracocentesis or tube thoracostomy, if the pleural space had been entered.

Hiatal Hernias

A hiatal hernia exists when part of the proximal portion of the stomach and/or the abdominal portion of the esophagus pass through the esophageal hiatus of the diaphragm into the thorax. This usually results from congenital laxity of the hiatus, although it may be acquired by blunt abdominal trauma or relaxation of the muscular structures of the hiatus. Sliding (bell or axial) and rolling (paraesophageal) hiatal hernias have been reported in small animals. In sliding hernias, the diaphragm can move cranially and caudally on the esophagus, so the abdominal esophagus, the caudal esophageal sphincter, and part of the stomach reside, intermittently, in the thorax. In rolling hiatal hernias, the cardioesophageal junction and the abdominal esophagus remain in their normal positions, but part of the stomach, surrounded by a peritoneal sac, herniates into the mediastinum adjacent to the esophagus.

Another congenital defect, eventration of the diaphragm, has been observed in conjunction with hiatal hernia in dogs. In eventration, the musculature of the diaphragm is aplastic, and the diaphragm is located more cranially in the thorax than normal. Gastroesophageal intussusception, which also can be associated with hiatal hernia, is discussed under diseases of the esophagus (see Chap. 12, The Esophagus and Stomach).

Clinical signs of hiatal hernia include intermittent or frequent vomition or regurgitation; no consistent time period elapses between ingestion and regurgitation. Excessive salivation may also occur. Dyspnea and exercise intolerance occur in severe cases. Signs are observed as early as the time of weaning to solid foods, and generally by 12 months of age. Cachexia, dehydration, and mental dullness may be associated with repeated vomition. Auscultation and percussion may reveal lung consolidation due to aspiration pneumonia as a result of inhaling refluxed material. This condition must be differentiated from other causes of vomition or regurgitation, such as cricopharyngeal dysphagia, megaesophagus, congenital or acquired obstruction of the esophagus or gastrointestinal tract, esophageal diverticulum, or peritoneopericardial hernia.

Plain radiography may show a radiodense mass cranial to the dorsal part of the diaphragm, in the area of the esophageal hiatus. Static barium contrast radiography may confirm that the mass is a portion of the stomach but because in sliding hernias the stomach can return to the abdominal cavity, this is not a consistent finding. Fluoroscopy with barium sulfate may demonstrate repeated reflux of contrast into the esophagus, in association with herniation of the stomach. Endoscopy helps assess the presence and severity of reflux esophagitis.

Medical management of sliding hernias includes antacids, which protect the distal esophagus and stimulate a gastrin-induced increase in caudal esophageal sphincter tone; cimetidine (Tagamet, Smith, Kline & French Laboratories, Philadelphia) or another histamine-2 antagonist (see Chap. 12, The Esophagus and Stomach) to decrease gastric acidity; and metaclopramide (Reglan, AH Robins, Richmond, VA) to increase caudal esophageal sphincter tone and speed gastric emptying.

Surgical correction usually is required, although in dogs and cats this has met with variable success. The hernia is reduced through a cranial ventral midline celiotomy. The hiatus then is tightened by plicating the tendinous portion of the diaphragm surrounding the esophagus with nonabsorbable monofilament synthetic suture material. An orogastric tube is inserted during the procedure to avoid a suture-induced constriction of the esophagus. In addition, for sliding hernias, a fundoplastic procedure (Nissen or Belsey) usually is performed in an attempt to eliminate esophageal reflux (see Chap. 12, The Esophagus and Stomach).

Traumatic Diaphragmatic Hernia

Etiology

Virtually all acquired diaphragmatic hernias in small animals result from traumatic tears caused by automobile accidents, falls, or penetrating wounds; the traumatic incident sometimes occurs without the owner's knowledge. Further, the animal may not immediately develop signs related to the presence of a hernia if the hernial opening is so large that abdominal contents easily move in and out of the pleural space or if it becomes plugged temporarily with omentum, liver, or another organ so that no abdominal contents can enter the chest. Therefore, traumatic hernias diagnosed months to years later have been reported in up to 40% of affected animals. Massive trauma often creates multiple injuries, including hemothorax, hemoperitoneum, and pulmonary contusions, which also can obscure the diagnosis of diaphragmatic hernia.

Diagnosis
Clinical Signs

A diagnosis of diaphragmatic hernia should be considered in patients exhibiting dyspnea or in patients with a history of recent trauma. Clinical signs of diaphragmatic hernia relate to four factors:

1. Dysfunction of the herniated organs may cause vomiting, diarrhea, or anorexia by

affecting the stomach or intestine, or icterus if hepatic incarceration with biliary obstruction has occurred.

2. As the herniated viscera fill the pleural space, they cause mechanical compression and displacement of the heart, lungs, and great veins, creating cardiovascular signs, including shock (from decreased venous return), and evidence of pulmonary decompensation (hypoxemia, due to atelectasis, leading to dyspnea, hyperpnea, and cyanosis).

3. Additional compression may be caused by pleural effusion from entrapped organs, due to passive congestion of the liver or, less commonly, the spleen, or dilation of the stomach or intestines.

4. Physical findings vary with the contents of the hernia. For example, muffled heart and lung sounds commonly are detected on auscultation of the thorax. Further, borborygmi are auscultable if the stomach or intestines are herniated, unless ileus exists (which often is the case in the first 24 hours after trauma). Decreased resonance and/or the presence of a fluid line may be detected on percussion of the chest, due to pleural effusion, and increased resonance may accompany gastric or intestinal distention.

Radiography

Often, the diagnosis of diaphragmatic hernia is confirmed on plain radiography. Radiography should be performed with care, as aggressive restraint and positioning can lead to respiratory failure by displacing abdominal organs or causing excitement. Loss of the diaphragmatic outline and cardiac silhouette, increased soft tissue density, and gas patterns in the caudal thoracic cavity all are common radiographic signs of diaphragmatic hernia. A dorsoventral or ventrodorsal view may indicate the side of the hernia. Major differential diagnoses include hemothorax in a recently traumatized animal and all other causes of pleural effusion. Occasionally, ultrasonography, a positive

contrast upper gastrointestinal study, or contrast peritoneography may be required to confirm the diagnosis. Removing pleural fluid often makes thoracic radiography more diagnostic.

Laboratory Data

Hepatic and renal function should be evaluated and a complete blood count should be obtained to search for anemia, hemorrhage, dehydration, or infection. Serum electrolyte and blood pH assessments are suggested if intestinal obstruction is present. A coagulation profile and serum protein measurements are indicated if liver incarceration is suspected. Blood gas values should be obtained if the patient's ventilatory capacity is in question. An electrocardiogram helps determine the presence of myocardial trauma or cardiac arrhythmias, particularly in acute cases. Pleural fluid should be evaluated to rule out other causes of effusion (see "Pleural Effusion," p. 233).

Treatment

Concurrent problems such as pulmonary contusions, pleural effusion, hemothorax, or hemoperitoneum often require emergency medical treatment before repair of the hernia is considered. Emergency herniorrhaphy is indicated by the presence of intrathoracic gastric distention, and speed is also essential if hepatic or intestinal strangulation occurs. Cardiopulmonary collapse does not necessarily call for emergency surgical treatment of a recently traumatized animal, however, as rib fractures, pulmonary contusions, pleural effusion, and acute blood loss may cause similar signs.

Although lateral thoracotomy and paracostal celiotomy approaches have been used to repair diaphragmatic hernia, the hernia is best approached through a cranial ventral midline celiotomy. This is the easiest and most versatile approach because it can be combined with either a median sternotomy or a paracostal incision to increase exposure. The entire thorax and abdomen should be prepared for surgery to allow possible extension of the incision. The abdominal contents should be examined for damage, and the extent of the hernia evaluated. Herniation usually occurs through the weakest portion of the diaphragm, one of the muscular segments. The liver tends to herniate through right-sided tears, the stomach through left-sided tears. The liver is the most common organ to have herniated, followed by the small intestine, stomach, and spleen. The rent can occur either parallel with the body wall, in a circumferential fashion, or radially from the body wall toward the center of the diaphragm. Combinations of these two types also occur, as do bilateral hernias.

Gentle retraction to reduce the contents of the hernia is the first step in repair. Occasionally it is necessary to enlarge the diaphragmatic tear to accomplish reduction, such as when a chronically incarcerated liver lobe has become swollen and friable. Particularly for repositioning traumatized liver lobes, it is preferable to extend several fingers (or the whole hand in large dogs) beyond the trapped tissues to push them back into place, rather than to pull on the pedicle. Cranial extension of the celiotomy to include a partial median sternotomy also may be necessary in some long-standing hernias to facilitate separating intrathoracic adhesions. After the hernia is reduced, the retracted organs should be inspected and the thoracic cavity should be examined carefully for evidence of hemorrhage, leakage of air or tissue damage. Any necrotic or damaged tissues, such as incarcerated bowel or liver, should be resected as indicated. The abdominal contents are retracted away from the hernial opening with moistened laparotomy sponges. Only necrotic tissue need be removed from the margin of the hernial ring prior to closure.

While both nonabsorbable and absorbable suture materials have been used for closure, we prefer monofilament nonabsorbable synthetics, such as polypropylene or nylon, because they are nonreactive and retain their holding power. A swaged-on taper needle should be used. The suture pattern should re-

lieve tension and completely appose the margins of the defect. Both one- and two-layer closures have been used successfully, employing a variety of patterns. We prefer two layers, the first of interrupted horizontal mattress sutures, which act as retention sutures, and the second of simple continuous sutures to appose the wound edges. It is easier to close the hernia by starting to suture at the most inaccessible (usually the dorsal) end. Sometimes, several tacking sutures may be placed first to partially close the tear, ensuring an anatomically correct closure. A series of interrupted pericostal sutures may be needed to reattach a diaphragm torn at its costal margin, again followed by a simple continuous layer. When repairing radial tears, it is particularly important to identify and avoid trauma, occlusion, or constriction of the aorta, esophagus, vagus nerves, or the caudal vena cava as they pass through the diaphragm.

Primary repair of a diaphragmatic hernia is nearly always possible. Occasionally, in a chronic hernia, scarring and contraction of the muscular diaphragm may occur, making closure difficult. In such cases, excising the scar tissue lining the hernia may allow greater mobilization of the diaphragm and primary repair. Rarely, it may be necessary to use reconstructive techniques to repair the diaphragm. A rotation flap of diaphragmatic tissue can be created by incising the diaphragm at its normal attachments and reattaching it to the body wall following closure of the defect. Autogenous pedicle grafts of the transversus abdominus muscle or omentum may be used for this purpose. Free fascia lata or synthetic mesh grafts also may be considered. An airtight closure is not necessary, because small openings tend to seal rapidly. Larger openings should be closed with additional sutures, however, to prevent reherniation of abdominal contents.

The abdominal wall is closed routinely. Because of contraction of the abdominal wall musculature, it may be difficult to fit the viscera back into the abdominal cavity once the diaphragm is closed. Care must be exercised not to injure the viscera during their replacement. Relaxation of the abdominal wall occurs after surgery.

Negative intrathoracic pressure is re-established by transdiaphragmatic aspiration after closure of the diaphragm and again by thoracocentesis after abdominal closure. A thoracostomy tube should be placed prior to herniorrhaphy (see "Chest Drainage (Thoracostomy) Tubes," p. 218) if breakdown of adhesions creates hemorrhage or pulmonary air leakage or if chronic pleural effusion had been present.

Perioperative antibiotics should be administered when there is evidence that the liver or gastrointestinal tract has contaminated the pleuroperitoneal space. Postoperative monitoring should include evaluation of cardiovascular, respiratory, and gastrointestinal function, and hydration. Radiography should be performed 24 to 48 hours after surgery to assess pleural effusion, pneumothorax, and pulmonary expansion.

The prognosis for animals with diaphragmatic hernia depends largely on concurrent injuries and the degree of dysfunction of the herniated organs. Mortality rates for this injury have ranged from 10 to 50%. Most deaths occur during the intraoperative or perioperative period and often are related to hypoventilation due to compression of the lungs, or to multiple organ failure. Re-expansion of atelectatic lungs may lead to pulmonary edema; this is an occasional cause of postoperative death, along with hemothorax or pneumothorax. Deaths occurring more than 24 hours after surgery are rare.

The Mediastinum

The mediastinum is the space separating the right and left pleural sacs. It extends from the thoracic inlet to the diaphragm and contains most of the thoracic structures, including the trachea and primary bronchi, the heart and great vessels, the esophagus, lymph nodes, nerves, and the thymus. The central position of the heart can be used to divide the mediastinum into cranial, middle, and caudal portions. These divisions are useful in developing a differential diagnosis, since certain conditions arise characteristically in specific portions of the mediastinum. There are few primary diseases of the mediastinum. More often, mediastinal changes reflect diseases of the structures lying within this space or are an extension of diseases of the adjacent tissues.

Mediastinitis

Mediastinitis is an inflammatory condition often caused by bacterial contamination. The most common cause of mediastinitis in the dog and cat is esophageal perforation and leakage (see Chap. 12, The Esophagus and Stomach). Extension of infection from deep wounds of the neck, migration of foreign objects such as plant awns, or mediastinal surgery also can cause mediastinitis.

Clinical findings are often dramatic and include thoracic pain, fever, and leukocytosis. Respiratory distress may be present when a pleural effusion occurs secondary to mediastinitis. Other clinical signs may reflect the underlying cause of the mediastinitis, such as regurgitation associated with esophageal rupture. The diagnosis of mediastinitis is based primarily on clinical and radiographic findings. Pneumomediastinum is seen frequently with mediastinitis due to visceral rupture, puncture wounds, or gas-forming bacteria.

Treatment of mediastinitis is directed toward resolving the primary cause. Surgical treatment may be indicated, particularly when the condition is localized. Surgery usually is performed through a lateral intercostal thoracotomy and includes establishing drainage of any loculated fluid within the mediastinum, obtaining samples for bacterial culture and antibiotic sensitivity testing, and thorough lavage of the mediastinum and pleural cavity. These procedures are followed by placement of a thoracostomy tube for drainage of the pleural cavity and initiating appropriate antibiotic therapy (see "Pleural Effusion," p. 233). The prognosis for an animal with mediastinitis depends on the underlying etiology.

Pneumomediastinum

Pneumomediastinum is the accumulation of free air or gas within the mediastinum. It is often associated with mediastinitis and may result from a number of traumatic or pathologic conditions, including blunt thoracic trauma, rupture of the trachea or esophagus, or penetrating wounds of the neck. Iatrogenic pneumomediastinum has also been related to transtracheal aspiration, traumatic jugular venipuncture, or overinflation of a cuffed endotracheal tube.

Although pneumomediastinum itself rarely produces clinical signs, the condition commonly occurs with pneumothorax or subcutaneous emphysema. Pneumothorax often causes dyspnea, and muted lung sounds are observed. Subcutaneous emphysema creates a characteristic palpable crepitance of the skin, which can be localized to the neck region or extend over the entire body. Signs of mediastinitis commonly accompany pneumomediastinum.

A diagnosis of pneumomediastinum is made when the presence of air produces an increased radiographic lucency around the normal mediastinal structures, thus increasing their visibility on thoracic radiographs.

While treatment of pneumomediastinum rarely is indicated, recognizing this condition and determining its underlying cause early is often essential for diagnosing and treating the primary disease.

Mediastinal Hemorrhage

Mediastinal hemorrhage most commonly results from trauma. Both penetrating wounds and blunt trauma can cause rupture of the major vessels contained within the mediastinum. Less commonly, mediastinal hemorrhage occurs associated with a hemorrhagic diathesis due to an acquired or congenital coagulopathy, or due to rupture of the thin-walled vessels of the involuting thymus in young dogs. Surgical treatment is rarely indicated.

Mediastinal Masses

Tumors may originate in any of the structures located in the mediastinum; fortunately, only a few of these are seen with any frequency in the dog and cat. Most of the masses occur in the cranial or perihilar regions of the mediastinum and arise from lymph nodes, thymus, esophagus, aortic body chemoreceptors, or ectopic thyroid or parathyroid tissue (Fig. 9–13).

The clinical manifestations of mediastinal masses vary widely and depend on:

1. the size and location of the mass,
2. the structures involved, and
3. the presence or absence of a paraneoplastic syndrome.

Many mediastinal masses cause no signs and are found incidentally on thoracic radiographs taken for other purposes. Clinical signs can occur due to involvement of several systems. For example, respiratory signs may occur secondary to obstruction or invasion of a major airway or the presence of pleural effusion, which often accompanies a mediastinal mass. Esophageal signs such as regurgitation occur when the mass invades or compresses the esophagus. Compression or obstruction of major mediastinal veins can cause forelimb and head edema when cranial veins are involved, or ascites and rear limb edema when caudal veins are affected. Lymphatic obstruction and chylothorax can occur if a cranial mediastinal mass obstructs the thoracic duct.

The most common neurologic signs include changes in vocalization due to invasion of the recurrent laryngeal nerve, or Horner's syndrome if the sympathetic trunk is involved. Systemic signs can occur when paraneoplastic

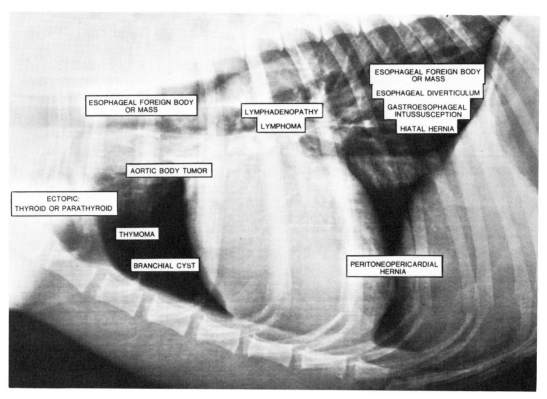

Figure 9-13. *The location of common mediastinal conditions as seen on a lateral radiograph.*

syndromes such as myasthenia gravis, poly-myositis, or hypertrophic osteoarthropathy develop secondary to certain tumors.

Diagnosis of a mediastinal mass can be as simple as recognizing a focal increase in density on a lateral thoracic radiograph, with mediastinal widening seen on the ventrodorsal view. Unfortunately, a small mass, or one obscured by a pleural effusion, can be considerably more difficult to define. Indirect radiographic signs, cytology of pleural fluid, contrast radiographic studies, ultrasonography, computed tomography, or scintigraphy can be used to define a mediastinal mass. The final diagnosis depends on biopsy of the mass; this can be obtained by a fine-needle biopsy directed by ultrasonography or fluoroscopy, or tissue can be obtained during exploratory thoracotomy.

Lymphosarcoma

Lymphosarcoma can involve the thymus and/or mediastinal lymph nodes. Thymic lymphosarcoma most commonly occurs in cats; a multicentric form of lymphosarcoma, sometimes involving the mediastinal lymph nodes, is more common in dogs. Diagnosis often can be made on fine-needle biopsy of the mass or cytologic examination of pleural fluid. Biopsy via thoracotomy is indicated only if less invasive methods fail to result in a diagnosis. Combination chemotherapy is the treatment of choice.

Thymoma

A thymoma is a multilobulated, encapsulated mass arising from epithelial cells of the thymus. It is rare and occurs most commonly in older cats and dogs. Thymomas often are associated with several paraneoplastic syndromes, including polymyositis, myasthenia gravis, and an increased incidence of nonthymic neoplasms. Clinical signs may be caused by the tumor itself or may be associated with a paraneoplastic syndrome.

Recommendations for treatment and estimates of prognosis are difficult to make because of the limited numbers of published cases. Thymomas have been said to be slow-growing and generally benign, but they often are invasive and at surgery are found to be nonresectable. Even when they are deemed resectable, rapid regrowth of the tumor is reported in some cases. In addition, resecting the thymoma does not always resolve the paraneoplastic syndrome it causes. The prognosis for surgical treatment of a thymoma, therefore, is guarded, particularly when a paraneoplastic syndrome such as myasthenia gravis is present. The muscular weakness and megaesophagus caused by this disease lead to chronic regurgitation and a high incidence of aspiration pneumonia, which complicates treatment. The prognosis is better in the absence of a paraneoplastic syndrome and when the tumor is resectable. Adjunctive chemotherapy should be considered along with surgical resection.

Branchial Cysts

Branchial cysts are thought to develop from the vestiges of the branchial arch system of the fetus. They can occur in the subcutaneous tissues of the neck or within the cranial mediastinum. Thymic branchial cysts have been reported rarely in the dog and cat. Dyspnea is the most frequent clinical sign. Radiographs typically show a variable amount of pleural effusion and a cranial mediastinal mass. Cytology of the pleural fluid and findings from fine-needle biopsies are nonspecific; thus, diagnosis typically is made at exploratory thoracotomy. The treatment of choice is surgical excision of the cyst, although close association with major vascular structures can make

complete resection difficult. The long-term prognosis is good when the cysts can be completely resected.

Ectopic Thyroid and Parathyroid Tissue

Ectopic thyroid tissue occurs infrequently in the dog and cat and usually is located in the cranial ventral mediastinum. Clinical signs exist only when the tissue becomes hyperplastic and produces excess thyroid hormone. Technetium 99m pertechnetate scintigraphy is a useful diagnostic aid for identifying ectopic thyroid tissue. Treatment alternatives include surgical resection of the hyperplastic thyroid tissue, antithyroid drugs, or I^{131} radiotherapy (see Chap. 8).

Ectopic parathyroid tissue also can develop in the cranial mediastinum. Clinical signs are related to the development of a mass lesion, usually a parathyroid adenocarcinoma.

Other Conditions

Lymph node enlargement other than lymphosarcoma should be included in the differential diagnosis of cranial and perihilar mediastinal masses. The causes of lymphadenopathy include systemic bacterial or fungal infections, or abscessation or metastatic invasion of the lymph nodes. Surgery may be indicated to obtain tissue samples for biopsy and culture.

Aortic body tumors and esophageal tumors also occur within the mediastinum. The diagnosis and treatment of these conditions are covered in Chapters 10 and 12.

Conditions causing radiographic and clinical signs similar to those of a mediastinal mass are gastroesophageal intussusception, epiphrenic esophageal diverticulum, hiatal hernia, esophageal foreign body, or diaphragmatic hernia. Recognizing these conditions is important in the differential diagnosis of caudal mediastinal masses (Fig. 9–13). The diagnosis and treatment of these conditions are covered above in this chapter, and in Chapter 12, The Esophagus and Stomach.

The Bronchi and Lungs

The Bronchi

Bronchial Diseases

Few primary diseases of the bronchi exist in companion animals. Traumatic injuries, neoplasms, and intraluminal foreign bodies all are rare, and most of these conditions also involve the lung tissue (see "Pulmonary Diseases," below). Further, treatment of traumatic injuries to the bronchi and resection of bronchial neoplasms generally are accomplished best by complete pulmonary lobectomy. Bronchoscopy and instrumentation is the preferred method of removing intraluminal bronchial foreign bodies. Bronchial surgery is indicated for removal of large foreign bodies that cannot be extracted by more conservative means, or when the bronchial condition does not involve the distal portion of the lung lobe and salvaging that lobe is essential.

Bronchial Surgical Procedures

Bronchiotomy is performed using a transverse incision, which is closed with simple interrupted sutures of fine-gauge nonabsorbable or slowly absorbable monofilament suture material. Sutures may be placed through or around the bronchial cartilages; in either case, the objective is to accurately align the edges of the bronchus and appose the bronchial mucosa. Resection and anastomosis of a bronchus can be performed using similar techniques.

Bronchial collapse as a result of atrial enlargement secondary to cardiac disease usually is treated by medical or surgical management of the cardiac disease. Rarely, bronchial banding has been used to treat bronchial collapse in dogs.

The Lungs

Pulmonary Anatomy

Each of the two lungs of the dog and the cat is divided into lobes based on the number of primary bronchi entering that lung. The right lung is composed of four lobes (cranial, middle, caudal, and accessory); the left lung has two lobes (cranial and caudal). Functional blood supply to the lungs is received through the pulmonary arteries, which divide to supply one branch to each lobe. One or more pulmonary veins drain each lung lobe. At the hilus of the lobe, a pulmonary artery lies cranial and a vein or veins lie caudal to each primary bronchus. Small bronchial arteries supply oxygenated blood to each lobe.

Pulmonary Diseases

Surgically treatable conditions of the lung generally are those localized to one or two lobes. Thoracic exploration may be useful to define the extent of pulmonary lesions when a condition is potentially treatable by surgical resection. The most common indications for pulmonary surgery in the dog and cat are discussed below.

Lung-Lobe Torsion

Lung-lobe torsion is an uncommon condition in the dog and cat. It occurs most commonly in large, deep-chested dogs and usually involves the right middle or cranial lung lobe. The mechanism by which the lung lobe becomes malpositioned is largely unknown. Several conditions that cause lung pathology, pleural effusion, and/or coughing have been associated with lung-lobe torsion and may be predisposing factors; among these conditions are chronic respiratory disease, pleural effusion, trauma, neoplasia, and prior thoracic surgery. Lung-lobe torsion also can occur spontaneously. Regardless of the etiology, torsion causes venous stasis and congestion of the lung lobe, followed by formation of an inflammatory or chylous pleural effusion that tends to become entrapped around the involved lobe.

Clinical signs typically include a variable degree of respiratory distress, tachypnea, and/ or coughing. Nonspecific signs due to pulmonary tissue necrosis and related pleuritis also may occur, including pyrexia, anorexia, and lethargy. Heart and lung sounds are muffled over the affected hemithorax due to the accumulation of pleural fluid.

A tentative diagnosis of lung-lobe torsion is based on the presence of a consolidated lung lobe that fails to reinflate after removal of a pleural effusion. The effusion is of a chylous or serosanginous, nonseptic inflammatory nature. In acute cases, a definitive diagnosis often can be based on plain radiographs in which the twisted bronchus is visible due to the presence of entrapped air. Later, the air is absorbed and bronchoscopy, bronchography, or exploratory thoracotomy may be necessary to confirm the diagnosis.

The treatment of choice is complete removal of the involved lung lobe, using a lateral intercostal approach. This procedure should be performed as soon as possible after the diagnosis is made. Since fibrous adhesions of the lung lobes to the thoracic wall are often present, particular care should be taken during the approach to avoid lacerating pulmonary tissue. Once the involved lobe is identified, an atraumatic cardiovascular or bronchus clamp is placed across the base of the lung before it is untwisted. This prevents shedding of necrotic or septic emboli from the damaged lobe into the systemic circulation, which can result in a shocklike syndrome within hours of the procedure. A routine lobectomy then is performed, followed by thorough lavage of the thoracic cavity and removal of fibrin and necrotic debris. All remaining lobes are examined to ensure they can expand and are properly positioned. A thoracostomy tube is placed prior to routine closure.

In addition to routine postoperative care for a thoracotomy, it is often necessary to treat the chylothorax that commonly develops after lobectomy for lung-lobe torsion. The cause of the chylothorax is ill-defined. Although the condition often is transient, resolving within 5 to 7 days, it may persist for a longer time. Treatment includes continued thoracic drainage and a low-fat diet (see "Chylothorax," p. 238).

Because of several potential complications, the prognosis for full recovery of a dog with lung-lobe torsion is fair to guarded. Complications include persistent chylothorax, development of a second lung-lobe torsion, or restrictive pleuritis.

Primary Pulmonary Neoplasms

Primary pulmonary tumors are relatively rare in both the dog and cat. They are nearly all malignant and tend to metastasize most often to pulmonary tissue, lymph nodes, and bone. Adenocarcinoma is the most common primary pulmonary neoplasm. Epidermoid (squamous cell) carcinomas and anaplastic carcinomas are seen less often; mesenchymal tumors are very rare. Lung tumors occur mainly in older animals (mean age at diagnosis, 10 years in the dog and 12 years in the cat). There is no consistent breed or sex predisposition. The most common clinical sign in the dog is a nonproductive cough. Nonspecific signs such as weight loss, lethargy, and anorexia also occur in the dog and are the most common signs in the cat. Occasionally, animals with these tumors are asymptomatic.

Dogs with lung tumors often have few or no abnormalities on physical examination. If the pulmonary lesion is large or if pleural effusion or pneumothorax develops secondary to the tumor, bronchovesicular sounds may be decreased and dyspnea may be detected. Lameness occasionally is seen in animals with primary pulmonary neoplasms and may be caused by metastatic bone lesions or hypertrophic osteopathy.

A tentative diagnosis of primary pulmonary tumor often is based on findings on thoracic radiographs. Left and right lateral, and ventrodorsal views are recommended to fully define the extent of the pulmonary lesion(s). In the dog, a primary lung tumor most often appears as a discrete mass, but may involve an entire lung lobe diffusely. Cavitation of the tumor is not uncommon. Rarely, multiple masses are present at diagnosis. Radiographic findings are much more variable in the cat. Pleural effusion occasionally is seen in both dogs and cats when the tumor has invaded the pleura extensively; this is a poor prognostic sign.

Animals are selected for surgical treatment based on the radiographic findings of a persistent or enlarging, solitary pulmonary mass with no evidence of nodal, pulmonary, or distant metastasis. Since these radiographic signs are nonspecific, several other conditions should be considered, including pulmonary abscess, granuloma (fungal, foreign body, or parasitic), pulmonary hemorrhage, or a solitary metastatic lesion. Regardless of the final diagnosis, the diagnostic and therapeutic method of choice for a persistent solitary pulmonary mass is surgical resection and biopsy. Percutaneous fine-needle aspiration biopsy can be used for diagnosis when the lesion(s) are thought to be nonresectable. This procedure can be followed by exploratory thoracotomy if the cytology results are nondiagnostic. Occasionally an exploratory thoracotomy also is indicated to delineate more accurately the extent and resectability of the lesions.

Wide surgical resection of lung tumors usually is accomplished by a complete lobectomy performed through a lateral intercostal thoracotomy, although partial lobectomy can be used to excise some peripheral masses. Following removal of the primary lung mass, the involved hemithorax is explored carefully to detect metastatic lesions. All accessible lung lobes and the pleural surfaces are examined visually and palpated. The tracheobronchial lymph nodes then are examined and appropriate biopsies are obtained. Closure and postoperative care are routine.

The prognosis for dogs with surgically resectable primary lung tumors is fair to guarded for short-term survival and poor for complete resolution of the disease. While resection of the tumor temporarily alleviates the clinical signs and seems to prolong the animal's survival, recurrence of the neoplasm and metastasis are common. The most valuable prognostic indicators in dogs with surgically treated primary lung tumors are:

1. the cell type,
2. the existence of metastasis, and
3. the presence or absence of clinical signs at the time of treatment.

Survival times vary from months to years, with the longest survivals occurring:

1. in dogs with adenocarcinoma (mean survival of 18 months, versus 8 months with squamous cell carcinoma),
2. in dogs with no evidence of metastasis at surgery, and/or
3. in dogs that were asymptomatic at the time of treatment.

Early detection and surgical treatment result in the longest survival times. The prognosis for cats with primary lung tumors is poor, because metastasis typically is present at diagnosis.

Foreign Body, Abscess, Granuloma

Pulmonary foreign bodies can be inhaled or can enter the lungs by migrating through the mediastinum or pleural space. Typically, they cause local atelectasis of the lung and abscessation or granuloma formation. The clinical course may begin with severe coughing episodes in the acute stages and progress to vague and intermittent signs, including coughing, pyrexia, anorexia, and lethargy. When the foreign body is radiopaque, the diagnosis can be made on thoracic radiographs. More often, the foreign body is not visualized, but radiographs show a local area of pulmonary consolidation consistent with atelectasis, abscess, or granuloma. Partial or complete lobectomy is the method of choice for removing pulmonary foreign bodies.

Pulmonary abscessation occurs more commonly in the cat than in the dog and can be associated with pyothorax. Other predisposing conditions include chronic pulmonary infection, foreign body, penetrating wound, and neoplasia. A pulmonary abscess may appear on radiographs as a cavitated lesion or as an area of localized increased density. Clinical findings are consistent with a systemic infection and often include lethargy, anorexia, pyrexia, coughing, and respiratory distress. Leukocytosis with a degenerative left shift also may be present. Appropriate antibiotic therapy directed by culture and sensitivity should be attempted before surgical intervention is considered. Excising the affected lobe is the treatment of choice in cases that do not respond to medical therapy.

Pulmonary granulomas can be caused by fungal infections, foreign bodies, or parasite migration. Clinical signs depend on the cause of the condition. The radiographic appearance of a granuloma often is similar to that of a pulmonary abscess or neoplasm. Surgical resection and biopsy is the treatment of choice, along with treatment of any underlying cause.

Pulmonary Trauma

Pneumothorax and hemothorax often are associated with pulmonary trauma. These conditions usually are best treated by establishing thoracic drainage and allowing the pulmonary laceration to seal spontaneously. However, the following situations indicate the need for surgical treatment:

1. Occasionally, a major bronchus is lacerated or avulsed, creating a tension pneumothorax that cannot be controlled even with continuous suction. In this situation, the bronchus should be sutured or the involved lung removed. Unfortunately, animals with major bronchial lacerations rarely survive to the point of surgical treatment.

2. A second indication for surgery exists when smaller volumes of air continue to leak into the pleural space for more than 5 to 7 days. In this situation, underlying lung pathology is likely and should be identified and treated via thoracotomy. Whenever possible, attempts should be made to identify the site of air leakage before surgery. If the pneumothorax is unilateral, a lateral intercostal thoracotomy can be used. In cases of bilateral pneumothorax in which the source of the air leak cannot be identified, a median sternotomy should be used to permit inspection and visualization of all lung fields.

3. A third indication for surgery involves treatment of traumatic lung cysts. These lesions, also referred to as traumatic bullae or pneumatoceles, may form secondary to pulmonary trauma. They consist of thin-walled accumulations of air or fluid within the lung. Most of these lesions resolve spontaneously within weeks of the initial injury; others rupture and are one cause of continuous pneumothorax after pulmonary trauma. Because of the likelihood that spontaneous rupture will cause life-threatening pneumothorax, traumatic lung cysts should be resected if there is no radiographic evidence of their resolution within 1 month of the inciting injury.

Pulmonary Lesions Causing Spontaneous Pneumothorax

Spontaneous pneumothorax results from leakage of air from nontraumatic pulmonary lesions. Pulmonary diseases associated with spontaneous pneumothorax include congenital and traumatic cysts, bullae, blebs, bullous emphysema, chronic obstructive pulmonary disease, bronchiectasis, granuloma, abscess, neoplasms, and pneumonia.

Congenital and traumatic cysts both consist of thin-walled, fluid- or air-filled sacs within the lung. Congenital cysts most often involve multiple lung lobes; severely affected animals die of respiratory disease at an early age. Rarely, congenital cysts are solitary or involve only one lung lobe. In these cases, the cyst or cysts are likely to rupture, causing pneumothorax. The diagnosis of a congenital pulmonary cyst is based on histopathologic evidence that the cyst has an epithelial lining. Traumatic cysts are similar structures, but are not lined by epithelium. The diagnosis and treatment of traumatic cysts is discussed above.

Bullae, blebs, and bullous emphysema all are pulmonary lesions that occur secondary to chronic obstructive pulmonary disease. The lesions tend to involve multiple lung lobes, and because of their small size are often difficult to identify before and during thoracic exploration. Bullae are thin-walled, air-filled sacs within the lung; blebs are small subpleural bullae. Bullous emphysema is an accumulation of air in the interalveolar tissue of the lung. Rupture of these lesions is a common cause of spontaneous pneumothorax.

Granulomas, abscesses, and neoplasms also have been associated with the development of spontaneous pneumothorax. These conditions are discussed elsewhere in this chapter.

Pulmonary Procedures

Lobectomy

Pulmonary lobectomy is the complete removal of a lung lobe at its primary bronchus. It is used commonly to resect solitary pulmonary lesions in both the cat and the dog. Optimal exposure for a lobectomy usually can be attained by a 5th intercostal lateral thoracotomy for the cranial and middle lobes and a 6th intercostal lateral thoracotomy for caudal and accessory lobes. A median sternotomy should be used when exposure of both hemithoraces is essential.

The lobe to be resected is identified and the remaining lobes are packed off from the surgical site with saline moistened laparotomy pads. Care should be taken to avoid excessive traction on the involved lung lobe; such traction may impair ventilation of the opposite lung by causing angulation of the trachea or bronchus or partial occlusion of the endotracheal tube. The lobe is mobilized by carefully severing the pleural reflections attaching it to the mediastinum. Pulmonary vessels are isolated within the pleural reflections on each side of the bronchus. They are triply ligated and transected between the two distal ligatures. The bronchus then is occluded with an atraumatic bronchus clamp and is transected about 1 cm distal to the clamp.

The bronchus is closed by placing a double row of continuous 2-0 to 4-0 nonabsorbable sutures in the free edges (Fig. 9-14). This procedure requires meticulous surgical technique, and leakage of air around the suture tracts is a common problem. In cats and very small dogs, simple double ligation of the bronchial stump is adequate. Prior to closure of the thoracotomy, the bronchial surgery site should be submerged in warm saline and observed for air leakage during gentle lung expansion by positive-pressure ventilation. If it occurs, gentle digital pressure may allow deposition of fibrin clots to seal the leaks. Occasionally, additional sutures may be necessary. A thoracostomy tube should be placed routinely following lobectomy and monitored closely for 24 to 48 hours. A less traumatic and more rapid method of bronchial closure involves the use of surgical stapling equipment, which is not widely available in veterinary practice.

Partial Lobectomy

A partial lobectomy is indicated for diagnostic biopsy or for excision of a small lesion in the periphery of the lung lobe. The procedure is performed by placing two noncrushing clamps along the line of transection (Fig. 9-15). A row of horizontal mattress sutures is placed proxi-

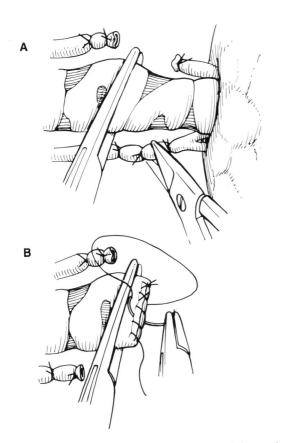

Figure 9-14. *Lung lobectomy is performed by triple ligation of the pulmonary vessels and closure of the bronchus using two rows of simple continuous sutures.*

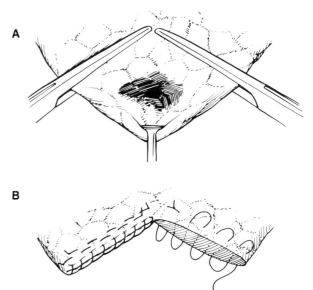

Figure 9-15. ***A,*** *Partial lobectomy is performed by isolating the lesion with noncrushing forceps.* ***B,*** *After resection, a double row of continuous horizontal mattress sutures is placed behind the forceps. The forceps is then removed and the edges are oversewn with a simple continuous pattern.*

mal to the clamp. Local ventilation of the sutured portion of the lung is controlled by digital compression applied by the surgical assistant. The clamps then are removed and the free edges are oversewn with a simple continuous pattern. Stapling equipment also can be used to perform a partial lobectomy.

Pneumonectomy

Pneumonectomy is the complete removal of either the right or the left lung; there are few indications for this procedure in veterinary medicine. The procedure is feasible only when the remaining lung is healthy and has adequate function to support oxygenation of the blood. Pneumonectomy is accomplished by performing multiple lobectomies on the affected lung or by amputating the lung at the level of the mainstem bronchus using the technique described for lobectomy.

Suggested Readings

Introduction

Crowe DT. Thoracic drainage. In: Bojrab MJ, ed. Current techniques in small animal surgery. 2nd ed. Philadelphia: Lea & Febiger, 1983:287.

Evans HE, Christensen GC. Miller's anatomy of the dog. 2nd ed. Philadelphia: WB Saunders, 1979.

Lee AH, Swaim SF, Henderson RA. Surgical drainage. Compend Contin Ed Pract Vet 1986;8:94.

Lipowitz AJ, Schenk MP. Surgical approaches to the abdominal and thoracic viscera. Vet Clin N Amer 1979;9:169.

Nelson AW. Bronchi and lungs. In: Bojrab MJ, ed. Current techniques in small animal surgery. 2nd ed. Philadelphia: Lea & Febiger, 1983:270.

Orton EC. Pleura and pleural space. In: Slatter DH, ed. Textbook of small animal surgery. Philadelphia: WB Saunders, 1985:536.

Wingfield WE, Blevin MT, Quirk PE. Use of continuous chest drainage in dogs and cats. J Am Anim Hosp Assoc 1985;21:29.

Chest Wall

Bell FW. Neoplastic diseases of the thorax. Vet Clin North Amer 1987;17:387.

Bjorling DE, Kolata RJ, DeNovo RC. Flail chest: Review, clinical experience and new method of stabilization. J Am Anim Hosp Assoc 1982; 18:269.

Bright RM. Reconstruction of thoracic wall defects using Marlex mesh. J Am Anim Hosp Assoc 1981;17:415.

Bright RM, Birchard SJ, Long GG. Repair of thoracic wall defects in the dog with an omental pedicle flap. J Am Anim Hosp Assoc 1982; 18:277.

Kolata RJ. Management of thoracic trauma. Vet Clin North Amer 1981;11:103.

Orton C. Thoracic wall. In: Slatter DH, ed. Textbook of small animal surgery. Philadelphia: WB Saunders, 1985:536.

Spackman CJA, Caywood DD. Management of thoracic trauma and chest wall reconstruction. Vet Clin North Amer 1987;17:431.

Pleural Space

Birchard SJ, Fossum TW. Chylothorax in the dog and cat. Vet Clin North Am 1987;17:271.

Brennan KE, Ihrke PJ. Grass awn migration in dogs and cats: A retrospective study of 182 cases. J Am Vet Med Assoc 1983;182:1201.

Christopher MM. Pleural effusions. Vet Clin North Am 1987;17:255.

Fossum TW, Birchard SJ, Jacobs RM. Chylothorax in 34 dogs. J Am Vet Med Assoc 1986;188:1315.

Holmberg DL. Management of pyothorax. Vet Clin North Am 1979;9:357.

Kramek BA, Caywood DD. Pneumothorax. Vet Clin North Am 1987;17:285.

Noone KE. Pleural effusions and diseases of the pleura. Vet Clin North Am 1983;15:1069.

Orsher R. Pleurodesis for chylothorax. Presented at the Annual meeting of the American College of Veterinary Surgeons, Tucson, Ariz., Feb. 5, 1988.

Orton EC. Pleura and pleural space. In: Slatter DH, ed. Textbook of small animal surgery. Philadelphia: WB Saunders, 1985:547.

Richardson DC. Trauma of the respiratory tract. In: Bright RM, ed. Surgical emergencies. Contemporary issues in small animal practice. Vol. 2. New York: Churchill Livingstone, 1986:89.

Scherding RG. Pyothorax in the cat. Compend Contin Ed Pract Vet 1979;1:247.

Smeak DD, Gallagher L, et al. Management of intractable pleural effusion in a dog with pleuroperitoneal shunt. Vet Surg 1987;16:212.

Diaphragm

Garson HL, Dodman NH, Baker GJ. Diaphragmatic hernia. Analysis of 56 cases in dogs and cats. J Small Anim Pract 1980;21:469.

Levine SH. Diaphragmatic hernia. Vet Clin North Am 1987;17:411.

Punch PI, Slatter DH. Diaphragmatic hernias. In: Slatter DH, ed. Textbook of small animal surgery. Philadelphia: WB Saunders, 1985:869.

Wilson GP, Hayes HM. Diaphragmatic hernia in the dog and cat: A 25-year overview. Semin Vet Med Surg (Sm Anim) 1986;1:318.

Mediastinum

Aronsohn MG, Schunk KL, Carpenter JL, et al. Clinical and pathologic features of thymoma in 15 dogs. J Am Vet Med Assoc 1984;184:1355.

Carpenter JL, Holzworth J. Thymoma in 11 cats. J Am Vet Med Assoc 1982;181:248.

Klopfer U, Perl S, Yakobson B, et al. Spontaneous fatal hemorrhage in the involuting thymus in dogs. J Am Anim Hosp Assoc 1985;21:251.

Liu S, Patnaik AK, Burk RL. Thymic branchial cysts in the dog and cat. J Am Vet Med Assoc 1983;182:1095.

Suter P, Zinkl J. Mediastinal, pleural, and extrapleural thoracic diseases. In: Ettinger SJ, ed. Textbook of veterinary internal medicine. 2nd ed. Philadelphia: WB Saunders, 1983;840.

Bronchi and Lungs

Aron DN, Kornegay JN. The clinical significance of traumatic lung cysts and associated pulmonary abnormalities in the dog and cat. J Am Anim Hosp Assoc 1983;19:903.

Kramek BA, Caywood DD, O'Brien TD. Bullous emphysema and recurrent pneumothorax in the dog. Vet Surg 1985;186:971.

Lord PF, Greiner TP, Greene RW, et al. Lung lobe torsion in the dog. J Am Anim Hosp Assoc 1973;9:473.

Mehlhaff CJ, Mooney S. Primary pulmonary neoplasia in the dog and cat. Vet Clin North Am 1985;15:1061.

Yoshioka MM. Management of spontaneous pneumothorax in twelve dogs. J Am Anim Hosp Assoc 1982;18:57.

10

Walter E. Weirich

The Cardiovascular System

Thirteen percent of dogs and nine percent of cats have heart or blood vessel disease, or both; most of these cases result in congestive heart failure due to cardiomyopathy or chronic valvular endocardiosis, and their condition is not amenable to practical surgical correction. In fact, less than 0.5% of all cases seen in general small animal practice are potential candidates for surgery. Many of these cases are complex malformations, and expensive, sophisticated equipment and skills are needed to reach an accurate diagnosis and prognosis. Therefore, it is not cost-effective for most veterinarians to develop the expertise and buy the equipment to provide complete care for these patients in their own facilities; clients and patients can be referred to a veterinary center where the capability does exist. When such a case arises, the veterinarian should provide information to help the client decide whether to accept referral or to pursue a more conservative treatment course with the local

veterinarian. This information should include realistic expectations from the referral and a reasonable idea of what course the disease might take without referral or surgery.

General Considerations of Cardiovascular Disease

Compensatory changes in the heart allow animals to survive congenital and acquired heart and blood vessel abnormalities. These changes proceed predictably and can be traced to the source of the problem.

Congenital cardiovascular disease is manifested in three basic anatomic forms. Anatomic changes lead to:

1. obstruction of blood flow,
2. overcirculation to one part of the cardio-

vascular system at the expense of normal channels, or

3. (infrequently) conduction abnormality and pump failure.

The basic principle is that the right and left ventricles of the heart must pump an equal amount of blood. Identifying any compensatory changes can narrow the list of differential diagnoses.

Evaluating the Cardiac Patient

Physical Examination and History

Take a thorough physical examination and history, even if the signs reported by the owner are highly suggestive of a cardiac problem. In young animals, the owner often is unaware that any problem exists. An accurate history and physical examination of the cardiovascular system provide a great deal of information. When taking the history, ask about exercise tolerance and other cardiovascular signs: this allows functional classification of heart failure (Table 10-1). Examine the character of the pulses for changes that may suggest abnormal cardiac function. The jugular veins should not be distended in dogs and cats in a normal sitting position, but they do distend when the patient is in lateral recumbency. Determine if fluid is accumulating in the peritoneal cavity and/or in peripheral tissues. Examine the mucous membranes for the intensity of color; they should be pink in nonpigmented animals. Palpate the rib cage and heart to determine the shape of the ribs and the location of the point of maximal impulse of the beating heart. Auscultation is essential. Note if a palpable thrill or a pulse deficit is present.

Laboratory and Special Clinical Evaluations

The clinical pathologic examination should include a complete blood count and chemistry panels, as poor cardiovascular function affects many organ systems. Thoracic radiographs should be taken to evaluate heart size and the pulmonary system. Ultrasound can be very helpful in evaluating a wide range of cardiovascular problems, and it significantly decreases the need for cardiac catheterization. An electrocardiogram provides information on the rhythm of the heart and also can support enlargement findings detected by radiographs or ultrasound. Typical results of each test are described under specific diseases.

Cardiac Catheterization

If noninvasive studies (ultrasound, radiography, and electrocardiogram) do not provide enough data for diagnosis, cardiac catheterization may be necessary. The goal of the procedure is to place the catheter near the suspected lesion, to allow abnormal pressures to be detected in a chamber of the heart and the vessels leading to and from the heart. Contrast media can be injected upstream from the suspected lesion; videotape or multiple spot films (3 to 12/second) are used to record the contrast medium flowing through or around the defect. This usually allows the defect to be visualized. Cardiac output also can be estimated and, if a shunt is causing blood to travel in abnormal pathways, the quantity of blood flowing through the shunt can be estimated.

Cardiac catheterization requires general anesthesia and a cutdown on the vessels in the thigh or the neck. Most of the information needed can be gained by catheterizing the left

---

Table 10–1. Functional Classification of Heart Failure

Functional Class I	Detectable cardiac abnormality only; no signs of pulmonary or systemic disease related to the cardiac abnormality; normal exercise tolerance.
Functional Class II	Clinical signs occur only after strenuous exercise.
Functional Class III	Clinical signs are present after ordinary exercise and may occur after a period of rest.
Functional Class IV	Clinical signs are present at rest.

carotid artery and the jugular vein. A pigtailed catheter is most convenient for the left ventricle, as this shape allows easy entry into the left ventricle, retrograde through the aortic valve. Straight-tipped catheters can hang up in the valve cusps and could damage the leaflets. A National Institutes of Health (NIH) catheter (closed, four side holes) can be used for the right side. If needed, this catheter usually can be maneuvered into the pulmonary artery. One helpful maneuver, when encountering a stenotic outflow tract or valve, is to measure the pressure gradient across it by pulling the catheter through the stenotic area as the pressure is being recorded (*i.e.*, "pressure pullback"). The magnitude of the gradient is proportional to the clinical severity of the problem.

Congenital Heart Disease

The most common types of congenital heart diseases and the breeds that are most often affected are presented in Tables 10-2 and 10-3.

Patent Ductus Arteriosus (PDA)

Anatomy

The ductus arteriosus is a shunt that allows blood to bypass the nonfunctioning fetal lung. In the fetus, blood flows through the ductus from the pulmonary artery to the aorta. The

Table 10–2. Congenital Cardiovascular Lesions (In Descending Order of Frequency of Occurrence)

Patent ductus arteriosus
Pulmonic stenosis
Aortic stenosis
Persistent right aortic arch
Ventricular septal defect
Tetralogy of Fallot
Atrial septal defect
Persistent left cranial vena cava
Mitral insufficiency

Table 10–3. Breed-Related Congenital Heart Disease

Breed	Disease
Beagle	Pulmonic stenosis
	Incomplete right bundle branch block
Boxer	Subaortic stenosis
	Pulmonic stenosis
	Atrial septal defect
Cocker spaniel	Patent ductus arteriosus
	Persistent right fourth aortic arch
Collie	Patent ductus arteriosus
Dachshund	Persistent right fourth aortic arch
Doberman pinscher	Bundle of His degeneration (sudden death)
German shepherd	Persistent right fourth aortic arch
	Patent ductus arteriosus
	Aortic stenosis
	Pulmonic stenosis
Keeshond	Tetralogy of Fallot
Labrador retriever	Pulmonic stenosis
	Ventricular septal defect
	Aortic stenosis
Newfoundland	Aortic stenosis
Poodle	Patent ductus arteriosus

lungs are not expanded, so high resistance to blood flow exists in the pulmonary vasculature. Blood follows the path of least resistance: to bypass the lungs directly into the aorta.

In normal puppies and kittens, the ductus is closed at birth. If it remains open when the animal is born and begins to breathe, the lungs expand and the vascular resistance drops precipitously (Fig. 10-1). The left ventricle begins pumping at a higher pressure as peripheral resistance rises. Blood flow reverses in the ductus, and the oxygen level rises to a much higher level than in the fetus. The higher oxygen levels in the blood flowing from the aorta to the pulmonary artery stimulate the smooth muscle in the ductus wall to contract, leading to functional closure.

Later, the ductus becomes a fibrous band, the ligamentum arteriosum. Prostaglandins play a role in closure of the ductus. Administering high levels of prostaglandin inhibitors, such as indomethacin, results in closure of the ductus if given before 11 days of age in

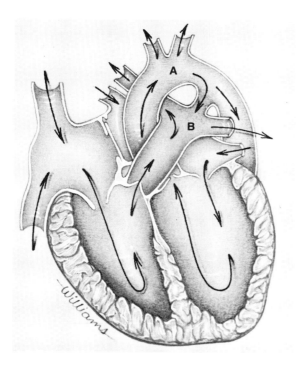

Figure 10-1. *Abnormal neonatal circulation. Blood flows from the aorta (A) to the pulmonary artery (B). This produces the continuous murmur that is classic in patent ductus arteriosus.*

humans. Dogs seldom are diagnosed that early; when the drug is given at 6 weeks or later, there is little likelihood of closure, even though the character of the murmur changes. This drug also may cause gastric ulceration in the dog.

In the dog, most of the ductus is in the wall of the aorta, leaving a very short length available for dissection and ligation. Table 3 provides information on PDA by breed prevalence. Females are more commonly affected than are males. PDA occurs in mixed breeds, but more often in purebred animals. PDA also has been shown to be hereditary in poodles. The mode of inheritance is polygenic.

Diagnosis

The classical continuous ("machinery") murmur (heard throughout systole and diastole) is auscultable, especially in the left 3rd or 4th intercostal space at the level of the point of the shoulder. Many dogs also have a holosystolic murmur of mitral insufficiency, due to dilation of the mitral valve ring. Possible confusion between a combination of rapid heart rate and systolic murmur, and a continuous murmur in a puppy can be differentiated by slowly moving the stethoscope back and forth between the base of the heart and the apex, as a purely systolic murmur has no diastolic component. The run-off of blood from the root of the aorta through the PDA into the pulmonary artery during diastole results in a very wide pulse pressure that can be detected as a water-hammer pulse in the femoral artery.

Radiography is very helpful in demonstrating the very enlarged left ventricle, which is compensating for the loss of blood flow to the systemic circulation by increasing the stroke volume. PDA produces the greatest dilation of the left ventricle of any of the common congenital heart problems of the dog. The lung receives more blood than normal because some blood recirculates through the lung via the ductus. This leads to vascular distention of the pulmonary vessels. Some lung damage results from this hyperperfusion; the longer the duration of the abnormal circulation, the greater the damage and the longer it will last following surgical correction.

On an electrocardiogram, the dilated left ventricle is seen as very tall R waves in lead II and aVf. R waves may be 4 mv. Hematologic findings are unremarkable, except for possible anemia. Ultrasound demonstrates the dilated left ventricle; if the puppy is large enough, the dilated arch of the aorta may be seen. The ductus itself, however, is too far dorsal to see because it is covered by the lung, especially in small puppies.

Treatment

Because of the damage caused by the hyperperfusion of the lung, surgery to ligate the ductus should be done as soon as the diagnosis can be established. This minimizes the damage to the heart and lungs. Treatment consists of ligating the ductus to stop the abnormal blood flow. Most patients and clients will be best served if they are referred to an experienced surgical specialist. Although the surgery often is very straightforward, it involves dissecting around blood vessels carrying 100% of the cardiac output, and the ductus is very short.

There are two common techniques for ligating the ductus, either direct dissection around the ductus, or dissection behind the aorta. Each is best approached via a left lateral 4th intercostal thoracotomy incision. The advantage of direct dissection is that the ligature is placed only around the ductus and complete closure is easily ensured. The danger associated with this technique is that it places greater stress on the pulmonary artery and aorta during dissection. The behind-the-aorta technique places very little stress on the major vessels, but it is difficult to clear all the connective tissue from the deep (right) side of the ductus. This could result in failure to completely close the ductus.

Prognosis and Management Without Surgery

If the owner rejects surgical correction, the animal will be at an increasing risk of left heart failure. Many animals do not survive to 6 months of age; rarely do any survive to 3 years of age, although one dog has been reported to survive to 15 years of age. Early surgery saves the lives of 92% of dogs; they then have the potential to live a normal life span.

Aortic Stenosis

Anatomy

In aortic stenosis, the subvalvular area on the left ventricular side of the aortic valve is encircled by a band of fibrous tissue that obstructs the free flow of blood into the aortic root (Fig. 10-2). The subvalvular area may have a nearly normal diameter at birth, but it does not enlarge at a normal rate as the animal grows, resulting in an increasing relative stenosis. A murmur may not be auscultable early in life, but as the relative stenosis increases, the increasing turbulence in the outflow tract results in a typical crescendo-decrescendo murmur. As the resistance to flow increases, the left ventricular myocardium hypertrophies. This can actually increase the degree of stenosis during systole, as the muscle bulges into the outflow tract. The mass of myocardium can cause severe arrhythmia and can reduce ventricular compliance, leading to an inability to increase cardiac output with increasing physical activity. The peripheral resistance drops as the skeletal muscles demand more blood. The central blood pressure drops because the delivery of blood cannot be increased commensurately with tissue demands. The brain does not receive sufficient blood pressure and flow to maintain consciousness, and syncope occurs. Severe arrhythmia can cause syncope and progress to sudden death.

Diagnosis

Most dogs with aortic stenosis have a systolic murmur by weaning age, while some are 4 to 5 months old before a murmur is noted. There may be no clinical signs at this time. The murmur is heard best over the left 4th intercostal space at the level of the point of the shoulder. The murmur radiates in the direction of the turbulent blood flow, so it often is heard at the thoracic inlet as it radiates into the carotid arteries. Loud murmurs may even be heard at top of the head. As the aortic root enlarges, the murmur may then be heard with greatest intensity on the right side of the chest. Pulses are weak and pulse pressure is narrow.

Radiographs show an enlarged left ventricle and dilated aortic root, with normal pulmonary vasculature. An electrocardiogram may show a prolonged QRS complex. An ultrasonogram shows the hypertrophy of the left ventricle. The obstructed outflow tract can be visualized, as most affected dogs are large. It is usually not necessary, therefore, to perform a cardiac catheterization to establish the diagnosis. Cardiac catheterization does allow mea-

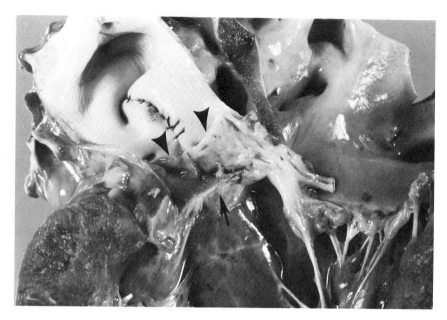

Figure 10-2. *Gross pathological specimens from a dog with subvalvular aortic stenosis. The stenosis is most often present in the subvalvular area (arrow). It may take the form of a diaphragm of tissue obstructing blood flow. As the left ventricular hypertrophy develops, the stenosis may be made more severe by muscular impingement on the outflow tract during systole. Note the aortic valve leaflets (arrowheads). They are slightly thickened by the jet of blood from the stenosis, but were functioning normally. (Gourley IM, Vasseur PB, eds. General small animal surgery. Philadelphia: JB Lippincott, 1985:824.)*

surement of the pressure gradient across the outflow tract.

Treatment

The hypertrophic subvalvular region can be seen and resected through the aortic valve under cardiac arrest conditions. Because of the hypertrophy of the left ventricle, the myocardium is very susceptible to oxygen deficiency and/or infarction. Also, the coronary arteries are widely dilated and the possibility that air emboli or clots will occlude a coronary artery is significant.

An alternative technique that preserves the myocardium can be performed on the beating heart. A valve dilator blindly tears the subvalvular area (Fig. 10-3) This is best done when the animal has achieved as much growth as possible, but before the heart has grossly enlarged or clinical signs become evident. Three to six months of age appears to be the ideal time for surgery.

If surgery is not done, the animal probably will die from an arrhythmia, usually very early in life.

Ventricular Septal Defect (VSD)

Ventricular septal defect (VSD) is the most common congenital cardiac defect seen in newborn humans and cattle. VSD may be the most common defect in dogs, but veterinarians seldom examine preweaning puppies, one third of which die before weaning. VSD most often is diagnosed at the puppy's first visit to a veterinarian. Clinical signs often are absent. VSDs sometimes close spontaneously at about 1 year of age, in an unknown percentage of dogs.

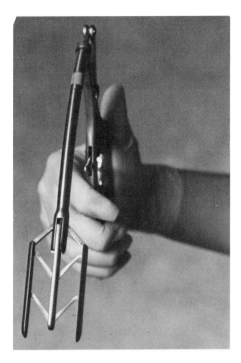

Figure 10-3.   *A valve dilator. The jaws of the valve dilator remain parallel to the shaft of the instrument as they are opened, thus keeping them within the valve as it is dilated. (Gourley IM, Vasseur PB, eds. General small animal surgery. Philadelphia: JB Lippincott, 1985:824.)*

Clinical Signs

The early clinical signs associated with a large VSD are related to left heart failure. Because of the overcirculation of the lung, the pulmonary vascular resistance rises to very high levels, requiring the right side to work very hard to pump blood through the lung. This leads to blood vessel rupture and severe hemorrhage into the lung parenchyma in the late stages of the disease.

Diagnosis is based on the presence of a holosystolic murmur, heard best over the right 5th to 7th intercostal space near the sternal boarder. Larger VSDs are heard further cranially and dorsally. Radiology reveals enlargement of both ventricles and the left atrium and hyperperfusion of the pulmonary circulation. The electrocardiogram is normal, or evidence

of mild right heart or biventricular enlargement may be apparent. Large Q waves are often present. An ultrasound study may suggest a VSD in the upper septum, though it is wise to perform an angiocardiogram via a selective catheterization of the left ventricle.

Treatment

No treatment may be needed if there are no signs of heart failure. It is important, however, to follow the animal closely to determine if the heart size enlarges out of proportion to its body growth. If the heart is not abnormally enlarged, the defect is probably small and may close spontaneously. If the heart enlarges rapidly, the animal should be referred for surgical repair using either cardiopulmonary bypass or hypothermia. If surgery is not performed to repair a large defect, the patient will die from heart failure and/or massive bleeding into the lung.

Pulmonic Stenosis

Anatomy

Pulmonic stenosis is the second most commonly detected congenital heart defect of dogs. The systolic murmur is evident at birth. The disease most often is diagnosed when the animal is presented for its first examination. Some affected puppies will show exercise intolerance, but right heart failure does not occur until later in the course of the disease.

The defect most often is of the valvular type (Fig. 10-4), in which the valve becomes a dome-shaped structure with a hole in the center. Some cases, usually those diagnosed later in the course of the disease, have a subvalvular component that may cause the right ventricular outflow tract to be closed off by bulging muscle during systole. This may coexist with valvular stenosis, or it can be secondary to a hypertrophic change resulting from a need for increased pressure to overcome the resistance to blood flow from the right ventricle.

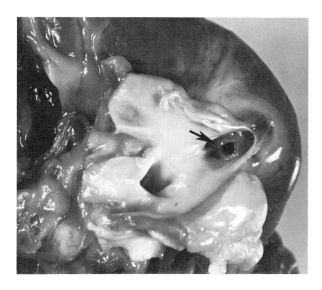

Figure 10-4. *Pulmonic stenosis in the dog is most often valvular. A stenotic pulmonary valve (arrow) as viewed from the pulmonary root is demonstrated in this photograph. The coronary blood flow in this animal was inadequate, and fatal subendocardial infarcts resulted after general anesthesia. (Gourley IM, Vasseur PB, eds. General small animal surgery. Philadelphia: JB Lippincott, 1985:814.)*

Diagnosis

This is based on physical findings of a systolic crescendo-decrescendo murmur, heard best in the left 3rd intercostal space just below the point of the shoulder. The murmur tends to radiate dorsally and caudally behind the left scapula. Radiographic features include a very enlarged right ventricle, due primarily to hypertrophy. Vascular patterns in the lungs are normal. Later in the course of the disease, prominent right heart failure signs may be evident, especially ascites. The electrocardiogram demonstrates severe right ventricular hypertrophy with a predominantly negative QRS complex in lead II and a W-shaped QRS complex in lead V_{10}. The results of clinical laboratory tests usually are unremarkable, although anemia is common in young affected dogs. An ultrasonogram clearly shows marked right ventricular hypertrophy; if the dog is large enough, the outflow tract can be visualized and the stenotic opening measured.

It may be difficult to distinguish the murmur of a VSD from that of pulmonic stenosis. If the evidence is equivocal, an angiocardiogram may be needed to establish the diagnosis. This should be a selective cardiac catheterization, with the contrast medium injected via a pigtail catheter in the left ventricle. If a VSD is pres-

ent, dye crosses the ventricular septum into the right ventricle and pulmonary artery. A second angiocardiogram also should be done with injection in the right ventricle to visualize pulmonic stenosis. An ultrasonogram provides adequate information for diagnosis in most cases.

Treatment

The most common method of treatment is a blind valvulotomy (Fig. 10-5), which is associated with very low surgical mortality or morbidity and provides sufficient relief from the obstruction for the size of the right ventricle to recede towards normal. This can be done via thoracotomy using a valve dilator to open the valve or a balloon catheter, which is inflated within the stenosis to dilate the valve. Some animals that have been followed clinically for as long as 9 years after blind valvulotomy have done well.

An alternate surgical procedure is to place a patch graft on the outflow tract to enlarge the valvular and subvalvular areas. This takes longer than valvulotomy and the potential for problems is somewhat greater, but in experienced hands the results are very good and the risks are low. This technique is rework is short. The risk of death from arrhythmias during surgery is somewhat greater than with valvulotomy.

Complications

The heart compensates for outflow obstruction by right ventricular hypertrophy. The end point of the coronary arterial circulation is in the subendocardium. Therefore, in animals with advanced disease, any compromise of the blood flow to the coronary arteries can result in myocardial ischemia. In all of these cases, the subendocardium is involved to the greatest extent, leading to ischemic hypotension and death in the most severely involved individuals. Once hypotension is manifest, there is so much myocardial damage that treatment is useless. Early surgery is required to avoid ischemic hypotension. If the owner does not wish to pursue surgical care, the animal should be treated for right heart failure. Most animals with pulmonic stenosis die before reaching 4 years of age, the most severely involved dying before one year of age.

Persistent Right Aortic Arch

Persistent right aortic arch is a malformation of the aortic arch. It is the most common of several vascular anomalies that result in digestive system signs. The right 4th aortic arch persists instead of the left, with the result that the ligamentum arteriosum encircles the esophagus between the aortic arch and the pulmonary artery. The patient shows signs of regurgitation as soon as it is offered solid food. This condition is discussed further in Chapter 12, The Esophagus and Stomach.

Tetralogy of Fallot

Tetralogy of Fallot is a complex congenital defect that consists of a severe pulmonic stenosis, usually subvalvular; a high ventricular septal defect; an aorta that overrides the ventricular septum, straddling the septal defect area; and severe right ventricular hypertrophy that de-

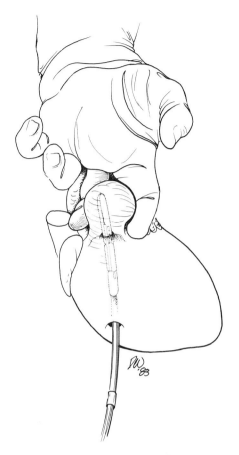

Figure 10-5. *Correction of pulmonary valve stenosis. The valve dilator, when closed, may be larger than the opening in the pulmonary valve. The valve dilator must be forced through the opening. To accomplish this, the index and second fingers of the surgeon's free hand are placed on the main pulmonary artery. The dilator can be felt as it passes through the valve. A smaller instrument, such as a straight Kelly hemostatic clamp, should be passed first so that the true pathway can be identified. Otherwise, the tricuspid valve septal leaflet could be damaged. (Gourley IM, Vasseur PB, eds. General small animal surgery. Philadelphia: JB Lippincott, 1985:817.)*

quired if a subvalvular component of the stenosis exists.

A pulmonary arteriotomy can be done to expose the stenotic pulmonary valve for plastic modification or removal of the valve. This produces a good result, but the venous inflow must be ligated temporarily and the time to

velops due to the high resistance against which the right ventricle must pump.

Clinical Signs

These become increasingly severe as the patient grows. The main problem is that venous and arterial blood mix, markedly reducing the blood oxygen concentration. The kidneys respond by releasing hematopoietin, causing an increase in the red cell mass that can be quite severe, with packed cell volumes rising to 70 to 80%. This leads to hyperactive clotting mechanisms; intravascular coagulation is a complicating factor, with packed cell volumes above 68%.

Diagnosis

An electrocardiogram, radiography, and ultrasound examination all show the very prominent right ventricular hypertrophy.

Treatment

Definitive repair is difficult to accomplish because of the position of the aortic root over the VSD. This results in great difficulty in suturing a patch with only the aortic valve ring in which to place sutures. Instead, palliative treatment is performed by using a piece of the jugular vein to fashion a shunt between the pulmonary artery and aorta (Fig. 10-6). The size of the jugular vein is ideal to provide increased blood flow to the lungs and yet not lead to pulmonary edema.

The shunt may close in the late postoperative period. To help prevent this, the animal must be maintained on some form of anticoagulant therapy for the rest of its life; 4 to 5 mg/kg of aspirin per day is sufficient. A normal life span following surgery is unlikely, but a reasonable quality of life is possible. The red blood cell mass returns toward normal after surgery.

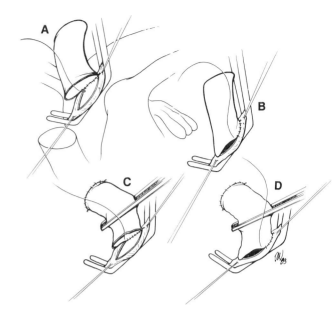

Figure 10-6. *Use of the jugular vein graft shunt for palliation of Tetralogy of Fallot.* **(A)** *Stay suture allows control of the aorta for the placement of a Satinsky clamp.* **(B)** *The back of the anastomosis is completed, followed by closure of the front.* **(C)** *The graft is cross clamped in its midportion and the Satinsky clamp is removed and placed on the pulmonary trunk.* **(D)** *The graft is sutured to the pulmonary trunk as previously described. (Gourley IM, Vasseur PB, eds. General small animal surgery. Philadelphia: JB Lippincott, 1985:832.)*

Acquired Cardiovascular Disease

Mitral Valvular Regurgitation

Mitral valvular regurgitation is the most common heart problem detected in dogs. Regurgitation is caused by an inadequate valve margin. Normally, the valve leaflets touch to prevent blood from escaping back into the atrium during ventricular systole. The lack of a tight seal results in a decrease in cardiac output. Regurgitation usually starts at 5 to 7 years of age. The heart compensates for this lesion by pumping more blood per stroke to keep up with the need for systemic blood flow.

This leads to dilation of the ventricle and further stretching of the valvular ring. Heart failure signs may appear at 8 to 9 years of age.

Treatment

Surgical replacement of the mitral valve is common in human beings. Because the dog has been the main research subject for the development of this technique, its performance on a clinical basis is feasible. However, the dog is not a good candidate for this surgery for several reasons, primarily because of the difficulty in preventing clots from forming on an artificial mitral valve. Clots that form on artificial valves can be disastrous on the left side of the circulation, as they can dislodge, block the atrial supply, and cause ischemia of important organs. In addition, most of these patients are old and often have multiple organ system problems that make them poor risks for the cardiac arrest surgery necessary to replace the mitral valve. The advanced age of the patients raises the question of whether the expense and pain resulting from the procedure justify performing it.

Clinical Signs

At 5 to 7 years of age, the dog may begin to have a systolic murmur heard best over the apex of the heart on the left side of the chest. At about 8 or 9 years of age, the dog will begin to show signs of congestive heart failure (Table 1, above). The earliest signs are coughing and vague discomfort after a period of rest. The dog sleeps for a period of time and then gets up and moves about and coughs, but produces no sputum. At this stage, the dog is in functional class II heart failure. As the condition progresses, as it tends to in every case, the dog begins to show clinical signs (usually a cough) after ordinary activity. At this time, the dog is in functional class III heart failure. In time, the dog progresses to functional class IV, in which it shows clinical signs at rest.

Diagnosis

Diagnosis is based on the history of clinical signs that can be referred to the left side of the heart. The most common sign is a cough, which appears with decreasing levels of exercise as the condition progresses. An electrocardiogram suggests left ventricular dilation, later progressing to severe arrhythmia. A radiograph shows a large left ventricle and left atrium and a congested pulmonary venous system. Pulmonary edema is seen in dogs with heart failure of Functional Classes III and IV. Ultrasonography provides information about myocardial contractility and the level of dilation of the left ventricle and atrium.

A late consequence is rupture of the left atrium. This can vary from splitting of the endocardium of the left atrium with no blood leaking into the pericardium, to splitting of the endocardium with a small leak and mild pericardial tamponade to the point that the heart cannot fill.

Mitral regurgitation can develop rapidly from the rupture of a cordae tendinae. Affected animals show a sudden onset of a systolic murmur and heart failure.

Acquired Changes of the Pulmonic Valve

Acquired pulmonic valve disease can result in either an insufficient valve or a nodular stenosis.

Acquired pulmonic valvular insufficiency has been seen in cases in which patent ductus arteriosus resulted in dilation of the pulmonary artery to such an extent that the valve became incompetent. This appears to be the result of very high pulmonary artery pressures and turbulent blood flow in the pulmonary arterial root due to the flow from the aorta to the pulmonary artery. Dogs with heartworm disease and secondary high pulmonary arterial pressure may also develop pulmonic valvular insufficiency.

Nodular pulmonic valvular stenosis is uncommon and is due to endocarditis or neoplasia. Because the pulmonic valve can be removed without serious consequences, nodular changes that lead to obstruction of blood flow are amenable to surgical correction. Once any infection is under control, the leaflet or leaflets with the offending nodule can be removed via pulmonary arteriotomy. If the cause is neoplastic, the benefit of surgery is significantly decreased because of the likelihood of metastasis. Primary tumors of the right side of the heart do occur, but metastatic disease is more common.

Heartworm Disease

Heartworm disease in the dog most often results in gradually increasing clinical signs. The condition is amenable to medical therapy with arsenicals. Younger, immunologically naive individuals are the most severely involved. If enough worms are present (usually more than 50), the more severely involved individuals may develop the vena cava syndrome. In this syndrome, the animal suffers a sudden increase in the severity of clinical signs over hours to a few days, due to obstruction of venous return to the heart because the worms have migrated into the right ventricle, right atrium, and the cranial or caudal vena cava. Unless this obstruction is removed, death may occur in as little as 72 hours. Because the cardiac output is hampered by poor venous return, the animal develops cardiogenic shock. Surgery is indicated to remove the obstruction quickly, or the animal will die of multiple organ failure and shock.

Treatment

Worms can be removed with relative ease and a minimum of equipment if they are in the right atrium, or the cranial or caudal vena cava. But if they are in the right ventricle, they move with ventricular systole, and so are very difficult to remove unless they are visualized with real-time ultrasound.

The worms are removed via a cutaneous cutdown over the jugular vein close to the thoracic inlet. Because animals with vena cava syndrome are moribund, only a local anesthetic at the cutdown site is usually needed. After incising the vein, an alligator forcep is used to remove as many worms as possible; 50 to 100 often can be removed. If most of the worms are in the right ventricle, they may be out of reach during diastole. Therefore, if ultrasound is available to visualize the worms, the forcep can be guided to the mass of worms as it is forced into the right atrium during systole. Usually, they can be removed easily.

Three to four weeks following surgery, dogs must be treated with an arsenical preparation (thiacetarsamide, 2.1 mg/kg IV at 12-hour intervals for four doses), as it is very unlikely that surgery will result in removal of all the worms.

Tumors of the Heart and Great Vessels

Some tumors of the heart and great vessels are amenable to surgery. Benign myxomas of the fibrous portion of the heart may be large enough to obstruct blood flow, and their removal often does not destroy valvular or other cardiac structures or functions. Some tumors occur outside the heart on or in the wall of a great vessel. Heart base tumors encroach on the blood flow as they enlarge. Some of these can be removed if the diagnosis is made early enough. Unfortunately, by the time they are usually diagnosed, these tumors have already grown around normal structures and are inoperable.

Diagnosis

To determine the tumor cell type and, therefore, the prognosis and therapy, a biopsy is needed. This should be done by percutaneous needle aspirate if possible, without opening the chest. In some cases, percutaneous Tru-cut needle biopsy may be possible with ultrasound visualization. However, the air in the lung often does not allow visualization of these masses by ultrasonography. If immediate evaluation of a frozen section is possible, an intraoperative wedge biopsy diagnosis can help the surgeon decide whether to remove the mass, and allows definitive surgery to be performed at the same operation. Biopsy forceps for removing tissue inside the heart are available, and a safe biopsy is possible if the mass can be seen on fluoroscopy or ultrasound. Some masses are close enough to an airway to allow bronchoscope-guided aspiration of a biopsy specimen through the wall of the airway.

Pericardial Sac

Pericardial Effusion

There are many causes of pericardial effusion, which can lead to very significant enlargement of the pericardial sac. If the effusion forms slowly, allowing the pericardial sac to stretch, a very large accumulation of fluid (400 to 1,000 ml) can develop with minimal signs of heart failure. Because large accumulations of fluid impede venous return, removing the fluid is necessary. The cause of the effusion must also be resolved, or the fluid quickly returns.

Pericardial Tamponade

Occasionally, in dogs with mitral regurgitation, spontaneous rupture of the left atrium results in bleeding into the pericardial sac. These episodes can be, but usually are not, fatal, but fluid around the heart prevents it from filling properly and limits cardiac output.

In pericardial tamponade, the pericardial sac does not have time to stretch, so a relatively small amount of fluid can very drastically compromise the function of the heart. With a slowly forming effusion, several hundred ml of fluid would be required to compromise heart function, but 50 ml of blood due to acute hemorrhage could cause nonconges-

tive heart failure. When the pericardial sac is filled with fluid, pressure is transmitted through the fluid to the great veins. This is seen as a prominent jugular pulse. Muffled heart sounds and inability to palpate the heartbeat also are commonly seen.

It may be necessary to drain the pericardial sac to relieve the pressure on the heart and allow it to fill properly. This procedure should be done under aseptic conditions, as the fluid in the pericardial sac is an ideal bacterial growth medium. The best site is low in the left 5th intercostal space, where the apex beat usually would be felt. The pericardial sac contacts the chest wall over a wide front in the lower left chest in benign effusion, but it is best approached at the costochondral junction in the left 5th intercostal space. An 18-gauge needle 1.5″ to 3″ long should be used, with a 35-ml syringe and a three-way stopcock. After the site has been prepared for aseptic surgery, the surgeon, wearing sterile gloves, should assemble the syringe, stopcock, and needle in a sterile manner. A basin should be available to collect the excess fluid if more than 35 ml is encountered. A sample of the fluid should be sent to a laboratory for analysis; most often, the fluid is defibrinated blood. (The action of the heart causes the fibrin to accumulate on the surface of the heart and visceral surface of the pericardium.) A sample of fluid should be submitted for both aerobic and anaerobic culture and antibiotic sensitivity testing. The animal should show improving clinical signs as cardiac output improves because of increased filling of the heart.

If the fluid reforms slowly and a specific cause is not apparent, a second pericardiocentesis should be performed as the fluid begins to compromise heart function. Diuretics and corticosteroids following pericardiocentesis have been successful in stopping the fluid formation in cases where no cause can be identified. If pericardial effusion continues to form, creation of pericardial windows or pericardiectomy may be necessary to allow drainage of the effusion into the pleural space.

Constrictive/Restrictive Pericarditis

Chronic pericarditis can cause the pericardial sac to thicken and severely restrict filling of the heart. It can progress to the point that the sac actually shrinks, due to fibrous changes, and constricts the heart. In these cases, the pericardial sac must be removed to allow the heart to perform properly.

Pericardiectomy allows the heart to fill normally. It is best performed via a median sternotomy. The phrenic nerves cross the base of the heart laterally on either side, and removing the pericardial sac below this point is usually sufficient to free the heart if no adhesions are present in the upper part of the pericardial sac. The most difficult part of this procedure is removing the portion of the pericardium caudal to the heart. This can be approached by retracting the heart craniad after the cranial portion of the pericardium has been removed. If fibrin coats the surface of the heart, some surgeons advise multiple incisions to relieve compression, but this could damage the coronary arteries. If the fibrin on the heart has a spongy appearance, it is probably not contributing to the constriction or restriction.

The surgeon must decide whether to close the pericardial sac or leave it open, and opinions differ on this point. I incompletely close the sac; the gaps between the edges of the closure allow drainage in the first few hours after surgery. The pericardial incision seals within about 24 hours.

Peripheral Vascular Disorders

Trauma

The most common cause of peripheral vascular disorders in small animals is trauma. This occurs most often when fractured bones lacerate vessels. In most of these incidents, the collateral blood flow is extensive enough or new vessels form quickly enough that specific vascular repair is unnecessary. Techniques for repair are discussed below.

Thromboembolism

Vascular occlusion occurs where mural thrombi form in the heart or on damaged walls of blood vessels, or where emboli, originating as thrombi in an upstream vessel or in the heart, break off and lodge, usually at a site of vessel bifurcation ("saddle emboli"). Vasoactive substances, such as serotonin, are released, causing vascular spasm that aggravates the vascular occlusion. When the occlusion occurs, the arterial pulse is no longer palpable, and the tissues served by the downstream portion of the vessel do not get enough oxygen, leading to severe pain as acidosis develops in the tissue. Dogs usually react very violently to this pain by vocalizing, causing the owner to seek help. Cats, however, often will hide; by the time the owner finds the cat, the painful stage is over and the affected part is cold, stiff, and nonfunctional. If the occlusion occurs in a limb, the nonfunctioning limb is readily apparent. If the occluded vessel was supplying an epaxial muscle, however, the loss of function may not be apparent. Occasionally, incomplete occlusion results in intermittent claudication, in which the animal may be normal at rest but lose ability to walk on the affected limb after exercise.

Thromboembolism occurs primarily as a result of cardiomyopathies in both dogs and cats, particularly if atrial fibrillation is present. However, any severely debilitative disease can lead to thromboembolism associated with cardiac failure, platelet clumping, or vessel wall fragility. In most cases of thromboembolism, the major problem is so great that surgically correcting the vascular occlusion often only adds to the morbidity rather than providing a long-term cure. In addition, recurrence is common. When they are fully aware of these factors, most owners do not request the surgery, which is caudal aortotomy and embolectomy.

Other Forms of Emboli

Cartilaginous emboli may affect the blood supply to the spinal cord (see Chap. 19, The Spine) and fat emboli are often released when long-bone fractures occur (see Chap. 21, Principles of Fracture Management), but most of the arterial circulation is protected from venous emboli by the capillaries in the lung. In humans, fat may occlude enough of the pulmonary arterial circulation to cause death from pulmonary insufficiency. In animals, this does not appear to be a problem, as the long bones contain less fat than those of humans.

Arteriovenous Fistulae

Occasionally, following injury, an abnormal connection develops between an artery and vein if they are in close anatomic proximity. Artero-venous fistulae fistulae occur most often in the extremities; the affected limb is larger than the opposite member and is warmer to the touch. A palpable thrill usually is present over the lesion and a continuous murmur can be heard on auscultation of the area. Most dogs show tachycardia and left ventricular dilation. If the shunting of blood is large enough, left heart failure may be evident. Confirmation is by angiography.

Theoretically, treatment of an arteriovenous fistula is straightforward, but in practice few are simple to correct. Because trauma is the prime cause of fistula formation, much scarring is usually evident in the area. The turbulent blood flow through the fistula causes the vessels to dilate over time. There may be multiple fistulae, making dissection difficult. Aneurysmal changes in the vessels may also be present, adding to the difficulty in dissection and increasing the risk of rupture. If the connections are small, they may be ligated; if the vessels are attached over a wide front, a linear suture line may be required to close both the artery and vein. The specifics are discussed below.

Vascular Surgery

Principles

To perform successful vascular surgery, the surgeon must keep in mind the special requirements of each structure to be operated on. The following principles and techniques are used to avoid thrombosis of the vessel and failure of the procedure:

1. Gentle handling of the tissue. The area of the vessel to be sutured should not be grasped with any instrument that may crush the vessel wall. Instead, stay sutures should be used. Thumb forceps may be used to grasp only the adventitia some distance from the suture line. The integrity and viability of the medial layer is vital; if the media becomes necrotic, the suture line will develop a large mural thrombus that could occlude the vessel.

2. Sutures should be placed only in normal tissue. If the reason for the vascular surgery is traumatic injury to the vessel, the damaged area must be debrided. One major cause of suture line failure is inadequate debridement back to viable tissue.

3. The media is the most important layer, and it must be carefully aligned anatomically across the suture line or failure of the suture line is likely.

4. Suture tension is critical. The tension on the suture cannot be so great that it leads to scalloping of the tissue. This can occur due to removal of a portion of the vessel because of trauma or disease or by merely tying the sutures too tight. A graft must be considered if tension on the suture line is too great. Short runs of continuous sutures usually are the most practical approach to suturing, as long as anatomical alignment can be achieved and a purse-string effect does not result (Fig. 10-7). In smaller vessels (less than 2 mm internal diameter), interrupted sutures must be used. Too many sutures may lead to necrosis of the media,

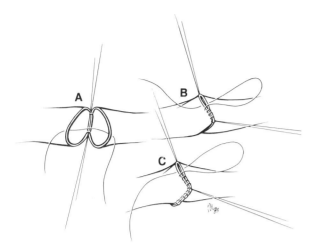

Figure 10-7. *Three-point suture technique (triangulation) for anastomosis of blood vessels. The vessel is sutured in three separate segments (**A, B,** and **C**) to ensure the vessel can expand. (Gourley IM, Vasseur PB, eds. General small animal surgery. Philadelphia: JB Lippincott, 1985:831.)*

and too few to bleeding. A general rule is to place sutures 1 to 2 mm apart and 1 to 3 mm from the cut edge of the tissue. The larger the vessel, the further apart and from the cut edge the sutures should be placed.

5. End-to-end anastomosis is preferred. End-to-side anastomosis may be unavoidable, but it will be more difficult to prevent thrombotic surfaces from coming in contact with the lumen.

6. The vessel ends to be sutured should be similar in size. Vessels that are up to 100% different in size can be anastomosed if the smaller vessel is cut obliquely. There is no advantage to cutting the vessels obliquely if they are the same size.

7. Arteries heal faster than veins. The strength of the suture line is not a factor, as the elastic properties buffer what little stretch may be applied. What is more important in the healing process is the time after surgery that the surgical site becomes covered with endothelium. Mural thrombi

are much less likely to develop after the endothelium becomes continuous. In arteries, this can be as early as 1 week; in veins, this may not take place until 4 weeks postsurgery. The incision line is always covered with a mural thrombus, which is minimal when correct principles have been followed. This prevents bleeding and covers the sutures that are exposed to the lumen.

Portosystemic Shunts

Etiology

When the portal system congenitally connects to the systemic venous system without passing the blood through the liver, products from the digestive tract that would normally be altered by the liver gain access to the general circulation. These products have direct effects, primarily on the brain, leading to encephalopathy and convulsions. Signs of poor nutrition also are evident, including stunted growth, vomition, and diarrhea.

Although human portosystemic shunts often are due to portal hypertension from cirrhosis of the liver, this condition most often is congenital in the dog. Portal hypertension also may be a cause in the dog, but cirrhosis of the liver occurs infrequently (Fig. 10-8)

Diagnosis

The presence of a portosystemic shunt is strongly suggested based on the clinical signs in a young patient. If surgery is contemplated, the abnormal connection must be located. If the shunt is within the parenchyma of the liver, the surgery is more difficult. If the shunt is outside the liver, surgical intervention is easier and carries a greater chance of success. The diagnosis is made by injecting contrast medium into the portal circulation, either by an injection into the parenchyma of the spleen with ultrasound guidance or by catheterizing a portal vein at the time of surgery. Ultrasound

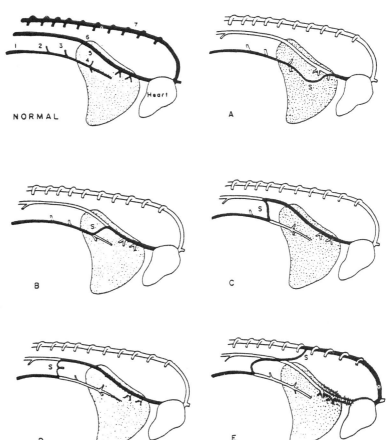

Figure 10-8. *Five types of portosystemic shunts. The veins involved are: (1) cranial mesenteric vein, (2) gastrosplenic vein, (3) gastroduodenal vein, (4) portal vein, (5) left branch of portal vein, (6) caudal caval vein, (7) azygous vein.* **A,** *Intrahepatic right patent ductus venosus.* **B,** *Intrahepatic left patent ductus venosus.* **C,** *Portocaval shunt via gastroduodenal vein.* **D,** *Portocaval shunt via gastrosplenic vein.* **E,** *Portoazygous shunt. (Gourley IM, Vasseur PB, eds. General small animal surgery. Philadelphia: JB Lippincott, 1985:428.)*

helps define the exact location intraoperatively. Shunts within the liver tissue can be partially ligated, resulting in improvement of the condition, depending on where the shunts are located (see Suggested Reading list).

Treatment

Affected animals have very poor liver function and are not good anesthesia risks, but they can be anesthetized safely if the agent used does not require detoxification in the liver. Surgery is performed to reduce the blood flow from the portal to the systemic circulation. Because it is impossible to determine accurately if there are sufficient pathways to accept the increased

portal blood flow within the liver, the shunt should only be partially ligated. A catheter is placed in a mesenteric venous branch to measure pressure (normal portal venous pressure is 8 to 12 cm H_2O) and for angiography. Ligation is gradual, and the pressure change is observed (a standard disposable central venous pressure manometer can be used) for at least 5 minutes before securing the knot on the ligature. If the pressure rises above 20 cm H_2O, the ligature should be loosened until the pressure remains no more than 20 cm H_2O. If the portal pressure remains between 8 and 20 cm H_2O after ligature, the ligature may be secured and the surgery is completed.

A postsurgical portogram confirms ligation and may demonstrate increased hepatic portal venous blood flow. This is a good prognostic sign. The patient is likely to do well postoperatively if it shows clinical improvement within 2 days.

Open Heart Surgery

During the development of human open-heart surgery, the dog was the primary laboratory animal. Therefore, a great deal of information exists that can be applied directly to canine open-heart surgery. However, the dog's red blood cells do not tolerate the trauma from heart-lung machines as well as those of other species, and the clotting time of dog blood is shorter. Further, small individuals are difficult to place on a pump because of their higher resistance to blood flow. Therefore, although cardiopulmonary bypass can be performed with reasonable success in large dogs, the success rate drops markedly in smaller dogs. Pumping red blood cells at flow rates necessary to keep tissues viable in small individuals damages the cells and produces fibrin, red blood cell fragments, and platelet debris that are trapped in capillary beds, causing the lung to sustain significant damage. Because most of the canine and feline cardiac patients are relatively small, this surgery is fraught with unacceptable risk except for highly selected patients.

Cost also is a factor. Dogs and cats with heart disease most commonly have either mitral valve disease or cardiomyopathy, so they would benefit from either an artificial mitral valve or a heart transplant. The costs of these procedures and their postoperative management are prohibitive for most clients. In addition, many if not most of these animals are near or beyond their anticipated life span, so the cost-benefit ratio does not generally warrant considering surgery.

Congenital heart disease, which occurs much less commonly, can be pursued on a sporadic basis. If the animal is large enough, cardiopulmonary bypass is possible; in small patients, hypothermia produces safe cardiac arrest for surgery (see Suggested Reading list).

Pacemakers

Older animals suffer from many heart conditions that lead to severe bradycardia and heart block. When the condition is clearly irreversible, implanting a cardiac pacemaker can provide a pacing stimulus to maintain at least a normal resting heart rate. Even after surgery, the animal will be severely limited in its ability to perform strenuous exercise, because the pacemaker will not increase the heart rate as the animal increases its activity. Therefore, moderate activity will be possible, but the animal will have to stop frequently to catch up with the oxygen demands.

The pacemakers most commonly used are the demand R wave inhibited generators, in which the artificial pacemaker shuts off if the natural pacemaker begins to function intermittently, but continues to sense the beat and begins to pace the heart if the natural pacemaker stops or drops back to less than the preset resting heart rate. Much research is being done to develop a rate-responsive pacemaker so that when demand for blood flow increases, the heart rate will automatically also increase.

A pacemaker lead can be implanted in the heart via the jugular vein, with the pacing electrode in the apex or the right ventricle, or be attached to the myocardium from the epicardial surface.

Transvenous pacemaker lead placement is carried out with fluoroscopic visualization so the lead can be positioned in the apex of the right ventricle. A pouch is made for the pacemaking generator on the lateral thorax behind the scapula. The lead is pulled under the skin and attached to the pacer to determine if the electrode tip is in a position where proper pacing results. The body of the pacing generator must be in contact with the tissues to complete the electrical circuit. If the unit is functioning properly, the lead then is sutured to the fascia in the neck and sutured to the wall of the jugular vein in such a way so the vein is not occluded. These sutures must not be too tight, or the vessel wall will become necrotic and the anchor point for the lead will be lost. At least four sutures should be used for this purpose. Slack must be sufficient in the lead between the pacer and the anchor point on the jugular vein, or the lead could be pulled out of the apex of the right ventricle when the animal turns its head to the right.

A better method is to place the electrode in the epicardium through diaphragmatic thoracotomy, via a limited midline celiotomy. The diaphragm is incised to place the electrode in the myocardium. The sternum usually does not need to be split in this procedure. The generator is placed in front of the liver and the lead is secured tightly to the diaphragm. This approach minimizes the complications associated with keeping the pacing electrode in contact with the myocardium. A disadvantage of this technique is that if the generator needs to be changed, the abdomen must be opened.

The patient must be monitored to ensure the pacemaker is continuing to pace the heart. Some human hospital pacemaker centers are willing to provide the monitoring if the animal is in an area where a veterinarian cannot provide this service.

Suggested Readings

Breznock EM, Whiting PG. Portacaval shunts and anomalies. In: Slatter DH, ed. Textbook of small animal surgery. Philadelphia: WB Saunders, 1985:1156.

Eyster GE, DeYoung B. Cardiac disorders. In: Slatter DH, ed. Textbook of small animal surgery. Philadelphia: WB Saunders, 1985:1069.

Eyster GE, Probst M. Basic cardiac procedures. In: Slatter DH, ed. Textbook of small animal surgery. Philadelphia: WB Saunders, 1985:1107.

Kittleson MD. Cardiovascular physiology and pathophysiology. In: Slatter DH, ed. Textbook of small animal surgery. Philadelphia: WB Saunders, 1985:1039.

Weirich WE. The heart. In: Gourley IM, Vasseur PB, eds. General small animal surgery. Philadelphia: JB Lippincott, 1985:803.

11

D. T. Crowe, Jr.

The Abdominal Cavity: Peritoneum, Retroperitoneum, Abdominal Hernias, and the Adrenal Glands

In clinical practice today the abdominal cavity is the body cavity most often opened surgically. Many important advances in the theory and practice of abdominal surgery have occurred over the past 10 years. For instance, suture closure of the peritoneal layer was previously recommended following celiotomy, but now such closure is known to lead to a higher incidence of intra-abdominal adhesions than when the peritoneal layer is left unsutured. It also was thought that continuous suture closure of the abdominal cavity would lead to an increased incidence of dehiscence, but this belief has been disproven.

The mesothelium of the peritoneal cavity is easily damaged within minutes by exposure to light, heat, and air; once desiccated, however, these surface cells protect the deeper layers. Following injury the desiccated cells slough, and viable exfoliated mesothelial cells proliferate and spread to heal the denuded surfaces. Complete re-epithelialization as a result of this seeding process occurs within 5 to 7 days, regardless of the lesion size. Historically, reperitonealization by suturing a peritoneal flap over the raw defect in the peritoneal surface was popular until it was observed that this method not only led to an increased incidence of adhesion formation but also was unnecessary.

Examination of the Abdomen

History

Clinical examination of the abdomen begins with carefully constructed specific questions related to historical data. Questions pertaining to the abdominal cavity and retroperitoneum most often are directed to the function of the organs contained within them. For example, a history of acute vomiting may suggest involvement with the gastrointestinal tract, liver, pancreas, kidneys, or the peritoneal cavity in general.

Physical Examination

Physical examination of the abdominal cavity should include inspection, first from a distance and then close up. This is followed by palpation, first shallowly then deeply, and then auscultation, and percussion.

Inspection

During inspection of the patient, its resting posture should be observed. Abdominal pain may be reflected by kyphosis, in which the animal attempts to relieve tension on the abdominal wall. Peritoneal irritation in dogs also may be reflected by a "praying" position in which the forelimbs are fully extended and the neck is outstretched, but the hindlimbs are in a normal standing position and the chest is lowered. This position appears to provide relief from pain.

Extreme changes in abdominal volume usually are obvious. Gross abdominal enlargement may be associated with pregnancy, neoplasia, benign cysts, obesity, or the accumulation of ingesta, gas or fluid in the gastrointestinal tract, or in the abdominal cavity. Gravity can cause large amounts of free fluid to collect in the dependent portion of the abdomen, which may produce an hour-glass profile when the animal is viewed from behind. A moderate accumulation of fluid is not detectable by inspection. A large accumulation of gas in the intestine tends to distend the lateral walls of the abdomen when the patient is sitting or standing. A decrease in the abdomen's volume is less obvious than an increase, but it should be considered, especially when a diaphragmatic hernia is suspected. Loss of fat deposits is the usual cause for decrease in abdominal volume.

Changes in the abdomen's volume can be more accurately evaluated by repeated measurement of its circumference at the umbilicus. A change of 2 cm in circumference measured at end-expiration in a 25-kg dog represents a change in volume of about 1 liter. A number of variables must be considered, however, when evaluating the abdomen's circumference. These include the depth of respiration, the amount of air in the stomach, the fullness of the bladder and colon, the degree of rigidity of the abdominal musculature, and the position of the animal.

Thorough visual inspection of the abdomen may require removal of hair over the ventral and lateral abdomen and the caudal thoracic area as far cranially as the sixth intercostal space, the cranial limit of the dome of the diaphragm. Removal of the hair enables inspection for bruising, puncture wounds, and cavitation or herniation; it often provides clues to a deeper injury.

The umbilical region should be examined closely for presence of discoloration or nodules. Symmetrically distributed red or purple discoloration has been observed in dogs with intra-abdominal bleeding, yellow discoloration of the skin with bile peritonitis and, in dogs and cats, firm nodules at the umbilicus with metastasis of abdominal neoplasms. This is explained by the fact that the umbilical scar is incomplete in many dogs and cats. This very small defect allows free peritoneal fluid and cells to find their way to the subcutaneous region of the periumbilicus. Although periumbilical subcutaneous infiltrates indicate an intraperitoneal disorder, subcutaneous infiltrates at the inguinal canals indicate retroperitoneal abnormalities. Red or bluish discoloration at the inguinal canal indicates retroperitoneal hemorrhage, a frequent occurrence following pelvic fractures. Expanding hematomas indicate continued retroperitoneal hemorrhage. Other swellings commonly may occur in this area due to hernias, free urine accumulation, trauma, and inflammation of the inguinal fat. Rarer causes include neoplasia.

Palpation

The abdomen can be palpated most effectively while the animal is standing. It is first palpated superficially, then deeply. Elevating the animal's forequarters assists palpation of structures in the cranial abdomen. In cats and smaller dogs, palpation can be performed successfully while the animal is in dorsal recumbency. Palpation should be gentle, systematic, and started away from the anticipated site of disease or tenderness. Animals that are severely depressed or suffering from cranial or spinal injuries may not respond to deep palpation despite the presence of peritoneal irritation. Examination of the caudal abdomen should include rectal palpation. This is best accomplished with one hand palpating the abdomen and a finger of the other inserted into the rectum. Muscle resistance should be judged before tenderness is elicited by deep palpation. If there is doubt about the significance of the patient's reaction, gentle palpation should be continued while the animal's attention is distracted. If signs of pain and guarding are elicited in a particular area, this may be an indication of localized peritoneal irritation. Localized tenderness may occur associated with superficial lesions in subcutaneous or muscular tissues. Referred abdominal pain due to thoracodorsal intervertebral disc protrusion also occurs and gives the false impression of an acute abdominal condition.

If abdominal palpation is difficult, because the abdomen is tense or because the animal resists, sedation or brief anesthesia may be required. Ballottement of an organ in a distended abdomen may also be useful in evaluating the presence of a large solid mass. This is performed by pushing deeply with fingertips into the abdomen to get any large and solid intra-abdominal structure to move away from the area of palpation. Then the fingers are quickly moved away a short distance; however, the fingertips remain in position for deep palpation. If a large and solid intra-abdominal organ is present, it may swing back to its original position and be detected by the tips of the fingers. Spasm of the abdominal muscles may result from a spinal reflex, direct stimulation of the muscle, or stimulation of the cerebrum, spinal cord, or thoracolumbar nerve trunk. It is important to determine the reason for abdominal rigidity, especially after an accident.

For example, abdominal rigidity may follow a thoracic wound, because the animal uses the abdominal muscles to immobilize the thorax.

Although abdominal rigidity may be associated with such conditions as peritonitis or pancreatitis, the rigidity also may occur merely as a response to deep palpation. Tranquilizers may produce relaxation of the abdomen; however, these drugs may be contraindicated because of their hypotensive effect in certain conditions. Rigidity over one area of an otherwise relaxed abdomen usually reflects acute pain in a specific organ. With severe local irritation of the parietal peritoneum, muscle rigidity may be marked. Generalized rigidity of the abdomen occurs with extensive peritonitis. In contrast, severe toxemia leads to abdominal flaccidity and signs of pain usually cannot be elicited.

Auscultation

Auscultation of the abdomen is part of a complete physical examination of the abdomen and can provide valuable information. Hypomotile, normal, or hypermotile high-pitched sounds usually are associated with gas under pressure, and may occur with acute, complete obstruction in a closed loop of intestine, and with small intestinal mesenteric volvulus. Early acute obstruction, or bowel irritation from many causes (*e.g.,* gastroenteritis) may also lead to loud and frequent bowel sounds due to hyperperistalsis. These sounds, also termed *borborygmi,* are often so loud they can be heard without the use of a stethoscope. Following abdominal surgery, auscultation of the abdomen can detect resumption of intestinal activity.

In a quiet room, the diaphragm portion of the stethoscope is placed on the ventral mid-abdominal region. In normal animals, intestinal movement is reflected by frequent crackling and gurgling noises at least several times per minute. A clinician should listen to the intestinal sounds for several minutes before characterizing them. The sounds are not diagnostic in themselves, and peristalsis may occur even though peritonitis exists. It is also possible for peristaltic sounds to be absent in a healthy animal. However, if bowel sounds are not auscultated after serious blunt trauma, it should be assumed that major intra-abdominal injury requiring surgery has occurred. Auscultation may enable detection of peritoneal friction when an irregular area of peritoneum moves against another peritoneal surface during respiration.

Percussion

Abdominal percussion is useful for detection of abnormal accumulations of gas within a viscus, (*e.g.,* the stomach), or of fluid within the abdominal cavity. A prolonged, low-pitched, resonant sound produced by percussion reflects the presence of air; a short, high-pitched sound with little resonance reflects the presence of fluid or a solid structure. The dull sound in ascites is noticeable in the ventral abdomen, but it is less obvious in the flanks, unless the volume of ascites is great. When the abdomen is distended and tense due to ascites, percussion on one side of the abdomen can cause a fluid wave that may be detected by placing a hand on the opposite side.

Special Examinations

Two special diagnostic procedures involving percussion and auscultation are useful for detecting fluid within the abdominal cavity. They are known as the shifting dullness test and the puddle test. The former refers to the change in location of the dull sound associated with ascites as the patient changes its position. This occurs because free fluid in the abdominal cavity moves to the lowest area. When percussion is performed with the patient in dorsal recumbency, dullness will be evident in the flanks and lateral abdominal wall. When the patient is placed in right lateral recumbency, the left flank and lateral regions of the abdomen will now be resonant, indicating a shift in the area of dullness.

The puddle test is helpful for detection of moderate amounts of free intra-abdominal fluid. It is performed by placing the animal in a standing position with its forelimbs elevated several centimeters. With a stethoscope placed on the abdominal midline just caudal to the umbilicus, the paralumbar region is percussed with a flicking motion of the middle finger of the opposite hand. The percussion is repeated in the same location with the same amount of force as the head of the stethoscope is moved dorsally on the opposite side of the abdomen. If at any point there is abrupt change from a dull to a resonant sound, a fluid line should be suspected. This test is sensitive enough for trained observers to detect as little as 50 to 100 ml of free fluid in the abdomen.

Paracentesis and Diagnostic Peritoneal Lavage

Paracentesis

Paracentesis often yields useful information when injury to abdominal structures, peritonitis, or any abdominal accumulation of fluid occurs. Physical and radiographic examinations should be performed before paracentesis to ensure that the latter procedure will not complicate an existing problem. Paracentesis can also inadvertently lead to a small amount of pneumoperitoneum. Finding pneumoperitoneum radiographically generally indicates the need for an emergency exploratory celiotomy. However, if paracentesis precedes the radiographs, interpretation of a finding of pneumoperitoneum is more difficult. Cytologic, microbiologic, and biochemical examinations of aspirated fluid may help to establish the diagnosis.

Attempts at abdominal paracentesis with a hypodermic needle often fail because of an inability to collect a fluid sample. This has been attributed to occlusion of the needle's lumen by omentum or other viscera. Use of a dialysis catheter will facilitate collection of fluid, because the catheter has small holes along the tip that are less likely to become occluded. A 4.5-cm, 14-gauge, plastic cannula with 3 to 5 side holes also can be used instead of a dialysis catheter.

Diagnostic Peritoneal Lavage

By injecting an isotonic solution into the abdominal cavity through a multiholed catheter, small amounts of free blood or other fluids can be detected more readily. This technique, known as diagnostic peritoneal lavage, has become established as the most reliable and accurate method for early detection of intra-abdominal injuries in dogs and cats.

Technique

About 2 cm caudal to the umbilicus, the skin is prepared as for surgery, and the area is infiltrated with a local anesthetic. A 3-mm incision is made through the skin on the ventral midline to facilitate penetration of the abdominal wall by the cannula. The bladder should be emptied prior to introducing the catheter to avoid damage to the organ during catheter insertion. With the animal in left lateral recumbency, the catheter's tip is gently thrust into the abdominal cavity with the aid of a metal stylet. To prevent injury to abdominal structures if an enlarged organ or adhesion is suspected, the cannula or catheter should be inserted into the abdomen without the stylet and only with direct visualization, via a full thickness incision (mini-celiotomy). This is best done using complete aseptic technique in an operating room.

After the catheter has been inserted, warm normal saline (22 ml/kg) is infused into the abdominal cavity by gravity flow. Then the patient is rolled gently from side to side to distribute the fluid and allow it to mix with other fluid in the abdominal cavity.

A small amount (20 ml) of fluid is removed from the cavity with a syringe or by gravity-siphon drainage, which usually is more successful. After a sample of abdominal fluid has been obtained, the catheter is removed, and a single suture is inserted to close the skin. Closure of the ventral rectus fascia also is necessary if a mini-celiotomy was performed to insert the catheter.

Strict hemostasis is essential when inserting the catheter to avoid contaminating the lavage fluid with blood from the skin incision. Scarred areas in the skin should not be penetrated, because these scars may indicate underlying old injuries and adhesions. The amount of lavage fluid withdrawn is limited to what is needed for examination (20 ml). If less than 3 hours have elapsed since an injury occurred, or if intra-abdominal hemorrhage is detected and immediate surgery is not planned, the catheter should be left in place and secured to facilitate future sampling. Repeated sampling of lavage fluid during the next 20 to 30 minutes is helpful in detecting whether a hemorrhage is continuing (indicated by a rise in lavage hematocrit greater than 5%).

When paracentesis is performed without lavage, the aspirate is examined and evaluated on the basis of its color, turbidity, cell content, and content of creatinine, urea nitrogen, bile or bilirubin, and protein. The same analyses are made of fluid aspirated after lavage, as well as other quantitative measurements, such as PCV, WBC, and enzyme concentrations, which enable a more accurate evaluation of abdominal disease or injury (Table 11-1).

An estimate of the amount of blood in the abdominal cavity can be made by observing the lavage sample. A red color reflects the presence of red blood cells; deep redness likely indicates that the hemorrhage is severe. If the fluid is opaque, so that newsprint cannot be seen through the plastic IV tubing containing the fluid, the hemorrhage is significant. If print can be seen through the tubing, only moderate or minimal hemorrhage has occurred; if the fluid is clear or slightly pink, it indicates no or insignificant bleeding. Pink fluid in the abdomen occurs when a blood to body weight ratio is as little as 0.8 ml/kg. When the volume of blood in the abdomen is greater than 2.0 ml/kg, the print on the syringe barrel cannot be seen through the sample.

When lavage samples aspirated 15 minutes apart reveal a 5% increase in hematocrit, surgical intervention is generally indicated. Such an increase may indicate the continuation of intra-abdominal hemorrhage before signs of shock appear. Surgical intervention also is indicated when the patients' signs remain or become unstable and the hematocrit of the lavage fluid is above 10%.

Retroperitoneal or diaphragmatic injuries may give false negative results, but rarely is the aspirate completely free of blood in these cases. In cases of diaphragmatic injury in which thoracic radiographs do not reveal a hernia, the diagnosis can be confirmed by aspiration of peritoneal lavage fluid from the thoracic cavity.

The aspirate's sediment should be examined microscopically if the fluid is not crystal clear. This assists the early detection of injury to a hollow viscus. Vegetable fibers, free and intracellular bacteria, and neutrophils may be found. In animals with bacterial peritonitis, free and intracellular bacteria and numerous toxic and degenerated neutrophils may be present. Cytologic examination of lavage fluid from animals with suspected abdominal neoplasia likewise is useful in diagnosis. Chemical analysis of the lavage fluid or bile can assist in establishing the diagnosis of biliary tract or hepatic injury. Bile in the lavage fluid will provide a positive Icto test (Ames Division, Miles Laboratories, Elkhart, IN). Chemical analysis of the returning fluid also assists identification of pancreatitis or pancreatic inflammation (amylase over 200 ka), urinary tract injury with urine leakage (creatinine or urea nitrogen greater than systemic circulation), perforation

Table 11–1. Interpretation of Chemical and Enzyme Analysis of Undiluted Peritoneal Fluid

Determination	Interpretation
Bilirubin test (Icto test*)	A positive result (bluish color change) is indicative of biliary or upper intestinal tract disruption; cannot be used in icteric animals.
Amylase activity (Amyloclastic method)	Increasing values or values greater than serum concentration indicate pancreatic inflammation or injury or intestinal ischemia.
Creatinine concentration	Values greater than serum concentration indicate urinary tract injury with leakage of urine.
Urea concentration	Values greater than serum concentration indicate urinary tract injury with leakage of urine. Because urea diffuses easily and rapidly, this test may be accurate only in the early stages of urinary leakage.
Alanine aminotransferase	Values greater than serum concentration are indicative of hepatocellular damage or inflammation.
Alkaline phosphatase and phosphate	Values greater than serum concentration are indicative of small bowel ischemia or perforation.

* Ames Division Miles Laboratories, Elkhart, Indiana

of the small intestine, (alkaline phosphatase above 150 SIU), and significant liver trauma (AAPT over 100 SIU).

Indications.   Diagnostic paracentesis is useful in detecting intra-abdominal injuries following blunt or penetrating abdominal trauma. Other indications include:

Shock without apparent cause
Severe thoracic trauma, especially in conjunction with pelvic hindlimb injuries
Cases in which the results of examination of the abdominal cavity for evidence of pain were inconclusive, as in patients with blunt blows to the head or spine
Signs of disease possibly involving the peritoneal cavity
Suspicion of postoperative gastrointestinal dehiscence

Moderate leukocytosis of peritoneal fluid is normal following uncomplicated abdominal surgery (up to 10,000 cells/mm^3), but without evidence of toxic or degenerative neutrophils. Toxic or degenerative cells occur with an overwhelming peritonitis, and their presence indicates prompt surgical intervention. The presence of intracellular bacteria also indicates surgery. Diagnostic paracentesis is not indicated when evidence suggests the need for exploratory celiotomy (*e.g.*, the presence of a large abdominal hernia following blunt trauma).

Complications seldom occur following diagnostic paracentesis. In a study of 129 dogs and cats subjected to the procedure, 1 suffered perforation of the bladder, 1 suffered a perforation through the mesocolon, and 3 had subcutaneous hematomas. Only the patient with a perforated bladder required surgery because of paracentesis.

Radiographic Examination

Radiographic delineation of most abdominal viscera is difficult if there is a large amount of ingesta within the gastrointestinal tract. Routine radiography of the abdomen generally should be preceded by a 12-hour fast, and an enema should be given unless the animal has been vomiting. With few exceptions, contrast radiography should be preceded by a 24-hour fast to ensure that the upper gastrointestinal tract is empty. Water can be given, but not in large amounts just prior to the radiographic examination. The large intestine should be emptied after the fasting period. This is performed with the use of multiple saline enemas and frequent trips outdoors if possible to encourage defecation. Severely debilitated animals that may not be able to tolerate fasting can be fed low-residue foods prior to radiographic examination. Such foods include commercial liquid diets, strained baby foods, and dietary concentrates. They should be lactose-free, because foods containing lactose frequently lead to lactose accumulation in the gut and osmotic diarrhea.

The following structures normally are identifiable on survey radiographs: stomach, small and large intestines, spleen, liver, kidneys, and urinary bladder. Because differentiation of viscera from other masses is important, pneumoperitoneography also may be performed to facilitate the diagnosis.

By using a horizontal beam technique (either lateral exposure with the animal standing or ventrodorsal exposure with the animal elevated by the pectoral limbs), free air in the abdominal cavity often is detectable. This technique also can be used to detect increased amounts of air or fluid in the small intestine.

Early radiographic diagnosis of peritoneal effusions can be difficult to make in dogs and cats, especially if the animals are dehydrated or emaciated, because this results in a diffuse increase in density. Lack of radiographic contrast, usually present due to extra- and intraperitoneal fat, also occurs in radiographs of animals with peritonitis and ascites. Because these conditions may co-exist, and they have a similar radiographic appearance, their differentiation by radiography may be difficult.

Contrast studies of the gastrointestinal tract may be made with air or positive-contrast materials, such as barium sulfate suspensions, iodinated materials, or metrizamide. Because metrizamide is a water-soluble, isotonic contrast material, it has advantages over barium and hypertonic, water-soluble, iodinated materials, especially in very small animals, debilitated and dehydrated patients, and animals suspected of having gastrointestinal leakage. Contrast studies of other organs (pancreas, urinary, genital) may be helpful, as well, in determining the cause of peritonitis.

Exploratory Celiotomy

The term *laparotomy* refers to any conventional incision that exposes the peritoneal cavity. By definition, however, laparotomy is a surgical incision in the flank. The term *celiotomy* correctly designates a surgical incision into the abdominal cavity from any site. Celiotomy is the term used throughout this text.

Exploratory celiotomy is necessary when other diagnostic procedures fail to provide the required information for a diagnosis and in life-threatening situations. Far more patients have died because an exploratory celiotomy was delayed, than because the procedure was performed without finding significant lesions.

Preoperative medical preparation is mandatory for animals requiring exploratory surgery. If the patient does not respond to supportive (fluid, electrolyte, *etc.*) therapy, a celiotomy may be needed on an emergency basis, despite the added risk. Carefully monitored and administered anesthesia and ventilatory support are essential in such cases.

For exploratory celiotomy, the patient is placed in dorsal recumbency, and the abdomen usually is opened from the xiphoid cartilage to the pubis on the ventral midline (see "Abdominal Incisions," p. 312). For additional exposure, the incision occasionally is extended cranially through or beside the sternum or caudally through the pubic symphysis. A symphyseal osteotomy can be effective in gaining the exposure required in an immature animal; but in a mature animal, a flap procedure and triple osteotomy is required. Preoperative skin preparation should include an area that will allow a possible extension of the midline incision in either direction and will fa-

cilitate lateral exits of feeding and drainage tubes. Exploration of the abdominal cavity requires a systematic examination of all the enclosed structures. This cannot be done thoroughly or safely through an incision that is too small, for instance an incision extending from the xiphoid to the umbilicus.

A suitable way to examine the intra-abdominal structures systematically is to examine the cavity quadrant by quadrant. The intestines should be palpated gently through their entire length. The mesocolon and mesoduodenum can be used to isolate structures in the left and right paralumbar gutters.

Following its exploration, the abdominal cavity should be lavaged with copious amounts of warm saline or Ringer's solution. Although including povidone–iodine solution (5%–10%), chlorhexidine solution 1:40 dilution, or an antibiotic solution, such as gentamicin (10 υg/ml), in the lavage fluid, has been advocated to decrease the possibility of peritoneal and surgical wound infections, there is no solid evidence that this is better than using saline alone. Furthermore, polyvinylpyrrolidone, the carrier of povidone–iodine solution, inhibits macrophage chemotaxis. Gentamicin also is potentially toxic. Lavage fluids in the abdomen should be removed thoroughly after celiotomy to prevent dilution of important small immunoreactive proteins and macrophages, a low concentration of which could predispose the abdomen to postoperative infection.

After a thorough inspection of the abdominal cavity to ensure that all foreign material and surgical equipment have been removed, the celiotomy incision is closed (see "Closing the Incision," p. 316).

Congenital Abdominal Wall Disorders

Hernias of the Ventral Abdomen

Congenital abnormalities of the ventral abdomen, in which some portion of the viscera lies outside the abdominal cavity, include: umbilical hernia, omphalocele, and gastroschisis. Hernial contents may be incarcerated (unable to be removed from the hernia) or strangulated (suffering from a severely impaired blood supply), or both.

Umbilical Hernia

Congenital umbilical hernias, the least serious and most common of the congenital defects involving the umbilicus, occur in dogs and cats, and result from failure of the rectus muscles to join at the umbilicus after the embryonic entry of the intestines into the abdomen. The abdominal viscera protrude through an enlarged umbilical ring and are covered by skin. The presence or absence of a peritoneal lining of the hernial sac depends on the size of the defect.

Although there is evidence that the size of the umbilical ring is governed by two or more recessive genes, breed predisposition for umbilical herniation has not been established. Occasionally, an entire litter is affected; there is no sex predilection for umbilical hernias. Some affected animals have poorly developed muscles surrounding the hernial ring. The rectus muscles and aponeuroses of the two oblique muscles are hypoplastic in these cases. The abdominal midline appears to consist solely of a wide, thin linea alba that may extend from the xiphoid cartilage to the pubis. This also may be associated with congenital anomalies involving the diaphragm (see "Diaphragmatic Hernia," Chap. 9).

Some umbilical hernias may be acquired. For example, the umbilicus may become enlarged or weakened and a hernia may occur if the umbilical cord is severed too close to the abdominal wall. This can occur if the cord is handled carelessly during cesarean section or when the bitch chews and pulls on the cord while cleaning the pup following parturition.

Umbilical hernias vary in size, but they usually are small. Palpation reveals a soft, fluctuating, painless mass that, by gentle manipulation, usually can be pushed into the abdominal cavity. After the hernia has been reduced, the umbilical ring can be palpated. Small firm hernias usually consist of a portion of the falciform ligament or a piece of omentum. These tissues may adhere to the underside of the skin and resist reduction. Large, fluctuant-to-firm masses may reflect concomitant cellulitis, abscess formation, or the presence of other organs, especially the small intestine. If signs of intestinal obstruction are present, hernial incarceration or strangulation should be suspected and is an indication for immediate surgical intervention. Very firm umbilical masses may also occur in patients with metastatic spread of intra-abdominal tumors. Such tumors should be suspected in middle-aged or older animals with a history of chronic anorexia, weight loss, and unthriftiness. Diagnosis is confirmed by cytologic examination of a fine needle aspirate of the mass.

Small umbilical hernias that are seen at birth often regress spontaneously, but large ones must be corrected surgically. Small hernias can be repaired when performing an ovariohysterectomy. Surgical repair is indicated for umbilical hernias that have not regressed by the time the animal is physically mature, and when a large or enlarging hernia involves more than the falciform ligament, properitoneal fat, or omentum.

Repair

The patient is placed in dorsal recumbency. For small hernias a midline incision is made through the skin directly over the hernial sac and extended past the cranial and caudal limits of the hernial ring. For larger hernias it may be necessary to make an elliptical incision and remove the redundant skin (Fig. 11-1).

The preferred method of repairing an umbilical hernia is to expose the hernial sac by making a longitudinal incision through the skin from a point cranial to the sac to a point caudal to it. The skin is then carefully dissected from the hernial sac, and the dissection is continued to expose the sac's neck and the hernial ring. The hernial sac is opened at a convenient place, and adhesions between it and the contents are severed between ligatures. The contents of the sac are then replaced into the abdominal cavity. The hernial sac is completely removed. The rectus fascia is

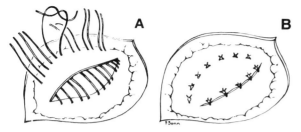

Figure 11-1. *A, An elliptical incision has been made around an umbilical hernia. The hernial contents have been returned to the abdomen, and the hernial sac has been resected. If the hernial opening is large or the adjacent fascia is thin, the fascia can be overlapped with horizontal mattress sutures.* *B, The edge of the external flap is sutured to adjacent fascia. (Gourley IM, Vasseur PB, eds. General small animal surgery. Philadelphia: JB Lippincott, 1985:757.)*

apposed with a series of interrupted or simple continuous sutures of polypropylene, nylon, or a synthetic absorbable material. Surgical gut may be used for only the smallest hernias. All fat must be removed from the internal and external rectus sheaths. Occasionally, the external rectus fascia may be mobilized to form flaps that can be imbricated or pulled medially to overlap the hernial site and reinforce the wound (see Fig. 11-1). It is advisable to take the tension off the skin edges and help obliterate the subcutaneous space between the skin and fascia by apposing the subcutaneous tissues with a series of interrupted synthetic absorbable or surgical gut sutures. The skin is closed with nonabsorbable sutures. For very large umbilical defects, a hernioplasty with synthetic patch material or fascia occasionally is required. Dead space in the subcutaneous tissues is then obliterated with a suction drain, placed at the time of closure. A circumferential dressing is also used to provide mild external counterpressure, which also obliterates dead space.

Postoperative Care

Possible complications of hernial repair, although uncommon, include seroma formation, wound infection, peritonitis, evisceration, and recurrence. Evisceration, or incisional hernia,

is best prevented by confining the patient and limiting its activity for at least 10 days following surgery. Seroma formation can be minimized by obliterating the subcutaneous dead space through the use of a suction drain or the application of a circumferential compressive dressing to immobilize the wound for the first 5 to 7 days after surgery. Although numerous studies have revealed that dead space cannot be adequately obliterated with the use of subcutaneous sutures, such sutures still are valuable for the apposition of the subcutaneous tissues that indirectly decrease dead space. Wound infections and peritonitis are prevented by following strict aseptic technique.

Omphalocele

An omphalocele occurs when most or all of the intestines and sometimes other abdominal organs lie outside the body in a thin, transparent avascular sac, on the apex of which the umbilicus inserts. The umbilical ring through which the hernial contents pass is enlarged to accommodate the base of these structures. Although the sac (derived from amnion) is always present, it may rupture before, during, or shortly after birth. Affected animals rarely are presented for diagnosis or surgical treatment, and the incidence is probably low. Omphaloceles reflect an arrest in development at the stage in which the growing intestines still are herniated into the umbilical cord. In the dog intestines normally return to the abdomen during the sixth week of gestation.

Although the occurrence of omphaloceles, especially in the presence of a congenital peritoneopericardial diaphragmatic hernia, has been reported in dogs and cats, there are no reports of their surgical repair. The only indication for surgery is in cases in which the omphalocele is small and can be closed, primarily by suturing (see "Diaphragmatic Hernia," Chap. 9). When tension on the suture line is considered excessive, some type of tissue or synthetic graft, such as the greater omentum, autogenous fascia, skin musculofascial autogenous grafts, fascial allografts, and synthetic muscles, can also be used.

Gastroschisis

This anomaly resembles an omphalocele, but the sac is absent and the defect is on a paramedian plane. Gastroschisis is a true eventration of the abdominal contents through a congenital muscular defect. The defect has been reported in cats and has resulted in early neonatal death. The repair, if considered, is similar to that for omphalocele. The defect in cats has been associated with schistosomus reflexus in other littermates.

Inguinal Hernia

Inguinal hernias are characterized by protrusion of intestine or other abdominal viscera through the inguinal canal. These hernias occur congenitally in both cats and dogs, alone or associated with midline abdominal defects. Although some inguinal hernias are first recognized in mature animals, there usually is evidence in such cases to suggest congenital predisposition and a hereditary basis for the defect. Inguinal hernias detected in mature animals are more frequently seen in females than males (in which they are usually scrotal —see "Scrotal Hernias," p. 292) for these reasons:

- Increased intra-abdominal pressure due to an enlarged organ occurs less frequently in the male.
- Estrogen and progesterone cause laxity of ligaments in females and less muscular development in the caudal inguinal region.
- The vaginal process, which remains open in the dog and cat throughout life, is larger in females than males.

Inguinal hernias often develop during pregnancy or in association with pyometra. In such cases the uterus may be found within the hernial sac; this is called an inguinal hysterocele. Theoretically, any structure that occupies space at the vaginal ring (testicular artery and vein, nerves, and ductus deferens) would tend to prevent entrance of other structures, but in females only the round ligament and a fat pad are present. Despite the persistence of an open vaginal process in both males and females, resistance to inguinal herniation may depend more on the neuromuscular reflex mechanism of the ventral abdominal wall than on the anatomy of the inguinal rings.

Inguinal hernias can be grouped as direct, indirect, and interstitial. Indirect hernias occur when the herniated structures pass through the inguinal canal and vaginal process. There is usually no history of trauma or abdominal stress, yet the patient's owner describes the sudden appearance of a fluctuating mass at the inguinal canal. Upon examining the animal for precipitating cause, none is found.

In some cases the herniated structures do not pass between all the layers of the abdominal wall after passing through the internal inguinal ring, and this is referred to as an interstitial hernia. These are rare in dogs and cats because the distance between the internal and external inguinal rings in these animals is small.

Direct hernias occur through a rent in the abdominal muscles and the hernial sac is external to the vaginal process. Usually, direct hernias are acquired, resulting from trauma. Obesity may predispose patients to the development of a direct inguinal hernia, as intra-abdominal force gradually causes stretching of structures that form the internal inguinal ring.

Inguinal hernias appear as protrusions of abdominal contents around the external inguinal ring. When the hernia can be palpated just at the external inguinal ring, it is called a bubonocele. Most inguinal hernias presented are unilateral. However, the opposite side is often weakened and predisposed for hernia occurrence. The hernial contents usually are soft, doughy, and insensitive when palpated, but these characteristics depend on the nature of the contents and length of time that the hernia has been present. A small swelling may be obscured by the caudal mammary glands. In other cases the swelling is large enough to contain a gravid or diseased uterus.

Diagnosis

If an inguinal hernia can be easily reduced, it usually is possible to palpate the hernial ring. Reduction of the hernia may be assisted by elevating the animal's hindquarters while it is in dorsal recumbency.

If it is impossible to reduce the hernia because of adhesions or size of the hernial sac, the diagnosis is not as easily made. Auscultation over the inguinal swelling occasionally reveals intestinal sounds that suggest the diagnosis. A swelling in the inguinal area, along with signs of intestinal obstruction, should arouse suspicion of incarcerated and strangulated intestine. An inguinal swelling also may consist of mammary tissue, fat, a neoplasm, hematoma, cyst, abscess, or a femoral or ventral hernia.

An abscess or cellulitis may be identified on the basis of warmth and sensitivity and the accompanying fever and leukocytosis. These swellings are not so freely movable as hernias. Cysts and hematomas are not warm to the touch, nor are they reducible. Evidence of contusion may be present in the inguinal skin following retroperitoneal hemorrhage, pelvic fractures, or sacroiliac luxations. Radiographic examination often is confirmatory.

Tumors often are identifiable by palpation because of their firmness and nodular conformation. Cytologic examination of an aspirate can be confirmatory. It may be difficult to differentiate an inguinal lipoma from a hernia, but deep palpation of the inguinal ring may be helpful. A mammary gland or tumor may obscure the presence of a small hernia.

Confirmation of bladder herniation can also be made by insufflating carbon dioxide or air through a urinary catheter while auscultating the inguinal swelling. Distinct bubbling sounds arising from within the sac during the insufflation will confirm the diagnosis. When air is used, the technique must be done care-fully because fatal air embolism can developed following pneumocystography. Such an embolism is most likely to occur when enough pressure is applied to significantly distend the bladder.

As a last resort in attempting to identify the origin of an inguinal swelling, the swelling can be aspirated. A needle puncture in normal intestine will seal spontaneously. If the intestinal blood supply is reduced, however, the needle hole may not seal and infection may occur.

Radiographic Diagnosis

Radiography is valuable in diagnosis, especially in determining whether intestine, gravid uterus, or urinary bladder has herniated. Barium sulfate can be used as contrast material when involvement of the digestive tract is suspected. If a gravid uterus has herniated, the fetal skeletons are visible on plain films in late gestation. At less than 43 days of gestation, a lobulated fluid density is apparent. When the bladder is involved, signs of cystitis may occur. A plain radiograph may reveal the presence of radiopaque calculi. If the bladder has herniated, radiographs taken following the instillation of air or carbon dioxide reveal a gas-filled bladder within the hernia. A decrease in the size of the hernia may be observed following urination or catheterization.

Plain radiographs may reveal a portion of the descending colon within the hernial sac. Fecal material and gas usually are apparent. Other structures that have been found in the hernial sac include the ovaries, retained testes, spleen, and omentum.

When only a small portion of intestine protrudes through the external inguinal ring, the bulge in the inguinal region may be so small that it is not noticed. Incarceration of only a small portion of the intestine may occur at the inner ring. Affected animals show signs of intestinal obstruction. The intestinal herniation in such cases may be discovered only by celiotomy performed to define the cause of acute abdominal pain.

Treatment

All inguinal hernias should be reduced and repaired surgically. When trauma has resulted in an inguinal hernia, it may be necessary during the herniorrhaphy to empty a hematoma, debride necrotic tissue, or sever adhesions. The repair involves making a skin incision cranial to the swelling and extending it caudally into the inguinal region. The skin and subcutaneous tissues are then bluntly separated from the fibrous capsule covering the herniated organs. The capsule is opened and resected, exposing the herniated tissues. If the bladder is included in the hernia, it should be emptied before attempting reduction. Tissue layers must be carefully apposed with nonabsorbable sutures.

The inguinal canal should be explored to estimate the number of sutures that will be required to close the canal sufficiently to prevent recurrence. During closure, the external pudendal artery and vein, the femoral artery and vein, and the genital nerves should be preserved (Fig. 11-2). Dead space is eliminated as discussed previously. It is not recommended to use Penrose (gravity) drains in this area as these drains predispose to infection, an increase in dead space, and subcutaneous emphysema due to the bellows-action of movement of the hind limb.

The usual approach to inguinal herniorrhaphy in males and unilateral hernias in females is via an incision directly over the hernia. In females, with inguinal hernias not associated with trauma, a better approach is to incise the skin on the ventral midline from the umbilicus to the pubis (Fig. 11-3). The inguinal mammary glands are dissected bluntly from their attachment to the rectus sheath and retracted laterally to expose the hernial sac and inguinal ring. The sac and its contents are handled in the same manner as described for the fibrous capsule associated with traumatic hernias. With this exposure the contralateral inguinal ring can be explored at the same time. If a hernia is present or impending, it can be corrected. The fascial tissue on either side of the hernial opening is sutured (Fig. 11-4), and the divided subcutaneous tissues and skin are apposed with both deep and superficial sutures.

Postoperative Care

Lymphedema in the pelvic limbs is common following inguinal surgery. Mild exercise is advisable to minimize this complication. Too much exercise, however, is associated with formation of a seroma. Gentle manipulation and elevation of the limbs assists in mobilizing the lymphatic fluid. Warm compresses applied

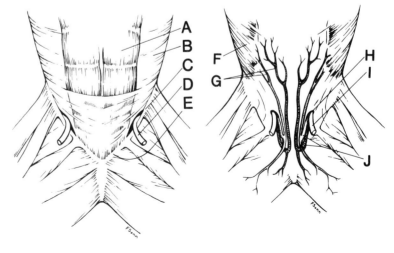

Figure 11-2. *Ventral abdomen of a dog, showing the rectus abdominis muscle (A) transversus abdominis muscle (B), inguinal ligament (C), vaginal process (D), prepubic tendon (E), external abdominal oblique muscle (F), caudal superficial epigastric artery and vein (G), superficial inguinal ring (H), vaginal process (I), external pudendal artery and vein (J). (Gourley IM, Vasseur PB, eds. General small animal surgery. Philadelphia: JB Lippincott, 1985:761.)*

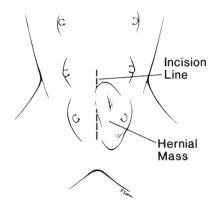

Figure 11-3. *Midline incision (dashed line) for correction of an inguinal hernia in a dog. (Gourley IM, Vasseur PB, eds. General small animal surgery. Philadelphia: JB Lippincott, 1985:762.)*

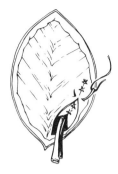

Figure 11-4. *Closure of inguinal hernia with two layers of sutures, leaving room for the pudendal vessels. (Gourley IM, Vasseur PB, eds. General small animal surgery. Philadelphia: JB Lippincott, 1985:762.)*

to the inguinal region also reduce the swelling. If a seroma forms, drains may be required. If suction drains are employed, the reservoirs are emptied and recharged as necessary. An Elizabethan collar or side brace is used to prevent the patient from disturbing the drains and suture line. The drains usually can be removed within five days as indicated by a significant decrease in the amount of drainage fluid collected.

Scrotal Hernia

When this rare hernia occurs in males, it is an extension of an indirect inguinal hernia. Strangulation of the herniated structures occurs frequently in untreated cases. Although evidence of inherited predisposition is lacking, affected animals should be castrated unless it is known that the herniation resulted from trauma. If bilateral castration is impractical, breeding should be discouraged on the basis that inguinal hernias can be hereditary.

A scrotal hernia often can be reduced through the inguinal canal when the animal is placed on its back with the hindquarters elevated. The spermatic cord, urogenital fat, omentum, and, occasionally, small intestine can be identified within the vaginal tunics by palpating the inguinal canal. Serous fluid

usually is present in the hernial sac. Occasionally, a large accumulation of fluid occurs in the distal process and tunica vaginalis (hydrocele).

Scrotal hernias often are bilateral. Testicular tumors and other causes of scrotal swelling should be considered before making a diagnosis of scrotal hernia. If, by grasping the upper part of the scrotum between the thumb and fingers, the skin on both sides can be apposed with nothing but the spermatic cord between it, a scrotal hernia is not present.

Repair of a scrotal hernia is similar to the repair of other inguinal hernias. If castration is not performed, the inguinal ring must accommodate the spermatic cord. As a consequence, the incidence of recurrence may be higher.

Repair

The skin is incised over the external inguinal ring to isolate the hernial sac, and its contents are reduced. Occasionally, adhesions prevent reduction by closed manipulation. In such cases the hernial sac must be opened to separate the adhesions.

If castration is to be performed, a double ligature of surgical gut is transfixed and passed around the spermatic cord and hernial sac as close to the internal inguinal ring as possible. The spermatic cord and enclosed vessels are severed distal to the ligatures. If the testicular vessels are large, they should be ligated separately; another ligature is used for the hernial sac. The edges of the inguinal ring are apposed with nonabsorbable sutures, and the skin and subcutaneous tissues are sutured in the usual manner. Recurrence is common unless the animal is castrated. If castration is not performed, the hernia is reduced and sutures are inserted in the neck of the sac, closing it without constricting the spermatic cord. If the inguinal canal is dilated, as it usually is, several sutures may be inserted into the fascia to close it partially. The skin is then closed in a routine manner. Attachment of subcutaneous tissues to underlying deep fascia helps to prevent the formation of seromas.

If inguinal and scrotal hernias coexist, the use of a synthetic or nonsynthetic material or fascia lata will be required to close the defects.

Postoperative Care

If the animal has not been castrated, testicular edema may be a problem. It usually is transient, however. Severe edema of the testes and pelvic limbs should be treated by gentle palpation, massage, and application of warm compresses. Mild exercise will help minimize postoperative edema.

Femoral Hernias

Femoral hernias are distinguished from inguinal hernias because they exit the abdomen within the femoral canal just lateral to the inguinal ligament (see "Inguinal Hernia—Treatment," p. 291).

The incidence of femoral hernias in dogs and cats is unknown but is believed to be very low. When an affected animal is stood on its hindlimbs, the hernial swelling is found to follow the femoral canal and the subcutaneous tissue of the medial thigh. The swelling is ventral to the inguinal ligament and ventral and lateral to the pubic brim. In contrast, inguinal hernias are dorsal and medial to the pubic brim.

The technique for repairing femoral hernias is similar to that used for inguinal hernias. Greater care must be taken to prevent injury to the femoral artery and vein. Repair also is complicated by the lack of a strong lateral boundary.

Repair with Prosthetic Materials

The materials used for repair include omentum, fascia, skin, and a variety of synthetic materials. When prosthetic materials are used to repair a hernia, it is called a hernioplasty.

Use of Omentum. Greater omentum has been used successfully as a transfer pedicle. The omentum must first be lengthened to close the defects. Either the left gastroepiploic or right gastroepiploic vessels are left intact to assure viability of the graft, which is then positioned and folded over itself repeatedly to cover the defect.

Use of Fascia. Autogenous fascia is obtained easily from the fascia lata or the lumbar area. It has the advantage of not causing a tissue reaction.

Use of Musculofascial Pedicle Grafts. Viable sections of the transversus abdominis and external and internal abdominal oblique muscles can be used for pedicle grafts. Parietal peritoneum–transversalis fascial pedicle grafts also have been used successfully to cover peritoneal defects.

Use of Synthetic Mesh. With very large defects synthetic nonabsorbable meshes have been used successfully to close the hernial defect, including stainless steel, nylon, polypropylene, woven Dacron, and silicone rubber sheeting. Sheets of various sizes up to 15×30 cm can be obtained in sterile packs ready for use. Larger sheets are available, but they must be cut to size and autoclaved or sterilized with ethylene oxide gas before use. They all cause minimal tissue reaction and provide adequate strength (see "Abdominal Wall Reconstruction," below).

After an abdominal wall defect or hernia has been closed with the mesh secured with suture material in a simple interrupted or continuous pattern, the skin and subcutaneous tissues are closed over it. If skin and subcutaneous tissues are not available, axial pattern grafts are made from nearby skin and subcutaneous tissues, or the defect is covered with omentum or sterile dressings. The mesh becomes incorporated in fibrous tissue and thus reinforces the suture line in the muscle fascia. Sharp ends and corners of the mesh must be removed, because they can cause excessive irritation or penetrate tissues with which they are in contact.

Acquired Abdominal Wall Defects

Injuries to the Abdominal Wall

Injuries to the abdominal wall are classified as blunt or penetrating. The examiner's first priority is to determine whether or not the abdominal wall has been penetrated. If penetration has occurred, further diagnostics are not necessary and expedient surgery is usually required.

The extent of injuries caused by blunt trauma is difficult to ascertain. Blunt injury can cause a surgical emergency when it results in rupture of vascular or hollow organs, and it can result in penetrating injury, caused by the tips of broken ribs. Blunt injury also may cause penetrating or lacerative damage to the abdominal muscles. Major trauma to deeper abdominal structures or muscle wall can occur with few or no evident external signs.

When the extent of a penetrating wound cannot easily be determined, the examiner should not probe the wound with the point of an instrument, because this may convert a superficial wound into one that penetrates the abdominal cavity. The wound can be explored under direct visualization and digital palpation to help ascertain the extent of damage to deeper structures. Radiography and peritoneal lavage are helpful in determining whether or not a serious intra-abdominal injury has occurred. These procedures are not required, however, if there is clear evidence of an internal injury or penetration of the peritoneal cavity.

If the peritoneal cavity has been penetrated, an exploratory celiotomy usually is indicated and should be performed as soon as possible. The celiotomy should be made on the ventral midline of the abdomen to provide best exposure of the abdominal structures regardless of where the injury is located. However, skin preparation of the inguinal area should also be done, because reparative surgery or placement of suction or gravity drains in this area is often required.

Ventral and Lateral Abdominal Hernias

These hernias are characterized by prolapse of abdominal contents through the abdominal wall at any point other than the umbilicus, femoral or inguinal rings, diaphragm, or perineal region. They are identified as ventral or lateral on the basis of their location on the abdomen. Hernias just caudal to the ribs are also referred to as paracostal hernias. Such hernias are usually acquired when an animal is kicked or struck by a car. These hernias have been described as false hernias because they do not occur through natural or potential body openings and because there is no true hernial sac. The herniated structures are covered only by subcutaneous tissues and skin. In paracostal hernias the origins of the external abdominal oblique and transversus abdominis muscles and the insertion of the internal abdominal oblique muscles have been torn from the ribs and costal cartilages. This allows the abdominal viscera to herniate into the lateral subcutaneous tissues. These hernias occur frequently in conjunction with acquired diaphragmatic hernias.

The abdominal muscles are likely to be contracted as an apprehensive animal is subjected to the blow that causes muscle separation. The blow imparts mechanical kinetic energy to the abdominal structures directly beneath it. The blow also causes a sudden increase in intra-abdominal pressure that may lead to bursting injuries of the abdominal wall and deeper abdominal organs. Herniation and injuries to deeper abdominal organs (spleen, liver, gallbladder, pancreas, or intestine) may result when small dogs are mauled by larger animals. In some cases it may take weeks after the original trauma occurs before the injury is recognized because of subcutaneous swellings and temporary sealing of perforations.

The incidence of ventral herniation is low. Such hernias occur most commonly just cranial to the pelvis, and often the prepubic tendons and inguinal ligaments are torn. They can occur, however, in any area of the ventral abdominal wall. Ventral hernias also may occur in conjunction with diaphragmatic and inguinal hernias.

Clinical Signs

The most obvious sign of ventral or lateral hernias is asymmetry of the abdominal contour. The consistency of the swelling depends on the hernial contents and the presence or absence of hematomas, tissue trauma, or infection. The swelling may become larger after a sudden body movement or during coughing. Signs unrelated to the hernia *per se* may also be present. For example, ventral hernias resulting from trauma may be accompanied initially by hemorrhage and signs of shock.

If the abdominal muscles are completely ruptured, it may be possible to palpate and identify intestine, spleen, a gravid uterus, or other abdominal viscera in the subcutaneous tissues.

An incarcerated hernia feels turgid, and its opening is difficult to palpate. When adhesions are present, it may be possible to reduce swelling, but overlying subcutaneous tissues and skin cannot be separated from the herniated structures. An incarcerated hernia must be differentiated from an abscess, hema-

toma, cyst, or neoplasm. Acute incarcerations usually appear painful to the patient on palpation, and the palpation often stimulates vomiting episodes. With strangulation, signs of shock and peritonitis usually occur.

Radiographs usually reveal gas-filled loops of intestine located subcutaneously in the lateral or ventral abdominal wall. Subcutaneous emphysema may be apparent if the intestine or skin has been perforated. Discontinuity of the *flank strip* that represents the musculature of the lateral abdominal wall should prompt suspicion of a lateral hernia. Injecting a small amount of sterile metrizamide or organic iodide contrast material subcutaneously or intra-abdominally will coat the loops of intestine and other viscera and thus assist in their identification.

In most cases a long-standing hernia is less serious than a recent one. The fact that a hernia has been present for some time without causing serious problems is in itself reassuring. Any ventral hernia is a potential hazard to the animal's health, however, because its contents are more vulnerable to injury than when they are protected by an intact body wall.

Irreducible hernias are likely to become strangulated. The danger of strangulation is increased if the hernial contents are large in relation to the size of hernial opening. If the strangulated tissues become gangrenous, the prognosis is poor. If herniation occurs close to the ribs, the continuous movement of the costal margin may interfere with healing. Spontaneous repair of ventral or lateral hernias does not appear to occur.

Treatment

In cases in which a ventral or lateral hernia has recently resulted from trauma, the animal should be examined for evidence of shock. If signs of shock are associated with hemorrhage, immediate surgical intervention may be necessary. Treatment for shock should be instituted first, however, and the surgery delayed, if possible, until the risks associated with anesthesia are decreased. During the course of shock therapy, strangulation of viscera may be prevented by reducing the hernia while the animal is unconscious or sedated. The abdomen should then be bandaged to temporarily prevent the recurrence of the herniation.

Abdominal wounds should be cleaned and debrided, and the site of the hernia prepared for surgery. Most of these hernias can be repaired following an exploratory celiotomy through the ventral midline. The deeper peritoneal and transversus muscle layers often are repaired from inside the abdominal cavity. Separations in the rectus muscles, oblique abdominal muscles, and attending fascia can be repaired from either within the celiotomy (preferred in many cases because the edges of the separations are often easier to find) or following celiotomy closure (i.e., from the outside.)

Repair of Ventral Hernias

When multiple hernias or a large hernia exist, an attempt should be made to expose them with as few incisions as possible. In most cases this can be accomplished with a ventral midline approach. After the abdominal cavity has been exposed, the organs should be inspected and repaired as necessary. The tear in the abdominal wall should be closed in layers. This can be simple when dealing with recent hernias, because the muscles are identified easily. With older wounds, however, the edges of the torn muscles may have retracted and become fibrotic and atrophic, making identification and apposition more difficult.

With traumatically induced ventral hernias, the rectus abdominis muscle often is avulsed from its attachment on the pubis and retracted cranially. To deal with this problem, first the rectus muscles are divided through the linea alba to enable inspection of the abdominal viscera. Then the avulsed muscle is attached to the pubis by preplacing nonabsorbable sutures that receive their holding power from insertion into the prepubic fascia and periosteum. These sutures are left untied. However, tears in the lateral, inguinal, and

femoral regions are repaired. The fascial edges of the deepest muscle layer are sutured first. This usually is the transversus abdominis muscle, which is identified by its dorsoventrally running fibers and the fact that the transverse fascia and peritoneum usually adhere to its deep surface. Fascia of the internal abdominal oblique muscle is sutured next; its fibers run cranioventrally. Fascia of the external abdominal oblique muscle, the fibers of which run caudoventrally, is sutured last.

Monofilament polypropylene or nylon sutures are recommended for the repair of ventral hernias. When torn fascia-muscle edges cannot be identified, they are apposed as well as possible with a series of interrupted sutures inserted into the fascial covering. These sutures are preplaced and then simultaneously tightened to avoid tearing the fascia. Because many ventral hernias also involve the inguinal area, care must be taken to prevent laceration or partial obstruction of the femoral and inguinal vessels. When apposition of large defects is impossible, or excessive tension must be exerted on the sutures placed to close the wound, the defect may be covered with synthetic mesh.

Postoperative Care. Occasionally either gravity or suction drainage of the subcutaneous tissues is necessary to prevent formation of a seroma. Because it often is necessary to reconstruct the femoral and inguinal canals, swelling of the pelvic limbs and the scrotal and inguinal areas may result. This is due to obstruction of lymphatics and blood vessels. Treatment includes mild range of motion and passive physical therapy, warm compresses, and elevation. Suction drainage is usually more successful in removing lymphatic fluid than gravity drainage, and therefore, is recommended here.

Repair of Lateral Hernias

Lateral (paracostal) hernias usually are repaired through a ventral midline incision, which enables exploration of the abdominal cavity for concomitant injuries and provides adequate exposure of the hernia. Positive-pressure ventilation should be provided while anesthetizing animals with lateral hernias, until it can be determined that their diaphragm is intact.

Lateral hernias are repaired by approaching them from within the abdomen, using monofilament suture material. Either a continuous or interrupted pattern can be used. If muscle and fascia are stripped from the caudal ribs, the exposed ribs can cause further trauma to the abdominal viscera or interfere with reduction of the hernia and may need to be removed. Withdrawal of herniated structures into the abdominal cavity may be difficult because mesentery and omentum are wrapped around an exposed rib. Gentle manipulation is required to reduce such hernias without injuring the herniated structures.

Occasionally, the herniated structures may be approached directly over the area where the injury has occurred. This approach is necessary when there is extensive separation of subcutaneous tissues and skin from the fascia of the abdominal wall. In these cases either gravity or suction drainage is necessary to prevent formation of seromas.

Postoperative (Incisional) Hernia and Evisceration

Postoperative herniation is a form of deep wound dehiscence in which the skin closure remains intact. The skin may be completely healed when the hernia is first recognized. Only a small amount of ligament, properitoneal fat, or omentum may herniate through the abdominal wall and lie subcutaneously. Most hernias of this type occur at the cranial end of ventral midline incisions. In more serious cases, abdominal viscera are displaced into the hernia.

Postoperative hernias must be distinguished from postoperative seromas and subcutaneous cellulitis. Palpation usually enables this differentiation. With incisional hernias, a rent in the abdominal wall usually can be palpated. Causes of incisional hernias include:

Vigorous or uncontrolled activity of the patient that results in breaking or tearing out of sutures from the abdominal fascia
Improper placement or selection of sutures
Improper handling of sutures or tying of knots
Delayed wound healing resulting from malnutrition, rough handling of tissues, or local infection

The incidence of incisional hernias can be reduced by proper selection and handling of the suture material, by correct placement of sutures, and by restricting of the patient's activity. If delay in wound healing and poor wound strength are anticipated, the use of a nonabsorbable, nonreactive monofilament suture material is recommended along with nutritional support.

The treatment of incisional hernias depends on their severity and duration. In most cases, surgical correction is indicated, especially when the hernia occurs 1 to 2 weeks after surgery or is large and includes more than fatty tissue. If only a small amount of fat has herniated, surgery may be postponed, but the animal must be examined frequently until a stage of healing has been reached that allows a prediction of no further herniation.

In a more serious form of incisional breakdown, the skin and underlying subcutaneous tissues are also separated, thus exposing the peritoneal cavity. This is called evisceration. This dehiscence usually occurs 1 to 5 days after surgery. Serous discharge from the skin incision and a palpable soft mass are often the first signs of dehiscence. If these signs are observed in any patient following abdominal surgery, it is advisable to recommend the placement of a circumferential dressing and careful transport to a veterinarian for examination. If the animal is allowed free activity, evisceration may occur within a short time. Evisceration may be fatal, and emergency surgery is required.

Repair of Incisional Hernias

The approach for repair of an incisional hernia is made through the old wound. Debridement of the wound's surface is limited to removal of necrotic and obviously devitalized tissue. After replacement of the hernial contents, the wound is closed with monofilament, nonabsorbable sutures placed through the external fascia of the abdominal muscles. In recent hernias the edges of the wound contain friable granulation tissue that does not hold sutures well. Rather than removing this granulating tissue that develops during the early stages of wound healing, the sutures are placed into fascial tissue lateral to this edge. This usually requires placing the sutures 1 to 1.5 cm from the wound edge instead of the normal 3 to 5 mm. The wound edges are debrided only if necrosis is evident. Gray to pinkish gray is the normal color for granulation tissue and should not be confused with necrotic tissue, which is dark or black.

Simple continuous sutures of monofilament nylon or polypropylene have been effective for closing abdominal fascia. The use of swaged-on, taper-point needles is preferred. Size 000 suture material usually is suitable for animals weighing 15 kg or less. Size 00 is used for animals weighing more than 15 and less than 50 kg. Those weighing more than 50 kg require size 0.

If infection is present, irrigation with 5% to 10% povidone–iodine solution, debridement of necrotic tissue, and placement of drains are required after closure of the fascia. Delayed closure of the skin may be preferred to the use of drainage tubes. In such cases, the skin and subcutaneous wound are kept open and treated with povidone–iodine packs and absorbent dressings for 3 to 5 days. The wound is then closed by suturing. If infection is not present, the wound can be allowed to heal by granulation. Closure of infected or badly contaminated wounds without drainage invites formation of abscesses.

Repair of Evisceration

The eviscerated structures should be covered with sterile saline-soaked laparotomy pads and a bandage applied promptly to prevent further damage. After inducing general anesthesia and preparing the skin for aseptic surgery, the laparotomy pads are removed in the operating room, and the exposed tissues are closely inspected and gently cleaned. Debridement and resection of tissues are performed as indicated, and the dehiscence is repaired following extensive copious lavage. In most cases the edges of the separated incision are only minimally debrided, if at all, and deep bites on each side of the separated incision are taken with each needle pass. Simple continuous or interrupted patterns are the most common suture patterns used for closure; the former is preferred in most cases. A nonabsorbable monofilament suture, slightly larger than might generally be used, is selected. Following fascial closure, extensive irrigation is performed and the skin and subcutaneous tissues are closed as indicated, generally without the subcutaneous sutures being buried.

Abdominal Wall Reconstruction

Loss of a portion of the abdominal wall due to trauma, infection, or neoplasia presents a difficult problem, because primary closure under tension can result in wound ischemia and increased intra-abdominal pressure that predisposes to dehiscence, evisceration, and ischemia and dysfunction of abdominal organs. When contamination of the abdominal cavity has not occurred, the transversus abdominis muscle or the internal or external abdominal oblique muscles and their aponeuroses may be used as a flap to cover the defect.

The transversus abdominis muscle has the advantage of including peritoneum and internal rectus and transversalis fascia, which provides a strong graft. A disadvantage is that its application is limited if very large defects need to be closed. Use of the transverse abdominis technique in the presence of infection may spread the infection; the technique is also time consuming. Note that failure of the flap, due to ischemia, is more likely in animals that have impaired cardiovascular and respiratory functions.

Polypropylene mesh is effective in restoring the continuity of the abdominal wall, and has been used successfully in contaminated and infected abdominal wounds. Favorable characteristics of the mesh include its durability, pliability, high tensile strength, and host tolerance when infection is present. With adequate drainage, granulation tissue will permeate the mesh and engulf bacteria, even in purulent infections. Chronic infections may occur, however, if there is a mesh-epithelium interface. For this reason it is recommended that the mesh be placed on the fascial side of the abdominal wall between muscle and the external fascia, rather than on the peritoneal surface. If there is no evidence of infection, the mesh can be placed on the peritoneal side of the abdominal wall. Whenever possible, omentum should be placed between viscera and mesh to prevent firm adhesions to vital structures.

Damage to the abdominal wall may be accompanied by loss of sufficient skin and subcutaneous tissues to preclude covering the mesh. In such cases, occlusive dressings should be used until granulation tissue covers the surface of the mesh. Otherwise, folds of viable omentum can be placed on the outer surface of the mesh. A skin flap then can be used to cover the defect.

Woven fabrics, stainless steel, plastic and celluloid meshes, and silicone rubber sheeting also have been used to reconstruct large ventral abdominal wall defects in dogs.

Acute Abdominal Pain

The term *acute abdomen* refers to the sudden onset of abdominal pain. Causes include acute systemic diseases, gastrointestinal obstruction, neoplasia, and urogenital diseases. Until proven otherwise, acute abdominal pain should be assumed to be caused by a disorder that can be corrected surgically. If the pain lasts more than 6 hours, it usually has surgical significance, especially when signs of shock or peritoneal irritation are present. Analgesics obscure signs that may have diagnostic value and, therefore, should be used sparingly until a definite diagnosis has been made.

The signs of acute abdomen include emesis, diarrhea, abdominal distention, and

evidence of pain and shock. An affected animal may be reluctant to walk and attempts to maintain the least painful position. Abdominal palpation reveals generalized tenderness. It is important that the cases requiring surgical treatment be identified quickly. The most common causes of acute abdominal pain requiring medical treatment are acute pancreatitis, nephritis, acute gastroenteritis, acute prostatitis, and acute hepatitis. Conditions requiring surgery include rupture of the urinary bladder; urethral obstruction; intestinal obstruction or strangulation; rupture of the spleen, liver, or kidneys; gastric dilatation or volvulus; uterine torsion or metritis; generalized peritonitis; and herniation of an intervertebral disc.

When evaluating a patient with acute abdominal pain, an attempt should be made to determine how the pain started, where it originates, and how far it extends. Although it may be possible to localize the area of maximum tenderness, old dogs and animals that are acutely ill or in shock may display less pain and abdominal rigidity than would be expected from the severity of the lesion. Tenderness and abdominal guarding may be difficult to localize in obese animals.

Laboratory tests should be performed promptly to determine the hemoglobin concentration, erythrocyte count, differential and total leukocyte counts, urine characteristics, and presence of occult blood in feces. As differential diagnoses are considered, other tests can be performed, including radiography, diagnostic peritoneal lavage, and ultrasonography. When the patient's condition is deteriorating rapidly and a diagnosis has not been made, an exploratory celiotomy is indicated.

The treatment depends on the diagnosis. Shock often is present and should be treated immediately. The intravenous administration of a balanced electrolyte solution often is required, because volume depletion is common.

Peritonitis

Inflammation of the peritoneal cavity is classified on the basis of its extent (diffuse or generalized, localized), nature (acute, chronic), and source (bacterial, viral); it is subclassified as primary or secondary. Primary peritonitis, often called idiopathic, accounts for less that 1% of cases. The causal organisms in primary peritonitis presumably gain access to the peritoneum hematogenously. Feline infectious peritonitis is an example.

Secondary peritonitis results from peritoneal involvement subsequent to a primary process, such as dehiscence of sutured intestinal wounds or perforation of the stomach or small intestine. The peritoneal cavity can also be contaminated by microorganisms that enter through a perforation in the abdominal wall. Penetration of the peritoneal cavity can result from animal bites or be caused by missiles or sharp objects. Such penetration usually is accompanied by the entrance of hair, dirt, or larger objects into the abdominal cavity. The gastrointestinal tract also may be the source of foreign objects in the peritoneal cavity.

Peritonitis may be a common cause of death following abdominal surgery in which aseptic technique is not used; an estimated 50% or more of the cases of septic shock in dogs and cats are caused by peritonitis.

Aseptic Peritonitis

Aseptic peritonitis results from various physical and chemical irritants that enter the abdominal cavity during surgery, despite the use of aseptic technique; bacterial infection (septic peritonitis) often complicates the inflammation.

Foreign bodies may cause localized peritonitis and granulomas. Causes include surgical equipment or supplies, such as sponges, suture material, powder from gloves, and debris from drapes and instruments. Some degree of localized peritonitis follows every surgical exposure of the abdominal cavity, because irritation and low-grade bacterial contamination inevitably result from ambient air, hair and skin from the patient, and foreign materials used during surgery. Such limited contamination is usually controlled by protective mechanisms of the peritoneal cavity. Occasionally, the degree of foreign body contamination is so great or the patient's defenses are so weakened by disease that diffuse peritonitis ensues. Foreign objects usually cause one of the following reactions:

- A localized inflammation by which the foreign material is removed
- A localized inflammation that results in a localized sterile abscess or granuloma
- A similar process with formation of a sinus or fistula
- Potentiation of the virulence of organisms that are present in the abdomen and the development of septic peritonitis

The clinical manifestations of sterile foreign bodies vary. A gauze sponge left in the abdominal cavity may stimulate formation of a sterile abscess. In such cases an intra-abdominal mass can often be palpated. Intermittent fever may result along with vomiting and diarrhea. Occasionally there is an intense local reaction and restrictive adhesions. Removal of the causal object often requires resection of intestine and other tissues.

Chemical irritants that can occasionally cause peritonitis include bile, blood, gastric juice, pancreatic juice, urine, antiseptics, antibacterial powders, enema solutions, and barium sulfate suspensions. Bile enters the abdominal cavity as a result of a biliary tract rupture or as a sequel to an operation on or near the biliary system. Sterile bile is a mild irritant. Bile is sterile when cultured from animals that do not have cholehepatic disease. Following the placement of sterile bile into the abdominal cavity, bacterial proliferation occurs. The bacteria cultured usually include *Staphylococcus aureus* and *Clostridium welchii; Streptococcus spp.* and various coliforms are less common. Death from bile peritonitis occurs when a sterile inflammation becomes complicated by bacterial infection. Administration of antibiotics significantly prolongs the lives of affected dogs.

Though blood is not irritating, it can serve as a nidus for bacterial infection and should always be removed from the abdominal cavity at the end of an operation.

Gastric and pancreatic juices are very irritating and their leakage into the abdominal cavity causes peritonitis. Within 6 to 8 hours, the spread of bacteria results in an infectious peritonitis. Sterile urine also is irritating and can cause peritonitis, though it is not nearly as irritating as biliary acids or pancreatic fluid. Occasionally bacteria that are present in the urine of animals with cystitis will complicate the chemical peritonitis.

Some antiseptic solutions and nearly all antibacterial powders and suspensions can cause a generalized peritonitis and granuloma formation. A virulent form of chemical peritonitis follows the accidental introduction of barium sulfate suspension into the abdominal cavity. This material is especially difficult to remove.

Talcum powder, composed mainly of hydrated magnesium silicate, can cause an intense fibroblastic reaction and dense adhesions within weeks or months. For that reason, different materials now are being used as surgical glove powders. Soluble starch powder, which is preferred at the present time, nevertheless produces granulomas if left within the peritoneal cavity. Therefore, surgical gloves always should be washed and dried before an operation. If a glove is torn during an operation, care should be taken to avoid spilling the glove powder into the wound. In humans, clinical signs of granulomatous peritonitis caused by starch are postoperative fever and abdominal tenderness that gradually subside after several days. In a few cases, dogs and cats presented with signs of depression, anorexia, and significant abdominal tenderness were found to have granulomatous peritonitis on biopsy or were found to have starch powder microgranulomas in peritoneal lavage fluids.

Septic Peritonitis

Septic (bacterial) peritonitis is caused mainly by enteric bacteria. There usually is a mixture of both anaerobic and aerobic organisms. Gram-negative bacteria predominate and *Escherichia coli* are cultured most commonly in both dogs and cats. In an early, acute stage of peritonitis, death is attributable principally to anaerobic bacteria.

Ischemia of the intestine, due to strangulation of the blood supply or obstruction, is an important cause of peritonitis. Although the intestinal wall may be grossly intact, its increased permeability enables bacteria to enter the abdominal cavity. Other common causes of septic peritonitis include rupture of the uterus and extension of infection from retroperitoneal or other intraperitoneal organs. Bacteria may also course retrograde through the oviducts in patients with pyometritis to cause peritonitis via the ovarian bursa.

Peritonitis following abdominal surgery usually is the result of dehiscence of a suture line in a hollow viscus. The stability of a suture line is endangered by tension, ischemia, hemorrhage, mucosal eversion, infection, excessive peritoneal fluid, and such systemic factors as hypoproteinemia and anemia.

Clinical Signs. The signs of septic peritonitis vary depending on the cause, location or generalization of the inflammation, and the patient's previous condition. The history usually is unrevealing, unless the owner observed a recent injury or abdominal surgery was recently performed. The signs include depression, diminished appetite, and vomiting. The patient may assume an unusual posture, such as a praying position, and may be unresponsive to pain on abdominal palpation.

Physical findings may include the presence of injuries in the caudal thoracic or the abdominal region; evidence of discomfort on abdominal palpation; inducement of vomiting by palpation; palpation of an intra-abdominal mass; and signs of shock, including congested mucous membranes and slow capillary refill time. The patient's temperature varies: it may be elevated due to infection, but it may become subnormal as shock ensues.

Radiography. Radiographs of the abdomen may reveal free gas resulting from a rupture in the gastrointestinal tract or from penetrating injuries of the abdominal wall. The presence of fluid in the abdominal cavity is reflected by the absence of normal definition of the viscera and by a "ground glass" appearance of survey films. The signs of ileus are common. Signs of localized inflammation may be apparent clinically or on radiographs. These include persistent localized tenderness, unthriftiness and weakness clinically, and a localized area on radiographs where there is loss of detail. Use of a contrast medium may help to confirm or exclude some possible causes such as loss of gastrointestinal mucosal integrity. In most cases of fulminating peritonitis, a radiological workup takes too much time. It is better to start preparing the patient for surgery and to perform an exploratory celiotomy early.

Cytology. A final preoperative diagnosis usually is based on the results of a cytologic examination of fluid obtained by paracentesis. The presence of degenerative neutrophils and intracellular and extracellular bacteria is confirmatory evidence of septic peritonitis. In aseptic peritonitis, cytologic examination of the peritoneal fluid reveals neutrophilia, but neither degenerative neutrophils nor bacteria.

Treatment. The treatment of peritonitis depends on its cause, severity, duration, and on whether the inflammation is diffuse or localized. Because generalized peritonitis results in rapid changes in fluid and electrolyte balances, correction of these imbalances and hypovolemia should be attempted first. A balanced electrolyte solution should be administered unless this is contraindicated by laboratory findings. Monitoring central venous pressure, urinary output, body temperature, and capillary perfusion time helps determine the amount of fluid to be given and the rate of its administration. The rate of administration may be as high as 40 ml/kg of body weight per hour in a cat (80 ml/kg in a dog) that is severely volume depleted due to the peritonitis.

A normal acid–base balance should be reestablished. In severely dehydrated animals, metabolic acidosis is a major problem. If the plasma bicarbonate level and the pH are unknown, sodium bicarbonate may be added cautiously to electrolyte solutions for these patients. The dose varies from 1.0 to 4.0 mEq/kg of body weight.

Appropriate antibiotics should be given in high doses. Because gram-negative aerobic and gram-positive anaerobic bacteria usually are involved in septic peritonitis, antibiotics often are used in combination. One commonly used combination includes gentamicin (2.2 mg/kg t.i.d.), sodium ampicillin or a first generation cephalosporin (22 mg/kg t.i.d.), and metronidazole (5–10 mg/kg t.i.d.) given by slow IV injection. Occasionally, the treatment of septic peritonitis is complicated by the presence of organisms not commonly implicated, such as *Actinomyces spp.* Therefore, aerobic and anaerobic cultures and antibiotic sensitivity testing of aspirated fluid should be done routinely, and antibiotic therapy may be altered based on the findings of the tests.

Corticosteroid therapy is recommended for its positive inotropic effect on heart muscle. Other beneficial effects include stabilization of lysosomal membranes, decrease in capillary permeability, protection against endotoxins, and restoration of normal permeability of the intestinal wall. Recently, the use of flunixin meglumine, to prevent liberation of thromboxane and prostacyclin, has been found to prolong the lives of dogs with septic peritonitis. It is given in conjunction with an antibiotic such as gentamicin.

After appropriate supportive measures for peritonitis have been instituted and the patient is hemodynamically improved, surgery is recommended to prevent continued contamination, to remove foreign material, and to provide for drainage of fluid. An additional measure adopted recently is the establishment of tube gastrostomies and enterostomies to keep the gastrointestinal tract decompressed while ileus is present. Later, in the early recovery stage, a jejunostomy tube provides fluids and nutrients. These procedures are important because animals treated in this way often are anorectic for several days and recover intestinal function prior to return of normal gastric motility and function.

A leak in a hollow viscus can be repaired in various ways depending on the extent and nature of the leaking material and the viscus involved. It may involve simple debridement and closure of a ruptured bladder, resection of an ischemic section of jejunum, or the use of a serosal patch (see below) to seal a perforated gastric or duodenal ulcer. Because of the high concentration of fibrinolytic enzymes induced by peritonitis, suturing a perforated lesion may not prevent leakage. The technique of serosal patching (using a loop of intestine as a patch over the defect) has been effective in providing a seal that is capable of withstanding increased intraluminal pressures.

All foreign material, necrotic tissue, and blood clots must be removed from the operative site. Copious irrigation with isotonic saline solution or Ringer's lactate solution significantly reduces the mortality and morbidity associated with acute diffuse peritonitis. The irrigation is continued until the aspirated fluid is clear.

Peritoneal lavage facilitates the removal of small pieces of necrotic tissue, blood clots, fat droplets, and bacteria, and it decreases the amount of endotoxin. Lavage also facilitates the dispersal of antibiotics and antiseptics intraperitoneally and helps to reduce peritoneal adhesions. The use of warmed fluids is recommended to treat or prevent hypothermia. This is especially indicated for small patients that have a greater proportion of peritoneal surface area per unit of body weight.

Antibiotics in lavage fluids are useful in the treatment of generalized peritonitis, but their concomitant intravenous administration is necessary to maintain therapeutic levels in serum and peritoneal fluid. On the other hand, some antibiotics given intraperitoneally may have some adverse effects, including irritation of the peritoneum, which causes the formation of adhesions (tetracycline, streptomycin); induction of an intensified catabolic state (tetracycline); hypersensitivity reactions (penicillins); respiratory arrest and hypotension due to calcium binding (aminoglycosides); and neuromuscular blockage (aminoglycosides, neomycin, kanamycin, and gentamicin).

When cephalosporins are administered intraoperatively, their concentrations in peritoneal fluid are higher than the concentrations obtained with intravenous administration of the same dose, and the therapeutic levels are maintained longer in the peritoneal cavity. Further, there is evidence that cephalothin administered intraperitoneally to dogs with experimentally induced peritonitis significantly increases the likelihood of survival. The use of such combinations as kanamycin, ampicillin, and metronidazole, or kanamycin, cephalosporins, and metronidazole also has been effective. Other drugs that have been used singly with favorable results include kanamycin, gentamicin, penicillin, ampicillin, sulfanilamide, chloramphenicol, bacitracin, streptomycin, neomycin, and noxythiolin. (Of course, the choice of drugs depends on the type of bacteria present.) Thus, the advantages of intraperitoneal administration of antibiotics in animals appear to far outweigh their disadvantages.

The addition of antiseptics such as povidone–iodine or chlorhexidine to lavage solutions has been effective in the treatment of peritonitis. Their use is controversial, however, particularly in regard to povidone–iodine, because the polyvinyl pyrolidone vehicle in povidone-iodine solutions may cause hypotension and inhibit macrophage chemotaxis. Chlorhexidine bigluconate (20%) diluted 1:1000 with sterile water or saline solution appears to be both safe and effective for intraperitoneal irrigation. Addition of 10 ml of povidone–iodine stock solution to 100 to 150 ml of warm saline solution has been recommended for use in a 12-kg dog. Following use of these agents, copious irrigation is performed until the fluid removed remains clear. Do not use diluted povidone–iodine or chlorhexidine surgical scrub solution in the peritoneal cavity, because these products contain detergents in addition to the antiseptic agent.

Although it is impossible to drain the entire abdominal cavity with tubes alone, sustained postoperative drainage is important in the treatment of peritonitis. Effective postoperative drainage can be achieved by continuous or intermittent lavage of the abdominal cavity or by keeping the abdominal cavity open and protecting against evisceration with sterile pads. Both of these methods have been used successfully in dogs and cats.

It is important to use drains that are effective in removing the peritoneal lavage solutions when continuous or intermittent lavage is being performed. A sump–Penrose combination drain appears to be the most efficient type. The drain is made by placing a double lumen (sump) drain inside a fenestrated latex Penrose drain. Use of silicone for the sump drain increases efficiency because of the lower thrombogenic and reactive properties of silicone, compared with common polyethylene or red rubber.

Continuous peritoneal lavage is difficult to perform in animals, but often can be accomplished in the early postoperative period when the animal is still under the effect of the anesthetic. Continuous low suction (40 to 70 mmHg) is applied to the sump drain as warmed physiologic saline solution containing antibiotics or an antiseptic solution is infused intraabdominally.

Intermittent lavage (2 to 4 times daily) also is an acceptable form of treatment. Patients weighing less that 15 kg should be given 500 ml of the lavage solution; heavier animals should be given 1 liter. The solution can include 1 to 2 g of cephalothin per liter. Simple tube, sump, or sump–Penrose drains can be attached to closed collection systems. Penrose drains alone cannot be attached to closed systems and therefore are used less frequently for this technique. As with all drains, protective sterile dressings are important to prevent an ascending infection.

Complications associated with lavage and drainage include anemia, hypoproteinemia, hyponatremia, hypokalemia, hypothermia (if the lavage fluids are not warmed sufficiently), ascending infection through the drainage tubing, and malfunction or dislocation of the drain tubing. Most of these complications can be prevented by using sterile occlusive dressings and povidone–iodine ointment around the drainage tube exits, and by administering blood, plasma, and appropriate electrolyte fluids as needed. Although

peritoneal lavage given postoperatively has proven to be lifesaving in cases of suppurative peritonitis, it failed to remove suppuration completely in over half the animals in one study, resulting in death of the affected animals.

In another method of draining the abdominal cavity, the abdomen is not closed following surgery. A loose continuous closure, leaving a gap of 1 to 2 cm, helps protect against evisceration. A large number of absorbent gauze pads are used to cover the abdominal incision and the abdomen is bound with circumferential bandages. These can be fashioned so that a "trap door" is all that is required to be opened to change the dressings. If the original abdominal incision extends to the pubic area, the caudal portion of the incision should be closed completely to facilitate bandaging. The sterile pads must be changed when they become saturated with fluid. This may require one to four changes daily (twice on average). The pads should be changed with the patient under sedation and in a sterile environment. Drainage of fluid usually is markedly decreased by the second or third day. The abdomen may be closed when the dressings have remained clean and dry for 24 hours, which usually occurs 3 to 4 days following surgery. With this method of drainage, the patient must be observed closely. Fluid, electrolyte, and protein losses should be replaced as indicated. A good way to estimate the amount of fluids lost is to weigh the dressings. Protein loss also can be estimated by sampling a portion of the fluid and obtaining a total protein concentration. Electrolytes also can be measured from a sample of the peritoneal fluid.

Urine Peritonitis

The escape of a small amount of urine into the abdominal cavity is of little consequence. Continued leakage of urine, however, can result in uremia, peritonitis, and death. In as little as 24 hours after the onset of urine leakage, uremia results from absorption of soluble toxic substances. If the urine is infected, septic peritonitis usually occurs.

The diagnosis of urine peritonitis often

involves the same procedures used in cases of suspected hemoperitoneum. Rupture of the urinary bladder due to blunt abdominal trauma or due to attempts to manually express a distended bladder are common causes of urine leakage into the abdominal cavity. Radiographs of affected animals often reveal evidence of fluid in the abdomen, ileus, abdominal adhesions, and peritonitis. In one series of cases, pneumocystograms revealed 72% of the ruptured bladders; positive-contrast cystograms revealed 100% of the ruptures. Increased BUN and serum creatinine concentrations and metabolic acidosis are common laboratory findings. Untreated animals develop serum electrolyte abnormalities and become dehydrated.

Treatment of urine peritonitis involves measures to correct fluid and electrolyte imbalances. The following procedures have been recommended:

1. A catheter should be inserted into the urethra, passed into the bladder, and, if the rent in the bladder is sufficiently large, passed into the abdominal cavity to drain the escaped urine. Alternatively, a peritoneal dialysis catheter can be inserted through the abdominal wall to remove the fluid.
2. Normal saline solution or lactated Ringer's solution should be administered intravenously. If peritoneal drainage or lavage and intravenous fluid support is given for 12 hours prior to surgery, the fluid and serum electrolyte, BUN, and creatinine levels often return to normal or near normal, and the risks of anesthesia to the patient are greatly reduced. Therefore, surgical repair of the source of escaping urine should be delayed, if possible, until the metabolic abnormalities have been corrected. Postoperative lavage or delayed closure of the abdomen seldom is necessary.

Escape of urine into the abdominal cavity often is complicated by infection with gram-negative bacteria. For this reason, the perioperative administration of a broad-spectrum an-

tibiotic, such as gentamicin, along with a synthetic penicillin or cephalosporin, is indicated. Empirical antibiotic therapy is usually required for only 72 to 96 hours while cultures are pending. Continued antibiotic therapy should be guided by the types and number of organisms cultured from the peritoneal cavity and by results of antibiotic sensitivity testing.

Chylous Peritonitis

This rare condition occurs in association with:

- Obstruction of intestinal lacteals
- Rupture of a chyle-containing cyst
- Injury to the cisterna chyli
- Blockage of chyle in the region of the cisterna chyli

Chyle may also enter the thorax.

Diagnosis of chylous peritonitis is confirmed by paracentesis. Affected animals commonly are presented after their abdomen has become distended. Microscopic examination of chyle stained with Sudan dye reveals fat globules; Wright's stain reveals a preponderance of lymphocytes. Chylous ascites may disappear spontaneously or after repeated aspiration of the chyle from the abdominal cavity. Special diets may also reduce lacteal flow and chyle production (see "Chylothorax," Chap. 9). If this treatment is unsuccessful, an attempt should be made to stop the leakage surgically. This begins with the performance of a lymphangiogram to identify the area of leakage and other lymphatic abnormalities. Closing off the leaking areas with hemostatic clips, if possible, is the simplest means of arresting the problem. Other means of treatment may include the injection of cyanoacrylate into the lymphatic tributaries where the leakage is occurring. In cases in which leakage is diffuse, due to major lymphatic blockages and lymphangiectasia, no treatment other than dietary is currently available.

Hemoperitoneum

Hemoperitoneum usually is associated with rupture of the spleen, liver, kidney, or a major abdominal vessel. Both blunt and penetrating blows are major causes of the hemorrhage, but it also may occur spontaneously when neo-plasms rupture or clotting abnormalities exist. Small amounts of blood within the abdomen are difficult to detect other than by peritoneal lavage. If a considerable amount of blood is present, it may be detected by palpation or auscultation–percussion (see above section, "Physical Examination"), although the fluid type will not be ascertained. Radiographs may be helpful in determining that a significant amount of fluid is present within the abdominal cavity. Confirmation is achieved by paracentesis and lavage.

Treatment
Most affected animals are presented shortly after the onset of acute signs of hypovolemic shock. Treatment involves replacing the blood volume that has been lost. In most cases fluid is initially replaced with a crystalloid-salt solution, such as lactated Ringer's. Whole blood or packed red cells are required if the hemorrhage continues or the hematocrit level drops below 20%. Autotransfusion has been lifesaving in cases of severe or continued hemorrhage (see Chap. 1). This should not be done if there is evidence of an abdominal malignancy.

If the appearance of the mucous membranes and the toe web temperature indicate that the animal's circulation is satisfactory, then careful monitoring may be is all that is required. Measuring the hematocrit alone will not assure detection of continued hemorrhage. Significant clinical signs and an increasing hematocrit in serial samples of lavage fluid are more reliable criteria of continued hemorrhage. If continuing hemorrhage is severe, whole blood and fluids should rapidly be given intravenously.

If significant hypotension does not respond to the rapid infusion of fluids or blood, abdominal pressure applied externally with a pneumatic tourniquet, or a circumferential abdominal bandage that also includes the rear limbs and pelvis may be helpful. The resultant increase in blood pressure occurs chiefly because the counterpressure increases peripheral resistance. There is also an increase in

preload to the heart due to autotransfusion of venous blood from the compressed area of the body. This causes venous pressure to rise. Abdominal counterpressure also is useful in controlling intra-abdominal hemorrhage and for this reason external counterpressure is recommended to be used on all patients with diagnosed intra-abdominal bleeding. As the counterpressure bandage is applied, respiration is watched carefully and, supported by positive pressure ventilation if necessary (although this rarely is required). A further complication of externally applied counterpressure (if applied to the abdomen) is venous engorgement and stasis of the hindlimbs. A pneumatic garment presently is being designed for use as a small animal "shock suit."

Abdominal counterpressure also can be created by rapid intraperitoneal infusion of a warm crystalloid solution. When internal counterpressure is applied, respiratory assistance may be required to prevent respiratory acidosis.

When there is evidence of continuing intra-abdominal hemorrhage, abdominal counterpressure may be applied as an emergency measure to buy time while preparations are made for surgery. Evidence of continuing intra-abdominal hemorrhage should prompt rapid exploratory celiotomy to identify the site of hemorrhage and control it. In these cases, the external counterpressure is maintained until the final section of the abdomen under the dressing must be prepared for surgery. Because the rate of hemorrhage is likely to increase when the dressing is removed, surgical instruments and other required materials should be laid out prior to releasing the counterpressure.

The abdominal section of the counterpressure is released, and the abdomen is rapidly prepared for surgery while digital pressure on the abdomen is continued. A midline skin incision is rapidly made using a scalpel blade. The blade is also used to penetrate the linea alba. A Mayo scissors is then inserted into the wound to extend the incision sufficiently to allow the surgeon's dominant hand into the peritoneal cavity. The left adrenal gland is palpated and then the hand is moved slightly cranial to this. By sweeping medially and probing dorsally, the aorta and celiac artery are identified and compressed. This stops all arterial hemorrhage in the abdomen. Then sterile towels, sponges, or laparotomy pads are packed into the abdomen to stop the major venous (retrograde) hemorrhage. The incision is opened further while the free blood is aspirated into a trap containing acid citrate dextrose (ACD) solution (1 ml for every 10 ml of blood aspirated, if antotransfusion is to be performed). Balfour retractors are then inserted and the packs are removed one quadrant at a time while looking for the sources of hemorrhage. Each source of hemorrhage must be found and controlled temporarily with tape tourniquets placed proximally or by the reinsertion of pressure packing. Only after all hemorrhage is controlled is definitive repair and hemostasis accomplished.

Pneumoperitoneum

Rarely is pneumoperitoneum of consequence, however it may reflect rupture of a hollow viscus, peritonitis caused by a gas-forming organism, a penetrating wound allowing entrance of air into the peritoneal cavity, and, occasionally, extension of the pneumothorax or pneumomediastinum. Minimal pneumoperitoneum can be expected following abdominal paracentesis and lavage, and following abdominal surgery, air may be seen in abdominal radiographs for several days to a week.

Radiographic evidence of free air within the abdominal cavity, without a history of recent surgery, paracentesis, or lavage, should arouse suspicion of a perforated hollow viscus and peritonitis. Tension pneumoperitoneum with intra-abdominal pressure exceeding 5 cm H_2O has been associated with rupture of the stomach. Air embolization interferes with respiration, and venous return to the heart may decrease significantly secondary to pneumoperitoneum and result in death. Emergency treatment of tension pneumoperitoneum is re-quired. A needle or multiholed catheter is inserted into the peritoneal cavity to allow the air under pressure to escape.

Intra-abdominal Abscesses

Intra-abdominal abscesses occasionally cause acute abdominal pain or intestinal obstruction. They have been classified in relation to their anatomic location as intraperitoneal, retroperitoneal, or visceral. Spaces in which intra-abdominal fluid may accumulate to become sites of abscess formation are the right and left omental sacs, right and left paralumbar gutters, perihepatic–diaphragmatic regions, and the periuterine or periprostatic area where a cul-de-sac of parietal peritoneum reflects onto structures in the pelvic canal. They may also form between loops of intestine or mesentery.

Abscesses may be a complication of generalized peritonitis. They can also develop in the immediate vicinity of diseased organs. Other abscesses are sequelae of abdominal surgery or trauma when there is leakage of gastric or intestinal contents. Bacteria that commonly are isolated from intra-abdominal abscesses include gram-positive anaerobes and gram-negative aerobes. Some abscesses do not contain bacteria.

Clinical Signs
The formation of an intra-abdominal abscess may not be accompanied by significant signs, making its diagnosis and localization difficult; however, inappetence, emesis, abdominal tenderness, and fever are common. The signs also vary with the extent of involvement of adjacent organs. For example, a peripancreatic abscess may cause jaundice by blocking the bile duct, or intestinal obstruction may be caused as well. A well-encapsulated abscess may be palpated as an abnormal mass or a discrete area of abdominal tenderness. Vigorous palpation can cause rupture of an abscess. If one should rupture spontaneously, signs of acute generalized peritonitis and shock occur.

Radiographic evidence of an intra-abdominal abscess depends on the size of the lesion and its location. When the abscess is within the peritoneal cavity, it usually appears as an area of decreased detail. Occasionally, encapsulated abscesses are well-defined in radiographs and pockets of intra-abdominal gas or pneumoperitoneum may be seen. Retroperitoneal abscesses may result in localized thickening of the abdominal wall, absence of the outline of the psoas muscle shadow, absence of the outline of retroperitoneal fat, or renal displacement. Visceral abscesses may be reflected by local or diffuse enlargement of the involved organ.

The diagnosis of an intra-abdominal abscess is assisted by blood cell counts and cytologic examination of peritoneal lavage fluid. Ultrasonography and nuclear scintigraphy also have been used for diagnosis and localization of abdominal abscesses.

Treatment

Treatment of intra-abdominal abscesses includes administration of antibiotics and fluids before, during, and after surgery; surgical drainage; and, perhaps, partial or complete removal of the abscess. Resection of a portion of an involved abdominal viscus occasionally is necessary. Intestinal bypass procedures may be necessary to relieve an obstruction when the location of the abscess prevents its removal. In such cases the abscess is drained and irrigated thoroughly. Identifying the responsible organisms will facilitate selection of an effective antibiotic. Following intraoperative surgical drainage and actual removal, when possible, the placement of silicone rubber multiholed suction drains has been recommended. The drains are placed in the bed of the abscess, brought out through the abdominal wall through a small stab incision and attached to a compressible reservoir that continues to exert negative pressure through the drains when activated. A syringe with a needle placed through its plunger can also be used to exert the continuous negative pressure. The drains are usually used for at least a few days to ensure that the abscess bed stays void of blood clots or reaccumulating serum or exudate. If the active portion of the drain is very

near a delicate hollow structure, such as a ureter, bile duct, or small intestine, the suction drain is placed inside a fenestrated latex rubber Penrose drain. This is to prevent direct suction being applied to these structures, which could lead to their injury.

Other concerns in the treatment of intra-abdominal abscesses include nutritional support and the use of drugs to decrease the effects of toxins liberated during the manipulation of the abscesses. A jejunostomy catheter is inserted. This allows nutritional support to be started in the immediate postoperative period, leading to more rapid recovery. Drugs that theoretically decrease the effects of the liberated toxins, such as rapid-acting corticosteroids, a thromboxane inhibitor (ketoconazole), oxygen-radical scavengers (DMSO), and oxygen-radical production blockers (Allopurinol, deferoxamine) may be used.

Adhesions

Serosal adhesions develop from a fibrinous exudate that is not dissolved by enzymes and becomes organized. Serosal injuries accompanied by hemorrhage may result in adhesions. These are classified as viscerovisceral or visceroparietal, based on their location, and restrictive or nonrestrictive, based on their mechanical properties.

Adhesions result from rough handling of tissues, infection, closing the peritoneal layer in sutures, and the presence of other foreign materials, such as glove starch powders and lint from gauze sponges.

In both cats and dogs, adhesions most commonly involve the omentum. Permanent adherence of omentum to ovarian pedicles is common following ovariohysterectomy. Such adhesions rarely result in intestinal strangulation, remaining loose and pliable and nonrestrictive. In some cases, adhesions of omentum or other serosal-to-serosal surfaces are lifesaving, by preventing or containing leakage from hollow organs following their injury or incision. Adhesions may be created intentionally between two or more loops of bowel to prevent an intussusception or strangulation from recurring (see Chap. 13, The Small and Large Intestines), between the stomach and abdominal wall to prevent recurrence of gastric volvulus and gastroesophageal intussusception (see Chap. 12, The Esophagus and Stomach), or between the colon and abdominal wall to prevent recurrence of rectal prolapse (see Chap. 14, The Rectum, Anus, and Perianal and Perineal Regions).

Clinical Signs

The signs caused by adhesions depend on their effect on visceral function. There usually are no clinical signs because most abdominal adhesions do not interfere with the lumen size, vascularity, or movement of viscera (*i.e.,* they remain nonrestrictive). When adhesions are restrictive, limiting movement of the gastrointestinal tract, the signs may include evidence of abdominal discomfort, anorexia, emesis, and debility. Peristalsis may be irregular or sporadic. The severity of signs depends on the degree of luminal obstruction, the location of the obstruction, and the lessening of blood supply to the area. In some cases, mild signs may occur periodically for months or years.

Restrictive adhesions following abdominal surgery have resulted in obstruction of a ureter or the colon following a localized reaction to the ligatures placed while performing an ovariohysterectomy.

Adhesions occur, rarely, as wide sheets of fibrous tissue that connect all of the abdominal organs from one wall to the other. Such generalized adhesions are impossible to remove surgically. If clinical signs are present, they usually reflect partial or complete intestinal obstruction. It has been hypothesized that such adhesions are the result of a lack of normal fibrinolytic enzymes.

Prevention

There is no reliable way to totally prevent the formation of adhesions. Postoperative adhesions can be kept to a minimum, however, if atraumatic surgical techniques are used.

Drying of serosal surfaces and the presence of blood clots have been implicated in the

pathogenesis of adhesions. If an area has been denuded of its peritoneal lining, it should be left uncovered. In areas where adhesions are inevitable, such as the site of an intestinal anastomosis, covering with omentum will create a less rigid adhesion.

A number of measures involving the use of chemicals have been suggested to prevent adhesions. Those chemicals include heparin and trypsin compounds, protoporphyrin, oxyphenbutazone, streptokinase, and glucocorticoids. Some of these have been effective experimentally, but they also have delayed wound healing and facilitated the spread of infection. One of the more successful methods of preventing adhesions in dogs involves parenteral administration of dexamethasone and promethazine (1.0 mg/kg of each) beginning 3 to 6 hours preoperatively and continued every 4 to 8 hours postoperatively for 24 to 36 hours. Gastrointestinal ulceration may be associated with the use of these drugs, however.

Adhesions also may be inhibited by infusing the abdominal cavity four times daily with physiologic saline solution at a daily volume that is about 10% of the patient's body weight. This is a common treatment for generalized peritonitis.

If necessary, strictures caused by adhesions can be relieved surgically. Intestinal resection or bypass procedures occasionally are indicated.

Neoplasms

Primary Tumors

The primary peritoneal tumor of dogs and cats is the rare mesothelioma. The clinical signs caused by mesotheliomas depend on their size and location. Listlessness, emesis, and progressive abdominal swelling of a few days' duration have been observed in affected animals. Ascitic fluid commonly is present, and nodular or diffuse abdominal masses may be palpable, as well. The ascites is caused by tumor cells that block the lymphatic vessels draining the peritoneal cavity. Mesotheliomas can spread to the pleural cavity by direct extension through the diaphragm or by hematogenous or lymphatic routes. Pleural effusion is common is such cases.

The diagnosis of intra-abdominal neoplasia is based on cytologic examination of ascitic fluid, exploratory celiotomy, and histopathologic examination. By the time a diagnosis is made, the tumor often has spread throughout the abdominal cavity. Surgical excision may be possible if a tumor is found early and is localized.

Secondary Tumors

Most secondary tumors of the peritoneum are metastatic sarcomas or carcinomas. The tumor reaches the peritoneal surface by penetrating the wall of a viscus, by hematogenous or lymphatic distribution, or by inadvertent inoculation of tissues during surgery. After a tumor has entered the abdominal cavity, it may become widely disseminated over the serosal surfaces.

The gross appearance of secondary tumors reflects the primary lesion and the mode of spread. Often they are accompanied by ascites. The ascitic fluid usually is bloody and may contain exfoliated tumor cells. Tumor nodules generally range from 1 mm or less in diameter studded diffusely over the peritoneal surfaces to large masses of neoplastic tissue. The omentum may be so infiltrated that it becomes a hard mass termed an *omental cake.* Some secondary tumors spread into the pleural cavity. This occurrence should be suspected when metastatic nodules are found on the surface of the diaphragm or near the lumbocostal arch.

Animals with metastases to the peritoneal cavity usually are presented with advanced signs associated with the primary lesion. The signs related to secondary tumors are weight loss, weakness, abdominal distention, anorexia, abdominal pain, and a palpable abdominal mass. Occasionally, a metastatic tumor nodule up to 2 to 3 cm in diameter will be present at the umbilicus.

The treatment of secondary tumors is usually palliative. Lesions that are causing intestinal or circulatory obstruction are removed surgically, if possible. Adjunctive chemotherapy and radiation therapy have been valuable in some cases, but in most cases, progressive deterioration is inevitable. Prognosis is very guarded, and euthanasia should be considered.

Abdominal Surgical Procedures: General Considerations

Anesthesia

The choice of an anesthetic for intra-abdominal surgery depends on the patient's age and condition, the nature of the surgical procedure, the presence of concurrent disease, the experience of the surgeon, and the facilities and assistance that are available. Inhalation anesthesia is preferred for abdominal surgery. Respiratory assistance with positive-pressure ventilation is necessary for many animals under general anesthesia and undergoing abdominal surgery. General anesthesia always should involve placement of an endotracheal tube. A combination of a narcotic, ataractic, nitrous oxide, and a muscle relaxant, or the use of epidural morphine or even acupuncture has been used to improve the results for poor-risk patients.

Positioning for Surgery

The patient is positioned according to the surgical approach to be used. For a ventral approach the animal is placed in dorsal recumbency. The patient's legs should not be stretched to the point that the ventral abdominal muscles are tightened. Pulling the forelimbs too far forward decreases tidal volume and can result in hypoventilation.

If hypotension occurs when the animal is supine, it usually is due to impeded venous return caused by the weight of abdominal viscera on the vena cava. When this occurs, the animal should be rotated to the left to relieve direct pressure on the vein.

A flank approach requires that the animal be in lateral recumbency. This position is better tolerated than dorsal recumbency, because the weight of the abdominal viscera is not directly on the vena cava, and excursions of the diaphragm are not compromised.

The dorsal recumbent, head-down position has been advocated for surgery involving the caudal abdominal cavity. When the table is tilted to a 30° angle, the viscera move cranially, which facilitates manipulation and inspection of fixed organs in the middle and caudal abdominal cavity. This increases the pressure on the diaphragm, however, and decreases tidal volume about 25% unless ventilation is assisted. Tilting the patient in this manner also increases the possibility of gastric fluid reflux into the esophagus, therefore this position should be avoided whenever possible. In dogs anesthetized and lying horizontally on a table, the lateral and ventral recumbent positions cause the least changes in cardiopulmonary function.

Maintenance of Fluid Volume, Electrolyte Balance, and Hematocrit

Unless the surgery is elective, most animals that require abdominal surgery have fluid volume and electrolyte deficits. Because of the large surface areas of the peritoneum and intra-abdominal organs, a slight increase in thickness in these structures, which would not be noticed on casual observation, may result in a loss of up to several liters of fluid. Such deficits should be corrected, at least partially, prior to surgery. If preoperative replacement of fluid is inadequate, hypotension may develop quickly following induction of anesthesia. Fluids also should be administered intravenously during and following the operation. Intravenous administration of appropriate isotonic crystalloids, at the rate of 5 to 10 ml/kg/hour of anesthesia plus the estimated blood volume loss, is also indicated for animals undergoing elective surgery. Dogs undergoing complicated procedures may require up to 20 ml/kg/hour of anesthesia of an appropriate fluid, such as lactated Ringer's solution. Animals that do not receive such therapy gradually develop acidosis and deficits in fluid volume.

When considerable hemorrhage occurs or when surgical patients are anemic (packed cell volume—PCV—below 20% or hemoglobin below 7.0 g/dl), whole blood transfusions are indicated. When there is considerable intra-abdominal hemorrhage, autotransfusion may be lifesaving (see Chap. 1, Principles of Companion Animal Surgery).

Prevention of Infection

Presurgical administration of a suitable antibiotic is recommended when the gastrointestinal tract is to be opened and contamination is likely. In addition, the intravenous administration of an antibiotic during surgery is recommended when contamination occurs or is possible. It is unwise to wait until the operation is completed to begin antibiotic therapy, because the best effects occur when tissue levels of antibiotic are optimal prior to exposure to infectious agents.

Preparation of the abdomen for surgery should include irrigation of the prepuce if a ventral approach is planned. For all abdominal operations, the use of drapes that are impervious to fluids is desirable because this decreases the amount of bacterial contamination.

Instruments

Self-retaining abdominal retractors, suction equipment, laparotomy sponges, and other special items often are required for abdominal surgery. Use of Balfour retractors provides greater exposure of the viscera and is equalled only by an assistant's manual retraction. The use of electrosurgical coagulation allows more complete and faster control of hemorrhage as the surgical approach into the abdomen is made.

Abdominal Incisions

The incision should cause minimal damage to the abdominal wall and yet be large enough to enable easy access to the surgical site. Placement of drapes should allow for enlargement of the incision if necessary. When making a ventral abdominal incision, it is important that the median plane of the patient be vertical. Rotation of the patient's body may not be noticed when it is completely covered with drapes and the relative positions of skin and muscles will be changed. Rotation makes identification of the patient's ventral midline more difficult.

When the patient is in dorsal recumbency, the right paracostal region overlies the duodenum, and the xiphoid region lies over the gallbladder. The left paracostal region overlies the stomach and spleen. The kidneys and ovaries lie in the lateral abdominal regions (the so-called paralumbar gutters) at about the level of the umbilicus. The cecum on the right and the beginning of the descending colon on the left are near the same level. The urinary bladder, prostate gland, and body of the uterus are on the midline in the prepubic region.

Although ventral abdominal incisions can be made directly over any abdominal organ or area, some provide only limited exposure. The most uniformly useful abdominal incision is made on the linea alba (midline, median incision) or just next to it (still considered median if the rectus muscle belly is not cut—Fig. 11-5). With such incisions there is no damage to the ventral abdominal muscles and resultant hemorrhage. An incision through the linea alba also can be extended cranially or caudally to obtain greater exposure. The incision can be extended into the thorax with a sternal or parasternal incision or caudally through the pubis.

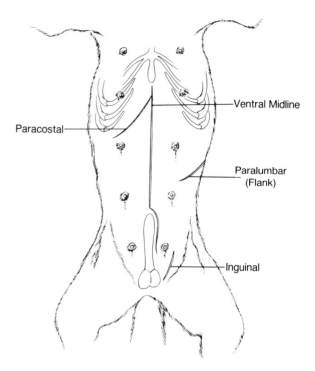

Figure 11-5. *Surgical incisions for abdominal procedures.*

In many instances after the abdomen has been entered, a thorough examination of the entire abdominal cavity is required to determine the presence of injury or disease. A linea alba incision is ideal for this purpose. In other instances this incision is the only one through which large cysts or tumors can be removed or through which many other reparative procedures can be accomplished (e.g., diaphragmatic herniorrhaphy).

Other abdominal incisions include: the paralumbar or flank incision, made to expose the retroperitoneal space, kidneys, ovaries, uterus, and mesenteric lymph vessels; the paracostal–retroperitoneal incision, made to expose the kidneys, renal pelvis, proximal ureters, and adrenal glands; and inguinal incisions made to repair inguinal or femoral hernias. Limited but specific approaches to the peritoneal cavity also include the unilateral or bilateral paracostal, thoracic–trans-diaphragmatic, and the perineal–pararectal approaches. These can be used to reach the diaphragm, stomach, and pelvic organs respectively.

Median (Midline) Incisions

To describe a ventral median or midline incision, the umbilicus, xiphoid cartilage, and brim of the pubis are used as reference points. These incisions can be made cranial or caudal to or directly through the umbilicus, and they can be extended in either direction as far as necessary. In many instances the incision will extend from the xiphoid region to the pubis. This is recommended whenever complete exploration of the abdominal cavity is necessary for diagnostic purposes.

A median or midline incision is the most useful and common abdominal incision in both dogs and cats, because it provides easy access to the abdominal viscera and is easiest to close. This incision does not require cutting through muscles, major vessels, or nerves. The midline is best identified by locating the umbilicus.

If a midline incision is made, the abdomen is entered through the linea alba. In the dog the linea alba can be located by following the raphe through the subcutaneous tissues. Condensed subcutaneous fascia in both the male and female can be used as a landmark to locate the linea alba. The preputial ligament in the male and the suspensory ligament of the mammary glands in the female also help guide the surgeon to the linea alba. Continuation of the skin incision caudal to the tip of the prepuce in males involves deviating from the midline to the parapreputial incision, ligating the preputial branches of the caudal superficial epigastric vessels, and severing the preputial muscle and suspensory ligament. This enables retraction of the prepuce and visualization of the linea alba.

Because of the loose attachment of the subcutaneous tissues to the superficial rectus fascia in cats, the linea alba can be located eas-ily by simply moving the skin until it can be seen. In both dogs and cats the linea alba is seen more easily at the cranial end of the incision. It is widest cranial to the umbilicus.

An incision through the linea alba can be made directly with the curved portion of the scalpel blade, while the thumb and index finger of the opposite hand are used to tense and stabilize the abdominal fascia. The depth of the incision must be controlled carefully to avoid injuring underlying viscera; control requires practice. When properitoneal fat or glistening peritoneal serosa is seen, the incision if sufficiently deep; it has penetrated the linea alba but has not entered the peritoneal cavity. In another acceptable technique, the linea alba is elevated with tissue forceps and punctured carefully with the tip of the scalpel blade. Following this puncture, the resistance to incision is lessened, and air moves into the abdominal cavity. During this procedure the tip of the scalpel blade often penetrates the properitoneal fat and peritoneum.

After the linea alba has been penetrated, the thin peritoneal layer is punctured bluntly, if this penetration has not already occurred. The incision is lengthened with a scalpel. A grooved director or thumb forceps is used to prevent injury to viscera. A Mayo or Metzenbaum scissors may also be used to lengthen the incision. To avoid injuring viscera, the instrument is lifted upward as the linea alba and peritoneum are severed.

After opening the abdominal cavity on the ventral midline, the falciform ligament and its related fat cranial to the umbilicus and the middle ligament of the bladder caudal to the umbilicus will be encountered (Fig. 11-6). Although these structures usually are not hindrances, they can be removed without harm. Branches of the cranial deep epigastric vessels may require ligation as the falciform ligament is severed. Some surgeons advocate removal of the falciform ligament to facilitate closure of the abdomen and to prevent wound dehiscence. This rarely is necessary, however, because properly placed sutures do not include

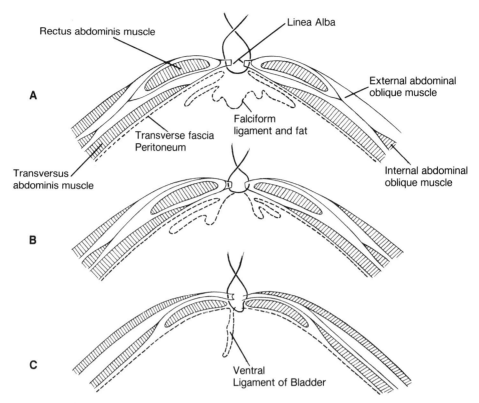

Figure 11-6. *Placement of sutures for closure of midline incision and structures forming the ventral abdominal wall in a dog.* **A,** *Cranial abdomen;* **B,** *Mid-abdomen;* **C,** *Caudal abdomen.*

the falciform ligament. To expose the cranial abdominal cavity the incision may be extended into the thorax by median sternotomy or parallel to the xiphoid cartilage and parasternally (see Chap. 9, The Thorax). By extending the incision cranially to the third or fourth sternebra, good exposure of the liver and other cranial abdominal structures is obtained, following incision of the diaphragm and use of a self-retaining retractor.

A midline abdominal incision also can be continued caudally through the pubis by separating the symphysis pubis with a scalpel blade or osteotome. This is done primarily in young animals whose pubic symphysis is not ossified. The pubic bones are then separated with Gelpi self-retaining retractors. In older animals, exposure of the pelvic cavity may require an osteotomy of the pubic rami. This involves elevating a bone flap to expose the underlying pelvic canal. The bone flap is reattached with stainless steel sutures.

Paramedian Incisions

These incisions are made in the ventral abdomen beside the midline. They may be made medial to the rectus muscle (pararectus) or through the rectus. As with a median incision, the umbilicus is a useful landmark. Pararectus incisions are made 0.5 to 1.0 cm lateral and parallel to the midline; they may be cranial or caudal to the umbilicus, and extend as far as necessary for sufficient exposure. The external lamina of the rectus sheath is incised in the direction of the underlying rectus fibers. The rectus muscle itself is not incised, but it is retracted laterally to expose the internal lamina of the sheath and the peritoneum. These structures then are incised to enter the abdomen.

A rarely used variation of the pararectus incision is made lateral to the lateral edge of the rectus muscle. After the external lamina of the rectus sheath is incised, the rectus muscle is retracted medially to expose the internal lamina, which is incised with the peritoneum to enter the abdominal cavity.

Per-rectus incisions are made longitudinally through the rectus muscles at varying distances lateral to the midline. The external lamina of the rectus sheath is incised in the direction of the underlying rectus fibers. The muscle is opened by separating its fibers. When the muscle is incised, hemorrhage occurs, and ligation or electrocoagulation may be required. The internal lamina and peritoneum are opened to enter the abdomen. Disadvantages of this approach are the additional trauma to the rectus muscle and subsequent hemorrhage. There are no advantages to a per-rectus incision, other than the possibility of being more directly over a particular structure. The previously held belief that this type of incision provides for a more secure closure and better healing than a median incision has been refuted.

Closure of a ventral paramedian midline abdominal incision is facilitated if the incision through the internal rectus sheath and its attached peritoneum is shorter than the incision in the external rectus sheath, which, in turn, is shorter than the incision in the subcutaneous tissue and skin.

Although the umbilicus often serves as a landmark in determining the length and location of median and paramedian incisions, its location between the xiphoid cartilage and brim of the pubis can vary considerably. As a consequence, the 12th or 13th rib rather than the umbilicus has been recommended as the landmark for the cranial limit of a midline incision for ovariohysterectomy.

Transverse Incisions

These incisions are made across muscle fibers, usually those of the rectus. The incision may be unilateral or bilateral and may be made at various levels of the abdomen. Compared to longitudinal incisions, transverse incisions create more hemorrhage and trauma and place more tension on sutures following closure, and therefore are seldom used.

When the abdominal cavity has been entered through a paramedian or transverse incision through the rectus abdominis, the internal lamina of the rectus sheath and the attached peritoneum are grasped and elevated with a tissue forceps and incised with a scalpel. The incision is then enlarged with scissors by inserting the blunt tip into the peritoneal cavity and incising the fascia and peritoneum. When using scissors to cut tissue, the blades need never be completely closed. They can be held partially open and pushed along the proposed line of incision in areas where the fascia is thin. (Hold the tips open only slightly to prevent catching deeper tissues or organs between the blades.)

Flank Incisions

These incisions may provide ready access to specific organs or areas of the retroperitoneum or the peritoneal cavity. Exposure beyond the specific areas is severely limited, however. These incisions have been used successfully for access to the kidneys, ureters, ovaries, uterus, adrenal glands, and stomach. It has been stated that an advantage of a flank approach is the lower incidence of postoperative herniation or evisceration compared to ventral abdominal incisions, however this has not been documented. Herniation at either site can be avoided by careful technique. There is more hemorrhage during standard "grid-iron" flank incisions, because large muscles often are transected. The amount of postoperative scarring also is greater with these incisions, and the length of the incision is limited. It also can be difficult to appose surfaces of transected muscles accurately.

A standard flank incision may be made on either side below the lumbar region and midway between the last rib and level of the tuber coxae. After the skin has been incised, the external and internal abdominal oblique and transversus abdominis muscles are transected. Care must be taken to avoid injuring the cranial abdominal or caudal circumflex iliac arteries and veins. If these vessels are severed, they should be ligated. The peritoneum and transversalis fascia closely adhere to the deep surface of the transversus abdominis muscle and usually are penetrated when the muscle is transected. When performing surgery on the adrenal glands or kidneys, it is not necessary to open the peritoneum. Although the thin parietal peritoneum often is torn inadvertently, this is of no consequence and the peritoneal layer should not be sutured. Separate approaches to the retroperitoneal space can be made if care is taken not to injure the parietal peritoneum and transversalis fascia in this region.

Flank incisions also can be made using a muscle-separation technique. This is a preferred modification of the standard flank incision (Fig. 11-7). It is less traumatic, causes less hemorrhage, and disturbs muscle function less. Its disadvantage is that the skin and fascial incisions must be larger to provide sufficient space for manipulation of abdominal structures.

The skin may be incised in either a dorsoventral, oblique, or craniocaudal direction. The muscles encountered are the external abdominal oblique, internal oblique, and the transversus abdominis. The fascia overlying each muscle is incised in the direction of the muscle fibers. A closed forceps then is inserted successively into the body of each muscle, and the jaws are spread in the direction of the fibers. Another closed forceps can be used to pull in the opposite direction from the first to enlarge the separated portion. In this incision, no muscles are transected, and when the tension of retraction is released, the muscle fibers return to their normal position. Hemorrhage and scar formation are minimal when muscles are separated in this manner.

Closing the Incision
The Peritoneal Layer
The peritoneal layer is thin and has little ability to hold sutures. Attempts to close it separately usually are unsuccessful and of little

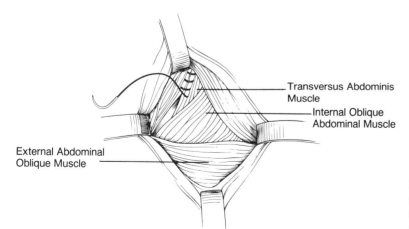

Transversus Abdominis Muscle

Internal Oblique Abdominal Muscle

External Abdominal Oblique Muscle

Figure 11-7. *Closure of a muscle-splitting approach to the flank of a dog. The deepest layer (transversus) is closed first.*

value. Abdominal adhesions are more frequent when the peritoneum is sutured than when it is not.

Because of its close adherence to the internal rectus sheath in dogs and cats, the peritoneum usually is included in the abdominal closure. If the incision is directly on the midline, the closure often does not include the peritoneum, because fat separates the deep surface of the linea alba from the peritoneum. If only the external rectus fascia is sutured, the peritoneum is not included. There are no adverse effects if the internal rectus sheath and peritoneum are not sutured. Reperitonealization occurs naturally, and few adhesions result. Formation of disabling intra-abdominal adhesions is not a frequent complication, regardless of the method of closure, if closure is done meticulously.

The Muscle and Fascia

Muscle has a minimal ability to hold sutures and its apposition is best achieved by placing sutures into its fascial covering. For longitudinal incisions in the ventral abdomen, these coverings are the internal and external laminae of the rectus sheath. Penetrating the muscles slightly during insertion of the sutures may enhance their apposition. If too much muscle is included in the fascial sutures, apposition of the fascia may be prevented by a ridge of interposing muscle. Furthermore, necrosis of the muscular tissue leads to loosening of the sutures, possibly resulting in hematoma.

Accurate apposition and secure closure of the abdominal fascia, especially the external rectus sheath in median and paramedian incisions and the external abdominal oblique fascia in flank incisions (see Fig. 11-7) are important in preventing wound dehiscence. Closures of incisions through the linea alba hold well, and it is not necessary to close the thin transversalis fascia and peritoneum. Recent studies have also indicated that it is not necessary to close the intimal rectus sheath

when a secure closure of the external rectus closure is performed.

Though the suture pattern and material used to close the fascia may be a matter of personal preference, studies have been made that aid selection. The use of either monofilament or multifilament, absorbable, or nonabsorbable synthetic sutures in either a continuous or simple interrupted pattern has proved acceptable. The strength of abdominal fascial wounds increases slowly during the first weeks of healing. Conversely, the tensile strength of surgical gut decreases during the same period. Studies have indicated that closure of aponeurotic incisions with surgical gut in dogs may be accompanied by wound dehiscence rates as high as 10%. There have been no reported studies in the cat. Slippage of knots due to swelling of the suture material and loss of friction as the suture material imbibes tissue fluids have been implicated as primary causes. Rapid loss of tensile strength of surgical gut (within 2 weeks) also has been implicated as a cause of dehiscence. Therefore, it is generally recommended that ventral abdominal closure in the dog not be performed with surgical gut. Even though this material was used extensively for abdominal closure in the 1940s to mid-1960s, the biology of wound repair and the physical characteristics of surgical gut now strongly support the selection of other materials that maintain better tensile strength and cause less tissue reaction.

When wound healing may be delayed because of malnutrition, hypoproteinemia, infection, or neoplasia, the use of nonabsorbable monofilament sutures is recommended to reduce the incidence of incisional hernias and wound dehiscence. In a clinical study involving the use of polypropylene to close the abdominal cavity of 550 dogs and cats (at least 220 of which had hypoproteinemia, infection or contamination), there were only 2 cases with major wound complications, 1 of which was a dehiscence. All wounds were closed using a simple continuous pattern in the abdominal fascia. With this simple continuous pattern of synthetic nonabsorbable material, size 2, is suitable for patients weighing more than 100 kg, size 1 for those from 40 to 100 kg, size 0 for those between 20 and 40 kg, 00 for those between 5 and 20 kg, and 000 is suitable for patients weighing 5 kg or less. Six throws should be made in each knot to prevent slippage. Long incisions should be closed by beginning the sutures at each end and joining them at the middle. With this closure, an effort is made not to include muscle tissue. A simple continuous pattern can be inserted more rapidly than simple interrupted sutures (Fig. 11-8). There appears to be more tissue reaction, incisional swelling, and seroma formation in dogs when an interrupted closure is used (compared with use of a continuous closure), and the rate of dehiscence is not different.

Sutures should be inserted into healthy tissues and in sufficient number to avoid dehiscence. A distance of 5 to 7 mm between sutures is satisfactory for closure of ventral abdominal wounds (see Fig. 11-8). The suture material should not be crushed with needle holders nor

creased with the point of a needle to avoid suture breakage and dehiscence. Interposition of fat or muscle between the fascial edges should be avoided. Although it is unnecessary to remove the falciform ligament, properitoneal fat, or the middle ligament of the urinary bladder prior to closing the abdomen, care should be taken to avoid interposing these structures between the fascial edges of a sutured incision.

Skin and Subcutaneous Tissue

In male dogs in which the preputialis muscle and suspensory ligament have been divided, these structures should be joined before closing the skin. In obese animals it is often necessary to approximate the subcutaneous fat with fine absorbable or nonabsorbable sutures to bring this tissue back into apposition. This helps eliminate dead space and reduce the tension necessary to suture the skin. The subcutaneous sutures should not simultaneously involve the deeper fascia or more superficial subdermal layer, because these sutures would artificially join the subdermal tissues to the abdominal fascia, leading to inversion of the skin in this area and predisposing to irritation and infection. Subcutaneous tissues should be closed over the knots of sutures that have been inserted into fascia, which serves to minimize irritation of the overlying skin and subdermal tissues by the cut ends of the knots and to prevent the cut ends of the knots from projecting from the skin incision. Such irritation may lead to infection, acute cellulitis, and formation of a granuloma or fistula, which would necessitate removal of the knot after sufficient fascial healing has occurred (1 month or more postoperatively).

In relatively thin dogs and cats it may not be necessary to close the subcutaneous tissues separately from the skin. A skin suture that incorporates the subcutaneous tissues can be used very effectively, thus eliminating the burying of another layer of suture. To help ap-

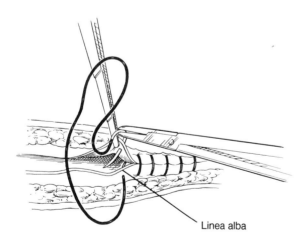

Linea alba

Figure 11-8. *Closure of a ventral midline (linea alba) incision with a continuous suture. (Lipowitz AJ, Schenle MP. Surgical approaches to the abdominal and thoracic viscera of the dog and cat. Vet Clin North Am 1979;9:177.)*

pose the skin and subcutaneous tissue during this type of closure, the drapes, which often contribute to the tension holding the wound edges apart, are squeezed together.

The skin has considerable ability to hold sutures and contributes greatly to the strength of the superficial wound. The skin should be closed accurately and without undue tension. If necessary, closure can be achieved with subdermal (subcuticular) sutures. Skin is usually sutured with nonabsorbable material, using one of a variety of suture patterns.

Retroperitonitis

Retroperitonitis can present in two major forms: acute and relatively diffuse and chronic and more localized. Causes of retroperitonitis are similar to those for peritonitis: puncture wounds and infections secondary to the introduction of foreign bodies and bacteria are most common. Extensions of infections involving the lumbar lymph nodes, kidneys, pancreas, and prostate gland are other causes. Retroperitonitis has also been documented following orchidectomy in the cat in which infection occurred at the stump of the ligated spermatic cord.

Acute retroperitonitis may present with the same clinical signs as seen with acute peritonitis: fever, anorexia, depression, vomiting, reluctance to move, and abdominal pain. Pain in the sublumbar and inguinal regions may be more pronounced. Swelling in these areas is usually not appreciated. Radiographs of the abdominal cavity may reveal a loss of detail around the kidneys and a ventral expansion of the psoas line. On rare occasions air may be seen in the ventrolumbar regions on the lateral radiographic projections. Clipping of the hair in the flank region may reveal bruising, penetrating injuries, or a hint of swelling. Laboratory workup usually indicates the presence of

an acute inflammatory process (*e.g.*, neutrophilic leukocytosis), a left shift, and hemoconcentration, although results may vary depending on the stage of the retroperitonitis.

On the basis of presenting signs of acute abdominal pain, as well as those cited above, an exploratory celiotomy is indicated. Acute retroperitonitis without extension into the peritoneal cavity and not resulting from infection localized in the peritoneal cavity is uncommon. In most cases the same approach for the treatment of diffuse peritonitis is followed for acute retroperitonitis. The retroperitoneum is exposed, local areas of necrosis and exudate are debrided or drained, and foreign bodies or gross contamination are removed. Extensive irrigation is then performed and suction drains are placed if residual suppuration is suspected. Gram staining of the exudative material, bacterial culturing, and sensitivity testing are performed. Systemic antibiotics are administered following sample collection or immediately if the patient's condition so warrants. Other methods of management are similar to the management of generalized peritonitis, including nutritional support, possible open abdominal drainage, and gastrointestinal protectants, such as cimetidine and sucralfate administration.

Chronic localized peritonitis often presents with a draining tract in the flank region (*e.g.*, due to the use of contaminated nonabsorbable and reactive suture material). Treatment involves the removal of the localized process and curettage of the draining tract. Fusiform bacterial infections are common and can be resistant to treatment. Abdominal exploration should be performed to rule out the extension or origin of the inflammatory process from any intra-abdominal organs (*e.g.*, ovarian pedicle ligation with contaminated reactive suture material and secondary tract formation with localized retroperitonitis, involving the parietal peritoneum). Long-term antibiotic treatment is often necessary, and recurrence can be a major problem.

Adrenal Glands

Hyperadrenocorticism

Spontaneous hyperadrenocorticism or canine Cushing's syndrome (CCS) results from chronic overproduction of cortisol by the adrenal cortex. The clinical signs of CCS include polyuria and polydipsia (about 85% of cases), abdominal distension (75%), anestrus (70%), lethargy (70%), hepatomegaly (70%), polyphagia (70%), muscular weakness and atrophy (50%), bilateral symmetrical alopecia (40%), testicular atrophy (40%), comedones (35%), and calcinosis cutis (10%). It is associated most often with bilateral adrenocortical hyperplasia. The condition also is called pituitary-dependent hyperadrenocorticism, because it basically is due to excessive secretion of adrenocorticotropic hormone (ACTH) by the pituitary gland. Pituitary tumors are present in some cases, but careful dissection of the pituitary gland is necessary to find the microscopic adenoma. It is not known what role, if any, the hypothalamus plays in releasing excessive corticotropin releasing factor (CRF) and causing ACTH release.

Functional neoplasms of the adrenal cortex account for 10% to 20% of the cases of CCS. Both benign (adenomas) and malignant (carcinomas) tumors of the adrenal cortex may secrete excessive amounts of cortisol and other glucocorticoids. These tumors usually are unilateral and function autonomously, resulting in atrophy of the other adrenal gland. The term *adrenal-dependent hyperadrenocorticism* has been applied to this entity, which can be treated successfully by surgical excision of the involved adrenal gland.

Iatrogenic CCS is the result of chronic administration of exogenous glucocorticoids, usually given for allergic dermatitis or arthritis, leading to decreased secretion of ACTH, subsequent atrophy of the zona fasciculata, and resultant decreased cortisol levels. Although these dogs have signs of hyperadrenocorticism, they have profound adrenal cortisol suppression. Signs of hypoadrenocorticism may be manifested if steroid therapy is stopped suddenly.

Animals suspected of having CCS should be examined thoroughly prior to initiating any medical or surgical therapy. At a minimum, the examination procedures should include a complete blood count, urinalysis, liver (SGPT, SAP) and kidney (BUN, creatinine) tests, and tests for blood glucose, cholesterol, and calcium levels.

More specific tests are performed to confirm a diagnosis of hyperadrenocorticism. The ACTH stimulation test is the most widely used and reliable. Animals with pituitary-dependent hyperadrenocorticism usually have an exaggerated response to exogenous ACTH, and about 60% of animals with adrenal tumors have a response identical to patients with pituitary-dependent hyperadrenocorticism. The ACTH stimulation test thus enables identification of an animal with hyperadrenocorticism, but not differentiation of pituitary-dependent from adrenal-dependent hyperadrenocorticism.

Dexamethasone suppression tests have been recommended for diagnosis of hyperadrenocorticism. This corticosteroid suppresses secretion of ACTH from the pituitary and possibly CRF from the hypothalamus. The low-dose dexamethasone test enables identification of animals with hyperadrenocorticism, and the high-dose dexamethasone test allows differentiation of pituitary-dependent hyperadrenocorticism from cases related to adrenal tumors.

An assay for ACTH may help in differentiating functional adrenal tumors from pituitary-dependent CCS. Such an assay is not currently available to veterinary practitioners.

Treatment

The therapy of choice for adrenocortical neoplasms is removal of the affected gland. The remaining adrenal gland usually is atrophied and secreting inadequate amounts of glucocorticoids. Administration of an exogenous glucocorticoid should be started 24 to 48 hours before surgery and continued for 10 to 14 days postoperatively. Long-term glucocorticoid therapy is given on alternate days at a low dose until adrenal function returns to normal. Therapy may take as long as 6 months.

Surgical treatment of pituitary-dependent hyperadrenocorticism involves a bilateral adrenalectomy or hypophysectomy. After a bilateral adrenalectomy, daily treatment for hypoadrenocorticism (Addison's disease) is required. For bilateral adrenalectomy, I prefer the paracostal approach to a midline abdominal approach, because the possibility of wound dehiscence, pancreatitis, and peritonitis is reduced. Considerable surgical skill is required to perform this surgery. Long-term results are good if careful postoperative monitoring and management are provided.

Hypophysectomy results in control of pituitary-dependent hyperadrenocorticism. Following this surgery, cortisone and thyroid supplementation is required daily. Signs of diabetes insipidus may occur transiently following hypophysectomy. Considerable surgical expertise is needed to perform a hypophysectomy, which is performed only at referral centers. Short-term survival and long-term stabilization following adrenal or pituitary surgery require intensive nursing, medical care, and monitoring.

The preferred treatment for pituitary-dependent hyperadrenocorticism is the administration of o,p″-DDD (Lysodren). This is a potent cytotoxic agent that causes atrophy of the zona fasciculata and zona reticularis. Overdosage or prolonged administration of o,p″-DDD can result in complete destruction of the adrenal cortex. A medical text should be consulted for further discussion of this treatment.

Injuries

Injuries to the adrenal glands are rare because of their location. They may be crushed when animals are struck by cars and are occasionally penetrated by a foreign body.

Medullary Neoplasia

In addition to functional adrenocortical tumors, pheochromocytomas of the adrenal medulla and sympathetic paraganglia are occasionally found in animals. These tumors arise from the embryonal neuroectoderm of the neural crest, and they contain chromaffin tissue. The clinical signs of pheochromocytomas reflect the excessive amounts of catecholamine hormones that they secrete, including dopamine, norepinephrine, and epinephrine. Paroxysms of panting, anxiety, depression, and restlessness are common. Tachycardia, weakness, and collapse may occur. Arterial hypertension may be demonstrated.

Pheochromocytomas usually are benign and do not metastasize. They can invade the caudal vena cava, however, and cause its obstruction. Ascites, edema of the limbs, and distention of superficial abdominal veins occur subsequently. Invasion of the vena cava may cause the pheochromoctomas to spread to the liver, lymph nodes, and lungs. The diagnosis of a pheochromocytoma often is delayed because clinical signs are not recognized and hypertension is not demonstrated. Recognition of an adrenal mass in a plain radiograph may not be possible, but arteriography, intravenous pyelography, or femoral venography often may demonstrate the mass. After an adrenal mass has been found, an exploratory celiotomy is indicated. Measuring excess catecholamine metabolites in a 24-hour urine sample is one way of confirming the diagnosis, but normal values for canine catecholamines have not been established. The detection of arterial hypertension supports a diagnosis of pheochromocytoma.

The treatment of an adrenal pheochromocytoma involves surgical removal of the tumor. This is not indicated, however, when there is evidence of metastasis or local extension of the tumor. Administration of α-adrenergic blocking agents (phentolamine) and β-adrenergic blocking agents (propranolol) may be needed during surgery to control hypertension and tachycardia.

Suggested Readings

Crowe DT, Bjorling DE. Peritoneum and peritoneal cavity. In: Slatter DH, ed. Textbook of small animal surgery. Philadelphia: WB Saunders, 1985:571.

Eigenmann JE, Lubberink AAME. The adrenals. In: Slatter DH, ed. Textbook of small animal surgery. Philadelphia: WB Saunders, 1985:1851.

Hayes HM. Congenital umbilical and inguinal hernias in cattle, horses, swine, dogs, and cats. Am J Vet Res 1974;35:839.

Henderson RA. Controlling peritoneal adhesions. Vet Surg 1982;11:30.

Lipowitz AJ. Peritonitis and intraperitoneal drainage. In: Bojrab MJ, ed. Current techniques in small animal surgery. Philadelphia: Lea and Febiger, 1983:240.

Lipowitz AJ, Schenle MP. Surgical approaches to the abdominal and thoracic viscera of the dog and cat. Vet Clin North Am 1979;9:169.

Orsher RJ, Rosin E. Open peritoneal drainage in experimental peritonitis in dogs. Vet Surg 1984;13:222.

Ripley WA, McCarnan HR. Umbilical hernia repair with mersilene mesh. Can Vet J 1974;15:357.

12

Ronald M. Bright

Esophagus and Stomach

The Esophagus

Surgical Anatomy and Physiology

The esophagus begins at the pharynx and terminates at the cardia of the stomach and consists of cervical, thoracic and abdominal portions. The esophagus is enveloped by pleura and peritoneum in the thoracic and abdominal cavities respectively. However, no true serosa is present. The esophagus has four layers—loose areolar adventitia, muscularis (two oblique layers of striated muscle in the dog), submucosa, and mucosa. The submucosa has mucous glands and loosely holds the mucosa to the muscular layer. The mucosa is made up of stratified squamous epithelium and is considered to be the layer contributing the most to suture holding capacity. The cat's esophagus

has striated muscle that slowly changes to smooth muscle in the caudal 3 to 4 cm of the organ.

The role of the esophagus is to transport food and liquid from the pharynx to the stomach. It has no absorptive or digestive functions.

In general, the signs of esophageal disease are related to loss of function or inflammation of surrounding structures. Mediastinal structures or portions of the lung can be secondarily involved in esophageal diseases. Functional disturbances usually result in dysphagia (proximal esophagus) or regurgitation.

Surgical Principles

Precise surgical apposition of esophageal tissues is of great importance, because this organ lacks a serosal layer and omentum, both of which help seal small leaks in the lower gastrointestinal tract. When suture line reinforcement is necessary, however, the surgeon can use adjacent muscle, diaphragmatic tissue, or pericardium. Omentum can be used by mobilizing it from the peritoneal cavity to the esophagus via an incision in the diaphragm.

The longitudinal elasticity of the esophagus is slight but enough to help overcome a small amount of tension across a suture line. Excessive tension or the constant motion of the esophagus, however, can lead to dehiscence or predispose to stricture formation. Meticulous dissection of the adventitia cranial and caudal to a proposed suture line will help reduce tension somewhat. Additional tension-relieving techniques include performing a partial thickness circular or spiral myotomy (only the outer muscle layer) above or below a line of anastomosis, or the cardiac and fundic portion of the stomach can be mobilized cranially into the thoracic cavity.

A good blood supply to the edges of an esophageal wound is critical to assure an optimal healing environment. The blood supply to the esophagus, especially the thoracic portion, may be compromised if there is too much tension across suture lines. Damage to the vascularity can delay healing, resulting in leakage, or can kill oxygen-sensitive ganglion cells, which has been shown to result in transient esophageal hypomotility.

The preferred method for closure of an esophagotomy or for anastomosing two segments of esophagus is a two-layer technique, using a simple interrupted suture pattern (Fig. 12-1). I prefer 3-0 or 4-0 nonabsorbable synthetic monofilament suture material for the inner layer of sutures, which incorporates the holding layer (mucosa) and the submucosa. The knots usually are tied to lie within the lumen to decrease the likelihood for intramural abscess and to increase the probability that the suture will slough into the lumen during the healing process. The outer layer is closed similarly, except I prefer synthetic absorbable sutures (3-0 or 4-0 polydioxanone); the knots are placed on the outside surface of the adventitia. Atraumatic tissue handling is mandatory when placing the sutures to minimize tis-

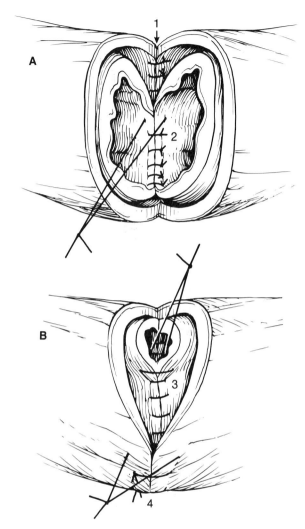

Figure 12-1. *Esophageal anastomosis.* **A,** *The muscular and mucosal layers have been dissected apart to enable more accurate suturing. The muscular and adventitial layers on the far wall are apposed with the knots placed on the outside, followed by closure of the inner mucosal layer with the knots placed in the lumen.* **B,** *The mucosal layer is completed (near side) with all knots in the lumen. Closure of the muscle and adventitia on the near wall completes the anastomosis.*

sue necrosis and scarring. Inverting and everting conventional and mechanical stapling suture techniques also have been employed for esophageal surgery. Sutures are meticulously placed approximately 2 to 3 mm deep and at 2 to 3 mm intervals to provide a watertight closure. Trauma to the esophagus is reduced if an assistant's fingers (rather than intestinal clamps) hold the segments together, while the sutures are placed to reappose two segments of the esophagus.

Access to the cervical esophagus is via a ventral cervical midline approach. The cranial portion of the thoracic esophagus (T2–T6) probably is best approached through a right lateral thoracotomy at the third or fourth intercostal space. The caudal thoracic esophagus can be approached by an incision on either side of the chest, somewhere between intercostal spaces 7 and 10. I prefer a left-sided seventh intercostal space thoracotomy in most instances.

A median sternotomy allows a maximum amount of esophagus to be exposed at one time, but it generally does not afford easy access to the esophagus, because of its dorsal location in the mediastinum. This median approach sometimes is indicated, such as for approaching the thoracic esophagus cranial to the heart near the thoracic inlet.

The bacterial flora in the esophagus usually is the same as that found in the oral cavity. Contamination of periesophageal tissues during surgery is best avoided by packing off surrounding tissues with moistened laparotomy pads and employing liberal irrigation of the surgery site after esophageal closure and prior to closure of the periesophageal tissues or the thorax. It is also best to change surgical instruments, gloves, and drapes prior to closing the wound.

When entering the esophagus, some contamination always occurs, regardless of precautions taken by the surgeon. For this reason, antimicrobial prophylaxis is employed perioperatively, using an injectable form of trimethoprim-sulfa, a cephalosporin or ampicillin.

Esophagotomy

Cervical Esophagus

The most common indication for an esophagotomy is to remove a foreign body. A cervical approach, via a ventral midline incision similar to that used for cervical disk surgery, allows access to a foreign body in the cervical and cranial thoracic portions of esophagus. The trachea and both carotid sheaths are retracted gently to the right side, allowing access to the esophagus, which lies to the left of the midline in the neck. Special care is necessary to protect the recurrent laryngeal nerves and the carotid sheaths. The esophagus is isolated and packed off well with moistened laparotomy sponges to minimize contamination with oral flora. A large-bore tube is inserted *per os* to aspirate esophageal contents just prior to the esophagotomy, to help immobilize the esophagus, and to serve as a "cutting board" to protect the deeper layer during the incision. Incising the esophagus for removal of a foreign body should be done just caudal to the foreign body in healthy tissue. The closure of the esophagotomy is done in two layers, as described above (see Fig. 12-1). The surgical field is irrigated liberally with saline. If infection is present or tissue trauma is excessive, drainage is performed with a silicone drain attached to a closed suction system.

Thoracic Esophagus

The cranial esophagus (T2–T6) usually is best approached through a fourth intercostal space incision on the right side to avoid the aortic arch. After entering the thoracic cavity, the cranial and middle lung lobes are retracted cranially. If necessary for exposure, the azygous vein is dissected free of the underlying mediastinal pleura, ligated, and divided. The mediastinal pleura over the esophagus is incised over a length sufficiently cranial and caudal to the proposed site of esophagotomy to allow adequate exposure; care is taken to avoid the vagal trunks running laterally along the esophagus. An esophageal tube is placed as discussed (see "Cervical Esophagus," above). The esophagus is packed off with moistened laparotomy pads, and the incision is made. The esophagus is closed as described above (see Fig. 12-1) following pleural irrigation, a chest tube is placed, and the thoracotomy incision is closed.

Caudal Thoracic Esophagus

After a left seventh intercostal space incision, the pulmonary ligament is transected and the caudal lung lobe is packed off cranially. A transdiaphragmatic approach to the abdominal portion of the esophagus also can be accommodated via a left-sided thoracotomy through either the seventh or eighth intercostal space. Closure of the esophageal incision, chest tube placement, and thoracotomy closure completes the procedure.

Postoperative Care

Following an esophagotomy, patients are not allowed to eat or drink for 48 hours; they are maintained on intravenous fluids. Water mixed with baby food or canned food to form a gruel can be administered on the third to the sixth or seventh postoperative day in small amounts. The diet is gradually returned to normal between days 7 and 10. Antibiotics are not given beyond the perioperative period unless indicated by the presence of infection at the time of surgery. Aerobic bacterial culture and antibiotic sensitivity testing is recommended if infection is present to assure more precise antimicrobial therapy.

Esophageal Resection and Anastomosis

When anastomosing two segments of the esophagus, the far (outer) layer (to include the adventitia and muscular layers) is closed first using a simple interrupted appositional pattern, as described above and in Figure 12-1. Then sutures are placed first in the far and then near mucosa and submucosa layer, and the last step is to close the adventitia-muscle layer of the near wall. Excessive tension across the suture line following resection of a segment of esophagus can be avoided by a circular myotomy. The myotomy should include only the outer muscular layer, because the

submucosal arterial network may be destroyed by a deeper incision. Injecting saline between the muscle layers can delineate the separation of these layers prior to myotomy.

Mobilizing the proximal portion of the stomach through the esophageal hiatus also can reduce tension across an anastomosis. Careful periesophageal dissection is done at the hiatus. The vagal nerves and blood supply to the distal esophagus must be preserved. A small portion of the cardia and fundus is then pulled cranially through the hiatus and fixed securely to the diaphragm with nonabsorbable sutures. This technique may result in gastroesophageal reflux, because the gastroesophageal sphincter (GES) is moved into the pleural space where it is subject to negative pressure.

Suture Reinforcement and Grafting Techniques

The esophageal suture line can be reinforced using omentum, cervical "strap" muscles, diaphragm, intercostal pedicle grafts, and pericardium. The omentum is advanced on a vascular pedicle developed by using one of the gastroepiploic arteries. The pedicle is then brought through a small incision in the diaphragm and wrapped around the anastomotic line. Diaphragmatic, pericardial, or intercostal musculature can be used not only to reinforce an esophageal suture line, but also to graft a full-thickness defect in the distal esophagus. By 8 weeks the mucosa completely covers the inner surface of the defect. In the cervical region the sternothyroideus "strap" muscle has been used to reinforce suture lines or repair defects following resection of a diseased portion of esophagus. The belly of one of the paired strap muscles (sternohyoideus or sternocephalicus) is separated from its attachment to the other belly and reflected laterally. The muscle is then mobilized deep to lie against the esophageal defect and subsequently is sutured to the mucosal incision. The suture bridges the end of the mucosal suture line. The muscle graft must be mobile enough and of sufficient width to prevent postoperative stricture. Gastric flaps also have been used successfully to repair defects involving the distal esophagus near the cardia.

Esophageal Replacement

When radical excision of the esophagus is indicated for neoplasia or for extensive damage due to accidental or surgical trauma, the methods available are technically very difficult, are associated with a high level of morbidity and mortality, and should be managed by a surgical specialist. Options to replace a segment of cervical or thoracic esophagus include the use of colonic or jejunal interpositioned segments, the formation of a gastric tube moved cranially into the thorax, or free grafts of intestine (using microvascular anastomosis techniques). In the dog and cat, movement of a pedicled segment of jejunum or colon is more difficult than in humans because of shorter blood vessels in these species. The canine colon has some advantages over the jejunum for this purpose, because the blood supply is more predictable and larger in size.

Failure of segment replacement most often results from necrosis of the interposed segment due to loss of blood supply, leakage from an anastomosis, or delayed postoperative stricture. In those instances in which the interposed segment surgery either fails or is impractical, a permanent tube gastrostomy may be considered, following resection of the diseased segment of esophagus.

Esophageal Obstruction

Obstruction of the esophagus in the dog and cat usually is due to foreign bodies. Strictures and neoplasia are much less common. The obstruction may be either partial or complete. Esophageal foreign bodies occur with greatest frequency in dogs, are usually bones, and most often lodge in the thoracic esophagus just caudal to the base of the heart.

History and Clinical Signs

Young animals, especially puppies, are predisposed to consuming foreign bodies. The owner may have noted the animal eating an object, or may be aware that something is "missing". Initial signs include dysphagia (in higher obstructions), excessive salivation, gagging, retching, and regurgitation. In incomplete obstruction, regurgitation of only solid foods may occur, and liquids often are retained. Later signs may include fever, lethargy, anorexia, coughing (associated with aspiration pneumonia), cranial abdominal pain, and dehydration.

A bolus type foreign body may cause only a partial obstruction, and if smooth and irregularly shaped, it may be present for weeks or months before signs appear. When signs do begin, regurgitation is a prominent feature.

The interval between eating and regurgitation depends on the location of the obstruction and the degree of dilatation cranial to it. A large foreign body can produce more rapid changes either from pressure necrosis or from complete obstruction. If complete obstruction is present, water and electrolyte losses can become severe over a short period of time.

Sharp foreign objects can cause additional signs related to perforation (see "Esophageal Perforation," p. 332). The sharp point of a fish hook or needle may eventually lead to mediastinitis and pleuritis (thoracic esophagus) or cellulitis (cervical portion). Cats with needles lodged in the esophagus often have an attached thread that may be wrapped around the base of the tongue. One always should examine the mouth of cats with suspected ingestion of a foreign body. Aspiration pneumonia frequently occurs associated with esophageal obstruction of any cause. This is because pooled esophageal contents cannot be completely swallowed, so they are aspirated, often while the animal sleeps.

Diagnosis

Esophageal obstruction caused by a foreign body is suspected on the basis of history (an object missing from the animal's environment), signs, physical examination findings, observation of the animal in the act of eating, and the results of endoscopy and radiography. Endoscopy delineates the amount of mucosal irritation present and helps identify the foreign body. A perforation or esophageal tear also may be seen.

Plain film radiography can confirm the presence of a foreign body if it is radiopaque. Megaesophagus cranial to the obstruction usually is present. Pulmonary changes often occur in the form of aspiration pneumonia. Hydropneumothorax or mediastinal thickening signal perforation. A positive contrast esophagram is necessary to identify a radiolucent foreign body. In the rare case of esophagobronchial or esophagotracheal fistula, the contrast material may be seen passing directly into the pulmonary tree.

Treatment

Prior to attempting removal of a foreign object, water and electrolyte disturbances must be corrected (Fig. 12-2). Parenteral antibiotic therapy should be initiated as well, especially when perforation or aspiration pneumonia has been confirmed.

The preferred method of relieving simple foreign body induced esophageal obstruction (without perforation) is forceps removal via esophagoscopy. This can be done with a rigid or fiberoptic gastroscope. Some surgeons attempt to remove nonsharp foreign bodies by inserting a Foley catheter to a point caudal to the foreign body. After the balloon is expanded, the catheter is retracted, pulling the foreign body with it. A second Foley catheter inserted cranial to the foreign body dilates the esophagus, allowing easier passage. Lubrication with an aqueous lubricant is beneficial to passage.

If removal of the foreign body via the oral route is too risky or difficult, then repelling the object into the stomach should be attempted. If the foreign body is a bone, removal from the stomach is usually not necessary, unless gastritis-related signs (vomiting with or without blood) persist. Sharp or large metal objects pushed into the stomach should be removed by gastrotomy.

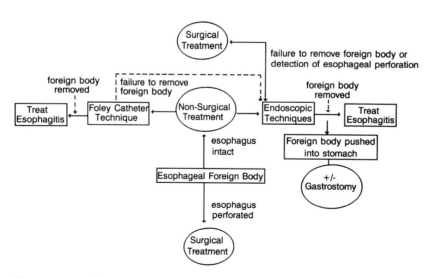

Figure 12-2. *Algorithm for treatment of foreign body obstruction of the esophagus. (Modified from Mehlhaff-Schunck CJ. Removal of esophageal foreign bodies. In: Bojrab JM, ed. Current techniques in small animal surgery. 3rd ed. Philadelphia: Lea & Febiger, in press.)*

If forceps manipulation is considered to be too dangerous or is unsuccessful, or if perforation is observed on endoscopy or radiography, surgical exploration and esophagotomy are necessary. A cervical esophagotomy usually allows good access to a foreign body lodged in the cranial thoracic esophagus. Fish hooks usually lodge within the cervical esophagus and are managed successfully by cutting the hook behind the barb and forcing the remaining shaft of the hook to the outside of the esophagus or into the lumen where it can be withdrawn by an endoscope.

Esophagotomy is performed as described previously. Silk stay sutures are placed above and below the proposed esophagotomy incision to help manipulate the esophagus. If extensive damage to the esophagus is observed at the time of surgery, resection and anastomosis of the diseased segment may be indicated. Careful periesophageal debridement should be performed if an abscess is present. Tissue samples should be taken for bacterial culture and antibiotic sensitivity testing. A chest tube is placed in all cases where a thoracotomy is used to approach the esophagus. It must remain in place until treatment for mediastinitis or pleuritis is complete.

Following simple removal of a foreign body, the patient is fasted and given intravenous fluids for 48 hours. Return to a normal diet is by the regimen discussed above for esophagotomy aftercare. In the more difficult cases requiring longer periods of convalescence and esophageal healing, postoperative management may include the need for aggressive nutritional support via the parenteral or enteral route. A tube gastrostomy, nasogastric tube, or tube pharyngostomy is ideal for providing short-term or long-term caloric needs.

Esophageal Stricture

Strictures usually are acquired and occur following reflux esophagitis, foreign body obstruction, esophageal surgery, or ingestion of caustic materials. Reflux erosive esophagitis occurs most often following anesthesia. For unknown reasons, acidic gastric contents are refluxed into the esophagus and pool in the esophagus during anesthesia, resulting in severe burns and strictures that usually are located at the level of the thoracic inlet.

History and Clinical Signs

Signs of partial obstruction usually develop 2 to 6 weeks following an anesthetic episode. Regurgitation of food occurs early, followed later by regurgitation of liquid as the disease progresses. The animal may be dysphagic if the stricture involves the proximal esophagus. The patient may drool and, on occasion, will indicate pain over the thorax when the rib cage is palpated. The patient also may be dyspneic due to secondary aspiration pneumonia.

Diagnosis

The diagnosis of stricture is based on history, signs of variable degrees of obstruction, radiography, and endoscopic findings. Plain radiographs of the esophagus usually reveal a dilated esophagus cranial to the stricture. A positive contrast esophagram demonstrates a narrowed segment of the esophagus. Endoscopy confirms the diagnosis as well as the location of the stricture. Radiography and endoscopy also may help assess the extent of the stricture.

Treatment

The preferred method of treatment is to use bougienage or balloon dilation. Dilating the esophagus is relatively risk free and is simple to perform. Bougienage now is considered a riskier method of dilation than is balloon dilation. Precise placement of a bougie within the strictured lumen is very difficult, increasing the likelihood of esophageal perforation just cranial to the stricture. Dilation is usually repeated every 7 to 14 days for a total of 2 to 4 times. Corticosteroid therapy is recommended between dilations using prednisolone at a dosage of 2 mg/kg b.i.d. Success can be measured best by assessing the clinical results, as radiographic signs do not always correlate well with the degree of clinical improvement.

Surgical correction of a stricture may be necessary if dilation is unsuccessful. An esophagoplasty procedure (longitudinal incision over the strictured area with transverse closure) or resection and anastomosis may be helpful if the lesion is not too diffuse. Tension-relieving procedures may be necessary if the segment resected is long. A patch graft technique may be employed to treat a stricture as well. Depending on the location of a stricture, pedicled or free (by microvascular anastomoses) intestinal grafts, or gastric tube grafts may be attempted. Long-term feeding gastrostomy is another alternative.

Esophageal Diverticulum

A diverticulum is a circumscribed pouch or sac of variable size created by herniation of the mucosal lining through a defect in the muscular coat of a tubular organ. This is a rare occurrence in companion animals, almost exclusively occurring in dogs. Generally, it occurs either cranial to the thoracic inlet or, most often, just cranial to the diaphragm (epiphrenic diverticulum). Diverticula may be congenital or acquired and are either of the pulsion or traction type. A pulsion diverticulum is a true diverticulum, whereas the much rarer (in dogs and cats) traction type has a wall that contains all layers of the esophagus. The latter type occurs in human beings when a periesophageal inflammatory lesion results in scarring. Contraction of the scar pulls the wall laterad. The majority of esophageal diverticula are associated with other lesions of the esophagus or diaphragm, such as hiatal hernia. Digested material can become impacted within the diverticulum, and chronic esophagitis, ulceration, and possible stricture formation may be associated with a diverticulum. The thin wall of the

diverticulum may become ulcerated or may weaken and rupture, resulting in mediastinitis. As is true with most esophageal disorders, aspiration pneumonia may be a sequela.

History and Clinical Signs

The owners of affected animals report a history of progressive dysphagia, regurgitation, and coughing. Weight loss may accompany prolonged cases.

Diagnosis

The diagnosis is confirmed via a positive contrast esophagram, which demonstrates outpouching and sacculation of the esophagus. Endoscopy adds to the information gained by radiography, but this requires anesthesia, and probably is unnecessary. Fluoroscopy may be helpful, although in most cases motor function remains normal.

Treatment

Treatment usually involves an epiphrenic diverticulectomy performed through a left eighth intercostal approach. The diverticulum is isolated by blunt dissection down to its base, and a noncrushing clamp is placed across the diverticulum at this level. The diverticulum is excised below the clamp, and the esophagus is closed in an open, two-layer technique as previously described. A chest tube is placed, and the thoracotomy incision is closed. Postoperative care is similar to that described earlier for esophagotomy aftercare.

Esophageal Neoplasia

Esophageal tumors are rare in the dog and cat, and when they occur, they usually are in geriatric patients. Metastatic tumors are more common than primary esophageal tumors in the dog. Most primary tumors are squamous cell carcinomas, whereas most of the metastatic tumors arise from thyroid, pulmonary, or mammary gland tissue. Leiomyomas, osteosarcomas, and fibrosarcomas may occur, the latter two in association with spirocercosis in the southeastern part of the United States.

History and Clinical Signs

The signs of esophageal tumors often are minimal. In advanced cases, however, they can include dysphagia, anorexia, regurgitation, weight loss, hematemesis, and signs of aspiration pneumonia.

Diagnosis

When an esophageal tumor is suspected, radiography and fluoroscopy should be performed, followed by endoscopy for biopsy. Radiography often reveals an enlarged air-filled esophagus. A barium esophagram may help outline masses or define ulcerations. *Spirocerci lupi* eggs may be detected by a fecal flotation.

Treatment

Treatment involves surgical resection of the involved portion of the esophagus. In those instances in which stenosis of the esophagus results from the tumor, temporary palliation of signs may be possible by bougienage or balloon dilatation of the affected segment.

If the tumor is small and requires minimal esophageal resection, a successful anastomosis of the remaining portions of the esophagus may be possible. Radical excision usually is necessary, however, because the neoplasms usually are large by the time of diagnosis. Interposing a pedicled or free segment of jejunum or colon may be attempted. A long-term feeding tube gastrostomy may be used in patients in which the integrity of the esophagus cannot be reestablished.

Vascular Ring Anomaly

Megaesophagus cranial to the base of the heart in a young dog or cat usually is due to the extramural pressure of a constricting band formed by a vascular ring anomaly. A persistent right aortic arch (PRAA) accounts for 95%

of these anomalies. Other anomalies include aberrant subclavian arteries or a double aortic arch. Coexisting anomalies often exist, such as a left cranial vena cava, patent ductus arteriosus, or abnormal origin of the subclavian artery. There is a breed predilection for PRAA in German shepherd dogs and Irish setters. There is no breed predilection known in cats.

History and Clinical Signs

Most animals affected with vascular ring anomaly are presented to the veterinarian between 4 and 8 weeks of age as a result of persistent regurgitation seen when weaning to solid food. Regurgitation occurs shortly after eating, usually within 1 hour. Affected animals usually are underweight, have a ravenous appetite, demonstrate poor growth, and have some degree of cervical ballooning, especially during a cough. The coughing is chronic in nature and is due to aspiration pneumonia.

Diagnosis

The tentative diagnosis of PRAA is made on the basis of signalment, clinical signs of esophageal disease at an early age, physical examination findings, radiography, and esophagoscopy. Plain radiographs of the thorax demonstrate an enlarged, air-filled and fluid-filled esophagus cranial to the heart with some ventral displacement of the heart. A contrast esophagram demonstrates precardiac saccular dilatation of the esophagus that narrows abruptly at the base of the heart. Occasionally, aspiration of some of the barium into the larynx or trachea may occur. Esophageal dilatation infrequently occurs caudally to the base of the heart because of concomitant idiopathic megaesophagus. Therefore, fluoroscopy always should be done prior to surgery, to evaluate esophageal motility both cranial and caudal to the constricted portion.

Treatment

Aggressive supportive medical therapy should precede surgical intervention and is aimed at correction of hydration and nutritional deficits. This may take several days. Antibiotics are given to treat coexisting aspiration pneumonia.

In PRAA, the esophagus is trapped between the aorta, the main stem pulmonary artery, and the ligamentum arteriosum. Surgical therapy is based on severing the ligamentum arteriosum and associated fibrous constricting bands. A left-sided thoracotomy through the fourth intercostal space allows good access to the ligamentum arteriosum and the esophagus. Occasionally, the ligamentum is a patent ductus arteriosus (PDA). Thus, it is best to place at least two ligatures (see "Patent Ductus Arteriosus," Chap. 10) of 3-0 silk followed by transection. The mediastinum and adventitia are dissected gently away from the esophagus for a distance of 1 to 2 cm above and below the constricted portion beneath the ligamentum. A large Foley catheter or a balloon dilator may be placed into the esophagus *per os* and passed down to the site of constriction. The dilator is then inflated to expand the lumen at this location. Fibrous restricting bands may then be severed carefully. Alternatively, repeated dilation may aid in breakdown of these bands.

Postoperatively, the patient is fed a gruel mixture three to four times daily for 48 hours. Water is given *ad libitum*. It is recommended that a normal diet be restored over the next 7 to 10 days. During this early convalescent period most animals need to be fed while standing on their hind legs with their forelegs and food on an elevated platform (see "Primary Megaesophagus," p. 334).

The prognosis is guarded to poor following surgery. The younger the patient is at the time of surgical correction, the more likely it is that some or all of its signs can be ameliorated by surgery. If preoperative fluoroscopy demonstrates poor peristaltic activity of any portion of the esophagus, the prognosis following surgery is worse. If peristaltic activity appears normal, and megaesophagus cranial to the heart is not severe, the prognosis following surgery is better.

Regurgitation may occur early in the postoperative period, because of stenosis at the surgery site (inadequate transection of fibrous bands) or, later, because of the formation of extraluminal scar tissue. In these cases, bougienage or balloon dilation may be attempted. If the latter fails to improve the signs, reoperation may be necessary. If stenosis is due to an intramural or mucosal stricture, an esophagoplasty procedure (longitudinal incision–transverse closure) to widen the esophagus at the site of stenosis is indicated. Ultimately, surgical resection of the strictured segment may be necessary.

In more chronic cases, esophageal dilatation may be so severe that muscular function is gone and does not return, and signs persist even if no restriction to esophageal flow exists at the surgery site. In such cases, longitudinal resection of the sacculation may be performed, usually using a mechanical stapler, to minimize esophageal accumulation of ingesta and to facilitate their passage by gravity. Even with this surgery, signs may persist.

The animals whose signs improve following surgery still may require feeding from an elevated position indefinitely. In addition, constant monitoring for signs of aspiration pneumonia is necessary.

Esophageal Perforation

History and Clinical Signs

Perforation of the esophagus can occur as a sequela of the ingestion of a sharp foreign body or may result from the chronic presence of a hard foreign body. It also can occur iatrogenically during esophagoscopy or intubation. In the cervical region it often results from a penetrating wound caused by a bite or bullet.

Cervical esophageal perforations result in periesophageal swelling, abscess formation, cervical drainage, crepitus, fever, pain, and anorexia. Morbidity is less than that associated with perforation of the thoracic esophagus. Unless thoracic esophageal perforations are recognized early, a high mortality rate results. Mediastinitis, pleuritis, mediastinal abscess, or empyema complicates intrathoracic esophageal perforations. Generally speaking, perforation should be suspected when a patient with an esophageal obstruction concurrently demonstrates leukocytosis, coughing, dyspnea, cervical soft tissue swelling, and fever.

Diagnosis

The diagnosis of esophageal perforation usually can be confirmed by esophagoscopy or radiography. An area of increased mediastinal density adjacent to a foreign body, pneumomediastinum, or a mediastinal mass on radiography suggests a perforation with mediastinitis or abscess. If a perforation cannot be substantiated on plain film radiography, the use of a water soluble (organic iodide) agent may improve its visualization. Barium better defines the nature and extent of the tear, but it should be used only in those cases that undergo surgery immediately, because it causes an intense inflammatory response.

Leakage of esophageal contents and bacteria from an esophageal perforation can result in empyema. If perforation is suspected, tube thoracostomy to drain the chest should be followed by radiography. Alternatively, methylene blue (5 ml of 1%) may be given *per os.* The presence of the dye in fluid drained from the chest tubes confirms the diagnosis of an esophageal perforation.

Treatment

The intensity of therapy depends on the extent and duration of the perforation and the nature of associated signs. A small tear may be treated successfully by antibiotic therapy alone. More severe injuries, without systemic signs or secondary problems, may require that no food or water be given *per os* for 5–7 days, while giving enteral (tube gastrostomy, pharyngostomy) or parenteral nutritional support.

If a leaking perforation exists and if clinical findings include fever, mediastinal air, and an abnormal esophagram, immediate exploration and primary repair is the procedure of choice, followed by thorough irrigation, and subcutaneous or pleural drainage. Repair of an esophageal perforation involves debridement of the edges and a two-layer closure. With cervical perforations it may be beneficial to debride, irrigate, and drain the pleuroesophageal tissues and treat with an antibiotic for several days before attempting primary repair of the perforation. If the defect in the esophagus created by the debridement of necrotic tissue at the time of primary closure is large, a transverse closure should be performed so as to increase rather than decrease the lumen, or, if this is not possible, onlay patch-grafting with sternothyroideus muscle is possible in the cervical region. If the distal esophagus is compromised, an onlay patch using a flap of the stomach, diaphragm, or a pedicled section of omentum drawn through a small incision in the diaphragm may be used. If over 30% of the esophageal circumference is compromised, resection and anastomosis usually are indicated.

Regardless of the location of the tear, if surgery is indicated, bypassing the esophagus with a tube gastrostomy is highly recommended. A pharyngostomy tube may be used instead, although its use in this situation is somewhat controversial because of possible interference with healing of the wound by the intraluminal tube. Providing enteral nutrition postoperatively enhances esophageal wound healing and may help improve resistance to wound infection.

The prognosis associated with thoracic esophageal tears is poor because of the serious nature of secondary problems. Cervical tears carry a better prognosis, but in either case, a successful short-term outcome may be followed later by stricture formation.

Esophagobronchial–Tracheobronchial Fistula

Fistulae forming between the esophagus and the tracheobronchial tree are rare in the dog and cat. Most often they are sequelae to the chronic presence of foreign bodies and occur most often at the base of the heart or esophageal diverticula.

History and Clinical Signs

The disease may go unnoticed for a period of time, because nonspecific clinical signs usually are present. Early signs are typical of esophageal obstruction (see above). After the fistula has formed, coughing, regurgitation, lethargy, anorexia, pyrexia, dyspnea, and weight loss are common. Coughing is the most characteristic sign of a fistula, observed especially after eating or drinking.

Diagnosis

A presumptive diagnosis is based on the history (coughing after drinking) and clinical signs. Radiographic signs include bronchial, alveolar, and interstitial localized patterns of infiltrate, the presence of an esophageal foreign body (if it is radiopaque), and, sometimes, pleural effusion. An esophagram is the most reliable means of confirming the diagnosis of esophagotracheal or esophagobronchial fistula. A very thin mixture of barium sulfate (20%–30% weight/volume) should be used. Large fistulae are easily demonstrated, but small ones may not be outlined. Placing the animal in dorsal, right and left lateral, and then ventral positions may assist the migration of the barium fluid through smaller fistulae.

Treatment

The surgical approach of choice is to isolate the esophagus and the trachea or affected lung lobe around the fistula. The fistula is severed near its respiratory attachment, and the tracheal or bronchial opening is debrided and sutured. A partial pulmonary lobectomy may have to be performed, if the pulmonary parenchyma is involved. The hole in the esophagus may be extended to allow the removal of the foreign body, if present. The esophagus is closed following debridement of the wound edges.

The prognosis is good if the degree of pulmonary involvement and esophageal trauma are minimal. Animals with concomitant empyema, severe pneumonia, or septicemia have a guarded to poor prognosis.

Primary Megaesophagus

Primary megaesophagus is caused by neurogenic, myogenic, or myoneurogenic disease. It is characterized by generalized enlargement of the esophagus with inadequate or no peristaltic activity. Generally, it is divided into primary (idiopathic, congenital) or acquired forms. Primary megaesophagus can be congenital and often is an hereditary disorder occurring most often in German shepherd dogs, great Danes, dachshunds, and miniature schnauzers. The exact etiology remains obscure. Primary megaesophagus rarely occurs in cats.

History and Clinical Signs

Clinical signs usually begin during puppyhood, with the majority of dogs showing such signs at less than 10 weeks of age. Weaning to solid food often results in oral and nasal regurgitation of undigested food, a ravenous appetite but poor weight gain, distension of the cervical esophagus (more pronounced when the dog coughs or when the chest is compressed), mucopurulent nasal discharge, coughing and, on occasion, dyspnea.

Diagnosis

The diagnosis of megaesophagus is based on clinical signs and contrast esophagography. A dilated esophagus filled with variable amounts of air and fluid or ingesta can be seen on plain films. The contrast study is necessary to define the extent of the disease and rule out other causes of megaesophagus, such as a stricture due to a vascular anomaly.

Because this is a disorder of motility, a definitive diagnosis requires fluoroscopy or esophageal pressure studies, which usually demonstrate little to no peristaltic activity and may show asynchronous relaxation of the gastroesophageal sphincter (GES).

Treatment

The congenital form of megaesophagus is treated by feeding small amounts of food to the animal from an elevated platform, while it stands in an upright position on its rear legs. Results may vary depending on the consistency of the food. This form of megaesophagus may reverse spontaneously over a period of several months. Approximately one third to one half of affected dogs respond to medical management, and, by the time they are mature, they appear normal clinically and radiographically. The fact that many of these animals improve with age suggests that this condition is a developmental disorder in which maturation of esophageal function is delayed.

Most puppies that die from congenital megaesophagus, do so because of the aspiration pneumonia. Supportive antibiotic therapy may be necessary for a prolonged period of time.

Acquired Megaesophagus

History and Clinical Signs

Acquired megaesophagus is a spontaneous disorder seen most frequently in adult dogs. It can be an idiopathic disorder or a disease secondary to other conditions, such as myasthenia gravis, hypoadrenocorticism (Addison's disease), hypothyroidism, immune-mediated polymyositis, or polyneuritis, as reported in dogs with systemic lupus erythematosus. It also has been seen related to the occurrence of acute gastric dilatation–volvulus syndrome in large and giant breed dogs and pyloric hypertrophy in cats. At times it is impossible to differentiate between acquired megaesophagus and congenital megaesophagus, in which the disorder existed from puppyhood, but signs

did not appear until after 1 year of age. Clinical signs are similar to those of the congenital form, plus loss of weight.

Diagnosis

The diagnosis of acquired megaesophagus is similar to that of the congenital form, relying mostly on clinical signs, radiography, and fluoroscopy. Searching for an underlying disorder is recommended, because correcting the underlying problem may allow esophageal-related signs to go into remission.

Treatment

Treatment of secondary megaesophagus is aimed at correcting the underlying etiology, after which the megaesophagus may resolve spontaneously. Feeding from a height as described previously may be necessary on a temporary basis.

When no cause of spontaneous megaesophagus is found in the adult (acquired idiopathic form), feeding from a height for an indefinite period of time is usually attempted first. The prognosis for this form of megaesophagus is poor, because recovery is rare once the disease is present. For this reason, a cardiomyotomy may be indicated as a last resort, and in some instances, this has proved beneficial. Following a cardiomyotomy it may still be necessary to feed a special diet or to feed from an elevated position for the duration of the animal's life.

Cardiomyotomy
The purpose of a cardiomyotomy is to reduce the functional obstruction associated with hypomotility of the esophagus, asynchrony of the peristaltic wave in the caudal esophagus, and opening of the gastroesophageal sphincter (GES). The goal is to allow the esophagus to empty more easily. Although this technique does not cure the esophageal motor disturbance such as that seen with megaesophagus, some animals appear to benefit from its use.

This procedure can be performed via an abdominal approach, although it is best done through the left eighth or ninth intercostal space. The caudal lung lobe is isolated and packed cranially. The mediastinal pleura is incised, and the caudal thoracic esophagus is dissected free of surrounding tissue. The vagus nerve is dissected free from the caudal esophagus so that umbilical tape may be placed around the esophagus. Cranial traction on the tape brings the gastroesophageal junction into the surgical field. A modified cardiomyotomy (Heller technique) requires incising the phrenicoesophageal ligament and exposing the cardia of the stomach. The outer longitudinal and inner circular layers of the tunica muscularis are incised for a distance of 2 cm above and below the gastroesophageal junction. The mucosa bulges out between the edges of the incision following gentle undermining of the muscle layer. Care must be taken not to penetrate the esophageal lumen, as leakage can be disastrous.

After completing the myotomy, the diaphragm is sutured to the cranial portion of the myotomy in a transverse plane so that the mucosal bulge now lies within the abdominal cavity. This is done to attempt restoration of the GES. Routine thoracotomy closure is performed.

Prognosis
This procedure is not curative, and although the results are variable, it is indicated more often in the acquired than primary form of megaesophagus in the adult dog, in which spontaneous remission of signs is uncommon. Its use in treatment of the congenital form usually is unsuccessful.

Reflux esophagitis may be a problem following this procedure because of disruption of the GES. Therapy with antacids and gastric motility modifiers (*e.g.,* metoclopramide) is warranted for at least 10 to 14 days and, in some instances, indefinitely.

On rare occasions, puppies with megaesophagus benefit by having a cardiomyotomy performed. This may be because the procedure decreases the pressure gradient needed to propel food from the esophagus into the stomach.

Gastroesophageal Intussusception

This is a rare condition seen in young dogs. The forward movement of the stomach into the distal esophagus follows prolonged periods of vomition, especially if there is concurrent megaesophagus. Most affected dogs present with a history of regurgitation or vomiting, dyspnea, coughing, abdominal discomfort, and hematemesis. The rapid course of this disease results in shock, severe abdominal discomfort, dyspnea, and usually death.

Although antemortem diagnosis is rare, the best diagnostic tool is radiography, in which gastric rugae may be seen within the lumen of the distal esophagus. This problem is differentiated from esophageal hiatal hernia by its acute onset and the rapid deterioration of the patient.

Treatment involves a left-sided gastropexy. If enlarged, the esophageal hiatus should be tightened with sutures. These two procedures prevent the stomach from moving cranially into the distal esophagus.

Because this disease seldom is diagnosed in time for surgical correction, only a few cases are described in the literature. The prognosis for reported cases is poor.

Stomach and Pylorus

Gastric Foreign Body

Most ingested foreign bodies in the dog and cat do not cause disease; they pass through or are digested. Cats most often present with a linear foreign body including string or thread with or without an attached needle. Most of the clinical problems caused in cats with string foreign bodies are not directly related to their presence in the stomach but result from small intestinal obstruction and perforation.

History and Clinical Signs

A gastric foreign body is suspected if the owner witnessed the act of ingestion or if an object is missing from the environment. Foreign bodies that remain in the stomach and lodge in the pyloric antrum usually cause emesis. If the obstruction is complete, severe water and electrolyte loss develop rapidly. Gastric emptying is delayed or absent. Obstructive signs may be intermittent, if the foreign body spontaneously dislodges from the pylorus and returns to the fundus or antrum.

On occasion, melena or hematemesis may occur because of mucosal erosion or ulceration or necrosis caused by the foreign body. In cases of incomplete obstruction, vomiting is less frequent, and weight loss and anorexia may be the predominant signs.

Diagnosis

History, clinical signs, physical examination findings, and radiography usually confirm the diagnosis.

Physical examination may reveal dehydration and even weakness, depending on the extent of water and electrolyte loss. Weight loss may be significant in cases of incomplete, chronic obstruction. Occasionally a large fluid-filled stomach may be palpable. Laboratory findings often include metabolic alkalosis, hypokalemia, and hypochloremia, especially if the pylorus is obstructed.

If the object is radiolucent, negative or positive contrast gastrography may be necessary to outline the foreign body. Endoscopy is a valuable diagnostic aid as well.

Treatment

Treatment includes restoring electrolyte, water, and acid-base imbalances to normal. An antiemetic may be indicated during this period to control excessive vomiting. If hematemesis or melena occurs, gastric erosions or ulceration likely are present, and antiulcer medical therapy is indicated (see, "Peptic Ulcer Disease," p. 344).

Although gastrotomy usually is required, endoscopy is recommended as the initial method for attempting to retrieve certain gastric foreign bodies. A basket-type snare or grasping forceps is used to pull the foreign body from the stomach. However, some smooth-surfaced foreign bodies, such as balls, cannot be grasped, and other large foreign bodies or those with rough surfaces may cause too much trauma to the esophagus during retrieval and should be removed via gastrotomy.

At the time of the gastrotomy, the gastric mucosa is inspected for erosions or ulcers. If present, ulcer therapy should be given for 10 to 14 days postoperatively. The prognosis following foreign body removal is good to excellent. Careful exploration of the stomach is required, to exclude the presence of multiple foreign bodies.

Pyloric Outflow Obstruction

Gastric outflow obstruction can be partial or complete and can be caused by congenital pyloric stenosis, foreign bodies, granulomatous or eosinophilic gastritis, chronic hypertrophic pyloric gastropathy (CHPG), chronic ulcer disease, or neoplasia. All types are associated with vomiting of food with no bile, up to 8 to 24 hours after eating.

Congenital Pyloric Stenosis

In pups or kittens, pyloric stenosis may be congenital. This occurs most often in brachycephalic breeds of dogs and in Siamese cats. The pyloric musculature is hypertrophied, causing delayed gastric emptying due to gastric outflow obstruction.

History and Clinical Signs

The most common sign of this disease is vomiting, which occurs at regular intervals following the ingestion of solid food up to 24 hours after eating. Signs often first appear at the time of weaning to solid food.

Diagnosis

The diagnosis of congenital pyloric stenosis is based on the age at onset of the disease, the clinical signs, and radiographic confirmation. Plain film radiography demonstrates an enlarged stomach filled with food and fluid, and delayed emptying of ingesta into the small intestine, confirmed by positive contrast gastrography. The presence of barium in the stomach beyond 8 to 12 hours is abnormal. Antral motility should be evaluated with fluoroscopy, if contrast gastrography demonstrates no mechanical reason for delayed gastric emptying. It is possible that the delayed emptying may be due to antral hypomotility, although this condition is rare. Fluoroscopy will help detect any decreased rate and vigor of contractions. Endoscopy rarely is necessary, but it can be done to rule out other causes of pyloric outflow obstruction, such as foreign bodies.

Treatment

The treatment of choice is a Fredet-Ramstedt pyloromyotomy (see Fig. 12-9, below). This usually results in a prompt cessation of signs, and the prognosis is good. If the vomiting continues beyond 48 hours postoperatively, smaller and more frequent feedings are recommended. If vomiting continues in spite of these feeding practices, the surgery may have to be repeated, or a pyloroplasty procedure or partial gastric resection may be necessary to alleviate the signs. This is usually necessary when the pyloromyotomy is performed with incomplete separation of the muscle layers overlying the pylorus, or if formation of excessive scar tissue at the surgical site results in a stricture.

Chronic Hypertrophic Pyloric Gastropathy (CHPG)

CHPG is an acquired disorder that results in pyloric stenosis in adult dogs. It occurs in cats, as well, but is rare. Most frequently it is diagnosed in middle-age toy breeds with excitable personalities, particularly Lhaso Apsos and Shih-Tzus.

History and Clinical Signs

The presenting history includes sporadic vomiting, which may or may not be related to the recent ingestion of a meal. Over time the frequency of vomiting increases. Weight loss is common. Clinical signs include mucous membrane pallor, weakness, and dehydration.

Diagnosis

The diagnosis of CHPG is based on the signalment, history, and the observation of vomiting of food with no bile continuing up to 8 to 24 hours after eating. Plain film radiography demonstrates a large fluid-filled stomach. A positive contrast gastrogram reveals delayed gastric emptying, irregular mucosal surfaces within the pyloric antrum or canal, and, on occasion, a filling defect in the pylorus. Endoscopy may demonstrate hyperemia of the gastric mucosa, polypoid lesions, and, in some cases, the presence of an ulcer. Biopsies at the time of endoscopic evaluation will help rule out neoplastic or other inflammatory diseases affecting the pylorus.

Treatment

Surgical treatment is recommended for satisfactory resolution of this disease (see "Surgery of the Pylorus," p. 352). However, fluid, electrolyte and acid-base derangements should be corrected prior to surgery. A pyloroplasty procedure is recommended to widen the diameter of the pyloric canal. The Y-U antral flap advancement pyloroplasty consistently widens the pyloric outflow tract, while allowing the surgeon the option of resecting some or all of the hypertrophied mucosa (see Fig. 12-12 below). Another option is to perform a Billroth I pylorectomy (gastroduodenostomy) procedure (see Fig. 12-13).

The prognosis following surgery is good. During the immediate postoperative period, gastric stasis and emesis are common. Intravenous fluid therapy is advised for up to 48 hours following surgery. After 48 hours, a low fat diet of spaghetti, rice, or macaroni may be given in small amounts four to six times daily. Metoclopramide (0.2–0.4 mg/kg *per os* or subcutaneously—Reglan, A. H. Robins, Richmond, VA) can be given for 2 to 3 days to help stimulate gastric contractility. If emesis continues, it may be related to overfeeding; therefore, the owner should be advised to feed smaller amounts more frequently.

Should vomiting continue in spite of dietary management or use of motility modifiers, alkaline reflux gastritis may be the cause. This is an uncommon but important sequela to surgery to the distal stomach. Bile in the vomitus is a good indication of duodenogastric reflux. Giving a prokinetic agent such as metoclopramide may be necessary for several weeks. Antiulcer therapy should be initiated and continued for 2 to 3 weeks, because erosive gastritis is often a sequela to reflux gastritis. A coating agent such as sucralfate (Carafate, Marion Labs, Kansas City, MO) can be given and, in my experience, is best given just prior to bed time. Should emesis continue in spite of aggressive medical therapy, results of a complete biochemical profile may indicate another cause for the unresolved vomiting. Further diagnostic tests, including radiography and endoscopy, may be indicated. Ultimately, an exploratory coeliotomy may be necessary if vomiting continues.

Eosinophilic Gastritis

Eosinophilic gastritis is characterized by diffuse, granulomatous and eosinophilic infiltration of some or all layers of the stomach. The changes in the gastric wall can be so severe that the scirrhous thickening can resemble gastric neoplasia. On occasion, well-defined polypoid masses may be found. This disease is thought to be immunologically mediated, but thus far no specific cause has been identified. It may be a component of a more generalized disease in which a patchy or diffuse pattern of eosinophilic infiltration affects the small intestine as well.

Clinical Signs

Clinical signs of eosinophilic gastritis are ill-defined. Sporadic episodes of vomition are seen along with one or more of the following signs: anorexia, weight loss, melena, and, occasionally, anemia. If the pylorus becomes thickened to the point of partial obstruction, frequent vomiting becomes the predominant sign with a rapid development of electrolyte and water imbalances.

Diagnosis

There are no tests specific for this disease, although the diagnosis is suggested by a hemogram showing eosinophilia, combined with signs of gastritis. A good clinical response to corticosteroid therapy adds to the diagnosis of eosinophilic gastritis, but definitive diagnosis requires a biopsy.

Treatment

Medical therapy includes feeding a liquid gruel diet, corticosteroids (prednisone 2 mg/kg *per os* SID) and H_2 receptor antagonists to control any hyperacidity that may be present (see "Peptic Ulcer Disease," p. 344). Surgical resection of well-defined granulomatous or ulcerated areas may be indicated. If obstruction results in delayed gastric emptying, a pyloroplasty may be indicated. Partial gastrectomy is necessary if the lesion is diffuse.

Gastric Dilatation–Volvulus

Pathophysiology

Gastric dilatation–volvulus (GDV) initiates a cascade of events that result in dramatic and severe metabolic disturbances, which, if untreated, often culminate in death. Approximately 40,000 to 60,000 dogs per year in the United States alone are affected by this disease, with an associated mortality rate of approximately 35% to 40%. Although all breeds of dogs can have this disease, giant or large breed dogs such as the great Dane, German shepherd and Irish setter appear to be most commonly affected. Some smaller breeds that are more commonly affected than others include dachshunds, basset hounds, and beagles. There is no sex predilection for this disease, and most affected dogs are between the ages of 2 and 8 years.

The exact etiology of GDV is unknown, but it is likely multifactorial. The stomach of a dog affected with GDV demonstrates laxity of the hepatogastric and hepatoduodenal ligaments. This is thought to allow a high degree of gastric mobility and predispose dogs to the clockwise rotation (volvulus) of the distended stomach when viewing the dog caudally–cranially. Possible contributing factors are chronic overeating, single daily large feedings, consumption of large amounts of water, genetic predisposition, changes in environment, aerophagia, and delayed gastric emptying caused by motility disorders associated with general anesthesia, prolonged surgery, spinal cord injuries, or prolonged recumbency. Most cases occur after eating. No specific diet has been incriminated in causing this disease.

Gastric accumulation primarily is from aerophagia, although bacterial fermentation of carbohydrates in the food is thought to be contributory. It is unknown at this time if aerophagia contributes to GDV, or if GDV initiates aerophagia. Slight distension of the stomach is thought to interfere with the dog's ability to maintain an eructation reflex, which may allow further gas accumulation to the point of severe gastric distension.

Dogs that experience dilatation almost invariably have some degree of stomach rotation. Volvulus occurs when the dilated fundus moves from a left dorsal position to a right ventral one. The pylorus shifts simultaneously from its right ventral position to a left caudal and dorsal position. The spleen follows the greater curvature to the right. This twisting of the stomach usually prevents the spontaneous relief of gas and fluid accumulation by shutting off the cardia and pylorus. Furthermore, once volvulus complicates distension, the distended

fundic portion often gets "fixed" in its abnormal position.

The two major pathological changes that occur with GDV are gastric wall ischemia and circulatory shock. Increased intragastric pressure results in venous stasis and the occlusion of intramural gastric vessels. The gastric mucosa can hemorrhage, become edematous, and, in the presence of stomach acid, can undergo sloughing, necrosis, and ulceration.

GDV induces circulatory shock by occluding the caudal vena cava and the portal vein. Interference to the venous return to the heart dramatically decreases the cardiac output, resulting in lactic acidosis. Decreased coronary blood flow results, which may contribute to myocardial dysfunction.

Portal vein occlusion and splanchnic ischemia contribute to endotoxemia. The bacteria within the lumen of the gut release endotoxins at a greater rate under these conditions. These endotoxins then move across the mucosal barrier of the intestine, entering the circulation via the intestinal or diaphragmatic lymphatics or peritoneal surfaces. Due to decreased portal flow, many of these endotoxins escape destruction by the reticuloendothelial system of the liver. Thus, signs of endotoxic shock often accompany GDV.

Ischemic injury to endothelial cells causes an array of microvascular changes that enhance the increased capillary permeability and microvascular sludging. This may be associated with disseminated intravascular coagulopathy.

Hypokalemia is the most common electrolyte disturbance seen with GDV. It results from the sequestration of potassium in the gastric fluids during dilatation and, secondarily, from aggressive fluid therapy.

Most cardiac arrhythmias are ventricular in origin and consist primarily of premature ventricular depolarizations and paroxysmal ventricular tachycardia. Most of the arrhythmias develop within 6 to 24 hours after hospitalization. There is some suggestion that arrhythmias occur most often following definitive surgery, suggesting a reperfusion injury etiology. They likely occur from other factors, such as severe autonomic imbalance, electrolyte and acid-base disturbances, myocardial ischemia, or the release of toxins from the portal circulation.

History and Clinical Signs

Dogs with acute GDV often present with hypersalivation, nonproductive retching, abdominal distension, hyperpnea, or dyspnea. Animals may be relatively alert and ambulatory on presentation or may be in severe shock, comatose, and near death. Severely affected patients in shock demonstrate tachycardia, mucous membrane pallor, prolonged capillary refill time, and weak femoral pulses.

Diagnosis

The diagnosis of GDV is based on the signalment, history, and clinical signs. Radiography always should be delayed until the patient is stabilized, following decompression and therapy for shock. Radiographs are necessary to differentiate simple gastric dilatation from volvulus. Right lateral recumbency gives the best view for confirming the diagnosis of volvulus. The pylorus is located dorsally, cranially and to the left of the midline. After decompression, it may assume a classical upside-down appearance. Barium sulfate *per os* helps confirm the location of the pylorus. Abdominal radiography also may reveal signs of peritonitis or pneumoperitoneum, suggesting gastric necrosis.

Treatment

Emergency Care

The most urgent concern is the need for gastric decompression (Fig. 12-3). Decompression immediately improves cardiovascular hemodynamics (cardiac output, aortic pressure). In most cases decompression can be accomplished by passing an orogastric tube into the stomach while the dog is in the sitting position. If this fails, the dog is placed in several different positions to assist in tube passage. If decompression still is not successful, gastrocentesis is done with one or several 18-gauge hypodermic needles. This usually aids the passage of the orogastric tube. Occasionally, dogs resist orogastric tube placement, and although chemical restraint is not generally suggested, its careful use may be necessary.

Once the tube is in place, the stomach is lavaged with 3 to 6 liters (in large and giant breeds) of warm saline or water using gravity flow and a syringe or stomach pump. In the event that the orogastric tube cannot be passed, a temporary gastrostomy can be performed caudal to the last rib. Some surgeons prefer to take the dog directly to surgery for a celiotomy, if intubation is unsuccessful.

Shock therapy should be initiated simultaneously with gastric decompression. A balanced electrolyte solution is administered at a rate of 100 ml/kg during the first hour. Fluid therapy thereafter should be titrated in accordance with the animal's condition. Following the initial fluid therapy for shock, some surgeons add 20 to 40 mEq of KCl to the fluid to counteract the tendency of most affected animals to become hypokalemic. Correction of hypokalemia may decrease the occurrence of cardiac arrhythmias. Normokalemia also is necessary for lidocaine to be effective in controlling arrhythmias.

Although the use of corticosteroids is controversial, they should be used (prednisolone sodium succinate, 10 mg/kg or dexamethasone 4–6 mg/kg intravenously), because endotoxic shock usually is present. Intravenous antibiotics also should be given if endotoxic shock is present. Intravenous sodium ampicillin (10 mg/kg) or cephalothin (30 mg/kg) should be given, combined with gentamicin (4 mg/kg). This is an effective bacteriocidal combination. The efficacy of this combination and the potential nephrotoxic effects of gentamicin should be monitored closely on a daily basis.

Oxygen therapy should be considered in those patients in shock or those that are dyspneic because of the pressure of the distended stomach on the diaphragm. Use of an oxygen mask or nasotracheal tube is suitable.

THERAPEUTIC APPROACH TO ACUTE GASTRIC DILATATION

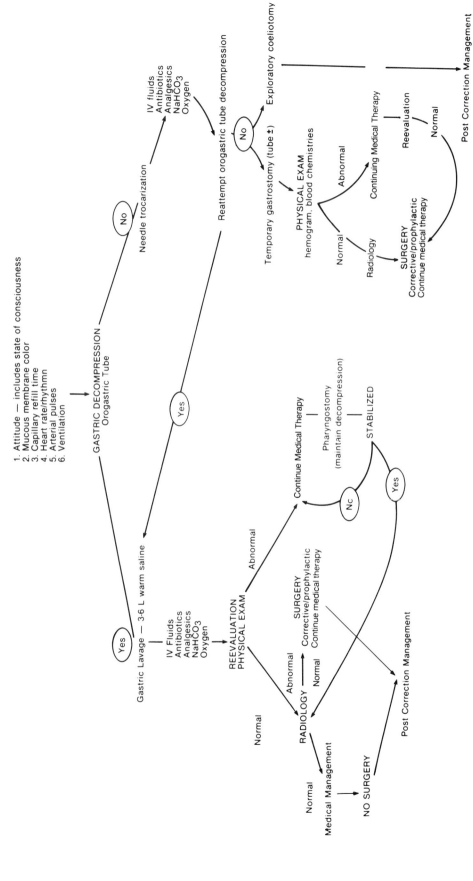

PATIENT EVALUATION

1. Attitude — includes state of consciousness
2. Mucous membrane color
3. Capillary refill time
4. Heart rate/rhythmn
5. Arterial pulses
6. Ventilation

GASTRIC DECOMPRESSION
Orogastric Tube

Yes

Gastric Lavage — 3-6 L warm saline

IV Fluids
Antibiotics
Analgesics
NaHCO3
Oxygen

REEVALUATION
PHYSICAL EXAM

Abnormal

Normal

Abnormal

RADIOLOGY

Normal

SURGERY
Corrective/prophylactic
Continue medical therapy

Continue Medical Therapy

Nc

Pharyngostomy
(maintain decompression)

STABILIZED

Yes

Medical Management

NO SURGERY

Post Correction Management

No

Needle trocarization

IV fluids
Antibiotics
Analgesics
NaHCO3
Oxygen

Reattempt orogastric tube decompression

No

Exploratory coeliotomy

Temporary gastrostomy (tube ±)

PHYSICAL EXAM
hemogram. blood chemistries

Abnormal

Normal

Continuing Medical Therapy

Reevaluation

Normal

Radiology

SURGERY
Corrective/prophylactic
Continue medical therapy

Post Correction Management

Figure 12-3. *A flow chart describing various alternatives for treatment of gastric dilatation–volulus.*

Not all cases of gastric dilatation have volvulus. Some dogs present with a simple dilatation that responds readily to orogastric intubation and gastric lavage. The need for fluid therapy in such dogs varies depending on the degree of shock. In some dogs, dilatation without volvulus resolves spontaneously by eructation or aboral movement of gas through the pylorus and into the small intestine.

Some dogs chronically demonstrate only the prodromal signs of GDV, including restlessness, belching, sporadic vomiting, excessive borborygmi, flatulence, occasional diarrhea, plus gradual weight loss. These "chronic bloaters" (also reported in dogs as chronic partial gastric torsion) do not always suffer from the severe signs usually associated with GDV. Radiographically, the stomach is displaced cranially, with some degree of rotation detected.

Gastropexy

It is accepted universally that most dogs presenting with GDV should undergo exploratory coeliotomy, because the recurrence rate of nonsurgically treated GDV is approximately 75%. Definitive management involves stomach and spleen repositioning, assessing the viability of the stomach and spleen, and some form of gastropexy procedure to prevent future volvulus. The abdomen of a dog is explored, and if gastric dilatation is present without volvulus, a gastropexy procedure should be performed anyway, because it is generally agreed that dilatation usually leads to volvulus.

The time after presentation that surgery is performed depends on the status of the patient, the response to initial therapy, and radiographic findings. Radiographic findings that dictate early intervention include the presence of fluid or air in the abdomen, suggesting gastric rupture. If the stomach is rotated but not distended, or if it has derotated into normal position, some surgeons prefer to observe the dog closely overnight, while maintaining fluid therapy and relieving any gastric distension that occurs. Other surgeons

advocate early definitive surgery (1–2 hours following decompression and stabilization), because GDV patients are at great risk of gastric rupture, and gastric viability cannot accurately be detected without surgical exploration.

A cranial ventral midline abdominal incision is used to allow excellent exposure of the abdominal viscera. With volvulus, the ventral surface of the dilated stomach often is covered with omentum. Passage of a stomach tube and gastric lavage is done by an assistant, to help evacuate the stomach of fluid and food contents. This also facilitates repositioning of the stomach and spleen. I prefer to stand on the right side of the patient and, while moving the pylorus ventrally counterclockwise toward the incision (the pylorus is often located just ventral and cranial to the cardia of the stomach), and then to the right, the fundus is pushed to the left and dorsally.

Following repositioning of the stomach and spleen, the viability of both organs should be assessed. Moderate to severe splenomegaly usually is apparent prior to repositioning. With the spleen returned to a normal anatomical position, the arteries are examined for pulsations and the arteries and veins for intravascular clots. If there are pulsations, and no clots are present, the spleen is retained. Splenectomy rarely is necessary; removal of the spleen does not prevent recurrence of GDV.

Gastric wall viability is assessed by color and palpation. The most common part of the stomach affected by ischemia is the greater curvature. Viable gastric tissue varies from hyperemic to dark red in color and has normal thickness. Gastric tissue that is dark blue to black in color and is considerably thinner than normal should be resected. Devitalized stomach wall is removed until bright pink tissue with bleeding edges is reached. A two-layer inverting suture pattern is used to close the stomach wall. I prefer to use a mechanical thoracoabdominal (T/A) stapler (United States Surgical Corporation, Norwalk, CT) in these critical patients, because it saves considerable surgical time. Unfortunately, regardless of the technique employed, the prognosis in dogs that require a partial gastrectomy is very poor —nearly 65% to 70% of these patients die.

The gastropexy technique entails fixing the pyloric antrum to the right abdominal wall. This can be done using either a tube gastropexy or a circumcostal gastropexy (see Figs. 12-7 and 12-8).

Gastropexy is designed to preserve the dog's ability to spontaneously decompress any future gastric dilatation episode via belching or aboral movement of gas through the pylorus, and to prevent volvulus. Although gastric distension still may occur occasionally following a gastropexy, it usually is mild and self-limiting.

Postoperative therapy for GDV includes 24 to 48 hours of fluid therapy, supplementation with potassium, and treatment of cardiac arrhythmias. Occasionally, dogs show signs of ulcer disease (hematemesis, melena, vomiting), requiring antiulcer therapy (see below) for 10 to 14 days.

When using a tube gastrostomy gastropexy technique, a small amount of antiseptic or antibiotic ointment is placed on the skin where the tube exits the abdominal cavity. The tube is capped and placed under a light bandage. If the dog has postoperative gastric distension, decompression is done by temporarily removing the cap. Water, oral medication, and liquid gruel may be administered through this tube if necessary. It is ideal to leave this tube in place for a minimum of 5 to 7 days. After removal of the tube, the skin wound is kept clean and allowed to heal by second intention. Antibiotic ointment can be applied to the wound until healing is complete.

Peptic Ulcer Disease

Pathogenesis

Benign peptic ulcer disease (PUD) results when the aggressive effects of acid–pepsin dominate over the protective effects of gastric or duodenal mucosal resistance. The pathophysiology of benign peptic ulcer disease fo-

cuses on three general areas: deficits in mucosal resistance to acid, abnormalities in gastric acid secretion, and defects in endocrine control mechanisms. All three are known to predispose dogs to PUD.

Aggressive factors causing injury to the protective mucosa include acid, pepsin, and bile acids. Mucosal disruption also can result from mechanical injury caused by foreign bodies or iatrogenic damage with an endoscope. Ulcer formation occurs because of one or more of the factors mentioned above, which allow the mucosa and underlying tissues to come into direct contact with pepsin and acid. It appears that gastric and duodenal ulcers may be associated with normal, hypoacidity or hyperacidity, and with variable degrees of gastritis.

The frequent use of nonsteroidal anti-inflammatory drugs (NSAIDs) is one of the most familiar and well-studied causes of PUD in the dog. Another common cause of PUD in the dog is hepatic disease. A specific hepatopathy cannot be implicated because of the wide variety of histopathological diagnoses being reported. Other causes of PUD in the dog include gastrin-producing tumors (gastrinomas, *i.e.,* Zollinger-Ellison syndrome), spinal cord disease, systemic mastocytosis (hyperacidity secondary to increased histamine levels), uremia, interference with regional blood flow to the gastric mucosa (GDV, shock), duodenogastric reflux (bile salts, pancreatic enzymes), and corticosteroids.

Clinical Signs

Vomition with or without the presence of blood is the most common sign associated with PUD in the dog. Melena, inappetance, abdominal discomfort, and pale mucous membranes are other common clinical findings.

Treatment

Medical
Identifying predisposing causes and understanding the pathogenesis of ulcer disease aids therapeutic decisions. The aim of ulcer therapy is to attack the disease by decreasing the

acid environment of the stomach (locally or systemically acting antacids) and affording cytoprotection to the sensitive mucosa. The purpose of antacids is to antagonize the hypersecretory state that occurs (*e.g.,* in systemic mastocytosis or Zollinger-Ellison syndrome) or to create an environment more conducive to ulcer healing.

Parietal cells contain receptor sites for histamine, gastrin, and acetylcholine. When the histamine (H_2) receptor is competitively blocked by an H_2 antagonist, acid production is markedly decreased. H_2 antagonists include cimetidine (Tagamet, Smith Kline Beckman, Philadelphia, PA), and ranitidine (Zantac, Glaxo, Triangle Park, NC). Cimetidine is given every 6 to 8 hours at a dose of 6 to 10 mg/kg. It comes in oral and injectable forms. Duodenal ulcers created experimentally in the dog that were treated with cimetidine showed a remarkable acceleration of ulcer healing, but there was little influence on the healing of experimental gastric ulcers. However, clinical use in cases of spontaneously occurring gastric ulcers has proven effective. Cimetidine is known to decrease hepatic metabolism of warfarin-type anticoagulants, phenytoin, propanolol, and diazepam in humans. It also interferes with the renal elimination of procainamide. The clinical significance of these drug interactions in the dog is not known.

The newer analogue to cimetidine, ranitidine, has the advantage of requiring only twice daily dosing, orally or by injection. It has very few drug interactions and is thought to be 5 to 10 times more potent in decreasing acid production than cimetidine. The useful dosage has not been worked out well in the dog, although I prefer 4 mg/kg orally and 2 mg/kg by injection b.i.d.

The dose of either drug should be decreased if there is renal impairment. Ranitidine has proven to be superior to cimetidine in decreasing ulcer recurrence in man, because of its effect on the quality and quantity of protein within the protective layer of mucus.

Cytoprotective drugs such as sucralfate (Carafate) are agents that derive their ulcer-healing capacity by virtue of their mucosal protective properties. Sucralfate also binds to bile acids at a lower pH and inactivates pepsin. It also has been shown to cause release of prostaglandins, which act as a barrier to back-diffusion of hydrochloric acid. Healing rates resulting from the use of sucralfate and cimetidine are comparable in human clinical trials. Concurrent use of cimetidine is to be avoided because of sucralfate's binding effect on cimetidine. Waiting two hours between sucralfate administration and giving cimetidine is recommended. Concomitant use of ranitidine, however, is acceptable because of its much lower binding capacity for sucralfate (less than 10%).

Sucralfate is safe at extremely high doses in the dog. It has no systemic effects and can be used as the sole drug for treatment of ulcers. The dosage and frequency of sucralfate administration is 250 mg/15 kg given 4 times daily.

Surgical

Surgical treatment of PUD is indicated for uncontrolled hemorrhage, gastric outlet obstruction, or acute perforation. Various procedures can be used, depending on the location and extent of the ulcer lesions. Ulcer resection with or without pyloroplasty is the most commonly used procedure; gastric resection and gastroduodenostomy or gastrojejunostomy are used when more extensive resection is necessary.

The prognosis for benign canine ulcer disease depends primarily on the number of predisposing factors and the severity of the underlying disease. With concurrent hepatic or renal disease, the prognosis is guarded. Dogs with ulcers secondary to mastocytosis or Zollinger-Ellison syndrome generally carry a poorer prognosis.

Neoplasia

Gastric neoplasia occurs infrequently in dogs and cats. Generally it is a disease of older animals with an average age at diagnosis of 9 years.

Benign Neoplasms

Leiomyomas and adenomatous polyps are benign tumors involving the stomach. Leiomyomas are the most common benign tumors in the dog. They seldom cause clinical signs. Polyps are a result of mucosal proliferation and probably are secondary to chronic mucosal irritation. These may occur as single or multiple growths and generally have no signs associated with them unless they are in the pyloric antrum, in which case, gastric outflow obstruction can result.

Vomiting is the most frequent sign of benign gastric tumors. The severity and timing of vomiting depends on the amount of gastric tissue involved and to what degree pyloric outflow obstruction occurs. If obstruction is complete, vomiting will be frequent, particularly following meals. Occasionally, the vomiting may be delayed 6 to 12 hours after eating, and it may be intermittent if the lesion is a polyp that occasionally is positioned at the pylorus where it acts like a ball valve. In rare instances, hematemesis or melena occurs.

Survey abdominal radiographs seldom show a lesion unless it is extensive. Contrast radiography may demonstrate thickening of the stomach wall (if the view is tangential at the right place), a filling defect, and delayed gastric emptying. Fluoroscopy demonstrates delayed gastric emptying if the antrum is involved. At gastroscopy, mucosal changes may be observed. Biopsy of abnormal tissue should help the veterinarian arrive at a definitive diagnosis.

Surgical exploration is necessary in most cases to better define the extent of the lesion. If involvement is limited to the corpus or fundus, local resection generally is curative. Involvement of the antrum necessitates partial gastrectomy followed by some form of gastric reconstruction. The prognosis following surgery for a benign tumor involving the stomach is good.

Malignant Neoplasms

Adenocarcinomas are the most common malignant tumors involving the stomach of the dog. These tumors account for approximately 1% of all malignant tumors in the dog and for 70% of all gastric tumors.

Adenocarcinoma is seen most often in dogs that are 8 years of age or older, and males are affected more often than females. These tumors arise most commonly in the distal stomach along the lesser curvature. Three configurations of adenocarcinoma occur: plaque-like mucosal lesions that are centrally ulcerated; polypoid masses that protrude into the lumen; or, an infiltrative lesion that results in a diffusely thickened stomach that becomes nondistensible (linitis plastica). The latter is also termed scirrhous adenocarcinoma.

Sarcomas are rare in the canine stomach. In cats, however, lymphosarcomas are the most common malignant gastric tumors. They can occur in FeLV negative cats. A lymphosarcoma may be a localized raised mass but, more frequently, it diffusely infiltrates the stomach wall. This tumor usually concurrently involves other abdominal viscera.

Clinical signs of canine gastric adenocarcinoma include weight loss, anorexia, hematemesis, melena, increasingly severe vomiting, and some abdominal discomfort. The gastric mass rarely is palpable. Older dogs with these clinical signs should be suspected of having gastric neoplasia.

Plain film abdominal radiography usually is not diagnostic unless the stomach wall is greatly thickened. If pyloric involvement is severe, the stomach may be dilated and full of fluid and gas. Positive contrast gastrography is most helpful in defining the extent and nature of the lesion, and fluoroscopy may demonstrate areas of the stomach that are thickened and lack significant motility. Decreased motility is suggestive of a scirrhous adenocarcinoma.

Polypoid masses or ulcerated tumors are demonstrable by gastroscopy. Neoplasia not involving the mucosa, however, may not be seen. When a lesion is visible, a biopsy should be taken. Tissue taken from the outer border of an ulcerated lesion is most likely to be diagnostic.

The "rule-out" list should include mycotic disease (phycomycosis), which often presents with lesions similar to the scirrhous form of adenocarcinoma, but usually in younger dogs. Benign gastric ulcer disease, adenomatous polyps, or eosinophilic gastropathy may present with signs similar to those associated with an adenocarcinoma. These benign diseases carry a more favorable prognosis and are usually treated surgically and medically with a good rate of success.

Surgical resection is the preferred treatment for malignant gastric tumors. It also allows further abdominal exploration and lymph node removal to stage the disease more accurately. Partial gastrectomy usually is indicated, along with some form of reconstruction to reestablish gastrointestinal continuity. On occasion, it may be necessary to perform a total gastric resection. However, given the poor to grave prognosis associated with advanced gastric adenocarcinoma, euthanasia should be considered. In less severe cases, surgery is palliative, allowing the animal to survive for several months with a better quality of life.

In cats, lymphosarcoma can be treated by surgical removal of the single or multiple masses followed by chemotherapy. In some cases, the response is favorable.

In general, the prognosis for malignant gastric tumors in the dog and cat is poor because of the degree of involvement at the time of diagnosis, the complications and morbidity associated with gastric resection, and the high rate of metastatic disease. If a lymphosarcoma or gastric adenocarcinoma is diffusely infiltrative, the prognosis is even poorer.

Gastric Phycomycosis

Phycomycosis rarely is reported in the dog, but it is an important consideration if a young dog is presented for vomiting and an abdominal mass that is thought to involve the stomach.

The genera of fungi that can infect the viscera include *Mucor, Absidia,* and *Rhizopus.* These organisms are ubiquitous in the soil and have airborne spores. They can become pathogenic after invading devitalized or ulcerated tissue. In humans, three factors contribute to the emergence of phycomycosis:

1. Lowered host resistance due to antecedent disease
2. Damaged tissue allowing a portal of entry
3. Disturbance of the normal flora due to the use of corticosteroids or antibiotics

Local tissue damage or a disseminated form of the disease can occur once the organism becomes established. Localized lesions may respond well to surgical excision. In dogs, however, lesions of phycomycosis rarely are well-defined and usually are nonresectable. The radiographic and gross appearance of the involved tissue mimics a neoplastic process. When the stomach is affected, a partial gastrectomy may be possible. Healthy margins are difficult to determine on gross inspection. Liberal resection of diseased tissue with apposition of healthy-appearing tissue will help minimize wound dehiscence. An omental or serosal patch placed over the suture line may be indicated.

Surgical Procedures

Gastrotomy

Gastrotomy in dogs and cats is indicated primarily to remove a foreign body, but also is used to explore for ulcer disease, neoplasia, or benign hypertrophy. The morbidity and mortality related to gastrotomy is very low.

A cranial ventral midline abdominal incision gives good exposure of the stomach, which is isolated from the rest of the abdominal cavity with moistened laparotomy sponges to decrease the likelihood of contamination. Two Babcock tissue forceps or 3-0 silk retention sutures are placed 10 to 15 cm apart on the relatively hypovascular area of the stomach, halfway between the lesser and greater curvatures. A stab incision into the gastric lumen is made with a #11 scalpel blade. Metzenbaum scissors are used to extend the incision to the desired length. Suction is used to remove and prevent spillage of gastric contents. Adequate visual and tactile exploration of the stomach and distal esophagus is possible through the gastrotomy incision.

Closure involves two layers of sutures. The first layer is a continuous inverting horizontal mattress (Connell) suture pattern involving all layers of the stomach. An alternative is to use a simple continuous suture pattern closing only the mucosa and submucosa. Surgical gut should not be used in this layer of the gastrotomy closure because of its rapid digestion by gastric enzymes and acid. Polyglactin 910 (Vicryl, Ethicon Corp., Somerville, NJ) or polydioxanone (3-0 or 4-0—PDS, Ethicon Corp., Somerville, NJ) is the ideal suture choice, although a nonabsorbable suture such as monofilament polypropylene or nylon is acceptable. The second layer of closure is done with a vertical (Lembert) or horizontal (Cushing) continuous inverting mattress suture pattern. This layer provides additional strength to the closure while giving more protection against leakage. A Halsted inverting mattress pattern may be substituted, but it has the disadvantage of being an interrupted pattern requiring more time.

The stomach is a highly vascular organ and heals rapidly. On occasion, however, the gastrotomy closure may incorporate diseased tissue in the suture line. In this instance, a piece of vascularized omentum or a serosal patch, provided by a segment of jejunum, should be sutured over the wound for additional reinforcement and protection against leakage.

Gastrostomy

The enteral route of alimentation is most ideal for the small animal patient. It can be provided via a pharyngostomy tube, needle jejunostomy, a nasogastric tube, or tube gastrostomy. Feeding via the gastrointestinal tract has been shown to have favorable effects on intestinal histology and structure, which are absent when the intravenous route is used. Parenteral hyperalimentation may be substituted for the enteral route, but it is riskier, more costly, and less physiologic. Furthermore, animals maintained intravenously are less able to overcome

a septic challenge compared to those fed by enteral means.

Percutaneous Tube Gastrostomy

A tube feeding gastrostomy may be employed to provide patients with their caloric, protein and water requirements. I prefer the percutaneous placement of a tube gastrostomy, but it requires endoscopy. A size 16 to 20 French mushroom-tipped catheter (Bard Urological Catheter, Bard Urological Div., CR Bard, Inc., Murray Hill, NJ) is used. The animal is placed in right lateral recumbency under a light plane of anesthesia or neuroleptoanalgesia (Fig. 12-4A). A 4 cm × 4 cm area behind the last rib is clipped and surgically prepared. A 3–4 mm stab incision is made through the skin at this site. An endoscope is placed into the stomach and the tip directed to lie under the skin incision. The stomach is inflated with air until the stomach bulges against the abdominal wall. A 16- or 18-gauge sheathed catheter is abruptly inserted percutaneously into the lumen of the stomach through the skin incision. Following stylet removal a length of #1 or #2 silk or polyester suture is passed into the stomach via the catheter sheath. A forceps or basket snare grasps the suture and the entire endoscopic unit is withdrawn from the stomach (Fig. 12-4C). The suture is passed retrograde through another 18-gauge sheathed catheter (Fig. 12-5A). The end of the catheter opposite the mushroom tip is modified to fit snugly within the flared end of the sheath catheter. A water-soluble jelly is applied liberally to the catheter, suture, and sheath. The catheter then is pulled into the stomach via the suture exiting the abdominal wall incision. Constant and steady traction advances the sheath and attached mushroom catheter through the stomach and abdominal wall until the mushroom tip is felt to rest gently against the mucosa (Fig. 12-5B, C). A traction suture affixes the tube securely to the skin (Fig. 12-5D). An abdominal wrap is applied to protect against self-mutilation or catheter removal. Twenty-four hours later and before using the tube to give

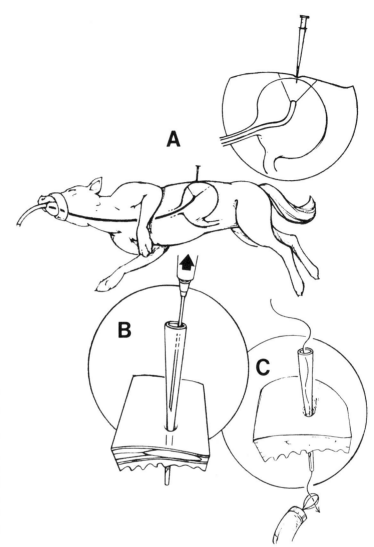

Figure 12-4. *Percutaneous tube gastrostomy.* **A,** *With the animal in right lateral recumbency, an endoscope is placed into the stomach, the stomach insufflated with air, and a sheathed catheter inserted abruptly into the stomach lumen through a small (3-mm) incision in the skin.* **B,** *The stylet is withdrawn, and a suture is passed into the stomach lumen and grasped by a 4-prong forceps or basket snare* **(C).** *The suture is then withdrawn to the exterior via the oral cavity.*

food or water, a small amount of water-soluble contrast material is injected into the tube and radiography or fluoroscopy is done to confirm intragastric presence of the tube.

Tube removal should not be done before the sixth or seventh day. In dogs 20 kg or larger, the tube can be cut free at the skin surface and the mushroom tip pushed back into the stomach. In smaller animals, the tip can be endoscopically retrieved, or it may be removed by pulling on the tube with steady traction. This latter technique should be limited to those cases in which the tube has been in for 3 weeks or longer.

Percutaneous tube gastrostomy can be used for either short-term or long-term nutritional support. I have used it for over 1 year in both dogs and cats.

Operative Tube Gastrostomy Without Separate Celiotomy

This technique does not require endoscopy but does necessitate a surgical plane of anesthesia and a small celiotomy incision. A left-sided 4 to 6 cm long paracostal skin incision is made just below the epaxial musculature with the

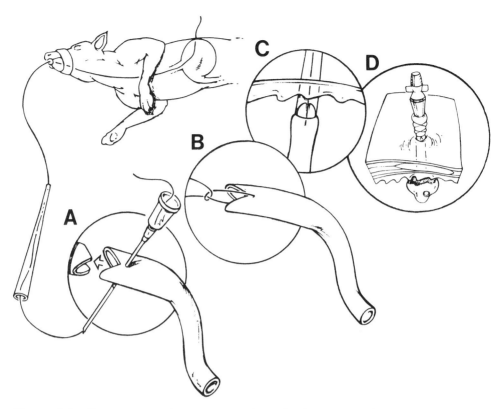

Figure 12-5. *Percutaneous tube gastrostomy (cont'd). The suture is placed retrograde through another catheter sheath. **A,** The end of the catheter is modified by cutting a v-shaped piece out of the tip. The suture is then placed transversely through the gastrostomy catheter using an 18-gauge hypodermic needle. **B,** The suture is then tied in a square knot, and with steady traction it is used to pull the modified catheter tip into the flared end of the catheter sheath. **C,** The suture exiting the abdominal skin incision gently pulls the well-lubricated catheter unit into the stomach and, with the tip of the catheter sheath acting as a dilator, is pulled through the stomach and abdominal wall. **D,** The tube is then fixed securely to the skin.*

animal in right lateral recumbency (Fig. 12-6). A grid incision through abdominal musculature allows entrance into the abdominal cavity. A portion of the fundus is exteriorized, and a Foley catheter (20–24 Fr) is placed into the stomach as described under the tube gastropexy section, below. The grid incision is closed with the tube and the long ends of the purse-string sutures exiting through the middle portion of the incision. Subcutaneous tissues and skin are closed routinely. The tube is then anchored to the skin using the free ends of the purse string suture. The suture is placed

through a tape butterfly with a slight degree of traction placed on the tube to get good apposition between the skin and stomach wall. The suture is tied into a bow. To remove the tube, the bow is untied and the ends of the suture are pulled free of the butterfly tape. The catheter balloon is drained, and the Foley catheter is withdrawn from the stomach. As the tube is pulled, the purse string suture is tightened simultaneously. The purse string knot is released into the abdomen. The wound then is closed primarily or is allowed to heal by second intention.

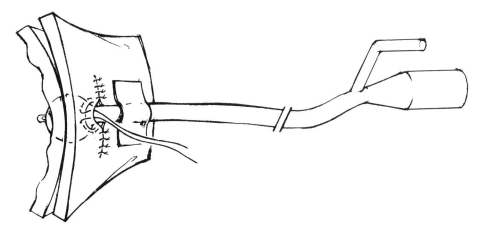

Figure 12-6. *Operative placement of a feeding tube gastrostomy. A Foley catheter is placed into the gastric fundus through an incision surrounded by a purse-string suture. The catheter is then sutured in place to the skin through a butterfly tape using the free ends of the purse-string suture. (Modified from Crane SJ. Compend Contin Ed Pract Vet 1980;2:773.)*

Tube Gastrostomy

A Foley catheter (20–24 Fr) is passed through a small paramedian skin incision caudal to the last rib. A purse-string suture is placed in the antrum followed by a stab incision into the lumen of the stomach. The tip of the catheter is placed into the stomach, the bulb is inflated, and the purse-string suture is secured (Fig. 12-7). The seromuscularis of the stomach is then sutured in four to six places to the abdominal wall using 1-0 or #1 nonabsorbable suture. Omentum may be interposed between the stomach and the abdominal wall to help decrease leakage. The Foley catheter remains in place for at least 5 to 7 days before removal. The presence of the tube allows for either intermittent or continuous gastric decompression postoperatively. The adhesion that forms is secure; recurrence of GDV is reported to be approximately 5% with this technique. Some surgeons feel it is the preferred technique when a partial gastrectomy is done for removal of nonviable tissue. The need to invade the gastric lumen to perform this procedure, with its attendant risk of leakage peritonitis around the tube, the potential for the tube to accidentally come out or be removed by the patient, and longer hospitalization time are the main disadvantages to this technique, when compared with circumcostal gastropexy.

Circumcostal Gastropexy

I prefer the circumcostal gastropexy technique for GDV (Fig. 12-8). It is easily performed, the stomach lumen is not entered, and it is thought to produce better anatomical alignment of the stomach. Two stay sutures of 1-0 or 2-0 polypropylene or nylon are placed proximally and distally in the antrum midway between the lesser and greater curvature. A 3 × 3 cm incision is made through the seromuscular layer between these stay sutures following in "I" configuration. Each flap is undermined to its base. The eleventh or twelfth rib is located below the costochondral junction and isolated with two towel clamps placed approximately 5 cm apart. The rib is exposed by incising the peritoneum and transversus abdominis musculature, and a circumcostal tunnel is created with a large curved clamp. The caudal arm of each stay suture is passed through the circumcostal tunnel. The gastric wall flap on the greater curvature side is pulled up and around the rib using another stay suture or Babcock

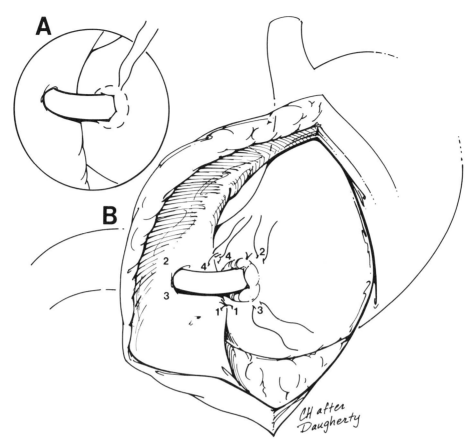

Figure 12-7. *Tube gastropexy technique. **A,** A Foley catheter is placed within the antrum and held in place with a purse-string suture. **B,** The catheter exits the right abdominal wall and is securely affixed to the skin. (Modified from Orton CE. Gastric dilatation—volvulus. In: Kirk RW, ed. Current veterinary therapy IX. Philadelphia: WB Saunders, 1986:860.)*

forceps. The two stay sutures then are tied securely around the rib cranial and caudal to the flap. The two flaps then are sutured to each other using 2-0 polypropylene or nylon, in a simple interrupted pattern. A second layer of sutures between the peritoneal wall and gastric seromuscularis completes the procedure. This technique has been proven to be biomechanically stronger than any of the other gastropexy procedures. The recurrence rate of GDV following use of this technique has been reported to be between 0% and 5%.

Surgery of the Pylorus

In general, most patients undergo pyloric surgery because of vomiting. The vomiting may be sporadic and infrequent, or it can be chronic and frequent, resulting in serious metabolic changes. A thorough clinical and biochemical assessment of these patients is mandatory. Hypochloremia, hypokalemia, metabolic alkalosis, and dehydration often accompany the vomiting episodes. Before surgery is per-

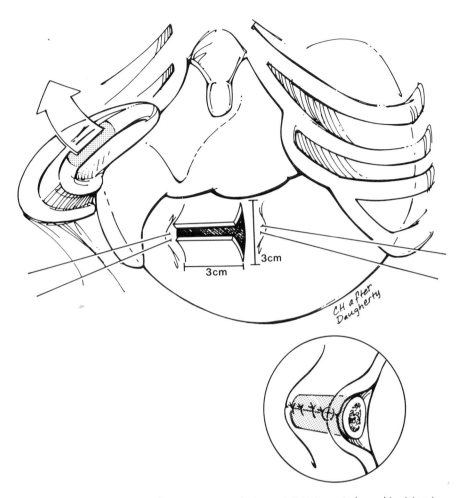

Figure 12-8. *Circumcostal gastropexy technique. A 3 × 3 cm I-shaped incision is made through the seromuscular layer of tissue overlying the antrum. The flap created on the greater curvature side is brought around the 11th or 12th rib below the costochondral junction and sutured back to the opposite flap. (Modified from Orton CE. Gastric dilatation—volvulus. In: Kirk RW, ed. Current veterinary therapy IX. Philadelphia: WB Saunders, 1986:859.*

formed, treatment should be directed towards correction of electrolyte and fluid imbalances. Total protein (albumin) and blood glucose levels should be monitored closely in young animals.

Fluid therapy should be started with an electrolyte and dextrose solution, usually 2.5% dextrose in saline 0.45%, at twice maintenance levels to correct water and chloride deficits. Potassium chloride can be added to these so-

lutions at a rate of 30 mEq/liter. Occasionally, plasma (10 ml/kg) is required in hypoalbuminemic patients.

A nasogastric suction tube should be inserted into the stomach following preoperative sedation. This will allow thorough evacuation of stomach contents, lessening the likelihood of aspiration pneumonia and peritoneal contamination.

Common problems after antral or pyloric

surgery include vomiting for 1 to 2 days and electrolyte imbalances. For this reason, intravenous fluids should be administered for at least 36 to 48 hours postoperatively. Frequent monitoring of blood glucose and albumin (especially in young animals) and electrolytes (in all animals) is recommended.

Pyloromyotomy (Fredet-Ramstedt)

This procedure is used to widen the outflow tract of the stomach to enhance gastric emptying. Its primary indication is in congenital pyloric stenosis. It should *not* be used when inspection or biopsy of the gastric mucosa is necessary.

After a cranial midline ventral abdominal incision, the greater curvature of the stomach is grasped to help elevate the pylorus out of the wound. The small gastrohepatic ligament is incised partially from mediad to laterad. Care is taken not to transect the common bile duct or the proper hepatic or right gastric arteries that lie dorsal to the ligament. Transecting this ligament allows more mobility of the pylorus. The rest of the abdomen is packed off with moistened laparotomy sponges, and two stay sutures or Babcock forceps are placed proximal and distal to the pylorus. An incision through the serosal and muscular layers allows the submucosal/mucosal layers to bulge (Fig. 12-9). The incision should extend into the antrum. All muscle fibers must be incised. Blunt dissection should be used to separate the mucosa from the muscularis over at least 180° of the pylorus. Should mucosal perforation occur, repair of the mucosal rent or conversion to a pyloroplasty should be performed. This pyloric procedure is simple and has few complications.

Pyloroplasty

In a pyloroplasty, the pyloric sphincter is transected surgically and reconstructed. Pyloroplasty originally was designed to relieve obstruction and the symptoms caused by duodenal ulcer in humans. Today, these techniques are employed in veterinary medicine for treatment of chronic hypertrophic pyloric gastropathy (CHPG), ulcer disease, some benign forms of neoplasia, and a functional (neurogenic) form of pyloric stenosis.

Heineke–Mikulicz Pyloroplasty

The Heineke–Mikulicz is probably the most frequently employed pyloroplasty technique in veterinary medicine today. A full-thickness longitudinal incision is made through the pyloric sphincter, extending 1 cm into both the antrum and duodenum. (Fig. 12-10A). The incision is then closed transversely starting in the middle and suturing laterally (Fig. 12-10B). Either a full thickness simple interrupted appositional or a Gambee suture pattern is used to close the wound (Fig. 12-10, inset). Either a synthetic absorbable or a nonabsorbable suture (3-0 or 4-0) is recommended. A two-layer inverting closure is contraindicated, because it invaginates too much tissue into the lumen, thereby diminishing the effect of the procedure. The Heineke–Mikulicz pyloroplasty allows limited exploration of the lumen of the stomach and proximal duodenum.

Finney Pyloroplasty

This technique actually results in a wider gastroduodenostomy than the Heineke–Mikulicz, with transection and inclusion of the pyloric sphincter (Fig. 12-11). It provides a wider stoma than other techniques and can be more securely closed, because multiple layers of closure can be used without compromise of lumen diameter. This procedure is technically more difficult and is associated with a higher rate of duodenogastric reflux in the dog than are other pyloroplasty techniques.

Y-U Antral Flap Pyloroplasty

This procedure is now used in the dog and cat with excellent experimental and clinical results. It involves the plastic surgery technique of conversion of a Y-shaped incision into a U-shaped closure (Fig. 12-12). Each limb of the "Y" incision should be 3 to 5 cm in length depending on the size of the animal. The base of

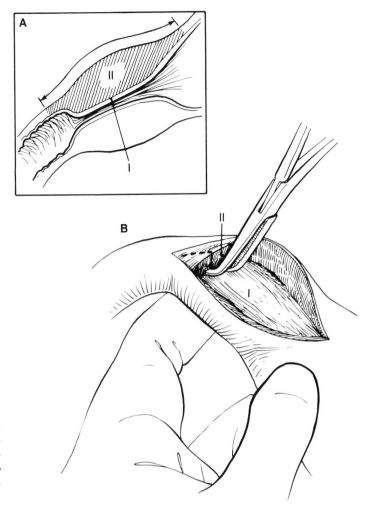

Figure 12-9. *Fredet-Ramstedt pyloromyotomy.* **A,** *The incision across the pylorus extends well into the distal stomach and proximal duodenum.* **B,** *All muscle fibers (II) are gently dissected free of the mucosa and submucosa (I) with a hemostat.*

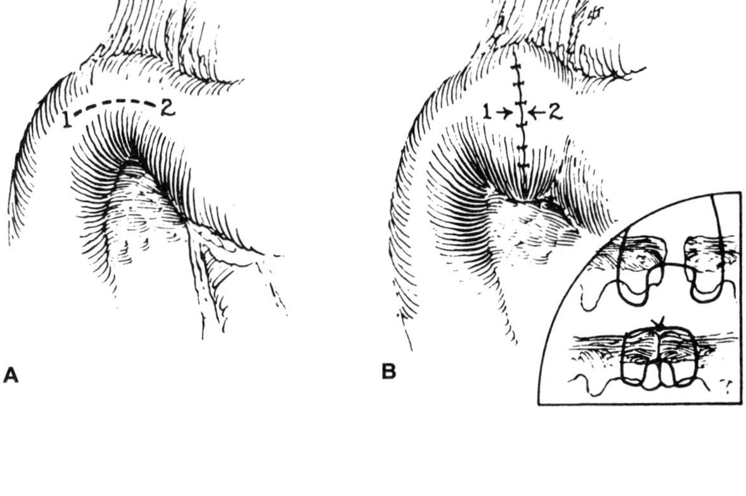

Figure 12-10. *Heineke-Mikulicz pyloroplasty.* **A,** *A longitudinal full-thickness incision is made extending into the antrum and duodenum, point 1 to 2.* **B,** *The incision is then closed transversely by apposing point 1 to point 2 using a simple interrupted appositional suture pattern. A Gambee suture can be substituted to more easily invert the mucosa* **(inset).**

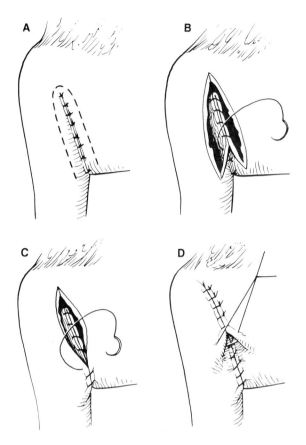

Figure 12-11. *Finney pyloroplasty. **A,** The medial wall of the duodenum is approximated to the antrum with simple interrupted seromuscular sutures. An inverted U-shaped incision is made across the pylorus. **B,** The mucosa is joined caudally by a continuous suture. **C,** This suture is continued across the front wall. **D,** Interrupted seromuscular sutures complete the procedure.*

the "Y" should always extend a small distance into the proximal duodenum. A flap of antrum is moved into the defect created by a longitudinal incision of the sphincter and duodenal wall. A double layer closure originally was described for this technique, but I prefer a simple interrupted appositional full-thickness suture pattern using 3-0 or 4-0 polypropylene. The tip of the flap is sutured first, followed by closure of the lesser curvature, and finally the greater curvature limb.

The Y-U pyloroplasty gives excellent exposure of lesions in the distal stomach. It also allows concomitant resection of hypertrophied mucosa as seen with CHPG, and can be used to resect ulcers and small tumors located in the antrum or proximal duodenum. Duodenogastric reflux, which is commonly seen following most pyloroplasty procedures, is minimal after use of this method.

Gastrectomy Procedures

Billroth I Gastroduodenostomy

This procedure was originally developed in humans to treat cancer of the pyloric region of the stomach. In the dog and cat it is used for treating neoplasia, ulcer disease, CHPG, and infiltrative inflammatory diseases. The Billroth I procedure for cancer should be used for tumors only if they are small, single polypoidal adenomas or carcinomas of the body or antrum of the stomach. Partial gastric resection with Billroth I repair can also be used to correct pyloroplasties that have failed.

The amount of stomach resected depends on the extent of the disease. Variable amounts of tissue above and below the pylorus can be removed. If the pathological changes are limited to the pylorus, such as seen in CHPG, a pylorectomy and gastroduodenostomy can be used. For ulcer disease, the entire antrum should be resected. Resection of a tumor that extends proximally into the stomach may require a Billroth I modification. Regardless of the indication for a gastroduodenostomy, 1 cm of duodenum must be available proximal to the opening of the common bile duct to allow an anastomosis of stomach to the duodenum.

Resection of the involved gastric tissue begins by ligating the vessels that supply the greater and lesser curvature and attached omentum. The pylorus is freed by partially incising the gastrohepatic ligament. The area to be resected should then be isolated from the abdominal cavity with moistened laparotomy sponges to decrease contamination by spillage. Large straight intestinal clamps are placed above and below the proposed lines of incision. After the tissue is resected completely, closure

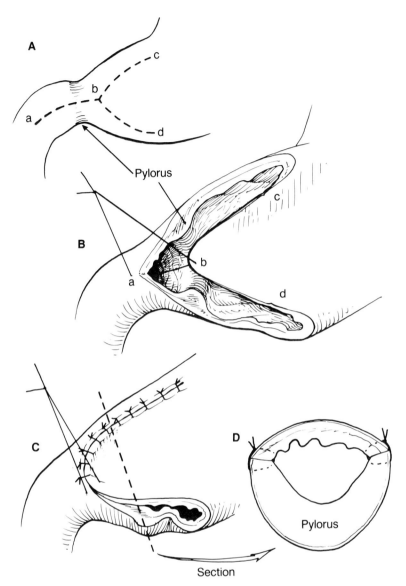

Figure 12-12. *The Y-U advancement flap pyloroplasty.* **A,** *A Y-shaped full thickness incision extends into the proximal duodenum and antrum; points a to b, b to c, and b to d are equal in length (approximately 4–5 cm).* **B,** *The tip of the antral flap is trimmed to a U-shape to avoid necrosis of a pointed tip. This flap is then advanced distally and anastomosed to the duodenum.* **C,** *The lesser curvature side is sutured, followed by the greater curvature side, using a simple interrupted appositional pattern.* **D,** *A cross section of the pylorus demonstrates the enlarged diameter provided by the antral flap.*

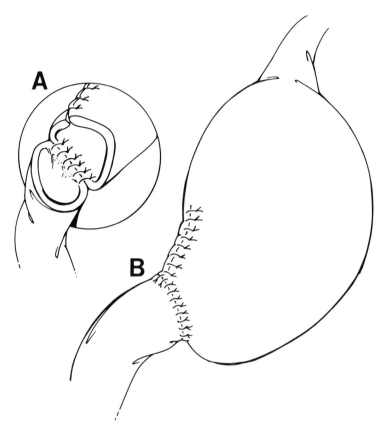

Figure 12-13. *A partial gastrectomy is followed by a gastroduodenostomy (Billroth I). Lumen disparity is corrected by partially closing the stomach* **(A)** *before anastomosing the stomach to the proximal duodenum* **(B).**

of the lesser curvature side is done until the gastric luminal opening is approximately equal in size to that of the duodenal segment (Fig. 12-13).

The Billroth I procedure is best used in the dog when distal stomach resection is done. It is preferred over the more radical Billroth II procedure, because the latter technique is associated more often with the postoperative "dumping syndrome" or marginal ulceration.

Billroth II Gastrojejunostomy

The term Billroth II describes various surgical procedures that have one common feature: following gastric resection, the duodenal stump (often distal to the point of entry of the common bile duct) is closed, and the stomach is anastomosed to a loop of jejunum. Gastrojejunal reconstruction can be used for extensive

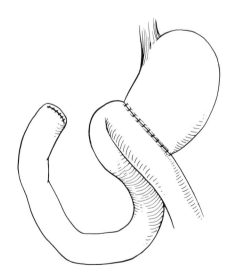

Figure 12-14. *Billroth II modification. An end-to-side gastrojejunostomy is performed using the entire width of the stomach to form the stoma. Partial closure of the stomach may be done prior to this anastomosis.*

ulcer disease or after resection of gastric tumors. It is also indicated for treatment of extensive infiltrative diseases of the stomach.

The original Billroth II technique in humans included closure of the stomach stoma followed by a gastrojejunostomy via a new incision on the ventral aspect of the stomach. For more extensive resections, it was found to be simpler to anastomose the entire width of the gastric stump stoma to the jejunum (Fig. 12-14). A subsequent modification involved partial closure of the gastric stump prior to the gastrojejunostomy, thereby decreasing the stoma size. Gastrojejunostomy involves ligation and diversion of the common bile duct and cholecystoduodenostomy and, possibly, amputation of a portion of the pancreas.

Suggested Readings

Boudrieau RJ, Rogers WA. Megaesophagus in the dog: a review of 50 cases. J Am Anim Hosp Assoc 1985;21:33.

Bright RM, Burrows CB. Percutaneous endoscopic tube gastrostomy in dogs. Am J Vet Res 1988; 5:629.

Bright RM, Richardson DC, Stanton ME. Y-U antral flap advancement pyloroplasty in dogs. Compend Contin Ed Pract Vet 1988;10:139.

Ellison GW. Vascular ring anomalies in the dog and cat. Compend Contin Ed Pract Vet 1980;9:693.

Ellison GW, Phillips L, Tarvin GB. Esophageal hiatal hernia in small animals: literature review and a modified surgical technique. J Am Anim Hosp Assoc 1987;23:391.

Fallah AM, Lumb WV, Nelson AW, et al. Circumcostal gastropexy in the dog: a preliminary study. Vet Surg 1982;11:9.

Parks JL, Greene RW. Tube gastrostomy for the treatment of gastric volvulus. J Am Anim Hosp Assoc 1976;12:168.

Stanton ML, Bright RM, Toal R, et al. Effects of the Y-U pyloroplasty on gastric emptying and duodenogastric reflux in the dog. Vet Surg 1987;16:392.

Walshaw R, Johnston DE. Treatment of gastric dilatation—volvulus by gastric decompression and patient stabilization before major surgery. J Am Anim Hosp Assoc 1976;12:162.

Walters MC, Goldschmidt MH, Stone EA, et al. Chronic hypertrophic pyloric gastropathy as a cause of pyloric obstruction in the dog. J Am Vet Med Assoc 1985;186:157.

Walters MC, Matthieson DT, Stone EA: Pylorectomy and gastroduodenostomy in the dog: technique and clinical results in 28 cases. J Am Vet Med Assoc 1985;187:909.

13

H. Jay Harvey

The Small and Large Intestines

Principles of Intestinal Surgery

Fluid Therapy

Most animals that need surgery of the small or large bowel are physiologically compromised to some extent. Structural disease of bowel, the only type of bowel disease amenable to surgical treatment, usually results in one or a combination of occurrences: the animal vomits, has diarrhea, develops local or systemic infection or toxemia, or malabsorbs nutrients. All of these may occur simultaneously or sequentially in a single animal. In such instances, a most significant event is the alteration of normal fluid and electrolyte balances. These may vary with the extent of disease and

with time, but are always present to some degree. Extracellular and intracellular fluids and their associated constituents are lost externally (through vomiting or diarrhea) or internally (through peritonitis, splanchnic sequestration, or ileus) and are unavailable to sustain the patient's normal physiologic processes.

The most obvious physical manifestation of this fluid loss is dehydration. Understanding that dogs and cats with surgical bowel disease always are ill, and that much of this illness results from fluid and electrolyte imbalances, is essential in planning effective perioperative care.

The principles of fluid therapy are discussed in Chapter 1, Principles of Small Animal Surgery. Ideally, the type and extent of fluid therapy needed for dogs and cats with surgical bowel disease should be individualized. Unfortunately, the occasional need for haste and/or the lack of adequate laboratory facilities for quickly determining imbalances forces the clinician to rely on clinical judgment, physical findings, and a knowledge of what imbalances are most likely. In general, using balanced electrolyte solutions is safest when specific abnormalities have not or cannot be determined. The choice of fluids can be based on losses predicted from the location of the lesion in the bowel, and clinical signs.

For example, pyloric or very proximal duodenal obstructions cause loss predominantly of gastric contents because of vomition, so the predominant losses include hydrogen and chloride ions (from hydrochloric acid). Thus, the principal acid-base alteration would be metabolic (hypochloremic) alkalosis, with some attempt at compensation by the respiratory system. The loss of hydrogen and chloride ions in the vomitus leads to their retention, along with sodium, by the kidneys. Potassium then is lost in exchange for the sodium and hydrogen. Therefore, the clinician preparing a patient with pyloric or high duodenal obstruction for surgery could assume that physiologic saline, perhaps with added potassium, would be the fluid most likely to restore predicted losses.

On the other hand, acute mid-duodenal obstructions result in vomition of the alkaline contents of the proximal duodenum (including that from the pancreas and biliary tract), as well as the stomach acids. Balanced electrolyte solutions, such as lactated Ringer's, would be the best to use in this situation. Distal jejunal or ileal obstructions or bowel obstructions of gradual onset at any site may produce relatively few imbalances until late in the course of disease, when obstruction becomes complete and effects become acute.

Thus, the safest course in a dog or cat with presumed surgical bowel disease is to assume that imbalances exist and to initiate treatment with solutions that will not worsen these imbalances. Fluid therapy at shock treatment dosage (up to 90 ml/kg) may be indicated during the first 3 hours of presentation if severe dehydration exists.

Antibiotics

Perioperative prophylactic administration of antibiotics is controversial, although the potential for peritoneal contamination by bowel contents, either from the disease process or from surgery, logically supports their use. The defense mechanisms of the peritoneal cavity in normal dogs and cats usually can deal with a minor single infectious insult. Unfortunately, many patients needing bowel surgery are either in no condition to mount an effective response to infection or have a source of continuous peritoneal contamination.

It is well accepted that antibiotics are most effective in preventing infection if adequate tissue concentrations exist at the time of an infectious insult. Broad-spectrum antibiotic therapy, preferably administered intravenously (*e.g.*, cephalothin, Keflex, Eli Lilly, Indianapolis, IN, 22 mg/kg every 6 hours), should be started 1 to 2 hours before surgery whenever feasible. As it is also generally believed that antibiotics are unnecessary once the potential for infection has passed, the drugs should probably be discontinued from 12 to 48 hours postoperatively, assuming there is no obvious indication of active infection. Another argument for discontinuing antibiotics promptly after bowel surgery is that it may ameliorate the clinical signs of suture line leakage and thus prevent the detection of peritonitis until the condition is advanced. Antibiotic use also predisposes to the generation of antibiotic-resistant hospital bacterial flora.

Instrumentation

Most instruments needed to perform bowel surgery are found in standard instrument sets. In addition, intestinal clamps of the Doyen type are useful to the surgeon who must operate without an assistant. However, intestinal clamps should be avoided if at all possible; it is better to have an assistant gently hold and compress the bowel by digital pressure. Both self-retaining abdominal retractors such as Balfours and hand-held retractors such as the malleable type are helpful.

Suture Materials and Techniques

Although arguments have been made that one suture material is superior to another, the type of suture material used rarely determines the success of bowel surgery; proper technique, attention to blood supply, and gentle tissue handling are much more important. Surgical gut, nonabsorbable and absorbable synthetics, and silk all work well when used properly. My preference for bowel surgery is to use 3-0 or 4-0 monofilament nylon with a swaged-on needle with a cutting point and a noncutting shaft. The cutting point penetrates bowel wall without requiring undue force; the shaft and the nylon slide through tissues without drag. The nonabsorbability and low reactivity of nylon is useful in the presence of inflammation or infection, in debilitated or hypoproteinemic animals.

The Small Intestine

Surgical Disorders

Intestinal Obstruction

Intestinal obstruction is a blockage of the flow of intestinal contents (chyme). Several generalizations about small bowel obstruction can be made:

1. The more orad the site of obstruction, the more acute the onset of clinical signs (*e.g.*, vomiting and dehydration) and the more rapid the patient's deterioration. Most of the intestinal fluid and electrolytes are secreted in the stomach and duodenum and absorbed in the jejunum. Obstructions near the pylorus and proximal duodenum negate resorption. Thus, electrolytes and fluid are effectively lost to the body by vomition and sequestration in the bowel. Because the secretory function of compromised bowel is among the last functions to cease, vast quantities of fluids and electrolytes are lost, and dogs and cats with obstructions of the proximal bowel can become seriously ill in a matter of hours. Conversely, obstruction at the level of the ileum may cause mild, nonspecific clinical signs for days or even weeks. Because of this, animals with high obstructions respond better to fluid and electrolyte therapy than do those with low obstructions.

2. Complete obstruction causes significant and early clinical signs; partial obstruction causes few or no signs, and signs arise later.

3. The most important initial physiologic effect of complete acute bowel obstruction is fluid and electrolyte imbalance. The most obvious physical finding in an animal with bowel obstruction is vomiting with progressive dehydration, leading to hypovolemia, poor tissue perfusion, and circulatory collapse.

4. Obstruction associated with disruption of blood supply to the affected segment of bowel (strangulated obstruction) is an acute life-threatening emergency requiring surgical correction while supportive therapy is being administered. When a segment of bowel wall becomes infarcted, with or without luminal obstruction, rupture of the bowel is minutes to hours away.

5. Obstruction can be mechanical or functional. A mechanical obstruction is due to an extensive intramural or intraluminal cause, such as a foreign body or tumor. A functional obstruction occurs without such a cause, often due to a hypodynamic

state such as ileus (see below), and less often due to strangulation of the blood supply to the loop of bowel (see "Intestinal Strangulation," p. 369).

Fig. 13-1 shows the continuum of events resulting from small bowel obstruction.

The diagnosis of small bowel obstruction is made by combining historical, physical, and radiographic data. Dogs and cats with complete obstruction of the proximal small bowel ("high" obstructions) usually have a history of acute vomition. In many instances, the vomiting will be the first obvious indication of illness, although owners often relate that their pet has been lethargic for several hours before the onset of vomition. Vomiting is often first

noticed as a postprandial event, but eventually continues independently of food intake. Anorexia ensues and the animal's general physical status rapidly worsens. The animal may moan, assume a "praying" position, and seem generally uncomfortable. Retching and vomiting may occur repeatedly.

Obstructions affecting the mid-jejunum, caudal jejunum, and ileum usually produce a more gradual onset of signs than the acute illness that obstruction of the duodenum or proximal jejunum produces. Affected animals eventually vomit, but may appear to be nonspecifically ill for several days before the onset of vomition. Owners often describe a progressively more lethargic pet with a gradually decreasing intake of food. Thirst often increases

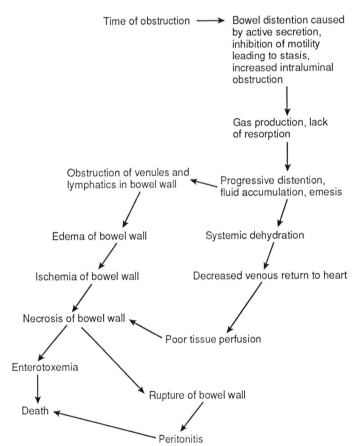

Figure 13-1. *Events associated with small bowel obstruction.*

initially, then decreases as the animal's condition deteriorates. Stools are scanty or nonexistent; indeed, many patients with complete obstruction of the distal small bowel are presented because of what the owner interprets as constipation.

In animals with partial obstruction caused by intussusception of the distal small bowel or of the ileocecocolic junction, vomiting may be delayed until after bloody diarrhea has developed. These animals are usually uncomfortable and restless. Once the intussusception progresses to complete obstruction, vomiting occurs. Bloody diarrhea is often present until the intussusception is surgically corrected; the diarrhea becomes fetid when the bowel mucosa begins to lose viability.

In most cases, owners will be unable to offer much more information than that their pet is sick and vomiting. Careful questioning may reveal helpful information about a missing toy, a bone the animal ate, a trash can it raided, or the disappearance of the string used to tie up last night's roast.

Tumors of the small bowel usually cause insidiously progressive signs. Adenocarcinomas are associated with slow, progressive weight loss and occasional vomition that gradually becomes more frequent. Malignant effusion may result from peritoneal metastasis. Leiomyomas and leiomyosarcomas are associated with partial obstruction, sporadic vomiting, and moderate to minimal weight loss. Bleeding into the intestine is common and eventually results in chronic anemia, lethargy, and fatigue. Lymphosarcoma of the bowel causes profuse, nonresponsive diarrhea and profound weight loss despite adequate or increased food intake; vomiting is rarely a feature of small bowel lymphosarcoma.

Clinical findings in dogs and cats with proximal small bowel obstruction include mental depression and lack of responsiveness, halitosis, poor capillary (mucous membrane) perfusion, dehydration (dry mucous membranes, lack of skin turgor, sunken eyes, and a rapid, thready pulse), moaning, a tense and painful abdomen, and frequent attempts to vomit. Retching may be precipitated by abdominal palpation. Dehydration may be severe.

Animals with a foreign-body obstruction of the distal small bowel eventually develop the same physical findings as those caused by proximal obstruction. However, early in the course of disease, animals with distal obstructions may be only mildly affected. Dehydration may be minimal or nonexistent, vomition may be sporadic or nonexistent, and some animals may retain their appetite.

Radiography is perhaps the most useful aid in diagnosing small bowel obstruction. The most telling radiographic finding is the presence of dilated loops of bowel. In some instances, the actual foreign body may be identifiable; in others, the evidence is circumstantial. Depending on the level of the obstruction, multiple loops of dilated bowel may be visible or only one or two segments of bowel may be dilated. Radiographs of animals with linear foreign bodies often show the bowel clumped together, with an intestinal gas pattern resembling rows of teardrop-shaped lucencies arranged in palisades.

Loss of abdominal detail, coupled with dilated loops of bowel and free gas in the peritoneum, is associated with peritonitis. Thoracic radiographs in severely dehydrated animals show a decrease in the size of the cardiac silhouette and in the diameter of the caudal vena cava, caused by reduced venous return to the heart.

Occasionally, the presence, degree, and site of the intestinal obstruction may be indistinct on plain radiographs. In these instances, contrast radiography of the gastrointestinal tract may be done. Contrast media may be either insoluble (barium sulfate) or water soluble (diatrizoate meglumine). Barium provides more detail and can show subtle abnormalities. Barium also has a soothing and mildly therapeutic effect on irritated bowel. The disadvantage of barium is that it is much more irritating to peritoneal surfaces if spilled during subsequent surgery or if it enters the peritoneal cavity through ruptures or perforations in the bowel wall. A water-soluble contrast medium provides poorer radiographic detail than barium, but is less likely to cause peritonitis. Water-soluble media are slightly hypertonic and tend to potentiate existing dehydration by pulling fluid into the lumen of the bowel.

Laboratory findings are supportive of the diagnosis of bowel obstruction and help determine how ill the patient is, but are rarely pathognomonic for bowel obstruction. However, laboratory values can occasionally identify diseases that produce clinical signs similar to those caused by bowel obstruction. For example, panleukopenia in a vomiting cat may indicate infectious rather than mechanical disease. Similar findings in dogs with hemorrhagic diarrhea might indicate parvovirus infection, whereas an elevated hematocrit with normal red and white cell counts might be associated with canine hemorrhagic gastroenteritis in dogs with bloody diarrhea. Elevated serum amylase and lipase concentrations in vomiting dogs are associated with pancreatitis.

The timing of surgery in a dog or cat with suspected small bowel obstruction is crucial. Correcting fluid and electrolyte imbalances before surgery is desirable, but while fluid therapy may be supportive, it is seldom completely corrective while the obstruction is present. The most efficient mechanism to correct imbalances is the animal's homeostatic system, which is ineffective until the obstruction is relieved. Thus, the surgeon is faced with a dilemma: should the patient's fluid and electrolyte imbalances be completely corrected before surgery, or should surgery be performed early so that the animal, with support, can correct its own imbalances? In general, a middle-of-the-road approach to the timing of surgery for *known* bowel obstruction is desirable; *i.e.*, supportive therapy is administered over a matter of hours, and then surgery is performed. In patients that are obviously benefitting from fluid and electrolyte therapy, surgery can be delayed. Those not responding

or continuing to deteriorate need surgery more quickly, no matter how poor their condition.

Adding to the surgeon's difficulty is the fact that the cause of acute gastrointestinal disease often is unclear. The decision to operate, then, becomes dependent on judgment and intuition. The fundamental rule is that in a questionable situation, performing an early exploratory celiotomy in which no lesion is found is better than delaying surgery until the need for it is unquestionable but the patient's condition has meanwhile deteriorated.

Etiology

Foreign Bodies

The most common cause of small intestinal obstruction in dogs and cats is an ingested object (foreign body). Round, smooth, foreign bodies such as balls tend to produce complete bowel obstruction if large enough, and they may cause pressure necrosis of the bowel wall. Balls that fill the lumen loosely are pushed down the bowel, leaving a trail of distended, edematous gut. Removal requires enterotomy, with resection and anastomosis of any severely compromised segments. Enterotomies to remove foreign bodies should always be long enough to allow removal of the object without further trauma to the bowel wall. Incision in dilated bowel proximal to the object is desirable if the wall is viable.

Foreign bodies with sharp edges, such as bones, rarely cause complete bowel obstruction but tend rather to perforate the bowel wall. Resection of perforated segments of bowel often is required. Some sharp foreign bodies, such as pins or needles without thread, may pass through the intestinal tract without causing perforation or even clinical signs. The passage of such foreign bodies may be followed radiographically.

Linear foreign bodies (string, tinsel, pantyhose, scarves) are more common in cats than in dogs. They cause vomiting, dehydration, and depression. If obstruction is not complete, signs still appear when the proximal portion of the linear foreign body becomes fixed at some point in the alimentary tract. A length of string or thread often loops around the base of the tongue or becomes wedged at the pylorus. A threaded needle also may be fixed in the pharynx or elsewhere. The remaining portion of the string or thread then passes into the small bowel, where peristaltic activity moves it anad. The result is that the bowel gathers along the string, becoming plicated, and sometimes an intussusception results. The mesenteric border becomes taut and edematous as the string embeds in the bowel wall. Eventually, perforation occurs at one or more points along the mesenteric border and peritonitis ensues. Multiple enterotomies, intestinal closure, or even resection and anastomosis may be required.

Animals with known linear foreign bodies and clinical signs should be treated as emergencies; once bowel perforation occurs, the prognosis is poor. If consumption of a linear foreign body can be confirmed but there are no signs, careful observation and radiographic follow-up, in the hope of natural passage, is acceptable. All vomiting cats should have a complete oral examination for the presence of string around the base of the tongue. Examination is facilitated by pushing a thumb upward in the intermandibular space to raise the base of the tongue. If string detected around the tongue of a severely ill cat cannot be pulled easily from the esophagus, it should be cut to minimize further damage to the bowel.

Tumors

Most tumors affecting the small intestine in dogs and cats are malignant. In general, bowel cancers affect middle-aged to older animals and have insidious courses. In older dogs and cats with chronic weight loss, progressively worsening vomiting, chronic diarrhea, or abdominal effusion, neoplasia should be suspected. An abdominal mass may or may not be palpable; the absence of a mass does not rule out intestinal malignancy. If plain or contrast radiographs or laboratory data suggest intestinal neoplasia, a search for distant metastasis is in order before surgery. Preoperatively, this investigation consists of thoracic radiographs to detect pulmonary metastases and ultrasonography to detect hepatic metastases. Detection of metastases by both techniques depends on the size of the nodules present. Elevated serum alanine aminotransferase and alkaline phosphatase concentrations are also suggestive of liver metastases. Intra-operatively, regional (usually mesenteric) lymph nodes should be biopsied; suspicious nodules in the liver or spleen should also be biopsied.

Adenocarcinomas of the intestine tend to be annular and eventually produce a 360° stricturelike effect on the bowel. Clinical signs usually are slow in onset because the tumor requires weeks or months to produce obstruction and because the most common site of occurrence is the distal jejunum and ileum. By the time clinical signs of obstruction occur, there is often evidence of metastasis. Palpably enlarged mesenteric lymph nodes, peritoneal effusion, ultrasonographic evidence of hepatic nodules, and radiographically evident pulmonary lesions may all provide evidence of metastatic disease. At surgery, the omentum and peritoneum are often riddled with metastases (carcinomatosis). Treatment consists of intestinal resection and anastomosis, with removal of wide margins of normal bowel (at least 5 cm on each side of the visible or palpable tumor). Mesenteric node biopsies help stage the disease and determine prognosis in animals without obvious metastasis. Average survival times of 9 to 12 months have been reported in cats with resectable adenocarcinoma grossly confined to the bowel. Treatment for animals with metastatic bowel adenocarcinoma is unrewarding.

Leiomyomas and leiomyosarcomas of the small bowel also may cause complete or partial intestinal obstruction. These tumors arise from the muscular layer of the bowel wall and produce obstruction by impinging on the bowel lumen. Affected animals may show a chronic low-grade anemia before obstruction becomes apparent, as these tumors tend to ulcerate and bleed into the bowel lumen. A positive test for occult blood in the feces is common. The treatment for leiomyoma and leiomyosarcoma is intestinal resection; the prognosis is good for leiomyomas and guarded for leiomyosarcomas. Regional lymph nodes should be evaluated, but this is of questionable benefit because lymph node metastasis is rare with these tumors.

Lymphosarcoma, another common bowel cancer, seldom produces bowel obstruction. The most common clinical finding is malabsorption, usually manifested as a protein-losing enteropathy. Intestinal lymphosarcoma occurs in two forms: a nodular type, with multiple granulomatous lesions throughout the small and large bowel, and a diffusely infiltrative type, in which the bowel appears to be grossly normal. In the latter circumstance, histologic examination of a full- thickness bowel wall biopsy specimen is necessary for diagnosis. Although dogs with malabsorption nearly always are hypoalbuminemic, I have noted few healing problems at the enterotomy sites used for biopsy. Intestinal resection and anastomosis is possible in the rare cases in which lymphosarcoma lesions are discrete, but chemotherapy is the usual treatment of choice.

Less common neoplasms include adenomas (polyps) and carcinoids. Adenomas are rare and may be asymptomatic throughout the animal's life. Adenomas are considered by some to be preneoplastic (though this is unproven in dogs and cats) and can produce irritation leading to intussusception in older animals. Carcinoids are carcinoma-like growths that occur anywhere in the gastrointestinal tract. In dogs and cats, carcinoids can produce effects consistent with space-occupying masses, but are often incidental findings at necropsy or celiotomy. In humans, a carcinoid syndrome is characterized by diarrhea and circulatory disorders such as flushing of the skin, hypertension, sweating, and abdominal discomfort.

Intussusception

Intussusception is the invagination of one part of the intestine into the lumen of an immediately adjoining part. An intussusception is composed of the intussusceptum (the portion of intestine that is invaginated within another part of the intestine) and the intussuscipiens (the portion of intestine into which the intussusceptum invaginates). Intussusception is a cause of complete or partial bowel obstruction, especially in young animals. The cause usually is unknown, but any condition that produces hypermotility of the bowel (enteritis, distemper, parasites, etc.) may result in intussusception. Affected puppies and kittens are presented because of diarrhea, vomiting, and abdominal pain. Palpation demonstrates the presence of a spindleoid, often mobile mass in the abdomen. The tentative clinical diagnosis is based on the age of the animal, clinical signs, and a palpable abdominal mass. Treatment consists of reducing the affected segment if the bowel is viable, and resecting the segment if reduction is not feasible. In young animals, the most commonly affected sites are the distal ileum and ileocecocolic junction.

On rare occasions, the intussusceptum travels anad far enough to protrude from the rectum. In these instances, the intussusception must be differentiated from a rectal prolapse. Differentiation is easily made by attempting to pass a blunt probe or thermometer along the wall of the evaginated portion. Inability to insert the probe more than a few millimeters indicates rectal prolapse, but the probe can readily be passed for its entire length if an intussusception is present. The clinical signs associated with intussusception (sporadic vomiting, hemorrhagic diarrhea, abdominal pain) also help in the diagnosis.

Intussusception cannot be ruled out in older patients, but is not as common as in puppies and kittens. In older animals, the intussusception can occur at any point in the intestine and is often associated with a structural abnormality such as a tumor or stricture. Because of the causes, treatment in older animals usually requires resection and anastomosis.

Volvulus

Volvulus of the small bowel, defined as a twisting of the intestine on its mesenteric root, is rare. Based on limited information, affected dogs often are German shepherds or mixed-breed dogs with German shepherd characteristics, weighing more than 25 kg. Fetid, bloody diarrhea usually is present. Vomiting is an inconsistent clinical sign. Clinical signs are notable by their peracute onset; the entire course of the disease, from onset of signs to death, is usually a matter of hours. Radiographs show massive dilatation of multiple loops of bowel. The gas-filled bowel loops often appear to be arranged in a stellate pattern originating from a central focus in the abdomen. The prognosis is exceedingly poor, regardless of how rapidly treatment is instituted.

Intestinal Strangulation

Strangulation of bowel implies a compromised blood supply to or within the wall of the bowel; this can occur with or without mechanical obstruction. However, the term "strangulated bowel" usually refers to bowel that has become entrapped in inguinal, diaphragmatic, umbilical, perineal, or ventral hernias or in "internal hernias" through a rent in the intestinal mesentery. Strangulation results from twisting or kinking of the arterial supply or venous drainage, or swelling of the bowel wall at a site of incarceration. Affected animals initially display signs of obstruction (vomiting, malaise), but as the bowel lumen distends and constriction of the blood vessels progresses, there is increasing abdominal discomfort and evidence of shock. Radiographs show segmental dilatation of bowel. Gas-filled loops of bowel in the thorax (diaphragmatic hernia), groin (inguinal hernia), or ventral abdominal subcutaneous tissue (umbilical hernia) are diagnostic. Peritonitis resulting from rupture or impending rupture of the bowel is represented by loss of regional detail, the "ground glass" appearance of effusion, and the presence of free gas in the tissues or the peritoneal cavity. Necrosis of the strangulated bowel follows and perforation occurs unless the strangulated bowel is removed promptly. Intestinal strangulation is an emergency of the highest priority.

Intestinal Trauma

Trauma to the small bowel may be blunt, in which the abdominal wall remains intact, or sharp, in which the abdominal wall is penetrated. Of the two, blunt abdominal trauma is the most dangerous, because the need for immediate and aggressive treatment is not always clear until the animal's condition has deteriorated. Blunt abdominal trauma rarely causes direct perforation of the bowel; more commonly, it causes tearing of the mesentery away from the bowel, leading to ischemic necrosis (infarction) of varying lengths of bowel. Affected animals commonly respond to initial treatment (fluids, corticosteroids, and antibiotics), only to deteriorate several hours later. Abdominal pain is progressive and severe. Bowel death commonly is demonstrated by fetid, bloody diarrhea. The prognosis is guarded even when the condition is suspected and treated promptly, and poor if the bowel ruptures.

Penetrating abdominal trauma always is an indication for exploratory celiotomy as soon as the animal's condition permits, or sooner if there is continued deterioration. There may be multiple sites of bowel perforation; a thorough examination of all portions of the bowel is mandatory. Small lacerations sometimes can be debrided and oversewn, but resection and anastomosis should be done unhesitatingly if there is any question about bowel viability. Severely damaged bowel should be removed rather than repaired.

Animals with penetrating wounds near but not directly over the abdominal wall also should be watched closely for signs of bowel damage. For example, the entry and exit wounds of bullets may bear little relationship to the actual trajectory of the missile through the body. Bullets entering anywhere from the eighth rib caudally may be deflected through the abdominal cavity. The course of the missile is altered by repeated contact with soft tissue and bone. Multiple bowel perforations are the rule rather than the exception.

Detecting a perforation sometimes is difficult. Radiography and physical examination are invaluable. Diagnostic lavage may help, but the results are sometimes difficult to interpret. The presence of enteric bacteria and plant fibers in abdominal fluid is an absolute indication for surgery. The presence of blood or inflammatory cells are relative indications, although degenerate neutrophils are highly suggestive of peritonitis (see "Diagnostic Peritoneal Lavage," in Chap. 10, The Abdominal Cavity). The surgeon's chief allies in these situations are a high index of suspicion and the willingness to be aggressive with diagnostic celiotomy.

Surgical Techniques

Celiotomy

The usual approach to the abdominal cavity is via a ventral midline incision; the length of the incision depends on the location of the involved organ(s). To prevent intestinal contents from spilling into the peritoneal cavity or on the edges of the incision, the site of incision or excision of the bowel must be isolated. This is done by applying moistened laparotomy sponges to the wound edges and the exposed tissues in the abdomen (this also keeps them moist). In addition, if the loop of bowel is mobile, it should be exteriorized and the incision "packed off," so surgery can be performed while the other abdominal tissues are protected from contamination.

The surgeon's next task is to determine the viability of the segment of intestine to be surgically manipulated. Viable intestine should be pink, with no segmental or punctate areas of bluish discoloration. The intestinal serosa should bleed readily when incised. Pulsating mesenteric vessels supplying the bowel segment are reassuring, but are not a reliable sign of intestinal viability. Conversely, lack of

pulsation, engorgement, or thrombosis of mesenteric vessels are obvious causes for concern. Peristaltic activity in the bowel segment is also reassuring, but lack of bowel wall motility, especially in dilated bowel, does not necessarily mean the bowel is nonviable.

Because the subjective evaluation of bowel viability is difficult, several methods have been proposed to allow more objective assessments. The most commonly used and practical method is to inject fluoroscein dye (1 mg/kg) into a peripheral vein. Directing an ultraviolet lamp at the questionable segment of bowel causes the adequately perfused portion of bowel to fluoresce. However, this method is not foolproof and requires some judgment in interpreting the margin of normal from abnormal.

There are two fundamental surgical manipulations of small bowel: enterotomy (opening and closing the lumen of the bowel) and resection and anastomosis (removing a segment of bowel and then re-establishing continuity).

The most important technical aspects of bowel surgery are gentle handling and attention to blood supply. Atraumatic manipulation of the bowel encourages an early return to function. The importance of blood supply to wound healing is an obvious feature of all surgery. However, the particularly devastating consequences of an ischemic enterotomy or anastomotic incision makes attention to blood supply especially critical.

Enterotomy

Bowel contents are gently manipulated away from the site of the enterotomy incision by digital stripping. The bowel lumen then is occluded orad and anad to the operative site. Although clamps or temporary ligatures of umbilical tape or latex drains can be used, it is preferred that an assistant gently occludes the bowel with saline-moistened fingers (Fig. 13-2A).

The surgeon gently holds the antimesenteric border of the bowel wall between thumb and forefinger; this increases tension on the wall and makes it rigid enough to be incised easily (Fig. 13-2*B*). Once the lumen has been entered, the incision is lengthened as needed with a scalpel or sharp scissors.

To close the enterotomy incision, almost any type of suture pattern or material is functional in healthy bowel. Many surgeons prefer to close enterotomy incisions with a simple interrupted appositional suture pattern. The sutures are placed through the full thickness of the bowel wall, 3 to 5 mm apart and 2 to 3 mm from the cut edge. Because it is an anatomical pattern (each layer of the two bowel ends is apposed), it facilitates healing. Because the luminal diameter is maintained, this suture pattern is especially useful in immature or small dogs and in cats.

A variation of the simple interrupted appositional suture pattern is the interrupted crushing appositional suture pattern. Crushing sutures are simple interrupted stitches tied tightly enough to cut through all layers of the bowel wall except the tough submucosa. Tied properly, the crushing suture releases the blood and lymphatic supply to the inter-suture bowel edge, possibly improving vascularity to that edge. Suture placement is important. The entire thickness of bowel wall is penetrated from serosa to lumen; placement is begun at least 3 mm from the cut edge to ensure all layers are included. Disadvantages of this technique are that the mucosa sometimes tends to become exposed between sutures, and exact alignment of the wound edges is more difficult than with the simple (noncrushing) interrupted technique.

In some cases, the bowel at the surgical site may have a poor blood supply, bowel-wall viability may be questionable, or the presence of peritonitis may reduce the likelihood of adequate healing. Hypoalbuminemia (*e.g.*, in cases with malabsorption syndrome) also results in poor wound healing, increasing the possibility of suture line dehiscence. For these cases, I prefer a vertical inverting mattress (Lembert) closure with nonabsorbable suture material. If Lembert sutures are used, they are placed at each end of the incision starting in normal, unincised bowel (Fig. 13-2*C, D*), and continuing through the remaining portion of the incision, placed 3 to 5 mm apart (Fig. 13-2*E*). The disadvantage of an inverting pattern is the narrowing of the bowel lumen that results (Fig. 13-2*F*), although this narrowing rarely causes problems in normal small bowel.

The surgeon should be gentle and precise. Multiple attempts to place a single stitch should be avoided; it is better to reinforce a questionable area with additional sutures. Although under ideal circumstances Lembert sutures should not penetrate the bowel lumen, the stitches must be placed deeply enough to penetrate the submucosa, which is the strongest layer of the bowel and is relied on as the "holding" layer. The sutures must also be placed deeply enough to avoid their tearing out; if suture material is visible through the serosa, its placement is superficial. In general, as no serious sequelae arise if the lumen is accidentally penetrated, it is better to place the suture too deeply than too superficially.

Non-crushing sutures are tied snugly, but not so tightly that the bowel wall blanches. Small clots that form on the suture line are left in place, because fibrin seals the incision for the first 24 to 36 hours. After the closure is completed, the isolated segment of bowel is gently filled with saline to check the integrity of the closure (Fig. 13-2*G*). Leaks are repaired by additional sutures. After the peritoneal cavity is lavaged with warm saline, the loop of bowel is thoroughly rinsed and replaced in the abdomen. Instruments, drapes, and gloves are changed and the abdomen is closed routinely.

Resection and Anastomosis

The abdominal incision is shielded with moistened laparotomy sponges. The segment to be removed is exteriorized and isolated between the fingers of an assistant, as described above under enterotomy. The blood supply to the ends of the bowel to be rejoined is determined; the integrity of these vessels must be maintained. Arteries and veins supplying the small

(text continues on page 374)

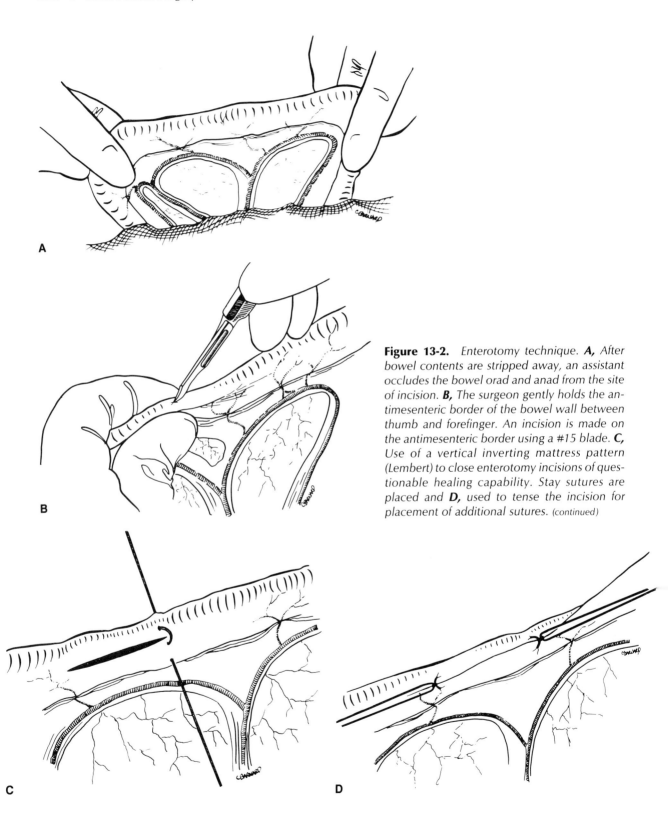

Figure 13-2. *Enterotomy technique. **A,** After bowel contents are stripped away, an assistant occludes the bowel orad and anad from the site of incision. **B,** The surgeon gently holds the antimesenteric border of the bowel wall between thumb and forefinger. An incision is made on the antimesenteric border using a #15 blade. **C,** Use of a vertical inverting mattress pattern (Lembert) to close enterotomy incisions of questionable healing capability. Stay sutures are placed and **D,** used to tense the incision for placement of additional sutures.* (continued)

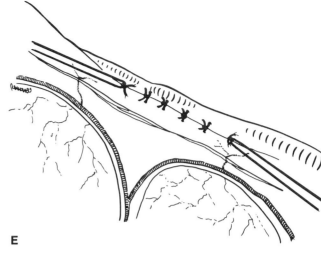

E

Figure 13-2 (continued)
E, *Sutures are placed 3 to 5 mm apart and deeply enough to penetrate the submucosal layer of the bowel wall.* ***F,*** *Some narrowing of the bowel diameter results from the inverting method of closure.* ***G,*** *The seal at the incision line is checked by filling the segment with saline with the lumen occluded above and below the incision site.*

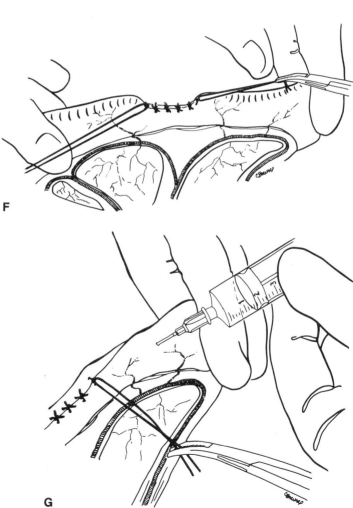

F

G

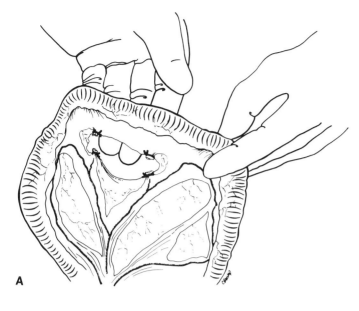

Figure 13-3. *Resection and anastomosis technique. **A,** Blood vessels supplying the portion to be removed are ligated and divided. **B,** Suture placement is facilitated by supporting the bowel wall with thumb forceps placed in the lumen. **C,** One suture is placed at the mesenteric border and one at the antimesenteric border. The ends are left long and used as stay sutures.* (continued)

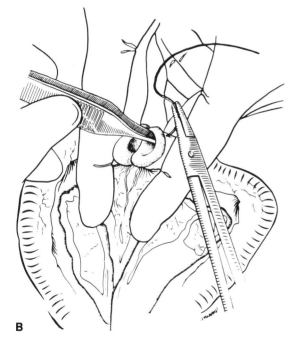

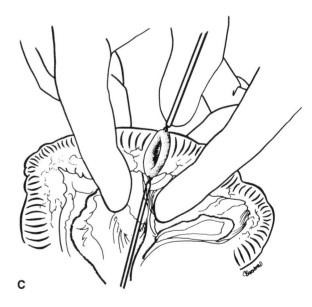

bowel arise from several mesenteric branches that connect through loops paralleling the mesenteric border of the bowel. Blood vessels supplying the portion to be removed are ligated and divided (Fig. 13-3A). The small connecting vessels along the mesenteric borders

are ligated just before resecting the bowel segment. (In some obese patients, excessive mesenteric fat prevents identification of the mesenteric vessels. In these instances, it may be necessary to sever the bowel first and identify and ligate the bleeding vessels.) If isolation and

Figure 13-3 *(continued)*
D, *The remainder of the incision is apposed with simple interrupted crushing stitches placed 3 to 5 mm apart. After one half of the bowel is closed, the stay sutures facilitate rotation so that the anastomosis can be completed.* **E,** *The defect in the mesentery is closed with care so that the mesenteric vessels traveling in the cut edges are not occluded or penetrated.* **F,** *The integrity of the anastomosis is checked by filling the occluded segment with saline.*

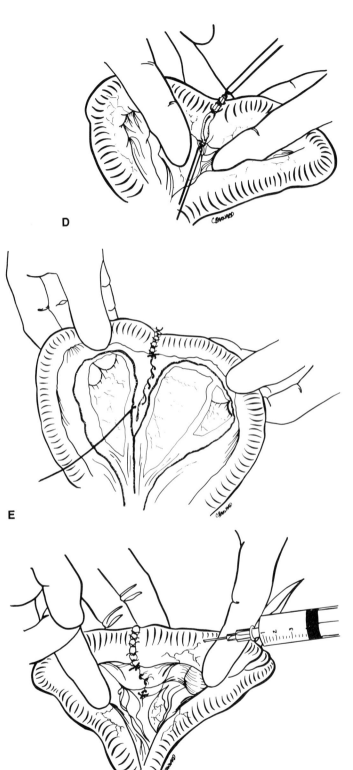

D

E

F

ligation of the blood vessels are done properly, the severed bowel ends will appear pink and healthy and the mucosal edge will bleed.

The bowel is severed using a scalpel or very sharp scissors. To ensure adequate blood supply to the antimesenteric border, the incision is angled so that the mesenteric border is left longer than the antimesenteric border. The angle on one segment can be made more acute to adjust to the diameter of the other bowel end. The diameter of the cut edge of the small segment severed at an acute angle may be increased to twice that of similarly sized bowel that is severed at right angles to the mesenteric border. But if cutting the smaller-diameter bowel at an acute angle will not increase its diameter sufficiently, the antimesenteric border of the smaller-diameter segment can be incised along the long axis of the bowel for a distance that increases the diameter enough to match the larger segment.

The bowel is then anastomosed end to end using standard techniques. The anastomosis that results is angled toward the antimesenteric border. Alternatives to end-to-end anastomosis include end-to-side anastomosis and side-to-side anastomosis. With the former, the end of the larger-diameter segment is closed using a two-layer inverting pattern. The small segment is then anastomosed to the side of the large segment using a simple interrupted appositional stitch, either crushing or noncrushing. The side-to-side anastomosis requires closing both ends of bowel, creating a stoma along the antimesenteric border or midway between the mesenteric and antimesenteric border, and anastomosis using a simple interrupted appositional pattern. The major disadvantage of end-to-side anastomosis and side-to-side anastomosis is that multiple suture closures must be made, two for the end-to-side anastomosis and three for the side-to-side. In contrast, end-to-end anastomosis requires only one suture line.

The mucosa of the remaining ends of the bowel protrudes and overlaps the ends of the bowel wall. Some surgeons excise the protruding mucosa to facilitate closure, but this is not essential. The assistant brings the ends of the bowel into position (Fig. 13-3*B*). If possible, the surgeon avoids grasping the bowel with forceps. Instead, suture placement is facilitated by supporting the bowel wall with thumb forceps placed in the lumen. One suture is placed in the antimesenteric border and one in the mesenteric border 180° apart. It is sometimes difficult to suture at the mesenteric border unless the fat is gently dissected away from the edge for 2 or 3 mm. The ends of these first two sutures are left long and are used as stay sutures (Fig. 13-3*C*). The rest of the incision is apposed with sutures placed 3 to 5 mm apart (Fig. 13-3*D*). Many surgeons use either the simple interrupted, the interrupted crushing appositional suture pattern, or the interrupted Gambee suture pattern for anastomosis (see "Enterotomy," p. 370); I prefer the crushing pattern. After half the bowel is closed, the stay sutures facilitate rotation of the bowel so that the anastomosis can be completed.

The defect in the mesentery is closed with care so that the mesenteric vessels traveling in the cut edges are not occluded or penetrated (Fig. 13-3*E*). A perfect anastomosis can be ruined if the mesenteric blood supply to the cut ends is accidentally compromised by a suture. This can be prevented at the time of resection by leaving an adequate width of avascular mesentery for suturing.

The integrity of the anastomosis is checked by filling the occluded segment with saline (Fig. 13-3*F*). Any protruding mucosa should be covered by a suture. Usually, however, as long as the anastomosis is water-tight and the bowel ends are viable, healing will occur uneventfully.

Up to 80% of the small intestine can be removed from normal dogs without serious sequelae; removing 90% of the normal small bowel causes severe morbidity and death in some dogs. Illness is caused by malabsorption, malnutrition, and fluid and electrolyte derangements. Fortunately, the veterinary surgeon rarely removes extensive portions of normal bowel.

The malabsorption exhibited by dogs after massive small bowel resection has been called the short-bowel syndrome. The malabsorption is actually maldigestion, in that nearly all the digestive processes influenced by the small bowel are affected. Reduction in the amount of various intestinal hormones results in pancreatic enzyme deficiency, the enterohepatic circulation of bile salts is reduced, resulting in altered digestion of fats and in steatorrhea, and transit time is reduced, resulting in less opportunity for the absorption of nutrients. The remaining portions of small bowel can compensate somewhat by increasing in diameter, by hypertrophy of microvilli, and by hyperplasia of mucosal cells. Until, and if, compensation occurs, affected animals appear malnourished (thin, unthrifty, poor hair coat) and have frequent malodorous soft to watery bowel movements. Serum albumin levels may be markedly low, resulting in edema that affects the ventral abdomen and limbs.

Intraoperative Considerations

Whether an enterotomy or resection and anastomosis has been done, the surface of the bowel is flushed with saline. Ideally, the surgeon and assistant replace gloves and change drapes and instruments. Because even a perfect bowel operation results in some spillage of contents, a thorough flushing of the peritoneal cavity with warm saline is advisable before closing the abdomen. Except in cases of preexisting peritonitis, abdominal drains are neither necessary nor desirable.

The omentum should be preserved whenever possible unless it is abscessed or infiltrated with tumor or has formed detrimental adhesions. As the scavenger of the abdomen, the omentum performs an important function: it brings its blood supply to areas of inflammation, localized infection, and recent trauma, including the sites of bowel perforation, or at suture lines. For this reason, surgeons often place the omentum on the surgical site, or even tack it to the site, before abdominal closure. However, there are functions that the omentum cannot be expected to do. It cannot effectively seal poorly performed enterotomy closures or anastomoses, nor can it effectively

compensate for inadequate blood supply when an enterotomy or anastomosis is performed in ischemic bowel.

Another means of protecting the suture line from leakage and improving chances of adequate vascularity at that location is the serosal patch technique. This involves suturing the antimesenteric surface of one or more uninvolved loops of jejunum to the area of suture line. This technique is suggested in cases of hypoproteinemia or other potential causes of poor healing.

Complications

Peritonitis

The most serious postoperative complication of bowel surgery is peritonitis, resulting from leakage at the suture line. Re-operation is imperative as soon as leakage is suspected, because waiting until leakage can be confirmed positively may result in death. Most animals that have an uncomplicated enterotomy or bowel resection recover quickly and show progressive clinical improvement over 4 or 5 days. Any postoperative bowel surgery patient whose clinical condition either does not improve promptly or improves and then shows signs of anorexia, fever, vomiting, or other signs of peritonitis should be suspected of having a leaking suture line until proven otherwise. Abdominocentesis and radiography may be difficult to interpret in the immediate postoperative period and may show relatively few abnormalities identifiable as peritonitis. For example, free gas in the peritoneal cavity may persist for 7 to 10 days postoperatively. The fluid obtained at abdominoparacentesis may, however, contain degenerate neutrophils, bacteria, plant fibers, etc., confirming presence of septic peritonitis and bowel rupture. Postoperative paracentesis in dogs without septic peritonitis reveals nondegenerative neutrophils without evidence of bacteria or plant fibers. Antibiotics may mask the signs of a leaky bowel suture line until illness is severe. In a case of postoperative morbidity, the surgeon always should first suspect problems with the integrity of the suture line.

Adhesions

Adhesions cannot develop without inflammation, such as peritonitis or trauma resulting in damage to serosal surfaces. In many instances, adhesions do not cause clinical problems and are incidental findings at surgery or necropsy. Clinically significant postoperative adhesions are rare in dogs and cats. Occasionally, however, adhesion of the omentum to an enterotomy or anastomotic site causes extraluminal obstruction of the bowel. More often, adhesions that cause clinical signs result from the original disease process rather than from surgery.

Ileus

Ileus is a lack of small bowel motility. It nearly always is a secondary condition, most commonly occurring proximal to a site of luminal obstruction in dogs and cats. Adynamic ileus is much rarer in dogs and cats than in humans. It consists of hypomotility or amotility of the small bowel, occurring in the absence of a mechanical obstruction. Adynamic ileus can result from peritonitis, electrolyte imbalances such as hypokalemia, the use of parasympatholytic drugs, and profoundly debilitating illnesses affecting other body systems.

The Large Intestine

Surgical Disorders

Megacolon

Megacolon is an abnormally large or dilated colon. It may be congenital or acquired, and primary or secondary. Congenital megacolon is a rare neuromuscular disease whose pathogenesis is unclear in dogs and cats. In humans, congenital megacolon is associated with deficiencies in myenteric plexuses located in a segment of the wall of the colon (Hirschsprung's disease). The essential functional deficit of congenital megacolon in dogs, cats, or humans is amotility of the large bowel, resulting in fecal stasis and constipation.

The most common form of megacolon in animals is acquired idiopathic megacolon observed in aged cats. Chronic constipation leading to obstructive constipation (obstipation) is the chief complaint. Treatment of idiopathic megacolon in cats requires complete or partial colectomy. The dilated segment of colon is removed from immediately anad to the ileocecocolic junction, if possible, to just orad to the rectum. Preservation of the ileocecocolic valve is desirable. Results usually are good, although moderate diarrhea can persist for weeks or months and can be permanent in some cases.

Secondary megacolon occurs because of complete or partial obstruction in the rectum or at the anus. Tumors, strictures, and perineal hernias are the most common primary causes. Treatment of secondary megacolon involves removing the cause of the obstruction. Adenocarcinoma of the colon, although rare, causes annular strictures just as it does in the small bowel. Adenocarcinoma of the rectum and anus is more common than carcinoma of the colon and usually causes other symptoms (bleeding, dyschezia) before megacolon develops (see Chap. 14, The Rectum, Anus, and Perianal and Perineal Regions). Extraluminal leiomyomas and leiomyosarcomas can obstruct the pelvic portion of the rectum enough to cause megacolon. These tumors are approached through a perineal incision and usually can be removed by blunt dissection along tissue planes (see Chap. 14). Secondary megacolon can resolve once the primary cause is relieved, although return to function may be delayed or absent when the colon has been dilated for prolonged periods.

Trauma

Trauma to the colon is nearly always the result of penetrating abdominal wounds. Blunt trauma seldom causes large bowel vascular injury because the colonic vasculature lies parallel to the longitudinal axis of the bowel; mesenteric disruption can occur without damaging colonic blood supply. Penetrating abdominal trauma or the discovery of fecal material in peritoneal fluid specimens always is an indication for surgical exploration. The surgeon's suspicion that colonic damage is present is of utmost importance to making a prompt diagnosis and providing timely treatment, as the bacterial concentration of colonic contents is high, leading to early severe peritonitis.

Nontraumatic Perforation of the Bowel

This can occur in association with chronic or subacute administration of corticosteroids. Affected animals may not show signs until peritonitis develops, although abdominal pain is present in some patients. A positive test for occult fecal blood is a consistent finding.

Cecal Inversion

This rare clinical condition causes low-grade clinical signs. The cecum inverts into the large bowel, causing a partial obstruction. Chronic intermittent and occasionally bloody diarrhea usually is present. The displacement of the dilated gas-filled cecum is usually evident on noncontrast radiographs or flexible fiber-optic coloscopy. Treatment consists of typhlectomy if possible or resection of the ileocecocolic junction if necessary.

Surgical Techniques of the Large Bowel

Preoperative Preparation

The value of preoperative preparation of the large bowel is one of the few noncontroversial areas in surgery. Although the bowel cannot be completely sterilized, the enteric bacterial population can be considerably reduced by a combination of cleansing soapy-water enemas and oral antibiotics. Phosphate enemas are contraindicated because they may induce electrolyte imbalances. When possible, enemas should begin 36 to 48 hours before surgery and stop by 24 hours preoperatively; solid food should be withheld. Enteric antibiotics, such as kanamycin, should be used in combination with metranidozole to kill both aerobic and anaerobic bacteria. If, due to an emergency, there is no time to pretreat with oral antibiotics, perioperative therapy with an antibiotic such as cephalothin (22 mg/kg IV) is suggested, repeated every 6 hours for the first 12 hours and then as indicated by the presence or absence of signs of infection.

Unfortunately, in many cases, optimal preparation of the bowel is impossible. For example, the presence of real or suspected colonic ulceration or colonic cancer contraindicates the use of enemas because of the risk of perforation. Annular carcinoma or colonic stricture may cause fecal impaction that cannot be relieved until the stricture is removed. The surgeon is thus forced to operate in the presence of fecal material and the risk of spillage is unavoidably high.

Colotomy

Compared to surgery of the small bowel, surgery of the large bowel is relatively rare. Colotomy is needed occasionally to remove foreign bodies, such as pins, needles, or bones that have become partially embedded in the wall of the colon. Colotomy to remove other kinds of foreign bodies is seldom necessary because foreign objects small enough to traverse the length of the small bowel without causing obstruction usually pass through the large bowel without difficulty. Colotomy is also indicated to obtain full-thickness biopsies of the bowel wall.

Ideally, colotomy is performed on a prepared bowel (see "Preoperative Preparation" above). If feces are present, they are pushed cranially and caudally from the site of incision. The segment is isolated and the lumen simultaneously occluded by the fingers of an assistant, by Doyen forceps, or by soft rubber drains passed around the bowel. The bowel is isolated from other abdominal contents with moistened laparotomy sponges. The incision is made longitudinally over the isolated segment for a length appropriate to the task at hand. I prefer to close the incision in two layers. The first layer consists of a simple continuous suture pattern of 3-0 surgical gut, placed in the mucosa. The second is an interrupted vertical inverting mattress (Lembert) suture pattern of 3-0 nylon placed in the seromuscularis.

Colon Resection

Colon resection is indicated for the removal of colonic neoplasms, for removal of colon damaged by trauma, and for treatment of idiopathic megacolon in elderly cats.

Colon resection begins by interrupting the blood supply at the margins of the segments to be anastomosed. It is preferable, if possible, to ligate and divide the vasa recti coming off the branches of the middle and caudal colic vessels that course parallel to the mesenteric border of the colon. The bowel is severed with a scalpel or sharp Metzenbaum scissors, leaving the mesenteric border slightly longer than the antimesenteric border. Anastomosis of the bowel is performed in two layers. I prefer the first layer to be placed in the mucosa-submucosa, using 3-0 or 4-0 surgical gut in a simple interrupted pattern. The second layer joins the seromuscularis with an interrupted Lembert pattern of 3-0 nylon. The integrity of the anastomosis is checked for water tightness, as described above in "Resection and Anastomosis," and the mesentery is loosely apposed with 3-0 surgical catgut. An alternative method of bowel anastomosis consists of a single layer of simple interrupted sutures apposing the bowel ends; 3-0 nylon is placed through the full thickness of the bowel wall and may be tied as a crushing stitch or as a simple appositional stitch. The single layer method of closure is especially useful when the anastomosis must be very caudal (*i.e.*, at the pelvic brim).

Immediate postoperative complications of complete or partial colectomy in cats are uncommon. Colonic resection performed because of colonic carcinoma in dogs also has a reasonably good immediate prognosis, although long-term survival data are lacking.

Typhlectomy

Typhlectomy (resection of the cecum) is rarely performed. Cecal tumors are rare and their presence usually requires removal of the ileocecocolic junction in addition to the cecum. Benign cecal tumors, usually leiomyomas, are observed occasionally and are amenable to local resection.

Typhlectomy requires isolation and division of the small cecal artery. An elliptical incision is made around the base of the cecum and the resulting defect is closed with 3-0 nylon placed in an interrupted Lembert pattern.

Complications

The major complications of large animal surgery are wound dehiscence, peritonitis, and adhesions (see "Complications," p. 377).

Suggested Readings

Dee JF. Common surgical techniques of the cecum, colon and rectum. Vet Clin North Am 1975;5:521.

Hutchen NE, Salzberg AM. Pre-ileal transposition of colon to prevent the development of short bowel syndrome in puppies with 90 percent small intestinal resection. Surgery 1971;70:189.

Lantz GC. The pathophysiology of acute mechanical small bowel obstruction. Compend Contin Ed Pract Vet 1981;10:910.

Richardson DC: Intestinal surgery: A review. Compend Contin Ed Pract Vet 1981;3:259.

Twedt DC, Grauer GF. Fluid therapy for gastrointestinal, pancreatic and hepatic disorders. Vet Clin North Am 1982;3:463.

Wilson GP, Burt JK. Intussusception in the dog and cat: A review of 45 cases. J Am Vet Med Assoc 1974;5:515.

14

Gert W. Niebauer

Rectum, Anus, and Perianal and Perineal Regions

General Principles of Anorectal Surgery

Most surgical conditions of the anorectal region are not emergencies; therefore, sufficient time usually is available for preoperative patient preparation. Thus, reduction of stool content in the large intestines can be attempted, and antimicrobial prophylaxis can be initiated prior to most surgical procedures that enter the rectal lumen. Such procedures include partial or complete resection of the rectum or rectal wall, and rectoanal, colorectal, and coloanal anastomoses. Other procedures, such as perineal hernia repair, perianal fistulectomy, or anal sacculectomy, do not necessarily require preoperative bowel preparation or antibiotic prophylaxis. In more urgent procedures, such as bowel resection for rectal or anal prolapse or in cases of traumatic rectal injuries, preoperative preparation usually is limited to perioperative chemoprophylaxis (see "Perioperative Antimicrobial Chemoprophylaxis" below).

Preoperative Reduction of Stool Content in the Large Intestine

When indicated and compatible with the animal's general condition, a low-residue diet (*e.g.,* lean meat and rice) may be fed for 2 to 3 days before surgery, and food may be withheld for 24 hours prior to surgery. In cases with constipation or partial rectal or anal obstruction (*e.g.,* stricture or tumor), a stool softener such as psyllium hydrophilic mucilloid (Metamucil, Procter & Gamble, Cincinnati, OH) can be added to the diet for several days before surgery. Cleansing enemas with warm saline should be given as often as deemed necessary, except when perforation of the rectum and leakage is suspected. Cleansing enemas should be stopped 24 hours prior to surgery to avoid spillage of liquid bowel contents into the surgical field. Liquid fecal material resulting from cleansing enemas may soil the perianal region, increasing the risk of perianal or perineal surgical wound contamination; therefore, many surgeons avoid cleansing enemas prior to performing perianal or perineal procedures that are unlikely to perforate the rectum. Nevertheless, the anal sacs should be evacuated prior to anorectal surgery to avoid soiling the perianal skin, and to lessen the chance of needle penetration of the anal sacs.

Perioperative Antimicrobial Chemoprophylaxis and Chemotherapy

The use of perioperative antibiotics is recommended in all surgical procedures invading the lower bowel and rectum. Of course, aseptic surgical technique is clearly essential in preventing infection. Although there are aerobic bacteria in the lower canine intestinal tract, the predominant microflora are anaerobic bacteria, such as *Bacterioides,* bifidobacteria, enterobacteria, streptococci, and lactobacilli. On the one hand, chemoprophylaxis and chemotherapy are aimed at reducing the intraluminal concentration of bacteria topically. On the other hand, these chemotherapeutic drugs also should reach sufficient concentrations in serum and interstitial fluid to reduce the risk of bacterial lodgement in tissues during and after surgery. The latter can only be accomplished by a combination of broad-spectrum antibiotics. For enteral prophylaxis, oral antibiotics with low intestinal absorption rates are given several days prior to surgery. For instance, the protocol of neomycin (25 mg/kg body weight) and erythromycin (10 mg/kg body weight) given every 8 hours, or metronidazole given alone (30 mg/kg body weight) once daily for 2 to 3 days, has given satisfactory results in dogs. Systemic prophylaxis should be initiated 1 to 2 hours prior to surgery, and chemotherapy should be continued for several days after surgery. Antibacterial combinations also can be used: for instance, cefoxitin sodium (15–22 mg/kg body weight) plus trimethoprim–sulfadiazine (30 mg/kg body weight); or gentamicin (4.5 mg/kg body weight) plus clindamycin (10–40 mg/kg body weight); kanamycin (7.5 mg/kg body weight) plus clindamycin (10–40 mg/kg body weight), or gentamicin (4.5 mg/kg body weight) plus metronidazole (30 mg/kg body weight).

Topical (oral) administration of antibiotics or antiseptics seems to be less important than systemic administration of antibiotics combined with extensive mechanical cleansing of a contaminated surgical field. Rinsing with warm saline alone is recommended. However, some surgeons prefer to add antibiotics to the irrigation solution. As an antiseptic, a 0.5% solution of chlorhexidine has been used.

Surgical Site Drainage

The use of surgical drains (*e.g.,* Penrose rubber drains, Davol Inc., Cranston, RI) is recommended when a communication between the rectal lumen and the perirectal tissues existed preoperatively or is created during surgery. A separate skin incision should be made for the drain as far ventral as possible to avoid compromising surgical wound healing and to allow gravity drainage. If the caudal perirectal tissues are contaminated, drains should exit in the perineal area. If the area cranial to the intrapelvic peritoneal reflection has been contaminated, drains also should be placed into the pelvic canal and the caudal abdomen, exiting in the prepubic region. Drains usually are removed after several days as determined by the quantity and quality of drainage: in selected cases they may be left in place for up to 2 weeks (*e.g.,* perirectal abscesses).

Postoperative Stool Softeners

Stool softeners may be used to help prevent straining to defecate after surgery. However, this benefit must be balanced against the increased likelihood of wound contamination by fecal soiling associated with stool softeners.

Congenital Anomalies

Congenital anomalies of rectum and anus are rare in small animals. They consist of either an inadequately developed or absent anal orifice (atresia ani, imperforate anus) or rectal aplasia (atresia recti, segmental aplasia), in which the anal orifice is developed normally, but the rectum is interrupted by an atretic segment. The mildest form of anal anomaly is congenital stricture. In females with rectal and anal atresia, rectovaginal fistulae also occur.

Clinical Signs

Pups or kittens with anal or rectal atresia usually are presented within the first days or weeks of life with signs of abdominal enlargement and discomfort. In longstanding cases, vomiting and dehydration develop. The severity of clinical signs corresponds to the duration of retention of meconium and does not necessarily correlate with the extent of the anomaly. In animals with rectovaginal fistulae, however, these signs are absent and feces are observed exiting from the vulva.

Diagnosis

Clinical diagnosis of atresia ani or recti depends on careful probing (*e.g.*, with a rectal thermometer) in the region of the anus. A dimple usually is apparent at the normal location of the anus. In some cases a thin bulge is visible at the anus, indicating that anorectal development probably is normal, except for a superficial anal membrane. A completely absent anal dimple may indicate that anal, and probably terminal rectal, atresia exist. Radiographic examination to evaluate the extent of congenital anomaly is recommended in all cases. Gas or feces in the rectum usually delineate the level of atresia.

Treatment

If imperforate anus (atresia ani) is partial, or a strictured anus exists, bougienage of the narrow opening may be attempted. Treatment of a completely imperforate anus depends on the extent of atresia. In some cases simple scalpel incision of the occluding membrane might be sufficient. Usually, there will be complete fecal continence, as anal sphincter development is likely to be normal. If atresia recti coexists, dissection in the perineum is necessary to locate the caudal, blind end of the rectum. The rectal mucosa then is incised and sutured to the skin. If there is a long segment of rectal atresia (segmental rectal aplasia) cranial to the atretic anus, surgical treatment is indicated only when the distance from the blind-ended rectum to the perineal skin is short and a rectal *pull-through* procedure (see "Rectal Pull-Through Procedure," p. 386) can be accomplished to bridge the defect without tension. In such a case, a combined abdominoperineal approach is necessary to identify and mobilize the intrapelvic blind end of the rectum. Descending colon and rectum are drawn through a bluntly created intrapelvic tunnel. A two-layered simple interrupted suture pattern is used; in the first layer, the subcutaneous tissues are sutured to the submucosa; and in the second, the perianal skin is sutured to the mucosa. Although the external anal sphincter muscle and its nerve supply are usually unaffected by the genetic defect, sphincter function may not develop satisfactorily after surgery.

Genitorectal fistula (rectovaginal fistula, anogenital cleft) is extremely uncommon in small animals, therefore clinical experience is limited. Rectovaginal fistula can occur in combination with anal atresia. Because soft fecal material usually passes through a fistulous opening into the vagina, animals might survive long enough to allow surgical repair. Successful closure of such fistulae is more likely if animals survive to adolescence. Anogenital clefts are seen in males. The urethra and anus form a cloaca-like opening. This defect generally is not repaired.

Trauma to Anus and Rectum

The anus or rectum can be injured from within or without. Ingested foreign objects, such as needles or pieces of bone, can become lodged in the rectum or anus and may penetrate the mucosa and underlying tissue layers because of sphincter contractions. Other causes of damage from within the lumen include improper rectal thermometry, rectal tearing during examination, improper use of enema tubes, impalement, or acts of sadism. Laceration of the anus and rectum from without can be due to severe trauma to the perineal region, such as from dog bites, or to pelvic fractures with dislocation of sharp bone splinters.

Clinical Signs

Depending on the extent of tissue damage, animals are presented with tenesmus, dyschezia, and hematochezia. Because peritonitis might develop in cases of deep rectal perforation, assessment of the extent of trauma is important in all perforating rectal injuries. Only the cranial half of the rectum is covered by visceral peritoneum; the rest of the rectum lies within the intrapelvic retroperitoneal space. The aspect most caudal to the peritoneal reflection, the pararectal fossa, is located lateral to the rectum, at about the level of the second coccygeal vertebra. Thus, only perforations cranial to and through the reflecting peritoneal sheets can lead to leakage of fecal material into the abdomen. Clinical and radiographic signs of developing peritonitis warrant immediate surgical exploration by caudal celiotomy, pelvic symphysiotomy, or pubic triple osteotomy (see Chap. 11, The Abdominal Cavity). Enemas (with or without radiographic contrast media) are contraindicated, because they are likely to spread fecal material beyond the area of leakage.

Treatment

Rectal lacerations should be closed with simple interrupted sutures, preferably with a synthetic monofilament, absorbable material (e.g., polydioxanone—PDS, Ethicon Inc., Sommerville, NJ). Drainage of the contaminated areas and intensive antimicrobial treatment with broad-spectrum antibiotics (see "Perioperative Antimicrobial Chemoprophylaxis and Chemotherapy," p. 382) is necessary to pre-

vent death from sepsis in cases of fecal spillage into the peritoneal cavity.

Most cases of rectal perforation are, however, retroperitoneal (in the caudal half of the rectum) and usually heal well by second intention. Closure per rectum of these defects should not be attempted, as this may lead to perirectal abscess formation by walling off drainage routes. Extensive perirectal tissue damage should be treated by debridement and flushing with saline via a perineal incision. One or more Penrose drains should be placed into the perirectal tissues, near but not through the torn rectal mucosa. Drains usually can be removed after 1 week. Broad-spectrum antibiotic therapy is indicated throughout this period.

Superficial internal injuries of the caudal rectum and the anus usually heal without the need for treatment, except for administration of a stool softener given to ease defecation (see "Postoperative Stool Softeners," p. 382).

External lacerations of the anus involving the internal or external anal sphincter muscles should be repaired by sutures. Care should be taken to evaluate whether anal sacs have been ruptured. In such cases excision of the affected anal sacs is recommended (see "Anal Sacculitis," p. 388).

Anorectal strictures due to scar formation or fecal incontinence due to damage to the anal sphincter muscles or their nerve supply may develop as sequelae to traumatic injuries.

Functional Anorectal Constriction (Rectal Spasm)

Anorectal constriction is a rare condition and can be either functional or anatomical in origin. Functional constrictions (anorectal spasms) can occur as transient or chronic spastic anal sphincter contractions, as a sequel to traumatic lesions, or in conjunction with any irritation of rectal, perirectal, or anal tissues.

Functional constrictions must be differentiated from strictures due to inflammation, fibrosis, or neoplasia, and from the normal narrowing of the rectal lumen, often found on rectal palpation, just caudal of the colorectal junction. Anatomically, this narrowed area is due to circular smooth muscle fibers of the muscularis mucosae that are distinctly thickened, forming a *functional sphincter ani tertius.*

Diagnosis

Rectal examination alone may not distinguish between functional and anatomical constricting lesions. General or epidural anesthesia relaxes functional sphincter spasms. In these cases palpation or a positive contrast radiographic examination (barium enema) under anesthesia generally reveals a normally shaped rectum. Because anorectal spasms can be seen in conjunction with any painful lesion in the anal region, an underlying inflammatory process should always be suspected and ruled out.

Pathologic idiopathic anorectal spasms are seen in nervous excitable animals, especially German shepherd dogs. In such dogs, most of the length of the rectum may remain spastically contracted at all times, and manual dilatation during rectal examination is painful. This disorder also has been described as *hypertrophy of the external anal sphincter.* The disease seems to be neurogenic in origin and does not have an inflammatory component. The functional spasms seem to originate in the autonomic nervous system dependent muscularis mucosae. Thus, complete or partial denervation of the external anal sphincter muscle by neurotomy of pudendal nerve branches does not completely reverse rectal spasm. In these cases, it is likely that the striated external anal sphincter might only be affected secondarily and myotomy of the muscularis mucosae in the area of the rectal spasm might be the best treatment.

Treatment

A caudal abdominal approach, combined with pelvic osteotomy is necessary for adequate exposure. The circular smooth muscle layers are transsected by two to three longitudinal, partial-thickness rectal incisions. Addition-

ally, partial denervation of the external anal sphincter can be performed. Irreversible fecal incontinence might develop after the denervation procedure, however.

Anorectal Stricture

True anorectal strictures occur as sequelae of traumatic or inflammatory lesions involving the rectum, the anus, or the anal sphincter. Chronic anal sac disease, perianal fistulae or previous surgical procedures often are part of the case history. Circumferential fibrosis constricts the rectal lumen in such cases. Clinical signs include tenesmus, dyschezia and chronic constipation, with or without secondary megacolon.

Diagnosis

Rectal neoplasms, which also can cause rectal constriction, must be differentiated from benign rectal or anal stricture. A careful rectal examination, proctoscopy, if available, and radiographic studies may help to distinguish between these two conditions. Usually, malignant rectal tumors present with hematochezia, and friable lesions may be palpable on rectal examination, or a characteristic circumferential constricting *(napkin ring)* lesion may be present. A biopsy is required for a definitive diagnosis, however.

Treatment

Treatment of strictures due to contraction of circumferential scar tissue involves either bougienage (in milder cases, by gentle dilation with the gloved finger or with dilators), surgical transection of the fibrous ring, with or without myotomy, or full thickness resection of the scar. Lesions located near the anus can be excised *per rectum,* by an intraluminal approach. For more cranial lesions, a dorsal or lateral pararectal approach may be necessary (see "Surgical Techniques," below). Fibrotic tissue can be incised or resected as necessary. In severe cases, involving the rectal wall beyond the mucosal layers, a full thickness

360° resection should be performed. The cranial end of the transsected rectum then is anastomosed either with the caudal end of the remaining rectum or with the anal canal. If an extensive excision is required, a *pull-through* procedure may be performed *per rectum* (see "Surgical Techniques," below). An abdominal approach, with or without pelvic osteotomy (symphysiotomy or pubic triple osteotomy), is indicated when rectal strictures extend cranially into the area of the rectocolonic junction.

A guarded prognosis should be given in all surgically treated cases of rectal stricture. These lesions usually develop as a sequela to trauma and inflammation and, thus, may recur after surgery.

Surgical Techniques

For all three of the following described approaches, animals are positioned in ventral recumbency with the hindquarters slightly elevated on a rectal stand, and with the tail fastened over the midline dorsocraniad.

Lateral Approach to the Rectum

A unilateral or bilateral curved dorsoventral incision of sufficient length is made just lateral to the hairless anal disk. Dissection proceeds craniad in a tissue plane between the external anal sphincter and the rectococcygeus muscles (medial), and the levator ani and coccygeus muscles (lateral). The approach is limited to a relatively small area of the lateral and ventral aspects of the caudal half of the rectum. Care has to be taken to avoid damage to the rectal nerves and the external anal sphincter, because fecal incontinence may ensue. In many cases a dorsal approach to the rectum is preferable.

Dorsal Approach to the Rectum

An inverted U-shaped incision is made dorsally around the anus half way between the root of the tail and the anus, ending just medial of the tubera ischii. Dissection dorsolateral to the anus reveals the levator ani and coccygeus muscles laterally, the rectococcy-

geus muscle dorsally, and the dorsal surface of the anus and external anal sphincter muscle. The rectococcygeus muscle is transsected near its vertebral insertion. The rectum is further exposed by separating, bluntly, the external anal sphincter muscle and portions of the levator ani muscle from the rectal wall. By careful dissection, avoiding damage to the caudal rectal nerves, the rectum can be mobilized enough to clearly visualize the peritoneal reflection dorsal and lateral to the cranial rectum. The autonomic nerve supply to the rectum is located in this area cranial to and within the peritoneal reflection and must be preserved to avoid postoperative fecal incontinence. The rectum can be separated from surrounding vessels enough to perform a 360° partial resection in the midportion of the rectum. After rectal anastomosis and closure, the rectococcygeus muscle is reattached with simple interrupted sutures of monofilament absorbable material, and subcutis and skin are closed by routine methods. If the rectal lumen has been entered, Penrose drains should be placed into the perirectal space.

Rectal Pull-Through Procedure

By gently retracting anal mucosa, four equidistant stay sutures are placed circumferentially into the rectal mucosa in the area of the anorectal junction. The rectal mucosa is circumferentially incised just cranial to the stay sutures, and, subsequently, the rectal wall is transsected. The severed cranial part of the rectum is then grasped with Allis tissue forceps or attached to stay sutures for better manipulation and traction. By blunt dissection between rectal wall and perirectal musculature (*i.e.*, external anal sphincter, levator ani, rectococcygeus) considerable latitude for retraction of the rectum is given. The cranial rectal artery can be seen dorsally and should be ligated. Sufficient retraction has to be achieved to allow tension-free anastomosis. For anastomosis, the freed rectal stump is pulled through the anal opening, and the lateral surface of the extracted bowel (serosa, in case the peritoneal reflection has been entered) is sutured circumferentially to the submucosal tissues just cranial to the transsected anorectal junction. The extracted part of bowel is then resected a few millimeters caudal to the first suture line to allow enough room to appose mucosa to mucosa in a second row of circumferential simple interrupted sutures. Monofilament absorbable material is recommended for both layers. The stay sutures are removed and Penrose drains are placed into the perirectal space.

Inflammatory Diseases of Anal and Perianal Regions

Proctitis and anusitis can occur as transient responses to internal and external stimuli, such as impacted anal sacs, enteroparasites, diarrhea and eczematous or seborrheic skin conditions. Itching and mechanical stimulus of the anal region by licking or rubbing aggravate inflammatory responses. Chronic irritation of the anal canal, the anus and the perianal region can lead to the development of various lesions described below.

Anatomy and Pathophysiology of Inflammatory Anorectal Surgical Diseases

A variable number of longitudinally oriented mucosal folds (anal columns), located in the columnar zone of the anus, form the anal sinuses. These sinuses are small, mucosa-lined, cranially opening pockets, acting under the tone of the constricting sphincter muscles as a valvelike mechanism, separating the rectal lumen from the anus. Tubuloalveolar anal glands (modified sweat glands) open their lipid-secreting ducts into the anal sinuses. Apocrine anal sweat glands are found in the cutaneous zone of the anus; together with sebaceous glands, they form a dense, subepidermal network of skin glands surrounding the anal orifice.

In the deeper layers of the perianal region lay the densely packed, lobulated circumanal

(perianal) hepatoid glands. They lack excretory ducts, and their development and growth are stimulated by androgens.

The third distinct glandular structures in the area of the canine anus are the anal sacs. Anal sacs are paired invaginations of the inner cutaneous zone of the anus. Their walls contain large apocrine, modified sudoriparous glands, and modified sebaceous glands, which produce a malodorous, pastelike secretion. This material is stored in the anal sacs and is expelled usually during defecation, extensive fear, or excitement by contraction of the external anal sphincter, which overlies the anal sacs.

Perianal Fistulation (Perianal Furunculosis)

This inflammatory disease is one of the commonly encountered anal disease in dogs. Although its etiology remains obscure, inflammatory involvement of specific glandular and epithelial tissues in and around the anus, such as hidradenitis and anal sacculitis, seem to play an important pathogenic role.

Hidradenitis

Hidradenitis is a pyogranulomatous inflammation of the anal glands, apocrine sweat glands, and sebaceous glands in the cutaneous zone of the anus and the hairless anal disk. Although initially superficial, the chronic inflammation involves the deep connective tissues surrounding the circumanal hepatoid glands and is thought to be one of the initiating lesions in the development of perianal fistulae. In fact, inflammation of the anal glands in the columnar zone, with subsequent fistula formation in the anal sinuses, in most cases is found concomitant with hidradenitis of the cutaneous zone.

Hidradenitis is present in about 50% of all dogs with perianal fistulation. Lesions can extend over the tail folds to the ventral surface of the tail. This condition most frequently is seen in German shepherd dogs, Irish setters, and other dogs with broad-based and low-slung tails. No sex predilection is apparent.

Treatment

Surgical treatment of hidradenitis consists of resection or fulguration of the affected anal cutaneous zone, including the paired tail folds, if affected. However, because hidradenitis most frequently is an early stage of perianal fistula formation, deeper hidden or developing fistulous tracts usually are detected during surgery. In these cases surgery is carried out as described below (see "Perianal Fistulae").

Anal Sacculitis

Anal sacs frequently are affected by inflammatory processes. In many cases it remains unclear whether inflammation is the cause or the result of anal sac disease. Anal sacculitis leads to an increase in secretory activity. Anal sac ducts can become obliterated. Infection aggravates the condition, and abscessation of the sac occurs. Anal sac rupture (Fig. 14-1) and chronic anal sac abscessation are common sequelae of anal sacculitis.

Clinical Signs

In milder cases of anal sacculitis and anal sac impaction, animals show signs of tenesmus, dyschezia and *scooting* (rubbing the anal region on the ground). In more severe cases, painful swelling and or abscessation in the area immediately lateral to the anus is apparent, with hemorrhagic or purulent discharge from the anal sac duct. Rectal palpation usually is diagnostic.

Treatment

In cases of chronic impaction, treatment consists of repeated manual expression of the anal sacs. A lubricated, gloved index finger is inserted into the anus, while the thumb applies pressure from outside. During this procedure it is important to avoid occlusion of the duct opening. Sedation or anesthesia usually is not

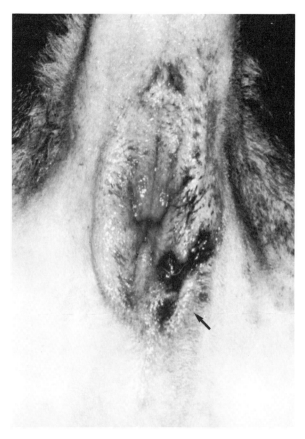

Figure 14-1. *Right-sided ruptured anal sac abscess (arrow) in a three-year-old German Shepherd.*

necessary. In cases of obliterated ducts, sedation might be required to allow cannulation of the ducts. Usually, initial non-surgical treatment is performed with an oil-based antibiotic and corticosteroid-containing ointment (*e.g.,* Panalog, E.R. Squibb & Sons, Princeton, NJ) injected via the ducts into the sacs after they have been expressed. Several treatments at 2 or 3 day intervals usually are curative, at least temporarily. An abscess is treated by warm moist packs until the abscess points, then it is lanced with a scalpel. The abscess cavity may be packed with iodoform gauze for 24 to 48 hours. Patency of anal sac ducts is reestablished by injection of an oily ointment into the ducts. The wound heals by second intention.

Complete surgical excision of the anal

sacs is indicated in cases of chronic and recurrent impaction or abscessation (during a quiescent period, if possible), non-healing abscesses, and in all cases of perianal fistulation.

Surgical Technique: Excision of the Anal Sac

In dogs, a short, dorsoventrally oriented incision is made about 1 to 2 cm lateral to the anocutaneous junction between 7 and 10 o'clock or 2 and 5 o'clock, depending on the affected side. The single anal sac ducts open at the inner cutaneous zone at 8 and at 4 o'clock relative to the anus. The anal sac is found beneath and between the fibers of the external anal sphincter muscle. Care should be taken to dissect between the muscle fibers, rather than sever them. The anal sacs usually are relatively easy to identify by their bluish gray tinged walls. The caudal rectal nerve and the caudal rectal artery and vein lie at the cranial pole of the anal sac. In this area, careful blunt dissection is mandatory. Injection of different dyes or polymerizing composite material into the anal sac has been recommended to facilitate resection. Of course, this injection is possible only in uncomplicated cases with patent ducts. If the duct is patent, a probe inserted into the anal sac is usually sufficient to identify its boundaries. The dissection is continued around the duct to its neck, which is severed where it joins the anocutaneous junction. After complete extirpation, the anal mucosa is closed with one or two absorbable skin sutures in the area of the excised duct. Likewise, the skin incision is closed with sutures. Some surgeons leave the ventral end of the incision open for drainage, or place a Penrose rubber drain, via a separate skin incision, into the cavity left after removal of the sac. The drain is removed when drainage stops, usually after 2 or 3 days.

Temporary or permanent fecal incontinence or anorectal stricture are rare potential complications of anal sac extirpation. Incontinence might occur when by extensive dissection the nerve supply to the external anal sphincter is inadvertently damaged (especially bilaterally), or if bilateral anal sacculectomy causes undue trauma to the anal sphincter muscles.

These same procedures can be used to resect anal sacs in cats, although they are rarely affected by inflammatory processes, and can be used in ferrets for descenting.

Perianal Fistulae

Perianal fistulae are chronic perianal inflammatory lesions of dogs. Their etiology is obscure. Pathogenically, infection, originating in the specific glandular structures, in and around the canine anus (see "Hidradenitis," p. 387) seems to be the most important initiating factor of the disease. Most commonly, mature dogs of either sex and of breeds with a long, low-slung tail are affected. The lesion most frequently is seen in German shepherds.

Clinical Signs

Depending on the extent of the disease, animals show tenesmus, dyschezia, bleeding, and malodorous purulent discharge from perianal fistulous tracts. Severe pain is present in most cases of extensive fistulation. Chronic constipation, with or without megacolon, lethargy, anorexia, and weight loss can occur as complicating factors.

Treatment

The disease is progressive in nature and conservative treatment is ineffective. Thus, surgical treatment should be initiated as soon as lesions are recognized. However, most cases are presented for diagnosis only after severe discomfort and bleeding have developed. Initial signs of abscessation are not easily detectable, and early recognition of developing fistulous tracts might be difficult. At surgery, a relatively small number of visible fistulous skin openings usually are found; however, during dissection, the fistulous tracts are commonly seen to be interconnected with an extensive subcutaneous, perianal, or perirectal network of sinuses. Most consistently, peri-anal fistulae are seen lateral to the anus in the area of the anal sacs. Although fistulae can extend dorsally to the ventral surface of the tail and beyond, connecting tracts are found more commonly ventral to the anus, resulting in a horseshoe-like fistulous ring encircling the anus.

Several methods of surgical treatment have been described. None is fully satisfactory. Healing without recurrence can be achieved in about 50% of severely affected animals. The various methods include excision or exterioration of all fistulous tracts, or their destruction by chemical or thermal means. The method of choice depends largely on the extent of fistulation and the preference of the individual surgeon. Regardless of the surgical method chosen, and because of the likelihood of involvement of the anal sacs in the disease, bilateral anal sacculectomy should be performed concomitantly (see "Excision of the Anal Sac," above).

Prior to surgery, broad-spectrum antibiotic therapy for about 1 week appears to decrease the degree of inflammation and may decrease the amount of actively infected tissues to be removed. Complete excision of all affected tissues using sharp and blunt dissection techniques is most desirable. Radical, yet careful, dissection allows excision of extensive fistulous tracts (Fig. 14-2). The following principles must be followed: complete anal sacculectomy; preservation of nerve supply to the external anal sphincter muscle (caudal rectal nerve and its arborization); and, preservation of large parts of the external anal sphincter muscle and drainage of larger wound cavities. Absorbable sutures are used to appose the skin, because suture removal usually can not be accomplished without sedation. Subcutaneous sutures are not necessary or suggested, because they obliterate drainage. Penrose drains are placed into the perirectal tissues via separate incisions ventral to the surgical site. They are removed when drainage subsides up to 1 week after surgery. A partial breakdown of the contaminated wound occurs in most cases after 2 to 3 days. An Elizabethan collar should be used to prevent the dog from reaching the anal area during the first week post surgery. Healing of the contaminated areas occurs by second intention. Hydrotherapy (gentle flushing with saline) has been beneficial, yet not all dogs tolerate manipulation in the anal region after surgery; and further, hydrotherapy might increase the likelihood of wound dehiscence. Although not routinely available as therapy, good results have been obtained when dogs have been encouraged to swim frequently or play in seawater during the first days postoperatively. A stool softener should be given *per os* until dogs defecate without pain. Continuation of antibiotic therapy postoperatively is unnecessary.

Some surgeons prefer not to attempt complete surgical excision, because they believe that in cases of extensive and deep-reaching fistulous tracts, surgery is potentially damaging to vital structures (nervous supply to the anal sphincter and the sphincter itself). Thus, a combination of fistulectomy and fulguration, or cauterization of remaining tracts by caustic agents such as 10% Lugol's solution, has been advocated. Although surgical excision alone is preferable, in very advanced cases, surgical procedures necessarily have to be a compromise between completeness of excision and minimization of trauma to prevent fecal incontinence. Thermal or chemical destruction leads to necrotic tissue and opposes the healing process, at least temporarily, and predisposes to postoperative stricture formation.

Cryotherapy to induce slough of infected tissues previously was advocated by many investigators, but it is not more effective than surgical excision and is potentially dangerous, resulting in more tissue destruction than necessary, and a higher incidence of post-treatment stricture than sharp and blunt dissection.

When perianal fistulae involve the anus and internal anal sphincter, complete excision of the anus and its surrounding tissue may be necessary. The procedure involves a 360° circumferential incision around the anus. Dissection progresses craniad in unaffected perianal tissues until a portion of the rectum, free of

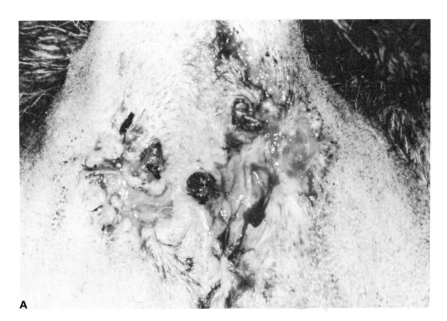

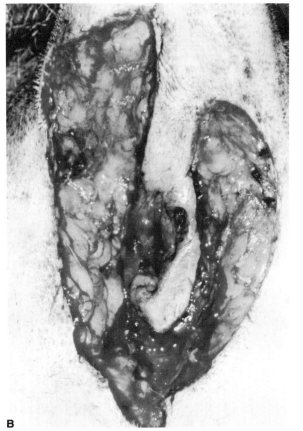

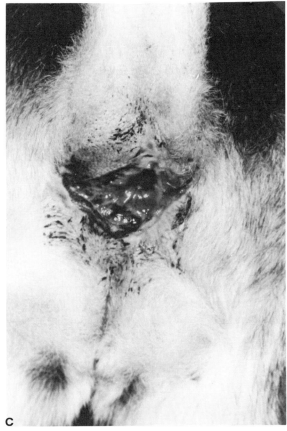

Figure 14-2.   **A,** Perianal fistulae with bilateral anal sac abscessation in an eight-year-old German shepherd. **B,** Same dog, intraoperatively after excision of fistulous tracts, bilateral anal sac resection, and partial resection of the anus. **C,** Same dog, six weeks after surgery. Healing by granulation and epithelialization is completed. The anal opening is slightly offset to the left. Full anal function has been restored.

lesions, is identified. The rectum then is separated transversely from the anus, and the rectal mucosa is sutured directly to the skin. During this procedure, the circular skin defect has to be narrowed with a few sutures on two or more sites to adapt to the narrower diameter of the transsected rectum. If major damage to the external anal sphincter and its blood and nervous supply is avoided, dogs usually remain continent. Animals with total resection of anus and internal anal sphincter lack the ability to separate the defecated feces from fecal material retained in the rectum at the end of the defecation process. Thus, complete cleanliness cannot be achieved after total anal resection, but animals are usually free of pain.

There is a hypothesis that a broad-based tail can prevent aeration of the anal region in certain breeds, and that this seems to contribute to the development and persistence of perianal fistulae. In these dogs, tail amputation has been proposed as treatment option. Results are not convincing, however, and only a few owners are ready to agree to such a procedure.

Rectal Fistulae

Rectal fistulae usually occur associated with severe forms of perianal fistulation. The fistulous tracts can extend cranially within perirectal tissues or submucosally within the rectum itself. The opening into the rectal lumen often is difficult to detect, requiring careful probing. In some cases of anal sac abscessation, particularly in German shepherd dogs, rectal fistulae develop without perianal fistulation. German shepherd dogs seems to have an anatomical predilection for rectal fistulae; their anal sacs extend farther craniad and are in closer proximity to the rectum than anal sacs in other breeds.

Solitary rectal fistulae (rectocutaneous fistulae) also can be found as sequelae to deep, perforating bite wounds in the perianal region.

Treatment

Whether of traumatic or inflammatory origin, rectal fistulae are treated by complete excision of the fistulous tracts via a pararectal ap-

proach, debridement of the mucosal lesion, closure of the rectal defect with simple interrupted, absorbable sutures, and placement of a drain. Depending on the extent of rectal fistulae and on the involvement of the external anal sphincter, anorectal stricture or incontinence may develop as sequelae to fistulation or surgical excision.

Hyperplasia of Hepatoid Circumanal (Perianal) Glands

Hyperplasia of hepatoid circumanal glands is a common phenomenon, usually seen in older male dogs. A moderate degree of hyperplasia, without accompanying lesions, is a physiologic response to androgenic stimuli. In cases of extensive hyperplasia, secondary irritation of the perianal skin with anusitis, hidradenitis, and tenesmus might develop. Frequently, hepatoid circumanal gland hyperplasia is seen concomitantly with perianal adenomas (Fig. 14-3).

Terminology and Pathogenesis

Hepatoid circumanal (perianal) glands are found in the hairless disk encircling the canine anus. They also appear scattered in the skin of the prepuce, inguinal area, hind limbs, sacral region, and tail of dogs.

The widely used term *perianal glands* is confusing. The perianal area contains three distinctly different glandular structures: apocrine sweat glands, sebaceous glands, and the deep, dermal, ductless circumanal (hepatoid) glands. *Perianal gland hyperplasia,* however, refers only to hepatoid glands. Thus, the term *hepatoid circumanal glands* is preferred to describe these specific canine glands.

Besides being located around the anus, hepatoid glands also are found concentrated within a characteristic plaquelike area on the dorsal surface of the tail. This so called *tail gland* is obvious in some (but not all) members of certain breeds (*e.g.,* English bull terriers, Irish setters, great Danes, Rhodesian ridgebacks, etc.). The canine tail gland is regarded as atavistic in nature. As do the hepatoid cir-

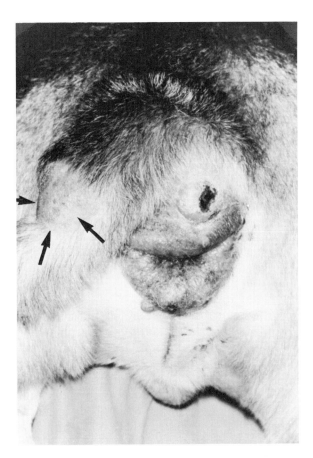

Figure 14-3. *Hepatoid circumanal gland hyperplasia, circumanal adenomas (the larger ulcerated tumor), and tail gland hyperplasia (arrows) in a 9 year old male Beagle. The tail is pulled to one side.*

cumanal glands, the tail gland also reacts to androgenic stimuli. Consequently, dogs exhibiting marked hepatoid circumanal gland hyperplasia alone may lack the tail gland.

Treatment

Because extensive hepatoid circumanal gland hyperplasia (with or without tail gland hyperplasia) is caused by androgenic stimulation, other diseases or lesions related to sex hormone imbalances may be present concomitantly (*e.g.*, prostatic hypertrophy). In male dogs, castration is the recommended therapy for extensive hepatoid gland hyperplasia, and testicles should routinely be submitted for his-

tological evaluation; androgen-producing tumors (commonly Leydig cell tumors) frequently are found. Occasionally, hyperplasia of the hepatoid circumanal glands may be detected in older, spayed bitches, probably associated with lack of estrogens and a relative increase in androgen hormone concentration.

Neoplasms of Perianal Glands and Anal Sacs

Neoplasms of the perianal glands originate almost exclusively from hepatoid circumanal glands. Only rarely do squamous cell carcinomas or other glandular tumors occur in the perianal region.

Hepatoid Cell Tumors

Hepatoid circumanal gland tumors are among the most frequently occurring canine tumors. All breeds are affected, although cocker spaniels seem to have a predisposition. Development and growth of hepatoid gland tumors is related closely to plasma androgen levels. Thus, 85% of hepatoid tumors are found in mature or aging male dogs. Most hepatoid circumanal gland neoplasms are benign and present as firm single or multiple nodular masses of variable size in the perianal dermis (Fig. 14-4). Occasionally, hepatoid adenomas also can be found in other areas of the skin where scattered hepatoid gland cells normally are found (tail, inguinal area, prepuce, thighs). Benign tumors appear well encapsulated and are not invasive. Yet, hepatoid adenomas often are ulcerated and infected secondarily. Mechanically irritated ulcerating tumors can cause considerable bleeding, and their appearance can mimic malignancy, so biopsy is indicated.

Hepatoid Adenocarcinoma

The rarer hepatoid adenocarcinomas show aggressive local invasion and occasionally cause severe hemorrhage. Extension of the malignancy into the perineal region and pararectally into the pelvic canal is common, yet metastasis to regional (sublumbar) lymph nodes often occurs slowly. Intrapelvic lymph node

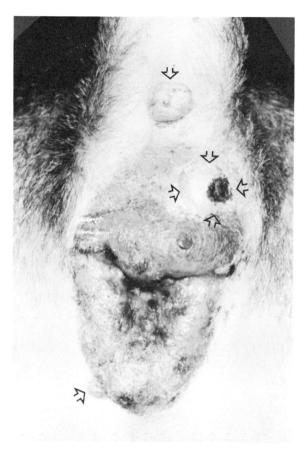

Figure 14-4. *Same dog as in Fig. 14-3. An ectopic hepatoid gland adenoma is visible on the ventral surface of the tail, and hepatoid circumanal adenomas are shown at 7 o'clock and 2 o'clock to the anus. This dog was treated by castration and excision of the hepatoid adenomas. By six weeks postoperatively (not shown), hepatoid circumanal gland and tail gland hyperplasia had disappeared.*

metastases also expand slowly, causing, in some cases, constipation and urinary stasis by mechanically compressing the colon and urethra. Spread of hepatoid adenocarcinomas to distant organs is very rare; however, I have observed a splenic metastasis.

Treatment

Several avenues for treatment of hepatoid gland neoplasms have been explored. Prior to treatment, however, benign and malignant tumors have to be differentiated. Due to ulceration of some benign hepatoid tumors, clinical distinction is not always easy. In these cases biopsy is recommended prior to surgical treatment. Surgical excision is necessary in cases of large ulcerating and hemorrhaging adenomas. They also can be treated by cryotherapy. Castration at the time of tumor excision usually prevents regrowth, enhances involution of remaining tumor nodules, and promotes regression of the frequently present hepatoid gland hyperplasia (see "Hyperplasia of Hepatoid Circumanal Glands," p. 392). A marked involution of hyperplastic or adenomatous tissues becomes apparent by 4 to 6 weeks after castration. Neither estrogen nor antiandrogenic long-term therapy are recommended as an alternative to castration.

Adenocarcinomas should be completely excised, which is achievable only when tumors are fairly small. The anatomy of the pelvic canal and the desire for postoperative continence restrict the options for radical surgical excision of intrapelvic tumors considerably. Local recurrence or lymph node metastasis can be expected. Radiation therapy as an additional treatment modality has shown some effect in selected cases. Hormone therapy or castration seem to be ineffective in cases of hepatoid adenocarcinoma.

Neoplasms of the Anal Sacs

Tumors involving the canine anal sacs almost invariably appear to be malignant. Adenocarcinomas arise from the apocrine glands of the anal sacs. Female dogs are affected in 95% of the cases. Anal sac adenocarcinoma is the most frequent neoplasm of the perianal and perineal region in older (>10 years) female dogs. Prior ovariohysterectomy seems not to affect the incidence. The most characteristic biological feature of anal sac adenocarcinomas (occurring in over 90% of the cases) is the occurrence of hypercalcemia and the resulting paraneoplastic syndrome. An idiopathic humeral mechanism (pseudohyperparathyroidism) is responsible for raising the serum calcium concentration.

Diagnosis

A presumptive clinical diagnosis of anal sac adenocarcinoma can be made reliably, based on the presence of a nodule in the perianal region in an older female dog with marked hypercalcemia. Although the tumors are metastatic, initially they seem to remain confined, possibly for several weeks, to the anal sac. At this stage they may be detected by routine rectal examination. In later stages, when dogs are presented because of related clinical signs (*e.g.,* dyschezia, ulceration, hemorrhage), lymph node metastasis to the sublumbar nodes and to distant organs usually already will have occurred.

Treatment

Surgical excision usually is not curative. Recurrence or metastasis, if not already present at the time of surgery, can be expected within weeks to months after surgery. Complete surgical excision at early stages, though not likely to prevent recurrence, reduces the elevated serum calcium concentration and thereby alleviates, at least temporarily, the metabolic effects of severe hypercalcemia.

Neoplasms of the Anus and Rectum

Nonglandular tumors arising from the cutaneous part of the anus are rare. Anaplastic squamous cell carcinomas (cloacogenic type) occur occasionally, as do melanomas and other skin tumors. Excision should be attempted as early as possible. Animals with malignant melanomas or cloacogenic-type carcinomas of the anus have a very poor treatment prognosis.

Primary neoplasms of the rectum also are relatively rare in dogs and cats. Rectal tumors occur more commonly in older dogs (mean age 8.5 years, range 2–14 years). There is a slightly higher incidence in male dogs, and poodles and German shepherd dogs appear to be affected more frequently than other breeds. Rectal tumors, whether benign or malignant, usually originate from the rectal mucosa. Other primary rectal neoplasms such as leiomyomas, hemangiomas, lymphomas, plasma-

cytomas, and sarcomas of the first three tumor types, occur occasionally.

Epithelial tumors are categorized as benign proliferative polypoid growths and infiltrative or ulcerative adenocarcinomas. Adenomatous polyps are raised, broad-based, sessile, multiple, or focal lesions of varied shapes and sizes. Distinct pedicles usually are absent. Some rectal polyps invade the muscularis mucosae histologically. In these instances, the polyp (histologically a papilliferous or tubular adenoma) is regarded as carcinoma *in situ.*

Both rectal polyps (adenomas) and adenocarcinomas can grow relatively slowly. Progressively intensifying clinical signs (*e.g.,* tenesmus, dyschezia, hematochezia) over a period of several months or even 1 to 2 years often are part of the case history. Based on these clinical observations and histologic reports, canine rectal polyps may be regarded as precancerous.

Adenocarcinomas feature a variety of growth patterns, including proliferative, friable masses that fill the rectal lumen and tumors that infiltrate the rectal wall, resulting in stricture. In these latter cases a fibrotic annular (napkin) ring can be digitally palpated or detected on positive-contrast radiography.

Clinical Signs and Diagnosis

The primary clinical sign is hematochezia. Digital rectal examination, proctoscopy, and positive-contrast (barium) radiographic studies usually are diagnostic. Infiltrative and anaplastic carcinomas bear a very poor prognosis. Thus, in cases suggestive of rectal cancer, a biopsy and thorough clinical staging is recommended prior to surgical treatment.

Treatment

Surgical treatment of invasive tumors circling the rectum usually (but not always) is only palliative, because these tumors frequently have metastasized to sublumbar lymph nodes or beyond by the time of surgery. In these animals, radiation therapy alone might be employed; this, however, most likely will result in only a moderately prolonged survival time. In all other cases with locally confined rectal tumors, radical excision, following prior biopsy, is recommended.

Depending on location, size, and extent, an intraluminal or a pararectal approach, with or without pelvic symphysiotomy or pubic triple osteotomy, can be employed. Resection of histologically confirmed malignant tumors usually requires a transpelvic or pararectal approach to maximize surgical exposure. In most cases of benign rectal polyps, however, an intraluminal approach will suffice.

Intraluminal Approach Technique

Epidural anesthesia, in addition to general anesthesia, is recommended to allow maximal dilatation of the anus. A speculum, proctoscope, or a vaginoscope is helpful to visualize the lesions. The rectum is relatively freely movable, and using long atraumatic clamps (e.g., Babcocks), the tumor or polyp, with its underlying mucosa, usually can be pulled near the anus, thus becoming accessible to surgical manipulation. Deep stay sutures, placed cranial to the lesion, are helpful to apply tension on the rectum throughout the procedure. Once seen, the tumors may be excised in different ways. Sharp submucosal dissection or full-thickness resection of rectal wall, depending on the extent of the lesion, followed by electrocoagulation, is recommended. Electrocoagulation or cryosurgery alone have been used rarely. Regardless of the surgical technique used, deep and wide excision of protruding masses or sufficient surrounding tissue destruction by freezing or coagulation appear to be important. In any case, the surgical specimen should always include at least the submucosal layer. After surgery, full-thickness defects of the rectal wall should be sutured with absorbable suture material, if accessible. Unsutured rectal wall defects usually heal by granulation, as long as perforations are in the retroperitoneal part of the rectum. Placing Penrose rubber drains lateral to the rectal wall in such cases may help prevent pararectal abscesses, whether or not the wall has been sutured.

A lateral or dorsal pararectal approach combined with a rectal pull-through procedure, as described above, is preferable in cases of lesions involving most or all of the circumference of the rectum. If the line of resection lies near the colorectal junction, a ventral pelvic (abdominal) approach combined with an anorectal approach should be used (modified pull-through procedure).

Modified Pull-Through Procedure

This procedure usually is performed best by surgical specialists. The rectum (or colon), severed by abdominal (transpelvic) approach, is pulled through the pelvic canal and anastomosed either by a second surgical team, or is temporarily transfixed with stay sutures to allow closure of the abdominal and pelvic cavities first, before the septic rectoanal (coloanal) anastomosis is performed (see "Rectal Pull-through Procedure," above). Placement of Penrose drains into the perirectal space and antimicrobial chemotherapy are mandatory (see "Preoperative Antimicrobial Chemoprophylaxis and Chemotherapy," above).

Despite attempts to preserve the sphincter mechanism, fecal incontinence frequently is seen as a sequel to extensive rectal resection. Sometimes incontinence is transient, however, lasting only for several days postoperatively. In other cases, severe anorectal stricture, and in some dogs, a combination of stricture and incontinence, might develop postoperatively. Thus, results of treatment are variable. In a study of 78 cases, the mean survival time of dogs with colorectal carcinoma was 15 months without treatment and 22 to 24 months after surgical excision, although other investigators report considerably shorter survival times. In cases with infiltrative anaplastic rectal carcinomas and annular lesions, the prognosis is very poor. In selected cases, radiation therapy has been used with moderate success to prolong survival.

Anal and Rectal Prolapse

Straining to defecate or urinate can cause anal or rectal prolapse. Prolapse occurs most frequently in malnourished pups and kittens with intestinal parasitism. However, any irritative lesion of the lower intestinal tract, usually associated with chronic diarrhea or uncoordinated peristalsis, can elicit prolapse. In animals of any age, rectal or anal prolapse also can occur in association with dystocia, prostatic disease, perineal hernia (especially immediately after its repair), rectal neoplasia, rectal foreign bodies, and so forth.

The difference between anal and rectal prolapse is a matter of degree. In anal prolapse, only anal mucosa protrudes. The bulging mucosa is usually engorged and edematous. Animals show tenesmus, are irritated, and inflict further damage to the protruding anal mucosa by licking or rubbing. In cases of rectal prolapse, an oblong, cylindrical mass protrudes from the anus. At the end of the cylinder, a dimple, marking the reflecting rectal wall, is visible. A palpating finger or a blunt probe can be inserted through this centered dimple into the lumen of the rectum.

Diagnosis

Rectal prolapse must be differentiated from prolapsed intussusception. In the latter condition, a probe can be inserted and advanced far craniad into a circular space between the cylindrical mass and the anal perimeter (see "Intussesception," in Chap. 13, The Small and Large Intestines). In anal or rectal prolapse, the probe cannot be inserted deep into the anus, lateral to the tubular mass.

Prolapsed mucosa is not appreciably sensitive to pain perception by superficial irritation. Thus, automutilation and necrosis of mucosal surfaces often occur.

Treatment

Treatment should include elimination of causes (*e.g.,* antiparasitic therapy, improved nutrition) in addition to reducing the prolapsed rectum or anus. In all forms of prolapse, protruding mucosa should first be cleansed with warm saline. Then, in the anesthetized animal (under general anesthesia and preferably in combination with epidural anesthesia), reduction is attempted by applying gentle circular

pressure on the protruding mass. Compresses soaked with cold saline can be helpful in shrinking the prolapsed tissues.

Reduction of an anal prolapse usually is simple. After reduction, a purse-string suture is loosely placed around the anus tight enough to avoid recurrence but loose enough to allow defecation of soft feces (about a pencil diameter opening). The purse-string sutures can be left in place for up to 1 week. In cases of repeated recurrence or severe swelling, the protruding mucosa can be trimmed surgically. Sutures are not mandatory after such a procedure; apposition of mucosal edges with absorbable suture material is preferable, however.

For rectal prolapse, the tubular structure usually can be reduced manually, and an anal purse-string suture placed as described above. In cases with severely damaged or necrotic prolapsed tissue, resection of the protruding mass may be necessary. Not unlike the above-described pull-through procedure, four stay sutures are placed in quadrants around the circumference of the protruding mass. Subsequently, the cylinder is transsected just caudal to the pre-placed sutures. The ends of the bowel segments, the telescopelike array of which is now visible, are anastomosed with simple interrupted monofilament synthetic absorbable sutures. Suturing around the circumference should proceed in quadrants, using the preplaced stay sutures as reference points. When the anastomosed segment inverts by replacing it craniad, knots will be situated intraluminally. Anorectal stricture, incontinence, or recurrence of rectal prolapse has occasionally been observed after amputation. Colopexy is recommended to prevent future prolapse when an extensive recurrent prolapse of healthy tissue has occurred (see below). This procedure is always preferable to resection, whenever possible.

In cases of prolapsed intussusceptions, no attempts should be made to reduce the protruding mass *per anum*. Reduction should be executed by laparotomy. The procedure is regarded as a surgical emergency, because affected animals may show signs of shock due to obstruction of intestinal circulation and fluid loss (see "Intussesception," in Chap. 13, The Small and Large Intestines).

Colopexy

To perform a colopexy, a ventrocaudal midline celiotomy incision is made. The descending colon is lifted and gently pulled cranially, with sufficient tension to stretch the rectum. This can be controlled by an assistant palpating the rectal lumen. While maintaining traction, the descending colon is sutured to the peritoneal surface of the ventrolateral body wall, adjacent and parallel to the linea alba, using horizontal mattress or simple interrupted absorbable sutures, avoiding penetration of the lumen. To fasten the colon securely, two parallel rows of sutures are suggested. Colopexy does not affect intestinal function adversely.

Rectal Diverticulum

Rectal diverticula occur unilaterally or bilaterally in the caudal rectum of dogs. Almost always, these lesions are seen in old male dogs in conjunction with perineal hernia, due to breakdown of muscular support (see below). Very rarely, diverticula may occur without apparent perineal herniation. Anal sphincter musculature and rectal muscularis mucosae most likely become atrophic, and muscle fibers are separated by bulging of the rectal mucosa during the slow and idiopathic stages of diverticulum formation. In rare instances, trauma with disruption of supporting muscular structures might cause a rectal diverticulum.

Clinical Signs

Clinically, dogs present with tenesmus, chronic constipation, and fecal impaction. In severe cases, when rectal diverticula are chronically impacted with fecal material, surgical repair should be attempted.

Treatment

Rectal diverticula can be approached surgically by a pararectal incision. In nearly all cases, the diverticulum is merely inverted into the rectum, without opening the rectal lumen, and the defect in the musculature is closed with absorbable sutures. Resection of the sacculated mucosa usually is not necessary. If, during dissection, the lumen is entered, a Penrose drain is placed to drain the wound. When the external and internal anal sphincters are severely affected, such as in cases of coexisting perineal herniation or when megacolon exists, the described procedure is unlikely to restore normal defecation. In most dogs, however, surgical reduction is attempted only when large rectal diverticula are encountered during the repair of a perineal hernia.

Perineal Hernia

Perineal hernia occurs spontaneously and almost exclusively in intact male dogs; animals between 7 and 13 years of age are at highest risk. Only a few cases are reported in older males that had been castrated during their first year of life, or in female dogs or in cats. In affected animals, an idiopathic process, probably associated with a hormone imbalance, progressively weakens connective tissues and muscles of the pelvic diaphragm. Subsequently, pelvic and abdominal structures and organs, lacking support, herniate through the pelvic canal and lodge in subcutaneous perineal pouches (Fig. 14-5). Perineal herniae can be unilateral, bilateral, or, less commonly, circumferential (in relation to the anus). In cases with unilateral perineal hernia (most commonly on the right side), however, the later appearance of a hernia on the opposite site is likely. Herniae usually contain some peritoneal fluid and characteristic fluid-filled or fat-filled cysts, attached to and covered by long fibrous strands of peritoneum. In severe cases, prostate, bladder, and occasionally intestines can herniate, and incarceration or strangulation can occur. The herniated tissues follow a route that is usually medial to the coccygeus muscle and lateral to the rectum: either lateral between the coccygeus and the levator ani muscle; or medial between the levator ani muscle and the rectal wall, coccygeoanalis muscle, and the sphincter externus muscle and

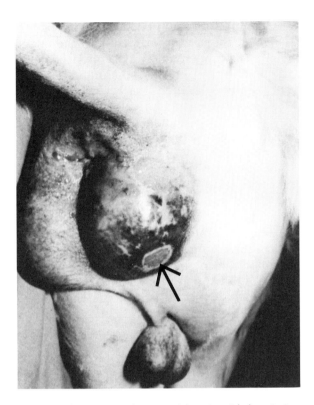

Figure 14-5. *Bilateral perineal hernia with herniation of the urinary bladder and prostate gland into the right sided hernia in an old male dog. Note the skin ulcer on the right side (arrow), signifying the chronicity of the lesion.*

the internal obturator muscle ventrally. The loss of lateral support to the rectal wall most likely occurs due to a degenerative process involving the supporting pelvic diaphragm, which is made up primarily of the levator ani and coccygeus muscles. Thus, rectal deviation (rectal flexure), or in particular, rectal sacculation (see "Rectal Diverticulum" above) is frequently present as well.

Clinical Signs

In addition to palpable and visible herniation, clinical signs of perineal hernia consist of tenesmus, dyschezia, and chronic constipation with or without megacolon, rectal impaction, or rectal sacculation. In cases of strangulation of herniated tissues, the hernial sac tends to be firm and painful and shows signs of inflammation. Also, depending on the organ involved,

anuria or ileus with or without organ necrosis might develop. Cases with a strangulated or incarcerated bladder or bowel segment must be treated as surgical emergencies. All other cases with reducible herniation can be prepared for surgery by manual removal of feces and optional cleansing enemas and by feeding a low residue diet for several days. In uncomplicated cases, antibacterial therapy generally is not necessary, but many surgeons employ perioperative antibacterial prophylaxis (*e.g.*, cephalothin sodium at 22 mg/kg IV just prior to surgery and at 6 hour intervals after surgery).

Treatment

For surgery, dogs are positioned in ventral recumbency with the hindlimbs over the end of the table and the tail pulled craniodorsally. Some surgeons prefer the table to be tilted with the dog's hindquarters elevated. If so, positive pressure ventilation is suggested during gas anesthesia. A urethral catheter may be placed to facilitate intraoperative palpation of the urethra and to minimize the risk of iatrogenic damage. A laparotomy sponge, secured with the long end of a suture, may be introduced into the rectum and pushed craniad to move fecal contents beyond the site of surgery and to lower the risk of fecal spillage *per anum*. Then, a purse-string suture is placed around the anus. The sponge not only will prevent fecal material from reaching the anus, but also will help to identify the rectal lumen during surgery. Furthermore, after completion of the repair, traces of fresh blood found on the extracted sponge likely indicate perforation of the rectal lumen by herniorrhaphy sutures. Such misplaced sutures may cause perirectal abscesses or fistula formation.

Several surgical techniques have been described for repair of perineal hernias. None of the methods is free of failures, because herniorrhaphy techniques rely on suturing and healing of tissues that are likely to be affected by a degenerative process. The repair recommended here (*i.e.*, transposition of the internal obturator muscle) has a much lower rate of complications than other described procedures.

Surgical Technique

A curved para-anal perineal incision is made extending from the base of the tail to near the midline over the ischium. Herniated structures are freed by blunt dissection and reduced craniad into and through the pelvic canal. Reherniation during surgery is prevented by tamponade with moistened laparotomy sponges that can be tagged via a long end to the outside. The sponge is pushed cranial to the site of surgery.

Then, the internal obturator muscle is elevated from its attachments to the pelvic floor. An incision is made through the periosteum along the dorsal side of the caudal brim of the ischium and about two thirds of the lateral aspect of the muscle is freed from the attachments by subperiosteal dissection (severing the tendon of insertion of the internal obturator muscle is not necessary). The caudal pudendal artery and pudendal nerve must be preserved. The caudally elevated internal obturator muscle is then used to close the ventral aspect of the pelvic defect (Fig. 14-6). Three lines of suture are placed to join the following structures in the form of an inverted Y: medially, the external anal sphincter muscle and fibers of the rectococcygeus and coccygeoanali muscles; laterally, the coccygeus and the levator ani muscles, and at times the sacrotuberous ligament; and ventrally, the freed edge of the internal obturator muscle (Figure 14-7). Different suture materials are preferred by dif-

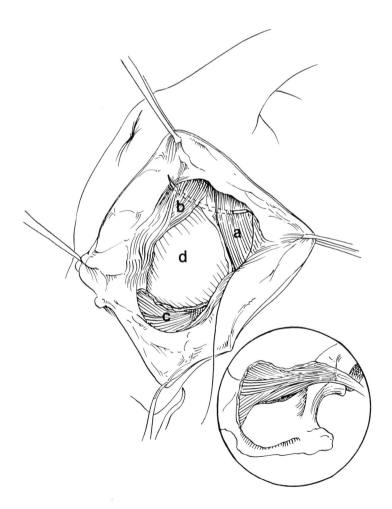

Figure 14-6. *Closure of a perineal hernia on the right side, using the internal obturator flap technique. a—the coccygeus muscle (and perhaps some residual strands of the levator ani muscle), b—the external anal sphincter muscle, and c—the transposed internal obturator muscle, d—rectum. The insert shows the obturator muscle being elevated from its insertion on the ischium. (Orsher RJ, Johnston DE. The surgical treatment of perineal hernia in dogs by transposition of the obturator muscle. Compend Contin Ed Pract Vet 1985;7:237.)*

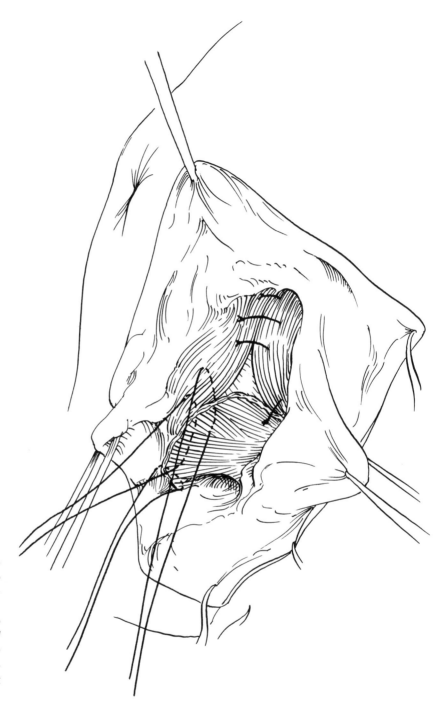

Figure 14-7. *Closure of the perineal hernia, using simple interrupted sutures between the anatomical structures. (Orsher RJ, Johnston DE. The surgical treatment of perineal hernia in dogs by transposition of the obturator muscle. Compend Contin Ed Pract Vet 1985;7:238.)*

ferent surgeons. Some use heavy surgical gut (#0 or #1, depending on the size of the defect), because such material is felt to stimulate a marked fibrous tissue response. Others prefer synthetic monofilament nonabsorbable su-

tures to insure long-term suture-holding power. Still others alternate suture materials to get both effects. All sutures are placed without tying, and the long ends are temporarily secured with hemostats. The laparotomy sponges are then removed prior to tying the preplaced herniorrhaphy sutures. After thorough flushing of the hernial cavity with warm saline, the incision is routinely closed with subcutaneous and skin sutures. Often, some excess skin has to be trimmed. Stool softeners are added to the diet until defecation is painless and effortless.

Castration of male dogs at the time of hernia repair is recommended. It is felt that androgenic hormones are pathogenically involved in perineal hernia formation, and castration may lower the rate of recurrence and may decrease progression of a nonoperated hernia on the opposite side. Many dogs with perineal hernia also have prostatomegaly; therefore, the benefits of castration are double.

Postoperative complications may include the following:

- Infection of the hernial region due to intraoperative contamination (proximity of the surgical field to the anus)
- Inadvertent partial or complete ligation of the sciatic nerve, if the sacrotuberous ligament is employed in the closure and sutures have been placed too deep
- Fecal incontinence, if the pudendal nerve is inadvertently damaged (especially if the nerves are damaged bilaterally)
- Rectal prolapse in animals intensively straining to defecate (see "Anal and Rectal Prolapse," p. 396)

The latter complication is more common when the sacrotuberous ligament, rather than the coccygeus muscle, is used as the lateral structure to anchor sutures, because more tension and discomfort seem to be induced. In the hands of the more experienced surgeons, the recurrence rate using the described method of repair is less than 10%.

References

Anderson GI, McKeown DB, Partlow GD, Percy DH. Rectal resection in the dog. A new surgical approach and the evaluation of its effect on fecal continence. Vet Surg 1987;16:119.

Church EM, Melhaff CJ, Patnaik AK. Colorectal adenocarcinoma in dogs: 78 cases (1973-1984). J Am Vet Med Assoc 1987;191:727.

Goring RL, Bright RM, Stancil ML. Perianal fistulas in the dog. Retrospective evaluation of surgical treatment by deroofing and fulguration. Vet Surg 1986;15:392.

Hardie EM, Kolata RJ, Earley TD, Rawlings CA, Gorgacz EJ. Evaluation of internal obturator muscle transposition in treatment of perineal hernia in dogs. Vet Surg 1983;12:69.

Hayes HM, Wilson GP, Tarone RE. The epidemiologic features of perineal hernia in 771 dogs. J Am Anim Hosp Assoc 1978;14:703.

McKeown DB, Cockshutt JR, Partlow GD, de Kleer VS. Dorsal approach to the caudal pelvic canal and rectum—effect on normal dogs. Vet Surg 1984;13:181.

Penwick RC. Perioperative antimicrobial chemoprophylaxis in gastrointestinal surgery. J Am Anim Hosp Assoc 1988;24:133.

Vasseur PB. Results of surgical excision of perianal fistulas in dogs. J Am Vet Med Assoc 1984;185:60.

White RAS, Gorman NT. The clinical diagnosis and management of rectal and pararectal tumours in the dog. J Small Anim Pract 1987;28:87.

Wilson GP, Hayes HM Jr. Castration for treatment of perianal gland neoplasms in the dog. J Am Vet Med Assoc 1979;174:1301.

15

Dale E. Bjorling

The Liver and Biliary Tract, Spleen, and Pancreas

The Liver and Biliary Tract

Surgical Disorders

Portal Hypertension

Portal hypertension (increased portal venous pressure) is categorized as posthepatic (caudal to the liver), intrahepatic, or prehepatic, depending on the location of the obstructive lesion causing the pressure rise. If portal hypertension lasts long enough, portosystemic shunts can develop to relieve pressure within the portal venous system. These vascular shunts directly connect the portal and systemic venous systems. Although ascites usually does not result from posthepatic obstruction, it is a common result of intrahepatic or prehepatic obstruction.

Etiology

Cirrhosis of the liver can cause intrahepatic obstruction of the portal venous system. Cirrhosis is the result of any toxic, infectious, or inflammatory process that causes replacement of normal hepatic parenchyma with scar tissue. The cirrhotic liver is decreased in size. The nondistensible scar tissue encroaches on hepatic sinusoids, restricting their luminal diameter and limiting their ability to dilate to accommodate increased blood flow.

In the presence of cirrhosis, the kidneys retain more sodium and water due to increased sodium resorption in the proximal tubules, further increasing ascites formation. Because of this, salt-restricted diets and diuretics can reduce the rate of production and accumulation of ascitic fluid in patients with cirrhosis of the liver.

Diagnosis

Animals with portal hypertension usually are emaciated due to chronic liver dysfunction and often have noticeable abdominal distention. Ascites usually is present, and a fluid wave within the abdomen is produced easily by ballottement. Abdominoparacentesis readily delivers fluid for laboratory analysis. The fluid is a transudate. The liver appears small radiographically. Laboratory tests (sulfobromophthalein [BSP] clearance or ammonia tolerance) confirm decreased liver function. Serum concentrations of alanine aminotransferase, alkaline phosphatase, and bilirubin are not increased unless inflammation or destruction of the liver is occurring.

Removing the abdominal fluid is of little therapeutic value, as it rapidly reforms. Creating a direct communication between the portal vein and caudal vena cava by performing a side-to-side anastomosis between these vessels may relieve portal hypertension; however, hepatic encephalopathy may be aggravated by the attendant decrease in portal blood flow to the liver. Valved conduits (LeVeen peritoneovenous shunt) have been used to drain fluid from the abdomen into the cranial vena cava, but complications resulting from the use of this device, combined with the initial cost of the shunt and the poor prognosis associated with advanced liver disease, limit the applicability of this technique.

Hepatic and Biliary Trauma

The liver usually lies cranial to the 13th rib and is therefore somewhat protected by the ribs. However, when the animal is subjected to blunt trauma, it is one of the most commonly injured abdominal organs. The most frequently observed injuries are tearing of the hepatic capsule and parenchyma, resulting in hemorrhage. The amount of hemorrhage associated with hepatic trauma depends somewhat upon the size of the vessels damaged, but profuse hemorrhage also can result from parenchymal injuries. Penetrating injuries seldom cause significant damage to the liver or associated vessels.

Animals with significant hemorrhage from hepatic injuries rapidly develop signs of hypovolemic shock. Continued intra-abdominal hemorrhage is reflected by a progressive decrease in the packed cell volume and plasma protein concentration. The presence of intra-abdominal hemorrhage is confirmed by retrieving, by abdominoparacentesis, blood that fails to clot (due to conversion of plasminogen to plasmin within the abdomen). If hepatic trauma is suspected and abdominoparacentesis fails to produce unclotted blood, diagnostic peritoneal lavage should be performed (see Chap. 11, The Abdominal Cavity). Abdominal radiographs may indicate the presence of intra-abdominal fluid, but are not specific in the evaluation of hepatic trauma. Injuries of the hepatic parenchyma often lead to significant increases in serum concentrations of alanine aminotransferase and lesser increases of alkaline phosphatase. Serum bilirubin may be increased, but significant increases in the concentration of bilirubin (and alkaline phosphatase) in peripheral blood are associated more often with obstruction or disruption of the biliary tract.

Blunt trauma may injure the biliary tract, but it is more commonly injured by penetrating trauma from gunshots, stabbings, or arrows. Leakage of bile results in a green-stained peritoneal effusion detected at abdominoparacentesis. The concentration of bilirubin is increased in the fluid; it often exceeds the bilirubin concentration in the plasma, especially immediately after the traumatic incident. Eventually, the bilirubin concentration within the abdominal cavity equilibrates with that in peripheral blood. Finding large quantities of bilirubin within the abdominal cavity is a strong indication for exploratory celiotomy. Bile is irritating, so it causes chemical peritonitis. Bile may normally contain bacteria (*Clostridia, Streptococcus,* or *E. coli*), and the development of bacterial peritonitis as a result of discharge of bile into the abdominal cavity is not necessarily an immediate consequence of biliary tract rupture (nor are signs of peritonitis always observed within the first few hours after the traumatic incident). Mixed (chemical and bacterial) peritonitis may follow entry of bacteria into the peritoneal cavity through disruption of the biliary system or concomitant injuries of the gastrointestinal tract. Portal venous blood has been shown to be an important route by which bacteria gain access to the liver, and bacteria may enter the abdominal cavity through the portal venous system after parenchymal injuries. Prolonged exposure of the gastrointestinal tract to bile or the presence of generalized peritonitis can impair the barrier function of the bowel wall, allowing bacteria to migrate into the abdomen.

Signs associated with bile peritonitis cannot be distinguished from those of peritonitis resulting from other causes (see Chap. 11, The Abdominal Cavity). Fever, anorexia, emesis, and abdominal pain all are commonly observed. In chronic bile peritonitis, jaundice may be present. The animal should be treated for endotoxic/septic shock, and exploratory celiotomy should be performed as soon as possible to eliminate the source of bile leakage. Bacterial cultures should be obtained and antibiotic sensitivity testing always should be performed, regardless of the duration of the problem. Gram-negative and gram-positive aerobic and anaerobic organisms may be isolated from the abdominal cavity. Antibacterial therapy for peritonitis is discussed in Chapter 11.

After recovery from the initial insult, the prognosis for recovery from traumatic injuries of the liver and biliary tract depends on whether the animal develops complications such as peritonitis, hepatic abscesses, or biliary obstruction.

Cholelithiasis

Cholelithiasis is the development of calculi in the gall bladder or bile ducts. The calculi are composed of cholesterol, bilirubin, biliverdin, calcium, phosphate, oxalate, magnesium, iron, fibrin, and bacteria. The causes of cholelithiasis in dogs and cats are unclear, but the definitive link between diet and cholelithiasis established in humans has been suggested by experimental work in animals. Some as yet undetermined biochemical abnormality in the individual dog or cat probably is the cause of development of stones. It is usually possible to culture bacteria (aerobic and/or anaerobic) from the bile of dogs and cats affected by cholelithiasis, but whether bacterial growth is the cause or the effect of the development of choleliths is unclear.

Stones may be present within the biliary tract for extended periods of time without causing clinical signs. When cholelithiasis results in clinically apparent disease, this usually is the result of obstruction or perforation of the biliary tract. Prolonged obstruction of the biliary tract due to cholelithiasis can result in necrosis and perforation of the gall bladder and bile ducts. Clinical and clinicopathological signs of biliary obstruction or disruption are present. The animals may appear jaundiced, and serum concentrations of bilirubin and alkaline phosphatase will be increased. Vomiting and abdominal pain also commonly are observed.

The definitive diagnosis of cholelithiasis is made by observing stones on radiography (positive contrast radiography may be needed to identify radiolucent choleliths) or at surgery. Intravenous or oral administration of contrast material may be used to opacify the biliary tract and outline choleliths on abdominal radiographs (contrast cholecystography and cholangiography). However, the results of these studies have been inconsistent and often inconclusive, so they are performed infrequently in animals. Ultrasound studies of the abdomen may demonstrate dilation of the gall bladder and bile ducts, but only rarely have they confirmed the presence of calculi. This lack of success may reflect a lack of experience on the part of the operator. Ultrasound may yet become a valuable technique for noninvasive diagnosis of cholelithiasis. Choleliths usually are found during surgery performed to determine the cause of biliary obstruction or perforation. They are removed by cholecystotomy and/or choledochotomy (see p. 412).

The prognosis for recovery after surgical treatment of cholelithiasis is good, unless the biliary tract is necrotic or peritonitis has developed. The frequency of recurrence of choleliths in dogs has not been determined.

Inflammatory Disorders

Infectious causes of hepatic disease include viral (canine adenovirus), bacterial (*Clostridium, Streptococcus, E. coli*), fungal (*Blastomyces, Histoplasma, Cryptococcus*), and parasitic organisms (*Opisthorchis felineus, Amphimerus pseudofelineus, Metorchis conjunctis*). Surgical treatment is required only when a focal or localized area becomes necrotic or abscessed or a granuloma forms. Some investigators have implicated a constant resident bacterial population within the liver, including both aerobic and anaerobic organisms as the source of bacteria; others argue that hepatic infections are the result of ascending migration of bacteria from the gut through the biliary tract or portal vein. Under normal circumstances, the animal is not susceptible to the development of infection within the hepatic parenchyma, so liver abscesses are uncommon in dogs and cats.

Signs associated with hepatic abscesses are similar to those seen in peritonitis. They include fever, anorexia, abdominal tenderness, and vomition. Abdominal fluid contains reactive and degenerative white blood cells, and bacteria usually are present in the fluid and within neutrophils. Evidence of localized or diffuse peritonitis is present on abdominal radiographs. Ultrasonography may suggest enlargement of a portion of the liver and the presence of cavitary lesions within the hepatic parenchyma. Liver abscesses usually are associated with significant increases in serum alanine aminotransferase and relatively smaller increases in bilirubin and alkaline phosphatase.

In cats, the biliary tract may become obstructed due to cholangiohepatitis (inflammation of the liver and biliary tract). It is not always possible to determine its cause. Bacteria, particularly *E. coli*, often are cultured from bile in cats with cholangiohepatitis. However, proliferation of bacteria within the biliary tract may occur subsequent to its obstruction. Biliary obstruction results from bile that thickens to the extent that it can no longer pass through the common duct. Affected cats have signs of biliary obstruction, including icterus, lethargy, and anorexia. Supportive therapy, including intravenous fluids, hyperalimentation, vitamins (B complex), and antibiotics (ampicillin, or amoxicillin) should be given until the flow of bile resumes. This is not uniformly successful, and surgical intervention often is required to restore patency of the biliary tract.

The prognosis for recovery often depends on how well the patient is supported during treatment; adequate nutrition, often requiring pharyngostomy or gastrostomy tubes, is critical to recovery. Tube alimentation may be required for several weeks before the animal recovers its appetite. The prognosis also depends on the response to treatment of the primary disorder.

Neoplasia

The liver is a common site for the development of both primary and metastatic neoplasms. Metastatic tumors (arising from the gastrointestinal tract, mammary glands, spleen, lymph nodes, adrenal gland, pancreas, prostate, bone, lungs, etc.) are more commonly observed than primary tumors. Primary tumors of the liver include hemangioma, hemangiosarcoma, fibroma, fibrosarcoma, hepatocellular carcinoma, hepatoma, and leiomyosarcoma. Clinical signs associated with the presence of tumors depend on their effect on the liver (*e.g.*, obstruction of the biliary tract or destruction of the hepatic parenchyma). When tumors result in destruction or necrosis of hepatic parenchyma, the signs observed are quite similar to those associated with hepatic abscesses. If hepatic neoplasia is suspected because of hepatomegaly or radiographic and/or ultrasound evidence of a mass, the animal should be evaluated carefully before exploratory surgery, to detect the primary site of neoplasia or additional areas of metastasis. Removing an isolated hepatic neoplasm may be curative if the tumor is benign and often gives prolonged relief from clinical signs even if the tumor is malignant. The entire abdominal cavity should be examined carefully for the presence of additional tumors when celiotomy is performed for treatment or evaluation of hepatic neoplasia.

The prognosis depends on the type of tumor present and the presence or absence of metastatic disease. Removing the primary tumor often eliminates the site of active hemorrhage and may result in partial regression of other tumors. In general, survival after removal of a malignant tumor of the liver will not exceed 6 months.

Surgical Procedures

Biopsy

Liver biopsies are obtained for diagnostic and prognostic purposes, and to allow formulation of a satisfactory treatment protocol. The liver may be biopsied using three approaches: percutaneous, laparoscopic, and surgical. Percutaneous liver biopsies, obtained by inserting a biopsy needle through a small incision, are most satisfactory when generalized liver disease is present, but may provide misleading information when only isolated areas of the liver are affected. The usefulness of the technique for diagnosing isolated hepatic lesions is improved by using ultrasound-guided biopsy needles. Laparoscopy allows direct observation and makes it easier to obtain a biopsy from a selected portion of the liver, although it is impossible to examine the liver or the abdominal cavity completely during laparoscopy. Surgical liver biopsy is by celiotomy. Biopsy samples can be obtained during surgery using a biopsy needle or by excising a small portion of the liver, and the liver and abdominal cavity can be examined and palpated completely.

Percutaneous Biopsies

Because the surgeon relies on the animal's ability to form a clot to stop hemorrhage associated with the biopsy procedure, a percutaneous liver biopsy should not be performed in an animal suspected of having a clotting abnormality. Ideally, the platelet count, activated clotting time, prothrombin time, and partial thromboplastin time should be determined before surgery. If this is impossible, the owner should be questioned about any history of prolonged bleeding and the animal should be carefully examined for evidence of continued hemorrhage after venipuncture or the presence of subcutaneous bruises. Other potential complications include perforating the gall bladder or large bile ducts with the biopsy needle. Radiographs should be taken before attempting a percutaneous liver biopsy to ascertain the liver's size and position.

A variety of needle types have been used for percutaneous liver biopsy; I prefer the Tru-cut needle. This needle consists of an inner specimen cutting rod that has a notch for retention of the sample and an outer cannula with a sharp point that severs the sample from the rest of the organ.

The animal should be fasted for 12 hours before the procedure, and a small amount of fat (20 to 30 ml of corn oil or whole cream) should be given orally 1 to 2 hours before surgery to cause the gall bladder to contract. Percutaneous biopsies commonly are obtained under tranquilization or narcotic sedation in combination with infiltration of the skin and body wall with a local anesthetic. A transthoracic or transabdominal approach may be used; I prefer the transabdominal approach. The transthoracic approach involves inserting the biopsy needle across the thorax, usually through the right 7th intercostal space, and can result in laceration of the lungs, pneumothorax, or leakage of abdominal fluid into the thoracic cavity.

The transabdominal approach is performed with the animal in dorsal recumbency. The area surrounding the xiphoid process is clipped of hair and prepared for aseptic surgery. A small incision is made in the skin between the costal arch and xiphoid process on the left side. The biopsy needle is inserted through the skin incision in a cranial and dorsal direction, angled slightly to the left of the midline. Once the needle is inserted beyond the resistance associated with the abdominal wall, it is advanced until further resistance is encountered, which is assumed to be the surface of the liver. The specimen cutting rod is inserted into the parenchyma of the liver, and the cannula is advanced. With the cannula in the closed position, the needle is withdrawn and the sample is examined to determine if enough tissue was obtained. Multiple attempts may be required to obtain a satisfactory sample, but the more attempts made, the greater the potential for hemorrhage or laceration of the biliary tract or other adjacent organs. Ultrasound-guided biopsy is associated with greater accuracy and safety in biopsying localized lesions.

"Keyhole" Technique

The keyhole technique is an alternative procedure. An incision just large enough to allow the surgeon to insert two fingers is made in the cranial ventral midline of the abdomen, just caudal to the xiphoid process. The liver is palpated and digitally stabilized against the body wall. The biopsy needle is inserted through a separate stab incision made lateral to the first and is directed toward the portion of the liver immobilized against the body wall. After one or more biopsy samples have been obtained as previously described, the surgeon continues to compress the liver against the body wall for a few minutes to promote formation of a clot. The incision is closed in a standard manner.

Laparoscopy

To perform laparoscopic examination of the abdominal cavity for biopsy of the liver, the surgeon must have the proper equipment and must know how to use it. The laparoscope is an endoscope inserted across the abdominal wall, allowing direct observation of the abdominal viscera. The abdomen is distended by insufflation of compressed gas (usually carbon dioxide or nitrogen) to facilitate separation and observation of the organs. Biopsy instruments then are inserted either through the laparoscope or via a second abdominal incision. The site of biopsy is selected and observed while the sample is obtained. The biopsy site is examined for hemorrhage after the sample has been taken.

Surgical Biopsy

Surgical biopsy of the liver allows the surgeon to examine and palpate the entire organ and permits thorough examination of the rest of the abdominal cavity. The midline incision should be long enough to allow complete examination of the abdomen, and it should extend to the xiphoid process; if necessary, the cartilaginous xiphoid may be incised. If generalized liver disease is present, the site from which the biopsy sample is obtained is not critical. The liver should be examined carefully and palpated for the presence of intraparenchymal nodules or cavities, and representative samples of focal lesions should be obtained.

Biopsies can be easily obtained from the edges of the liver lobe by isolating the biopsy samples with sutures. If a sample is desired from the tip of a liver lobe, this may be obtained by placing one or more encircling ligatures of absorbable suture (I prefer 0 or 2-0 surgical gut) around the liver lobe proximal to the intended area of biopsy (Fig. 15-1). The suture is tied and tightened, cutting through the capsule and much of the parenchyma, and encircling and occluding blood vessels and biliary ducts. The tissue should be excised with a scalpel at least 3 to 5 mm from the ligature to prevent its slippage. If hemorrhage occurs from the exposed surface of the parenchyma, the vessels may be cauterized or ligated with 3-0 or 4-0 surgical gut.

A larger sample may be obtained from the margin of the liver lobe by placing overlapping or interlocking sutures (0 or 2-0 surgical gut) across the hepatic parenchyma (Fig. 15-2). These sutures are tied tightly, occluding the entrapped vasculature and bile ducts. The tissue specimen is excised a short distance distal to the sutures. Larger biopsy samples may be obtained using the technique described below for partial hepatectomy.

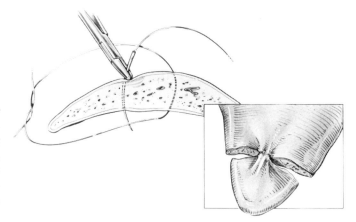

Figure 15-1. *A simple encircling ligature or two interlocking sutures can be placed to occlude the vessels and bile ducts when a biopsy is taken from the tip of a liver lobe. (Bjorling DE. Liver biopsy and partial hepatectomy. In: Bojrab MJ, ed. Current techniques in small animal surgery. 3rd ed. Philadelphia: Lea & Febiger, 1989, in press)*

Samples may be obtained from isolated lesions away from the periphery of the liver lobes using a Keyes or Baker cutaneous biopsy punch. These are available in a variety of sizes; depending on the size of the patient and the lesion, punches with a diameter of 2 to 8 mm are most useful. The larger punches allow more tissue to be obtained but carry a greater attendant risk of significant hemorrhage. Occasionally, small lesions may be completely removed with a cutaneous biopsy punch. Samples of larger lesions usually are obtained from the periphery of the lesion; the surgeon should attempt to remove some normal as well as abnormal tissue for evaluation. Hemorrhage can be minimized by carefully controlling the depth of biopsy: the punch should penetrate no deeper than half the thickness of the liver lobe. The defect created by the punch may be closed by deeply placed mattress sutures of surgical gut, or the defect may be filled with omentum or absorbable gelatin sponge (Gelfoam, Upjohn, Kalamazoo, MI).

Partial Hepatectomy

Partial hepatectomy is indicated to remove isolated tumors or abscessed liver lobes or to obtain a large biopsy. Crush injury or profuse, uncontrollable hemorrhage from the liver as a result of trauma may necessitate removal of one or more lobes. The left division of the liver

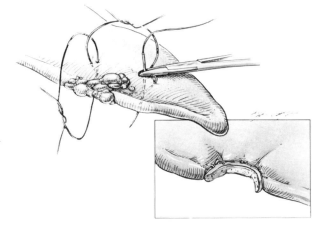

Figure 15-2. *A biopsy can be taken from the edge of a liver lobe by isolating the area to be biopsied with interlocking sutures. (Bjorling DE. Liver biopsy and partial hepatectomy. In: Bojrab MJ, ed. Current techniques in small animal surgery. 3rd ed. Philadelphia: Lea & Febiger, 1989, in press)*

(consisting of the left lateral and medial lobes) makes up about 40% of the liver mass; the central (quadrate and right medial lobes) and right divisions (right lateral and caudate lobes) each contain about 30% of the liver mass (Fig. 15-3). The left lateral and medial lobes maintain their separation from adjacent lobes near the hilus to a greater degree than the other lobes. Therefore, it is technically easier to remove either or both of these two lobes. The caudal vena cava is surrounded by the right lateral and caudate (and occasionally the right medial) lobes as it passes through the liver. The location of the caudal vena cava should be considered when operating on these lobes, because inadvertent damage to this structure results in profuse hemorrhage.

Partial hepatectomy is most commonly performed using some variation of a parenchymal crushing technique; most commonly described is the "finger-fracture" technique.

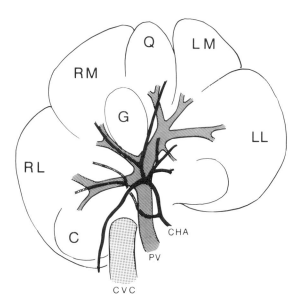

Figure 15-3. *The blood vessels and lobes of the liver as viewed from the caudoventral perspective. CVC—caudal vena cava; PV—portal vein; CHA—common hepatic artery; C—caudate lobe; RL—right lateral lobe; RM—right medial lobe; Q—quadrate lobe; LM—left medial lobe; LL—left lateral lobe; G—gall bladder. (Bjorling DE. Liver biopsy and partial hepatectomy. In: Bojrab MJ, ed. Current techniques in small animal surgery. 3rd ed. Philadelphia: Lea & Febiger, 1989, in press)*

To perform this procedure, the capsule of the liver is incised along the line of excision (Fig. 15-4). The hepatic parenchyma is compressed between the fingers along this line, causing separation of the tissues and isolating the still-intact vasculature and biliary ducts. Individual ligatures (2-0 or 3-0 surgical gut or silk) are applied to these structures, and the tissue is removed. Alternatively, a scalpel handle or forceps can be used to crush the parenchyma. Parenchymal bleeding, uncommon with this technique, can be controlled by applying pressure to the exposed tissue.

In extremely small dogs (and some cats), an entire lobe can be removed after placing an encircling ligature near the hilus. A separate ligature should be used for each lobe, and this technique probably should be used only when the left lateral or medial lobe is being removed. Although this technique has been recommended for removing liver lobes in larger dogs, there is a significant risk of hemorrhage due to the likelihood that the single ligature will be dislodged. This is because it is extremely difficult to excise the liver lobe far enough away from the ligature to ensure the ligature's security. A better technique is to crush the parenchyma near the hilus with fingers or a forceps, and to place a ligature in the crushed area. This decreases the amount of parenchyma contained within the ligature and facilitates direct placement of the ligature on the vasculature and bile ducts. My preference for ligature material is 0 or 2-0 silk, for knot security.

If an entire liver lobe is to be removed, it is preferable to isolate the blood vessels and biliary ducts near the hilus for individual ligation using sharp and blunt dissection. Simply crushing the parenchyma near the hilus may damage or obscure the ducts and vessels. Hemorrhage after liver lobectomy often is associated with dislodgement of ligatures encircling the hepatic veins, which are broad and short near the hilus and tend to retract from within ligatures. The surgeon should take every precaution, therefore, to ligate these vessels securely. Dissecting the vessels should continue until a length has been exposed sufficient to allow placement of ligatures and divi-

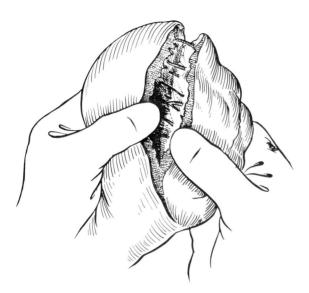

Figure 15-4. *Parenchymal crushing technique for partial hepatectomy. Following sharp incision of the capsule, the parenchyma is bluntly divided with fingers or a forceps, isolating vessels and bile ducts for subsequent ligation and division. (Bjorling DE. Liver biopsy and partial hepatectomy. In: Bojrab MJ, ed. Current techniques in small animal surgery. 3rd ed. Philadelphia: Lea & Febiger, 1989, in press)*

sion of the vessels 3 to 5 mm distal to the ligatures. Large vessels should be doubly-ligated or oversewn. The surgeon should be aware of the location of blood vessels and biliary ducts of the hepatic remnant, to avoid damaging these structures.

Continued capillary hemorrhage after removal of liver lobes can usually be controlled by direct application of pressure or ligation, or by cauterizing individual vessels. Sponges soaked with reconstituted thrombin also may be applied, or the greater omentum may be secured to the hilus with fine-gauge plain surgical gut sutures to promote hemostasis. In my opinion, the placement of even absorbable foreign materials (such as microfibrillar collagen, gelatin sponge, or oxidized cellulose) on the hilar region is undesirable, due to the inflammation associated with their reabsorption and the increased potential for infection due to their presence.

Hemorrhage, the most common complication of partial hepatectomy, most often re-

sults from slippage of a ligature. The animal should be evaluated for coagulopathies before reexploration of the abdominal cavity. If hemorrhage from the hepatic remnant is suspected, exploratory celiotomy should not be delayed.

Hypoglycemia is common after partial hepatectomy; it is more profound if larger amounts of the liver are removed. Postoperative hypoglycemia can be prevented after excising even 70% of the liver in dogs by intraoperative infusion of 10% glucose at a rate of 1 g glucose/kg/hour. Plasma proteins, particularly albumin, also are decreased after partial hepatectomy. Normal values should return in a few days. Hepatic function, as indicated by clearance of intravenously administered sulfobromophthalein (BSP) or indocyanine green (ICG), is decreased after partial hepatectomy, but improves as the liver regains mass. If the parenchyma of the hepatic remnant is normal, liver mass and function are normal 6 weeks after 70% hepatectomy in the dog. Restoration of hepatic mass primarily is the result of hypertrophy of the remaining parenchyma.

Bilirubin is not greatly increased after partial hepatectomy and should return to normal rapidly. Serum alkaline phosphatase (SAP) and serum alanine aminotransferase (SALT) usually show marked increases 24 to 72 hours after partial hepatectomy and remain slightly increased for up to 6 weeks. Prolonged increases in bilirubin and SAP indicate the presence of biliary obstruction or disruption. Increased SALT persisting beyond the first postoperative week suggests continued hepatic necrosis.

Management of Hepatic and Biliary Trauma

Hemorrhage associated with hepatic injuries usually is best managed conservatively. Surgical treatment of hemorrhage resulting from hepatic trauma commonly is undertaken only when the presence of bile in the abdominal fluid or ongoing intra-abdominal hemorrhage has been confirmed.

Abdominal exploration for treatment of traumatic injuries of the liver and biliary system can be extremely challenging. A liberal midline celiotomy incision should be made to allow thorough examination of the entire abdominal cavity for other sources of hemorrhage. Continued hemorrhage may obscure the operative field and impede the surgeon's ability to determine the source of hemorrhage and extent of injuries. Blood flow to the liver can be interrupted for up to 20 minutes by performing the Pringle maneuver: the index finger or one jaw of an atraumatic forceps is placed through the epiploic foramen, and the thumb or opposing jaw of the forceps is used to occlude the hepatic artery, portal vein, and common bile duct. Blood is removed from the operative field, and the liver and biliary tract are examined.

Severe crushing injuries of the hepatic parenchyma may necessitate partial hepatectomy. Diffuse capillary hemorrhage usually can be controlled by direct application of pressure. The omentum also may be applied with pressure to the surface of the liver to provide a surface for formation of clots. Injuries to the caudal vena cava or hepatic veins result in profuse hemorrhage that is extremely difficult to treat successfully. Treating these vascular injuries requires occluding the blood supply to the liver and occluding the caudal vena cava cranial and caudal to the liver. The caudal sternum (at least the xiphoid process) may be divided and the diaphragm incised to allow occlusion of the thoracic portion of the caudal vena cava.

The gall bladder and bile ducts should be examined carefully for damage during surgery. Small lacerations of the gall bladder or bile ducts can be repaired directly with a fine-gauge (5-0 to 7-0) monofilament nonabsorbable suture material (e.g., polypropylene), without further treatment. When the common bile duct is completely disrupted or the gall bladder is lacerated, surgical repair may be combined with some form of drainage of bile. Tubes of various configurations (including a T-shaped tube) have been used to stent the common bile duct to decrease the potential for stricture formation and direct the flow of bile into the duodenum or to the body surface. The

arms of the T are placed within the lumen of the duodenum, and the stem is placed within the common bile duct, with the tip extending into the gall bladder. Straight tubes also have been placed from the lumen of the duodenum, through the common bile duct, and into the gall bladder. These tubes become dislodged after a few days and are excreted through the bowel. Alternatively, the arms of a T tube are placed within the common bile duct and the stem of the tube penetrates the body wall. After several weeks to months, a fistulous tract forms, preventing contamination of the abdomen with bile when the tube is removed; the tract heals closed eventually. Another variation of tube drainage of bile involves placing a straight tube through the body wall and into the gall bladder, securing it to the body wall near the tube's entry point. External tube drainage of bile is uncommon due to complications associated with tube maintenance.

If destruction of the gall bladder or common bile duct precludes repair, the gall bladder may be removed (cholecystectomy), or the flow of bile may be rerouted from the gall bladder directly into the intestinal tract (cholecystenterostomy) (see below).

Cholecystotomy

A cholecystotomy may be required to remove choleliths or inspissated bile from the gall bladder and ducts. The gall bladder is isolated from the rest of the abdominal cavity with moistened laparotomy pads, and stay sutures of fine-gauge material (5-0 or 6-0) are placed at either end of the proposed site of incision. The incision should not extend into the cystic duct unless obstruction of the duct cannot be otherwise alleviated. Samples are obtained for aerobic and anaerobic microbial culture and antibiotic sensitivity testing. Bile is aspirated from the gall bladder and biliary ducts, and the ducts are probed with a catheter using a combination of gentle probing and flushing with sterile saline. The catheter is passed from the cystic duct through the common bile duct into the duodenum. If patency of the common bile duct cannot be re-established, an incision is made into the duodenum to allow retrograde catheterization of the common bile duct. Drainage tubes and stents may be placed as described above to maintain patency of the common bile duct. Their use should be combined with medical therapy to reduce the viscosity of the bile so as to decrease the potential for obstruction. I do not routinely use these tubes, but their use is recommended if the health of the tissues or security of the closure appears tenuous. Incisions into the gall bladder or bile ducts are closed with 5-0 to 6-0 monofilament nonabsorbable suture (*e.g.,* polypropylene) placed in a simple continuous pattern.

Cholecystectomy

Cholecystectomy (removal of the gall bladder) is performed infrequently in veterinary surgery. Indications include necrosis or destruction of the gall bladder due to traumatic or neoplastic causes or prolonged biliary obstruction. The gall bladder is dissected from the fossa between the quadrate and right medial liver lobes by a combination of sharp and blunt dissection. Care should be taken to avoid perforating the wall of the gall bladder. Hemorrhage during the dissection of the gall bladder from its attachments to the liver usually can be controlled by a combination of pressure and electrocoagulation. Ligation of vessels is required infrequently. The cystic artery, which accompanies the cystic duct, usually is small and may be ligated individually if identified. The cystic duct is short and should be ligated near the gall bladder proximal to its junction with the ducts leading from the central division of the liver (Fig. 15-5). Although drainage of bile may develop through auxiliary ducts, the surgeon should avoid obstructing the lobar ducts, which may result in stasis of bile within the corresponding lobes. Tube drainage of the fossa of the gall bladder to the body surface after cholecystectomy is not necessary.

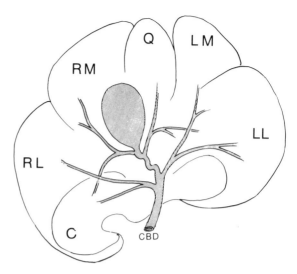

Figure 15-5. *The most commonly observed configuration of the biliary system in the dog is illustrated. The common bile duct (CBD) is formed by the junction of the short cystic duct and the ducts draining the central division of the liver (right medial and quadrate lobes). Separate ducts usually drain the left and right divisions of the liver and join the common bile duct closer to the duodenum. (Bjorling DE. Partial hepatectomy in dogs. Compend Contin Ed Pract Vet 1985;7:257)*

Choledochoenterostomy and Cholecystenterostomy

Obstruction of the common bile duct can result from inflammatory, neoplastic, or traumatic causes. If patency of the common bile duct cannot be re-established or part of the common bile duct has been destroyed, the surgeon should create a new opening between the small bowel and the common bile duct (choledochoenterostomy) or the gall bladder (cholecystenterostomy).

Choledochoenterostomy is feasible only in large dogs and cats and/or when the common bile duct is distended due to chronic obstruction. A linear incision is made in the common bile duct, and a corresponding incision is made in the antimesenteric surface of the duodenum. The incisions in the common bile duct and duodenum are placed at a 90° angle to one another. A primary anastomosis of the edges of the bile duct incision is then made to the edge of the duodenal incision using a single row of 5-0 monofilament nonabsorbable sutures. The anastomosis is facilitated by first placing four interrupted sutures to secure the ends of the incision in each organ to the corresponding midpoints of the incision in the opposing organ. The anastomosis is completed by placing interrupted or continuous sutures between the four initial sutures. Because the opening created by this procedure may become smaller in time, in dogs and cats this procedure may be inferior to a cholecystenterostomy.

In a cholecystenterostomy, the gall bladder may be anastomosed either to the duodenum (cholecystoduodenostomy) or the jejunum (cholecystojejunostomy). When a cholecystojejunostomy is performed, the most proximal available segment of jejunum should be used. Cholecystenterostomy results in chronic inflammation of the gall bladder and bile ducts due to reflux of intestinal contents into these structures. However, the most common complication after cholecystenterostomy is obstruction of the stoma. The surgeon therefore should take special care to create an opening between the two structures at least 2.5 cm long in a medium-sized dog. Usually, the gall bladder must be freed from its hepatic bed to diminish tension on the suture line between the gall bladder and bowel.

The gall bladder and bowel are placed in apposition, and stay sutures are placed through their serosal surfaces at either end of the proposed site of anastomosis to maintain them in this position during the rest of the procedure. The gall bladder is secured to the bowel along one side of the intended ostomy site with 5-0 monofilament sutures in a simple continuous pattern. The sutures are placed 2 to 3 mm from the intended location of the incisions into the small bowel and gall bladder. I prefer starting at the oral end of the suture line. Noncrushing intestinal forceps or finger pressure may be applied to the bowel proximal and distal to the anastomotic site to prevent intestinal contents from entering the incision during the procedure. It is difficult to use forceps to occlude the duodenum, as they may interfere with the procedure because the duodenum is relatively immobile. An incision is made in the gall bladder, and bile is aspirated. This incision is made parallel to, and 2 to 3 mm from, the initial suture line and should be at least 2.5 cm long. A corresponding incision (2 to 3 mm from the initial suture line) is made in the bowel. A primary anastomosis of the wall of the gall bladder to the wall of the bowel is then performed using 5-0 monofilament nonabsorbable suture in a simple continuous pattern. The edges should be carefully approximated to ensure that no gaps remain and to ensure that the length of the anastomosis is maintained at no less than 2.5 cm. The suture line between the serosal surfaces of the gall bladder and bowel is then finished, encircling the ostomy site completely. This is done using the suture remaining from the first serosal suture line. This suture line is completed by tying the suture to the free end of the suture from the initial knot or the stay suture. Two layers are used for closure to diminish the potential for leakage.

Leakage of bile, leading to peritonitis, and stricture of the anastomotic site are the most common complications of choledochoenterostomy and cholecystenterostomy. If postoperative free bile is detected within the abdomen, surgery should be performed to identify and repair the area of leakage. It is very unlikely that the defect will close spontaneously. Stricture of the anastomotic site causes clinical signs and laboratory findings indicative of biliary obstruction. Contrast radiographic studies may help confirm obstruction of the stoma, but they often are inconclusive. Surgical exploration may be complicated by the presence of adhesions and fibrin deposition, but should be undertaken to evaluate the anastomotic site and revise the stoma if necessary.

The Spleen

Surgical Disorders

Splenomegaly

Splenic enlargement (splenomegaly) is a common indication for surgery. It is classified as symmetrical or asymmetrical, based on whether all or part of the spleen is enlarged. The diagnosis of splenomegaly often can be made by abdominal palpation and/or radiographic or ultrasonic examination, sometimes requiring exploratory celiotomy for confirmation. Both symmetrical and asymmetrical splenomegaly may be caused by benign or malignant disorders, although symmetrical splenomegaly may not be pathological, such as when it is induced by administration of barbiturates or tranquilizers (Table 15-1). The prognosis for treatment of splenomegaly depends on the cause.

Volvulus of the Spleen

This condition is more accurately described as volvulus of the splenic pedicle. It can occur in the absence of other abnormalities within the abdominal cavity, but it occurs more often in conjunction with gastric dilatation/volvulus

(GDV). Isolated splenic volvulus occurs most often in large-breed dogs. Some investigators think that gastric dilatation (without volvulus) causes displacement of the spleen, somehow predisposing it to rotate on its pedicle. Isolated splenic volvulus also has been observed after trauma. Because the splenic veins are thinner-walled and more collapsible, the initial result of volvulus is obstruction of venous outflow while splenic arterial blood flow continues. The spleen therefore enlarges until intracapsular pressure equals arterial pressure.

Splenic volvulus causes signs of acute abdominal distress (pain). The abdomen may appear distended, and the animal usually is restless and may be in shock (rapid heart rate, weak pulse, decreased capillary refill time, and increased respiratory rate may be present). A symmetrically enlarged spleen may be palpated, unless abdominal splinting occurs due to pain. Abdominal radiography or ultra-

Table 15–1. Causes of Symmetrical and Asymmetrical Splenomegaly

Symmetrical Splenomegaly	Asymmetrical Splenomegaly

A. Congestive enlargement
 1. Drugs (barbiturates, tranquilizers)
 2. Venous obstruction
  a. Splenic volvulus*†
  b. Gastric dilatation GDV†
  c. Obstruction of the portal vein or caudal vena cava†
 3. Passive congestion†
B. Inflammatory diseases
 1. Bacterial†
 2. Fungal†
C. Functional causes
 1. Immune-mediated diseases (hemolytic anemia and thrombocytopenia)*†
 2. Extramedullary hematopoiesis
 3. Amyloidosis
D. Hemic neoplasia
 1. Myeloid†
 2. Lymphoid†
	A. Primary neoplasia
	 1. Hemangiosarcoma*
	 2. Fibrosarcoma*
	 3. Leiomyosarcoma*
	B. Metastatic neoplasia
	C. Nodular hyperplasia
	D. Trauma (hematoma)
	E. Torsion of the spleen or splenic pedicle*†
	F. Gastric displacement†
	G. Abscess/Granuloma*

* Indicates diseases usually treated by splenectomy.
† Indicates diseases usually managed by treatment of the primary disorder. (Perman V, Lipowitz AJ. The spleen. In: Gourley IM, Vasseur PB, eds. General small animal surgery. Philadelphia: JB Lippincott, 1985:465)

sonography usually allows detection of a symmetrically enlarged and often C-shaped spleen, with or without GDV.

Splenic volvulus is an emergency requiring immediate surgical treatment (*i.e.*, splenectomy, or derotation if there is neither splenic necrosis nor vascular thrombosis). Hypovolemia due to sequestration of blood within the spleen should be treated before surgery by intravenous infusion of crystalloid fluids, plasma, or whole blood. Untreated splenic volvulus is associated with high mortality, while early surgical treatment results in very low mortality.

Symmetrical Splenomegaly without Splenic Volvulus

This also often occurs in association with GDV in dogs. Following correction of the gastric volvulus, the decision to perform a splenectomy depends on the existence of thrombosis of the splenic vessels (see below). Symmetrical splenomegaly can result from any condition that causes increased portal venous pressure (such as cirrhosis of the liver or obstruction of the caudal vena cava cranial to the liver).

Neoplasia

Hemangiosarcoma is the most common primary malignant neoplasm of the spleen. The gross appearance of hemangiosarcoma is similar to that of hemangioma and may even be confused with a hematoma. Hemangiosarcomas of the spleen tend to have cavernous areas containing blood, and obvious areas of neoplastic tissue may not be observed. Fibrosarcomas and leiomyosarcomas, originating from the capsular or muscular elements of the spleen, also occur. These tumors tend to develop as large asymmetric masses within the substance of the spleen. When incised, they are found to be composed of densely compacted fibrous tissue, usually white or gray. Hemangiomas are benign tumors of the spleen that also cause asymmetric splenomegaly. Nodular splenic hyperplasia, another benign condition causing asymmetric splenomegaly, may be confused with malignant conditions of the spleen. These discrete areas of nodular swelling are the result of localized accumulation of lymphoid cells. The nodules are rarely greater than 2 cm in diameter; they vary from gray to pink and may be variegated red and white. Large nodules may have necrotic centers. Nodular swellings may also be associated with metastatic spread of tumors. A biopsy often is required to distinguish nodular hyperplasia from neoplasia.

Some neoplastic conditions of the spleen can result in either symmetric or asymmetric splenomegaly. For example, tumors of the lymphoid tissue, such as lymphosarcoma, usually result in asymmetrical splenic enlargement if the white pulp is involved, while symmetrical splenomegaly results if the red pulp (myeloid tissue) is the tissue of origin. Tumors of lymphoid origin are solid, and those arising from the white pulp are often discrete and multifocal. Mast cell sarcoma in the cat causes marked symmetrical splenomegaly; in the dog, mast cell sarcoma may lead to symmetrical or asymmetrical splenomegaly. The cut surface of mast cell tumors varies from white to pink or red. Mast cell tumors easily are diagnosed by cytologic examination of samples obtained from the spleen at surgery.

Malignant mast cells also occasionally (more commonly in the cat than in the dog) invade the bone marrow, and in advanced cases the presence of circulating mast cells can be detected by buffy coat smears of the peripheral blood. Feline systemic mastocytosis refers to the invasion of multiple organs by the neoplastic growth of mast cells. Signs of feline systemic mastocytosis include lethargy, loss of appetite, vomiting, and diarrhea. This disease affects the hematopoietic system (including the spleen and liver), and splenic enlargement is often detected by palpation, radiography, or ultrasonography.

It is not uncommon for primary or metastatic tumors of the spleen to enlarge to the extent that they distend the abdomen. Hemangiosarcomas and hemangiomas often are associated with the formation of large hematomas that may rupture, resulting in significant blood loss. Due to hemorrhagic shock, these animals may be severely depressed when presented. Examination of blood samples drawn from animals a short time after acute hemorrhage has occurred may show no signs of anemia (*i.e.*, normal hematocrit), while in chronic abdominal hemorrhage, signs of regenerative anemia and bilirubinemia may be present and bilirubinuria may also be detected.

Splenectomy is the treatment of choice for splenic tumors in dogs. The mean and median postoperative survival times following splenectomy of dogs for hemangiosarcoma have been reported as 80 and 65 days, respectively. The length of survival is increased slightly, but not significantly, by the use of adjunctive chemotherapy. Similar data are unavailable for cats. Splenectomy for treatment of systemic mastocytosis in cats is associated with survival for several months. Splenic mast cell sarcomas are uncommon in dogs, and survival data following splenectomy for this disease in dogs are unavailable.

Siderotic Plaques

Sometimes referred to as Gamna-Gandy bodies, siderotic plaques may be observed on the surface of the spleen and are often mistaken for neoplastic disease. They are brown or gold and consist of iron and calcium deposits. The development of siderotic plaques is a normal consequence of aging, so their presence in association with splenomegaly is coincidental.

Inflammatory Lesions

Splenic abscesses or granulomas, rare in dogs and cats, may result in asymmetrical splenomegaly, which may be associated with concomitant hepatic involvement. Septicemia (especially that associated with hepatitis or endocarditis) and parasitic or fungal disorders can lead to symmetrical splenomegaly. Signs associated with inflammatory disorders of the spleen may predominantly arise from the primary disease (*i.e.*, endocarditis, septicemia, histoplasmosis). Affected animals are often febrile and may show signs of acute or chronic peritonitis. The white blood cell count usually

is elevated and a left shift in the distribution of white blood cells toward more immature forms is observed. Treatment should be directed at correcting the inciting cause. Isolated splenic abscesses or granulomas usually carry a low mortality rate when treated early by splenectomy. The prognosis for treatment varies, depending on the nature of the primary disorder and how advanced the disease process is at treatment.

Traumatic Injuries

Splenic injuries most often result from blunt trauma, but the spleen also may be damaged by penetrating wounds or during surgery. Although large surveys of traumatic injuries of dogs and cats report a low incidence of splenic damage, evidence of healed splenic lacerations or fractures and/or splenosis (see "Splenosis," below) occasionally are seen during exploratory celiotomy for other problems. Intra-abdominal hemorrhage after traumatic injury most commonly is the result of damage to the spleen or liver. Splenic injuries vary from minor lacerations associated with few or no signs, to crushes involving most of the organ and causing significant abdominal hemorrhage. Asymmetrical splenomegaly due to the presence of subcapsular hematomas also may be seen after blunt trauma. Splenic injuries often do not result in unrelenting, life-threatening hemorrhage, but lacerations of large vessels may result in profound blood loss, shock, and death, so these injuries require surgical intervention. Penetrating injuries of the spleen seldom cause significant hemorrhage. Intra-abdominal hemorrhage may be detected by abdominal paracentesis or diagnostic peritoneal lavage (see "Peritonitis" in Chap. 11).

Hypovolemia should be treated by administering intravenous fluids or, occasionally, transfusion before surgery, unless immediate abdominal exploration is indicated by rapid, voluminous hemorrhage. In the latter case, blood should be administered rapidly as the patient is being prepared for surgery. Autotransfusion of abdominal blood may also be considered (see Chap. 1, Principles of Small Animal Surgery). The prognosis in cases of traumatic injury of the spleen depends on the amount of blood lost and whether hemorrhage is continuing.

Splenosis

Splenosis is the dissemination of multiple nodules of splenic tissue throughout the abdominal cavity, due to a prior rupture of the spleen. This condition is the result of revascularization of fragments of splenic tissue that adhere to peritoneal surfaces. All serosal surfaces and predominantly the greater omentum may be involved. Splenosis must be distinguished from a neoplastic disorder. This usually can be done presumptively at surgery, based on evidence of healed splenic trauma. Biopsy of a splenic nodule should be performed if there is any question about the diagnosis. The benign nodules of splenosis need not be removed.

Surgical Procedures

Biopsy

Biopsy of the spleen is indicated to determine the cause of symmetrical or asymmetrical splenomegaly. While the surgeon may elect to remove the entire spleen and submit it for histologic evaluation, splenectomy is not appropriate in all cases. Preserving the spleen should be considered whenever possible to avoid the complications of splenectomy discussed later in "Sequelae of Splenectomy."

Percutaneous Fine-Needle Aspiration

This may be performed to obtain a sample for cytologic analysis. Before the procedure, the surgeon should ensure that the animal has no coagulopathy; testing should include a platelet count, activated clotting time, prothrombin time, and partial thromboplastin time. Historical evidence of bruising or prolonged hemorrhage from minor lacerations should be con-

sidered contraindications for percutaneous aspiration of the spleen.

The spleen should be palpated and immobilized digitally against the abdominal wall (usually on the left side). Aspiration is performed with a 22-gauge needle 2.5 to 7 cm long, depending on the thickness of the abdominal wall. Significant hemorrhage usually does not occur unless there is a coagulopathy or if the spleen is lacerated by multiple punctures or movement of the needle once it is in the spleen. Smears of the aspirated sample are prepared on microscopic slides for examination.

"Keyhole" biopsies of the spleen, using biopsy needles or punches through a limited surgical approach, are inadvisable due to the high probability of significant hemorrhage.

Celiotomy

Celiotomy allows direct examination of the spleen and the rest of the abdominal viscera and permits direct treatment of any hemorrhage that occurs during the procedure. During celiotomy, biopsies may be easily obtained from the periphery of the spleen by isolating the desired area with interlocking mattress sutures of 2-0 or 3-0 absorbable material, similar to the technique used for the liver (see Fig. 15-2). The tissue should be excised at least 3 mm from the sutures to avoid dislodging them. A wedge or semicircular specimen may be obtained by compressing the parenchyma some distance from the lesion with fingers or an instrument. Absorbable sutures then are placed in the crushed area in an interrupted horizontal mattress pattern to isolate the biopsy sample and to control hemorrhage. The biopsy is removed by excising distal to the sutures. Solid lesions may be biopsied by removing a wedge-shaped piece of tissue by scalpel incision. Alternatively, a cutaneous biopsy punch can be used, as described under hepatic biopsy above. These punch biopsies should not create a full-thickness defect in the spleen. The defect is closed with absorbable material in a horizontal mattress pattern.

Splenic Trauma and Hemorrhage; Splenorrhaphy

Trauma may cause either parenchymal damage to a portion of the spleen or continuing hemorrhage that requires surgical exploration of the abdomen. Ischemic or necrotic areas of the spleen may be excised by performing a partial splenectomy. A partial splenectomy also may be required to control hemorrhage. Alternatives to partial or total splenectomy include ligation of the blood supply of the spleen, splenorrhaphy, or splenectomy followed by reimplantation of splenic tissue (see below).

In case of splenic hemorrhage, splenic blood flow can be occluded temporarily by digital pressure to facilitate exploration of the abdomen. The procedure is most easily accomplished by rotating the spleen, stomach, and greater omentum ventrally and to the right and applying vascular forceps or digital pressure to the celiac artery or the aorta cranial to the celiac artery. Because of increased afterload and ischemia of the kidneys and hindquarters, aortic blood flow should be interrupted for no more than 5 to 10 minutes; celiac flow, however, can be stopped for up to 20 minutes without adverse sequelae. The arterial blood supply to part or all of the spleen has been permanently ligated to control hemorrhage with no apparent untoward affects, although splenic devascularization without splenectomy is not advisable. The ischemic splenic tissue becomes revascularized, but function may not return. Necrosis of the spleen leading to peritonitis also is possible. Care should be taken to ligate splenic vessels distal to the origin of gastric vessels (Fig. 15-6). It is preferable to ligate segmental splenic vessels supplying only the damaged portion of the spleen near the hilus, to leave the rest of the splenic circulation intact. Temporary or permanent occlusion of splenic vessels should be followed by splenorrhaphy or, if this is impossible, by partial or total splenectomy.

Splenorrhaphy (suture closure) may be required to close lacerations of the splenic

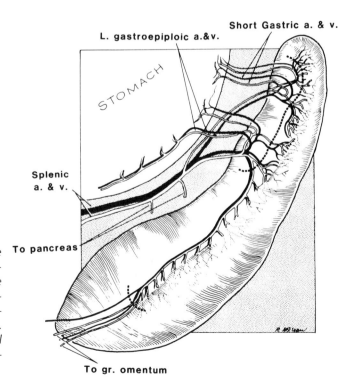

Figure 15-6. *The vascular anatomy of the spleen of the dog and placement of ligatures during splenectomy. The vascular supply to the spleen of the cat is similar. The broken lines indicate the location of ligatures for total splenectomy. (Bjorling DE. Partial and total splenectomy. In: Bojrab MJ, ed. Current techniques in small animal surgery. 3rd ed. Philadelphia: Lea & Febiger, 1989, in press)*

capsule (Fig. 15-7). Large, isolated bleeding vessels within the splenic parenchyma should be ligated individually with absorbable suture material. The splenic capsule is closed with 3-0 or 4-0 absorbable suture material in a simple continuous or interrupted pattern.

Partial Splenectomy

Partial splenectomy is indicated for removal of an isolated, benign lesion of the spleen (such as a hematoma or a crushed area secondary to trauma) or to obtain a large biopsy. It is preferable to total splenectomy because of the adverse sequelae of the latter.

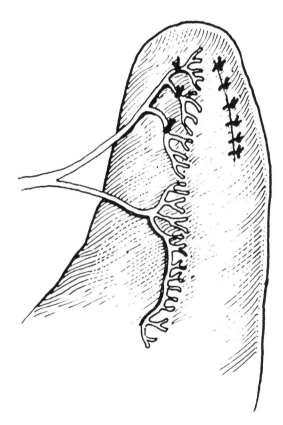

Figure 15-7. Splenorrhaphy. *Conservative treatment of a splenic laceration. Ligation of the segmental blood supply leading to the lacerated area of the spleen may be done before closing the splenic laceration. (Bjorling DE. Partial and total splenectomy. In: Bojrab MJ, ed. Current techniques in small animal surgery. 3rd ed. Philadelphia: Lea & Febiger, 1989, in press)*

To perform a partial splenectomy (Fig. 15-8), the segmental blood supply to the portion of the spleen to be removed is ligated near the splenic hilus and transected. The line of resection is determined by the obvious area of ischemia that develops after ligation. The parenchyma is compressed between the surgeon's fingers to remove splenic pulp from the proximal edge of the ischemic area. Two forceps are applied to the spleen about 10 to 15 mm apart. The line identifying the ischemic area of the spleen should be halfway between the two forceps. Atraumatic (large vascular or Doyen intestinal) forceps should be applied to the portion of the spleen not being removed; crushing forceps may be applied to the portion of the spleen to be removed. The splenic tissue is divided between the forceps 5 to 7 mm from the noncrushing forceps. Absorbable suture material (3-0 or 4-0) is used to place a double row of continuous horizontal mattress sutures distal to the atraumatic forceps, 3 to 5 mm from the cut edge of the splenic capsule. The edges of the splenic capsule are closed with the same suture material in a simple continuous or continuous cruciate pattern. If direct pressure does not control hemorrhage from the splenic parenchyma, ligatures should be applied as needed. Instead of using conventional sutures, a stapling device may be used both to crush and suture the spleen. It is applied at the location described above at which digital splenic compression is performed during the suture technique.

Splenectomy

Indications for splenectomy include splenic volvulus, thrombosis, neoplasia, large cavernous hematomas involving a majority of the spleen, and crushing injuries of the spleen, and as part of the treatment of immune-mediated thrombocytopenia or hemolytic anemia unresponsive to medical therapy (in which the spleen may be enlarged or of normal size). It also has been recommended that the spleen be removed from dogs intended for use as blood donors (see "Sequelae of Splenectomy," p. 422).

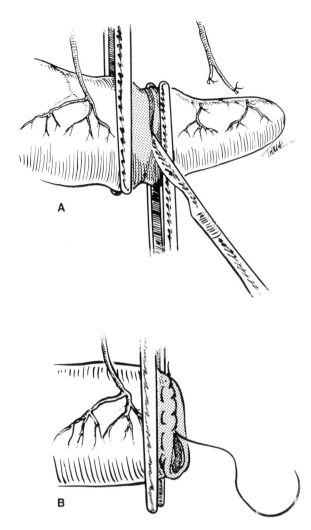

Figure 15-8. Partial splenectomy. **A,** *After deciding which part of the spleen will be resected, the surgeon ligates the segmental blood supply to that area. An ischemic area then develops. Digital compression centered over the line of ischemia moves the splenic pulp from the site of incision (hatched area). A noncrushing forceps is applied at the proximal edge and a crushing forceps to the distal edge of the compressed area, and the splenic specimen is excised, leaving 5 to 10 mm of emptied capsule distal to the noncrushing forceps. **B,** First, two rows of continuous horizontal (through-and-through) mattress sutures are applied distal to the noncrushing forceps, then the end of the capsule is closed with a simple continuous suture pattern. The forceps is then removed. (Bjorling DE. Partial and total splenectomy. In: Bojrab MJ, ed. Current techniques in small animal surgery. 3rd ed. Philadelphia: Lea & Febiger, 1989, in press)*

A cranial midline abdominal incision should be made of sufficient size to allow the spleen to be delivered from the abdominal cavity with minimal force. The spleen should be evaluated with minimal manipulation or palpation to avoid splenic trauma or the discharge of toxic products (present with splenic volvulus) or clusters of neoplastic cells into the venous circulation. Tugging on the spleen may result in rupture and hemorrhage, or dissemination of neoplastic tissue throughout the abdominal cavity.

When splenic volvulus alone, or splenomegaly or splenic volvulus in conjunction with GDV, is present, the decision to remove the spleen is made on the basis of its size and color. It often is difficult to tell by observation or palpation of the splenic vasculature whether complete thrombosis of the splenic vasculature has occurred. If the spleen is grossly distended and has become blue-black, it is unlikely that correcting the twist of the splenic pedicle and/or stomach will restore the spleen's normal circulation and function. The blood trapped within a devitalized spleen usually has a low pH and contains byproducts of anaerobic metabolism; these may result in the development of cardiac arrhythmias when discharged into the portal (and thus general) circulation. It is recommended, therefore, that splenectomy be performed without correcting the splenic volvulus. The spleen should not be excised if it appears viable and thrombosis is not apparent, or if correction of GDV or the splenic volvulus returns the spleen to a normal color.

The splenic pedicle never should be permanently ligated *en masse*, because this may lead to dislodgement of the vessels from within the ligature and massive postoperative hemorrhage. It has been recommended, however, that during splenectomy for treatment of splenic volvulus, the splenic pedicle can be temporarily occluded with an encircling ligature while the spleen is removed. Individual vessels subsequently should be identified and ligated. Sutures or staples may be used to ligate splenic vessels. My preference for ligation is 1-0 to 3-0 silk, depending on the vessels' size. If the spleen is being removed to treat autoimmune disorders or to reveal hitherto undetected parasitemia, 1 to 2 ml of a 1:100,000 dilution of epinephrine may be applied to its surface to cause contraction, preventing loss of the blood volume contained within the spleen. Epinephrine potentiates cardiac arrhythmias, so the dose should be carefully limited.

Ligatures should be placed near the hilus of the spleen to avoid compromising vessels supplying the stomach (left gastroepiploic and short gastrics) and the left limb of the pancreas. Individual vessels may be identified, ligated, and divided, or the vessels may be divided between forceps and ligatures applied proximal to the forceps after the spleen has been removed.

The abdomen should be thoroughly explored before or after splenectomy. If the spleen is being removed because of the presence of neoplasia and the owner is contemplating euthanasia, the abdomen should be explored before splenectomy for the presence of metastasis. After splenectomy, the splenic bed should be observed carefully for hemorrhage, and additional ligatures should be applied as needed.

Postoperative hemorrhage, the most common complication of splenectomy, is often first shown by increased respiratory and heart rate. The mucous membranes may appear pale, and capillary refill time is decreased. Rarely, the abdomen becomes distended early in the course of hemorrhage. A concurrent, progressive decline in the packed cell volume and plasma protein concentration indicates hemorrhage due to displacement of a ligature, although rapid, massive hemorrhage may result in shock or death before there is any evidence of a lowered hematocrit. Abdominoparacentesis or insertion of a peritoneal dialysis catheter usually confirms the presence of intra-abdominal hemorrhage (see "Peritonitis" in Chap. 11). Small quantities of serous fluid with a low packed cell volume (<10%) are sometimes seen after splenectomy. Retrieval of large quantities of bloody fluid with a packed

cell volume approximating or exceeding that of peripheral blood is an indication that the abdomen should be re-explored.

Ischemic necrosis of the stomach or pancreas due to inadvertent ligation of their blood supply, or the development of pancreatitis subsequent to intraoperative trauma, are other potential complications of splenectomy. The effects of loss of splenic function are discussed below under "Sequelae of Splenectomy."

Splenic Reimplantation

When the spleen has been removed because of traumatic injury, attempts have been made to retain splenic function by returning normal, undamaged splenic tissue to the abdomen. Splenic tissue will readily become revascularized when placed in contact with peritoneal surfaces. It appears that the pattern of revascularization is critical to maintaining splenic function. Homogenized aliquots of splenic tissue placed in the abdominal cavity retain the histologic appearance of splenic tissue without any discernible function. Placing slices of spleen 3 mm thick in a pocket created within the greater omentum appears to maintain splenic function in humans. Several other techniques of splenic reimplantation have been described, with varying degrees of success. It appears that implanted splenic tissue regains normal function only if total splenectomy had been performed first. Splenic reimplantation has not been widely applied clinically in veterinary medicine, but because there are very few complications associated with its use, this technique should be considered following excision of a nontumorous spleen.

Sequelae of Splenectomy

Overwhelming sepsis is relatively common after splenectomy in humans. This has not been observed in animals, but fatal septicemia after dentistry has been reported in a splenectomized dog. Splenectomy in dogs results in reduced IgM production and alters leukokinin synthesis so that the leukokinin produced no longer stimulates phagocytosis. Although prophylactic antibiotic administration is not routinely used perioperatively in conjunction with splenectomy in veterinary medicine, such use should be considered when splenectomized animals undergo procedures carrying a high risk of bacteremia (such as dentistry).

The spleen functions to remove abnormal red blood cells, and subclinical infections with blood-borne parasites may become apparent after splenectomy. Particularly in the cat (but also in the dog), macrophages in the spleen are able to remove *Hemobartonella sp.* from the surface of red blood cells. This may prevent detection of the parasite by normal screening methods. Anemia may not be observed in dogs infected with *Babesia canis* until the spleen is removed. The presence or absence of the spleen appears to have no effect on infection with *Ehrlichia canis*. Splenectomy of dogs intended for use as blood donors has been recommended to identify those with undetected infestation with *Hemobartonella* or *Babesia*.

Splenectomy results in several transient changes in blood components that may persist up to 15 weeks after surgery. For example, mild leukocytosis (primarily due to mature neutrophilia) is often seen. The spleen stores up to 30% of the body's platelets; thrombocytosis is common after splenectomy. The number of circulating nucleated red blood cells and red blood cells with Howell-Jolly bodies increases after splenectomy due to loss of the spleen's capacity to remove abnormal red blood cells from circulation. Anemia, reticulocytosis, and decreased serum iron concentrations occur after splenectomy and may continue for several months. Because the spleen acts as a reservoir of red blood cells in dogs and cats, splenectomy diminishes these animals' ability to maintain the circulating red blood cell volume during hemorrhage. Experimentally, dogs failed to respond normally when exposed to hypoxemia 2 weeks after splenectomy, suggesting a lessened ability to maintain cardiovascular homeostasis during anesthesia or stress. These changes may be transient and of no clinical significance.

The Pancreas

Surgical Disorders

Surgical treatment may be required for disorders affecting the endocrine or the exocrine portion of the pancreas. Surgical disorders of the endocrine pancreas are limited to neoplasia, while surgery may be required to treat inflammatory, traumatic, or neoplastic diseases of the exocrine pancreas.

Neoplasia of the Endocrine Pancreas

Carcinoma of the beta islet cells (insulinoma) is by far the most common neoplastic process affecting the endocrine cells of the pancreas. This is primarily a disease of older dogs, with mean and median ages of 9 to 10 years. Clinical signs of insulinoma are related primarily to decreased blood glucose, due to excessive production of insulin. Various combinations of the following signs may be observed: generalized convulsions, weakness or collapse, disorientation, muscle fasciculations, and ataxia. By the time of diagnosis, the signs usually have been present less than 6 months. The diagnosis of insulinoma is strongly suggested by low blood glucose (< 60 mg/dl) in an older animal displaying the previously mentioned signs, particularly if the animal has been fasted. The diagnosis may be confirmed by the presence of hyperinsulinemia, preferably determined during a hypoglycemic episode. Normal concentrations of immunoreactive insulin in canine plasma have been reported to be 9 to 20 μU/ml. The most definitive means for preoperative diagnosis of insulinoma is calculation of the amended insulin-glucose ratio; however, the validity of this test in all cases has been questioned. Other causes of hypoglycemia should be considered and ruled out, including hepatic failure, stress due to exertion, hypoadrenocorticism, hypopituitarism, hypothyroidism, sepsis, insulin overdose, or laboratory error.

Isolated pancreatic insulinomas are rare and can be treated successfully by extirpation of the mass. Metastasis is very common, and attempts to achieve permanent control by surgical excision of the primary pancreatic tumors are almost never successful. The metastatic foci often contain functional cells that produce insulin, and if the functional tissue is not completely excised during surgery, hypoglycemia will persist. If a substantial amount or even all of the grossly evident neoplastic tissue is resectable, signs may regress for a year or more, as the tumors generally regrow slowly.

Insulinomas may be found in any portion of the pancreas, but are less commonly observed at the pancreatic angle. The tumors may be small, requiring careful palpation to detect their presence. Unfortunately, metastatic foci may also be small, and metastases may be extremely difficult to confirm during exploratory surgery. The regional lymph nodes and liver should be carefully examined for metastasis. Biopsies should be taken from these structures, regardless of their appearance. Before surgery, the owner should be informed of the very guarded to poor prognosis for a cure, but a guarded prognosis may be given for temporary remission of signs after surgical treatment.

Hypoglycemia often can be controlled before surgery and in animals with recurrent or metastatic disease with dietary management and medical therapy. This should consist of feeding a high-protein, low-carbohydrate diet 4 to 6 times daily. Adrenal corticosteroids are gluconeogenic, so prednisolone or prednisone given at an initial dose of 0.25 to 0.5 mg/kg/day in divided doses may help raise the blood glucose concentration. The total daily dose may need to be increased to obtain a positive effect. Diazoxide (Proglycem, Schering Corp., Kenilworth, NJ) inhibits insulin release and may directly increase blood glucose. This compound is related to the thiazide diuretics and can be given orally; the dosage reported for dogs is 10 to 60 mg/kg/day divided into three doses. Chemotherapeutic treatment of this tumor has been largely unsuccessful.

Gastrinomas

Non-beta cell pancreatic islet cell neoplasms (gastrinomas) of the pancreas are extremely rare in dogs and have not been reported in cats. These tumors secrete large quantities of gastrin, which stimulates the stomach to produce massive amounts of hydrochloric acid. This results in peptic ulceration of the stomach and/or small bowel and can be associated with severe reflux esophagitis. This disease is referred to as the Zollinger-Ellison syndrome. It is treated by excision of the pancreatic and detectable metastatic tumors and by total gastrectomy to remove the parietal cells (which produce hydrochloric acid in response to gastrin). Medical treatment with cimetidine (Tagamet, Smith Kline & French Laboratories, Philadelphia, PA), ranitidine (Zantac, Glaxo Inc., Research Triangle Park, NC), or any of the newer histamine H_2-receptor antagonists is expensive in larger animals and is not uniformly successful in controlling hydrochloric acid production in response to high levels of circulating gastrin. Other types of ulcer disease treatment include the ulcer protectant sucralfate (Carafate, Marion Laboratories Inc., Kansas City, MO) or magnesium aluminum hydroxide antacids (*e.g.*, Maalox, Rorer, Fort Washington, PA). The prognosis for long-term survival is poor, regardless of the type of treatment.

Spontaneous Acute Pancreatitis

The etiology of spontaneous pancreatitis is unclear and is probably multifactorial. Experimentally induced reflux of gastrointestinal contents into, or obstruction of, the pancreatic ducts causes pancreatitis; these may contribute to naturally occurring disease in dogs and cats. Pancreatitis is common after prolonged ingestion of a high-fat diet or treatment with certain drugs (particularly glucocorticoids), and it is a frequent sequela of trauma due to excessive manipulation during surgical procedures or to other injuries. Regardless of the cause, once pancreatitis is initiated it often becomes a progressive disorder, due to continued leakage of digestive enzymes into the parenchyma of the organ. Bacterial colonization of damaged pancreatic tissue is often seen, and infection may be a predisposing cause in some cases. Pancreatitis causes intense local inflammation that can lead to abscess formation, generalized peritonitis, or both.

Animals affected with pancreatitis usually are presented for evaluation of vomiting, depression, and occasionally diarrhea. Owners often observe that the animal's abdomen appears tender. Concentrations of amylase may be increased in serum and abdominal fluid, but this is not absolutely specific (it is common with any abdominal disorder causing inflammation or disruption of the bowel). An increased serum lipase concentration is thought to be more diagnostic of pancreatitis. Serum glucose concentrations often are increased due to decreased production of insulin. The presence of pancreatitis may be suggested by radiographic signs, including loss of detail or the suggestion of a mass in the area of the pancreas, or the presence of ileus or peritoneal fluid. Patients with pancreatitis often are dehydrated due to vomiting. Because potassium, chloride, and hydrogen ions are lost in the vomitus, animals with pancreatitis may initially have hypokalemia and alkalosis. If dehydration is prolonged, acidosis develops, leading to hyperkalemia. The animal's hydration status and serum electrolyte concentrations should be evaluated before anesthesia and surgery.

Surgery may be required to allow drainage of a pancreatic abscess or to perform partial pancreatectomy to excise abscesses or granulomas. Acute pancreatitis can lead to septic peritonitis. Antibiotic therapy should be based on the results of microbial culturing and antibiotic sensitivity testing. Antibiotic therapy should not begin before obtaining samples for microbial culturing. Before obtaining these test results, broad-spectrum antibiotics (ampicillin, 10 mg/kg every 8 hours, and gentimycin, 2 mg/kg every 8 hours) should be given perioperatively.

The prognosis for recovery from severe, acute pancreatitis in the dog has been reported to be poor. In my experience, the prognosis depends upon how rapidly vomiting ceases (or is controlled) and how well the animal is managed relative to fluid and electrolyte therapy. Parenteral alimentation is advisable (but, unfortunately, often impractical) in animals that continue to vomit despite aggressive treatment.

Pancreatic Trauma

Trauma to the pancreas can occur from a blunt injury, but injuries of the pancreas more often are seen after penetrating trauma. Pancreatitis due to trauma may resolve spontaneously, provided the area of damaged tissue is limited. Autodigestion of the parenchyma due to leakage of digestive enzymes into the tissues can lead to progressive, fulminant pancreatitis. Traumatic injuries affecting the pancreatic ducts or major portions of the pancreas lead to signs associated with pancreatitis.

Pancreatitis, whether spontaneous or subsequent to trauma, can be fatal and requires aggressive treatment. Diabetes mellitus and/or pancreatic exocrine insufficiency due to widespread destruction of pancreatic tissue can occur after resolution of pancreatitis. If the pancreatic ducts are intact, and pancreatitis does not develop, the prognosis for recovery from pancreatic trauma is good.

Pancreatic Adenocarcinomas

These are the most common tumors affecting the exocrine tissues of the pancreas. They usually are difficult to diagnose, and they have a high rate of metastasis, primarily to the liver and draining lymph nodes. Clinical signs of pancreatitis or abnormal pancreatic function are infrequent with nonendocrine tumors of the pancreas. Rather, signs primarily are related to the development of metastatic foci. The prognosis for animals with pancreatic adenocarcinoma is poor due to the aggressive metastatic nature of the tumors and their advanced stage at the time of detection.

Surgical Procedures

Biopsy

Biopsy of the pancreas is indicated to determine whether the disease is disseminated or focal and to aid in deciding on the prognosis for treatment. Care should be taken to avoid damaging the larger pancreatic ducts when obtaining a biopsy (Fig. 15-9). Biopsies are obtained easily from the periphery of the pancreas by teasing apart the parenchyma with a fine-tipped forceps. This allows identification of the ducts and blood vessels supplying the area to be removed. Ligatures are applied to these structures before removing the sample. Although the capsule of the pancreas is extremely thin, it often can be sutured closed after removal of the sample by using fine-

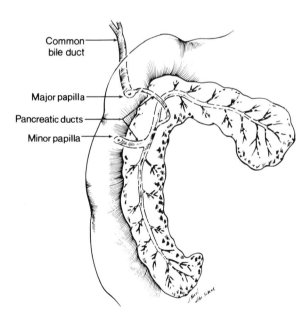

Figure 15-9. *The pancreas of the dog usually has two excretory ducts, the ventral (which joins the common bile duct and is small) and the dorsal (which has a separate opening into the duodenum distal to that of the common bile duct). There are other patterns, however, including only one duct (usually the dorsal one). (Rosin E. The pancreas. In: Gourley IM, Vasseur PB, eds. General small animal surgery. Philadelphia: JB Lippincott, 1985:438)*

gauge (4-0 or 5-0) absorbable suture material in an interrupted horizontal mattress pattern. Biopsies of isolated solitary masses can be obtained by using a Keyes or Baker cutaneous biopsy punch (as described for the liver, above) or by removing a wedge of tissue. The defect created by removing the sample can be closed with absorbable sutures in a horizontal mattress pattern.

Partial Pancreatectomy

Partial diagnostic or therapeutic pancreatectomy is indicated for removal of a portion of the pancreas that is affected by a traumatic, necrotic, or neoplastic process. The surgeon should be aware of the location of and variability of the anatomy of the major pancreatic ducts and the location of blood vessels, to avoid damaging them (Figs. 15-9 and 15-10). It is critical that the remaining pancreatic tissue be left with an adequate drainage system to convey pancreatic secretions to the small bowel. The mesentery is divided in the area of the portion of the pancreas to be removed, and the segmental blood supply is identified and ligated. The pancreaticoduodenal vessels should be protected during dissection of the right lobe of the pancreas to avoid devascularizing the duodenum. Manipulation of the remaining pancreatic tissue should be minimized to decrease the potential for postoperative pancreatitis. The pancreatic duct draining the portion of the pancreas to be removed is identified, isolated, and ligated (Fig. 15-11). Surgical gut suture should not be used for this ligature because exposure to pancreatic enzymes may accelerate its enzymatic breakdown. I prefer 2-0 or 3-0 silk. The limits of partial pancreatectomy should be identified before beginning the resection; these limits should be chosen with consideration for the location of the major (dorsal or accessory) and minor (ventral) pancreatic ducts. Referral to a surgical specialist is suggested for difficult cases requiring dissection near the angle of the pancreas.

Partial pancreatectomy is often performed to treat pancreatitis. Surgical place-

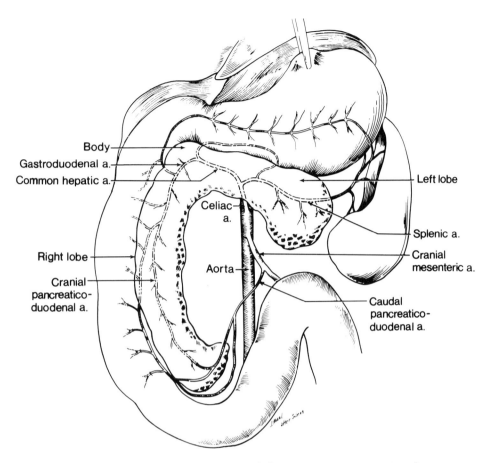

Figure 15-10. *The arterial blood supply of the canine pancreas arises from branches of the celiac and cranial mesenteric arteries. (Rosin E. The pancreas. In: Gourley IM, Vasseur PB, eds. General small animal surgery. Philadelphia: JB Lippincott, 1985:439)*

ment of abdominal drains and postoperative lavage as a form of treatment also has been recommended. Drains are not necessary unless large amounts of purulent or necrotic material are present after surgery, as they tend to become occluded rapidly (see "Peritonitis," Chap. 11). Further, intra-abdominal drains for postoperative lavage to treat pancreatitis are no more successful than resecting affected tissue and aggressive medical treatment. Treatment of severe peritonitis by open peritoneal drainage with delayed abdominal closure may have more merit, but it requires intensive care and frequent dressing changes and is asso-

ciated with significant sequelae (see "Peritonitis," Chap. 11).

Pancreatectomy

Removal of the entire pancreas is indicated for treatment of uncontrolled pancreatitis or widespread neoplasia. The procedure renders the patient diabetic and devoid of exocrine pancreatic function, and the implications of these changes should be discussed thoroughly with the owner before surgery. The techniques associated with this procedure are difficult un-

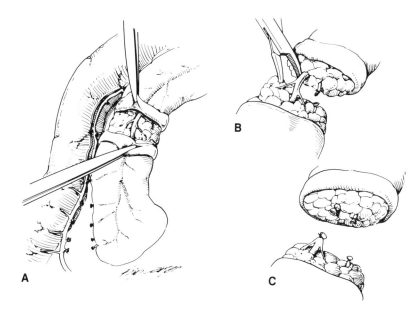

Figure 15-11. Partial pancreatectomy. *A, The vessels associated with the portion of the pancreas to be removed are identified and ligated, taking care to avoid damaging the blood supply to the duodenum and pancreatic remnant, and the pancreatic capsule is dissected at the intended resection line. B, The pancreatic parenchyma is bluntly dissected to reveal the intraparenchymal ducts and blood vessels, which are ligated (C). (Illustration by Kip Carter)*

less the surgeon is experienced, so referral should be considered.

The pancreas may be isolated and removed alone or in conjunction with the associated portions of the antral and pyloric regions of the stomach and/or the proximal duodenum. To remove the pancreas alone, the left limb of the pancreas is freed of its attachments to the greater omentum. Care must be taken to avoid the splenic artery and vein. Multiple small branches that supply the left limb of the pancreas should be identified and ligated near the pancreas. The right limb of the pancreas then is approached. The caudal pancreaticoduodenal vessels should be identified and preserved, as they supply and drain the duodenum. The pancreas can be dissected from its attachment to the duodenum with the tips of a forceps, allowing the surgeon to identify and ligate segmental branches of the caudal pancreaticoduodenal vessels without tearing them. Isolation of the remainder of the pancreas is difficult and requires careful dissection to avoid damaging the common bile duct and the blood supply to the duodenum and stomach. The mesoduodenum is incised, and the limits of the pancreas are identified and isolated by blunt dissection with forceps.

Individual vessels are ligated or electrocoagulated as they are encountered. The ventral pancreatic duct, which joins the common bile duct, may not be identified due to its small size or absence. The dorsal pancreatic duct is ligated if it is identified, although this is not essential. The defect in the mesoduodenum should be closed to prevent entrapment of viscera.

If the pancreas and associated portions of stomach and small bowel are to be removed, a gastrojejunostomy and cholecystoduodenostomy (Billroth II procedure) is performed (see Chap. 12, The Esophagus and Stomach).

Postoperative Care

Intravenous fluid administration should continue for at least 24 hours after pancreatic surgery. Small amounts of water may be offered 24 hours after surgery and, if vomiting is not observed, feeding of small amounts of an easily digested diet may begin 48 hours after surgery. The animal should be monitored closely for continuing signs of pancreatitis. Treatment of diabetes or exocrine pancreatic insufficiency should be initiated. Perioperative antibiotics should be administered until at least 24 to 36 hours after surgery. Antibiotic therapy can be discontinued at this time if signs of infection are not present.

Suggested Readings

The Liver and Biliary Tract

Bjorling DE. Partial hepatectomy in dogs. Compend Contin Ed Pract Vet 1985;7:257.

Blass DE. Surgery of the extrahepatic biliary tract. Compend Contin Ed Pract Vet 1983;5:801.

Drazner FH. The liver and biliary tract. In: Gourley IM, Vasseur PB, eds. General small animal surgery. Philadelphia: JB Lippincott, 1985:413.

Tangner CH. Cholecystoduodenostomy in the dog. Comparison of two techniques. Vet Surg 1984;13:60.

Walshaw R. Surgical diseases of the liver and biliary system. In: Slatter DH, ed. Textbook of small animal surgery. Philadelphia: WB Saunders, 1985:798.

The Spleen

Hosgood G. Splenectomy in the dog: A retrospective study of 31 cases. J Am Anim Hosp Assoc 1987;23:275.

Lipowitz AJ, Blue J, Perman V. The spleen. In: Slatter DH, ed. Textbook of small animal surgery. Philadelphia: WB Saunders, 1985:1204.

Pabst R, Kamran D, Creutzig H. Splenic regeneration and blood flow after ligation of the splenic artery or partial splenectomy. Am J Surg 1984;147:382.

Perman V, Lipowitz AJ. The spleen. In: Gourley IM, Vasseur PB, eds. General small animal surgery. Philadelphia: JB Lippincott, 1985:459.

Scher KS, Scott-Connor C, Jones CW, et al. Methods of splenic preservation and their effect on clearance of pneumococcal bacteremia. Ann Surg 1985;202:595.

Withrow SJ. Dental extraction as a probable cause of septicemia in a dog. J Am Animal Hosp Assoc 1979;15:345.

The Pancreas

Greenfield CL, Walshaw R. Open peritoneal drainage for treatment of contaminated peritoneal cavity and septic peritonitis in dogs and cats: 24 cases. J Am Vet Med Assoc 1987;191:100.

Rosin E. The pancreas. In: Gourley IM, Vasseur PB, eds. General small animal surgery. Philadelphia: JB Lippincott, 1985:437.

Walshaw R. Surgical diseases of the exocrine pancreas. In: Slatter DH, ed. Textbook of small animal surgery. Philadelphia: WB Saunders, 1985:830.

16

Elizabeth A. Stone

The Urinary System

Kidney

Anesthesia and surgery decrease the total renal blood flow and redistribute intrarenal blood flow away from the cortex because of the activity of the sympathetic nervous system and the renin-angiotensin system. Recognizing and treating renal disease is essential to prevent decompensation and further destruction of nephrons. Renal function should be assessed before renal surgery in any animal and before any surgery on an animal over 4 years old, with suspicious history or physical examination findings, or with concurrent disease that might affect the kidney secondarily (e.g., lymphoma, hypercalcemia, feline infectious peritonitis). A urine specific gravity greater than 1.030 indicates that at least one third of the renal mass is functioning. An elevated blood urea nitrogen and creatinine in a hydrated dog suggests a 75% reduction in renal function.

Prerenal azotemia from dehydration or hypovolemia should be corrected before surgery. Urine output is monitored by an indwelling urethral catheter, and a minimum of 2 to 3 ml of urine/kg/hr is considered sufficient. If urine flow is insufficient, physiologic diuresis is induced by rapidly administrating 10 ml/kg lactated Ringer's solution, and then maintained using the same solution at a rate of 5 ml/kg/hr. If the physiologic diuresis is unsuccessful, an osmotic mannitol diuresis (0.25 to 0.5 g/kg IV over 20 minutes) can be used to increase renal blood flow and the glomerular filtration rate. If urine output does not increase with this treatment, the animal's cardiovascular and renal status needs reassessment. After surgery, the diuresis is gradually decreased until the animal can maintain sufficient urine output from oral intake.

Hydronephrosis

Hydronephrosis results from outflow obstruction of the ureter, bladder, or urethra. Obstruction eventually destroys renal function because of elevated ureteral pressure and decreased renal blood flow leading to cellular atrophy and necrosis. Complete ureteral occlusion causes progressive dilation of the renal pelvis during the first few weeks, with concomitant atrophy of the cortex. Incomplete ureteral obstruction will destroy renal function more slowly, but even with mild obstruction, all measured renal functions (except urine dilution) are significantly impaired.

Causes of unilateral hydronephrosis include abdominal masses compressing the ureter, ureteral neoplasia, ureteral calculi, accidental ligation of the ureter during ovariohysterectomy, torsion of the renal pedicle, or ureteral stenosis or stricture. Hydronephrosis can also be associated with an ectopic ureter or pyelonephritis. Bilateral hydronephrosis can occur from the aforementioned causes, or from obstruction of the urinary bladder trigone or urethra by neoplasia, prostatism, calculi, or pelvic trauma.

Diagnosis

Unilateral hydronephrosis is asymptomatic unless the enlarged kidney distends the abdomen. If the kidney becomes infected, signs of pyelonephritis may occur (fever, leukocytosis, flank pain). Bilateral hydronephrosis is asymptomatic until signs of uremia associated with renal failure become apparent (polyuria, anorexia, vomiting, oral ulcers).

Radiographic evaluation may reveal a space-occupying mass in the region of the kidneys. During early hydronephrosis, an excretory urogram will show a dilated renal pelvis with loss of diverticula. Later, a thin rim of functioning cortex surrounds a fluid-filled mass. Radiographic visualization of kidneys after complete ureteral occlusion may continue for 2 to 4 weeks. Glomerular filtration continues at a rate of a few milliliters per minute after ureteral obstruction, so contrast material is still filtered into the tubules and renal pelvis.

Treatment

The decision to excise a hydronephrotic kidney depends on whether patency can be restored and how much renal function remains.

The kidney can recover normal renal function after 2 weeks of ureteral obstruction and may still recover some function after 3 or 4 weeks of obstruction. If the duration of hydronephrosis is unknown, the degree of residual renal function should be estimated. There may be a correlation between the ability to excrete and concentrate radiographic contrast media and the potential for recovery of function after relief of obstruction.

After release of bilateral ureteral or lower urinary tract obstruction, there is often an obligatory diuresis because of the animal's impaired ability to concentrate and absorb sodium. The animal's urine output should be monitored and fluid therapy administered as needed.

When the hydronephrotic kidney has minimal function or the obstruction cannot be removed, a nephro-ureterectomy is performed. A midline abdominal incision extending from the xiphoid to the pubis may be necessary to remove a very large kidney. The fluid is aspirated from the kidney to facilitate excision, and the renal vessels and ureter are ligated and severed (Fig. 16-1).

Pyelonephritis

Pyelonephritis may result from ascending infection from the lower urinary tract or from hematogenous seeding of bacteria. Vesicoureteral reflux of sterile urine may not damage the canine kidney, but reflux of infected urine causes alterations in renal structure and function. In addition, motile bacteria may ascend the ureter even without reflux. Ureteral aperistalsis, which occurs after ureteral anastomosis and with some *Escherichia coli* infections and hydroureter, as associated with urinary outflow obstruction, may further contribute to the retrograde spread of bacteria from the bladder to the kidney.

Hematogenous spread of bacteria to the kidney may also occur, especially when there is previous renal damage. In animals with an additional infectious site (*e.g.*, discospondylitis) it may be difficult to determine the initial lesion.

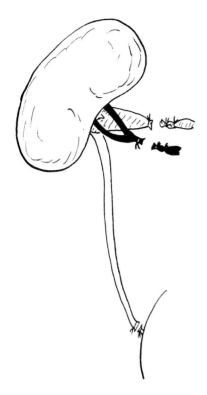

Figure 16-1. *The renal artery and vein are individually double-ligated, transfixed, and severed. The ureter is ligated and transected at its entrance to the bladder.*

Diagnosis

Dogs with pyelonephritis are usually asymptomatic unless systemic signs develop (fever, lumbar pain, anorexia, vomiting). There may be concomitant signs of cystitis (dysuria, hematuria). If the pyelonephritis has destroyed enough renal tissue, uremia will occur. Physical examination often is not helpful in the diagnosis.

Localizing urinary tract infection to the kidneys is very difficult. Leukocytosis often is present. Bacterial culture of a urine sample obtained by cystocentesis is a reliable diagnostic test for urinary tract infection, without differentiating between upper and lower tract infection. The presence of casts is indicative of renal disease, but their absence cannot be used to rule out pyelonephritis. Excretory urography may reveal dilation of the renal pelvis and

a decrease in renal size with chronic bacterial pyelonephritis. Resolved or unrelated disease may have similar radiographic signs.

Treatment

The objective of antibiotic therapy of bacterial pyelonephritis is to achieve effective tissue concentration within the kidney. The choice of antibiotic is based on urine culture and bacteriologic antibiotic sensitivity testing. Administration of antibiotics is continued for at least 4 weeks, and the urine culture is repeated 5 days after antibiotic cessation. In dogs with renal failure, the dose of drugs excreted by the kidney must be adjusted. Nephroliths should be removed and urinary tract obstruction relieved if possible.

If antibiotic therapy is unsuccessful in eradicating the infection in unilateral pyelonephritis, nephrectomy should considered, and the opposite kidney should be evaluated. In an azotemic dog, the pyelonephritic kidney should not be removed unless it is making no contribution to total renal function. In a referral center, individual kidney function can be assessed by renal scintigraphy.

For a nonazotemic dog in a practice situation, a laparotomy is performed and the opposite kidney is inspected and palpated. A ventral cystotomy is done and each ureter is catheterized. A urinalysis, including urine specific gravity, is done. A concentrated urine specimen from the opposite kidney would suggest adequate renal function. If possible, urinary excretion of phenolsulfonphthalein by each kidney can be measured to determine the relative contribution of each kidney.

If the opposite kidney has sufficient function, the pyelonephritic kidney with its ureter is excised. Care is taken to prevent leakage of purulent material and urine into the abdomen. It may be necessary to dissect through adhesions from the kidney to the body wall. It is better to remove some of the abdominal wall musculature with the kidney than to accidentally puncture the pus-filled kidney.

Nephrolithiasis

The true incidence of renoliths is unknown, since renal calculi are more difficult to diagnose and are less commonly removed than bladder or urethral calculi. Dogs with portovascular anomalies have an unusually high incidence of concurrent renal and urinary bladder urate uroliths. The likelihood of diagnosing renoliths in these dogs may be increased because of the extensive diagnostic or postmortem evaluation in dogs with portovascular anomalies.

The cause of a particular renolith depends on its mineral composition. Struvite, calcium phosphate, urate, oxalate, and silica uroliths have been removed from canine kidneys.

Diagnosis

Clinical signs of nephrolithiasis are often nonspecific. Whenever uroliths are diagnosed in other locations, the kidneys should be carefully examined with radiography (and ultrasonography, if available) and during surgery. Signs of persistent lower urinary tract infection suggest the need for a thorough investigation of the entire urinary tract for uroliths or other abnormalities. The animal should be evaluated to determine if any underlying metabolic defects are responsible for or contribute to stone formation. Plain and contrast radiographs should be evaluated for numbers and position of all uroliths throughout the urinary tract and to demonstrate any obstruction in the urinary tract. Renal function can be assessed by serum creatinine or urea nitrogen determinations.

Treatment

Antibiotics, selected on the basis of urine bacterial culture and sensitivity tests, are administered to establish adequate tissue concentrations. Medical dissolution can be attempted in adult dogs and cats with renoliths of known mineral composition. Surgical removal of nephroliths is indicated if there is no response to medical dissolution, or when there is obstruction of the renal pelvis, uncontrollable infection, progressive enlargement of the calculus, or deterioration of renal function.

Any fluid or electrolyte imbalances should be corrected before anesthesia. Urine output is monitored with a urinary catheter connected to a sterile collection bag. A mannitol osmotic diuresis is initiated before surgery to increase glomerular filtration rate, renal blood flow, and urine output and to help protect renal function during surgery.

A *bisection nephrotomy* is routinely used to remove large nephroliths from a normal-sized renal pelvis or to remove multiple calculi within the diverticula. A *pyelolithotomy* is done to remove a single, large calculus from a greatly dilated renal pelvis. The incision into the relatively avascular renal pelvis causes less parenchymal damage than a bisection nephrotomy. A *nephro-ureterectomy* is performed if the kidney is infected and has marginal function, and the opposite kidney has good function.

Nephrotomy

The cranial pole of the kidney is elevated by severing the cranial peritoneal attachments, and the renal vessels are located. A small mosquito hemostat or right-angle vascular clamp is used to separate the renal artery from the renal vein. A vascular clamp or a tourniquet is placed on the renal artery; double or triple renal arteries can be clamped separately. The duration of ischemia to the normothermic canine kidney should not exceed 20 minutes. Occluding only the renal artery allows venous drainage of the kidney and increases the pliability of the kidney.

The kidney is immobilized between thumb and forefinger and the renal capsule is incised on the midline sharply with a scalpel (Fig. 16-2) for about two thirds the length of the kidney. Extending the incision into the cranial and caudal poles unnecessarily increases parenchymal damage. The renal parenchyma is separated bluntly with a scalpel handle or a

Figure 16-2. Nephrotomy. ***A,*** *The renal capsule is incised sharply with a scalpel blade (insert). The renal parenchyma is separated bluntly with a scalpel handle or a blunt osteotome.* ***B,*** *The cut edges of the kidney are retracted with forceps (top). Any arcuate or inter-lobar vessels within the incision are ligated and then severed with scissors (bottom).* ***C,*** *The renal capsule is sutured with a simple continuous suture pattern while the cut edges of the kidney are apposed with digital pressure. (Stone EA. Canine nephrotomy. Compend Cont Ed 1987;9:883)*

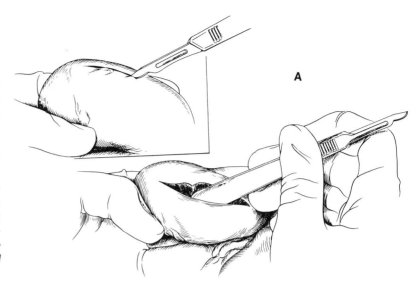

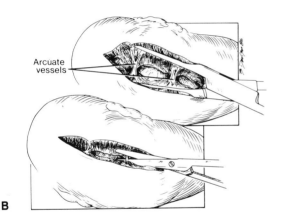

Arcuate vessels

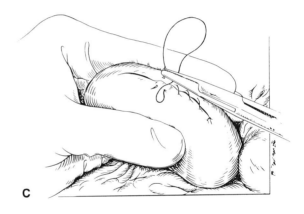

blunt osteotome. The cut edges are retracted with forceps. Arcuate or interlobar vessels within the incision are ligated and severed. Large calculi are carefully removed without fragmenting them. Each diverticulum is systematically explored with a small mosquito forceps and flushed with warm saline using a small soft catheter and syringe to ensure removal of all existing calculi. A 3.5 French gauge soft catheter is passed down the ureter to check for obstruction. The two sides of the nephrotomy incision are apposed with digital pressure from thumb and forefinger, while a simple continuous synthetic absorbable suture is placed through the renal capsule. Mattress sutures through the parenchyma are unnecessary.

The vascular clamp or tourniquet is removed. Bleeding collateral or capsular vessels can be ligated. If there is bleeding from the renal parenchyma, it may be necessary to reclamp the renal artery and apply digital compression for 5 to 10 minutes. After bleeding is controlled, the kidney is returned to its original position. Tacking sutures can be placed between the kidney and the body wall to prevent rotation if the kidney has been excessively mobilized. Abdominal closure is routine.

Pyelolithotomy (Fig. 16-3)

The kidney is freed from its peritoneal and fascial attachments and reflected medially to expose the dorsolateral surface of the renal pelvis. It is unnecessary to occlude the renal artery, since the pelvis is relatively avascular. The pelvis and ureter must be sufficiently distended by the calculus to allow removal through the pelvis without tearing the parenchyma or fragmenting the calculus. Otherwise, a bisection nephrotomy is necessary.

A longitudinal incision is made into the dilated renal pelvis and ureter, and the calculus is removed with forceps. The renal pelvis and ureter are flushed with saline using a 3.5 French gauge soft catheter. A ventral cystotomy is performed to remove any cystic calculi and to allow retrograde catheterization and flushing of the ureter.

The incision is closed with simple continuous synthetic absorbable sutures.

Postoperative Management

Intravenous fluid therapy is continued after surgery until the dog can maintain hydration. If urine production is questionable, urine output is measured. Radiographs are taken to compare with preoperative radiographs and to document removal of all calculi. Antibiotic administration, based on bacterial culture and sensitivity, is continued for 4 weeks. A week after antibiotics are stopped, a bacterial culture of a cystocentesis urine sample is performed. Long-term antibiotic therapy may be required to suppress bacterial growth in a damaged kidney. The calculi are submitted for quantitative mineral analysis, and appropriate medical management is initiated to help prevent recurrence.

Renal Neoplasia

Compared to other tumors in the body, renal tumors account for 1.7% of dog tumors and 2.5% of cat tumors. Carcinoma (adenocarcinoma, squamous cell, undifferentiated) is the most common cell type in dogs. Hereditary

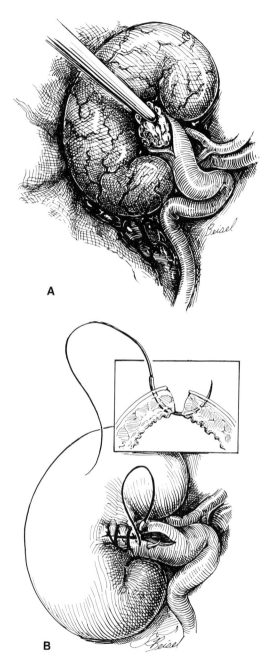

Figure 16-3. **A,** *After the kidney is reflected medially to expose the dorsolateral surface of the renal pelvis, an incision is made into the dilated renal pelvis and proximal ureter. The calculi are removed with forceps.* **B,** *After the renal pelvis and the ureters have been flushed with saline, the incision is closed with synthetic absorbable suture material in a continuous pattern. (Greenwood KM, Rawlings CA. Removal of canine renal calculi by pyelolithotomy. Vet Surg 1981;10:12)*

multifocal renal cystadenocarcinoma, associated with multiple nodular dermatofibrosis, has been reported in German shepherd dogs in Norway. Metastasis occurred in 10 of the 43 dogs examined. A common male ancestor was found for all the dogs with known ancestry. No breed predilection for other types of renal neoplasia has been reported. Embryonal nephromas (Wilms' tumor, nephroblastoma) have been reported in young dogs. Renal malignant lymphoma may originate in the kidney, especially in cats, or may be secondary to metastasis from other sites. Other tumors can also metastasize to the kidney. The kidney is occasionally invaded by tumors of the adrenal gland or the ovary.

Diagnosis

The signs associated with renal tumors are usually nonspecific (anorexia, weight loss, vomiting, polyuria/polydypsia, hematuria, and flank pain). Physical examination findings may include a cranial abdominal mass and fever. Secondary polycythemia because of erythropoietin release from a functional renal tumor may occur.

Urinalysis findings may include red blood cells and possibly tumor cells. Plain abdominal radiographs may reveal a cranial abdominal mass on the left or right side. If urine flow has been obstructed, hydronephrosis may be present. Excretory urography will show a distortion of the nephrogram and an irregular interface between the tumor and normal tissue. The renal pelvis may be distorted or have filling defects. Diffuse infiltrative tumors such as lymphosarcoma produce a generalized opacity of the nephrogram.

Definitive diagnosis is made with a fine-needle aspirate, needle biopsy, or exploratory laparotomy and biopsy. Cystic masses should not be aspirated percutaneously.

Treatment

Nephrectomy is the initial treatment, if possible. Surgery is complicated by extensive adhesions, local invasion, and the proximity of the caudal vena cava, aorta, and adrenal gland.

It may be difficult to identify and isolate the renal vessels. Preoperative embolization or balloon catheter occlusion of the renal artery is sometimes used in humans to reduce the size of the tumorous mass and to decrease hemorrhage. The renal vessels still require ligation.

The results of chemotherapy, radiation therapy, or immunotherapy for renal tumors have not been reported.

Renal Trauma

Although protected by the rib cage, the kidneys can be damaged by blunt trauma (such as an auto accident) or penetrating wounds (such as a fractured rib or a bullet). Types of trauma include contusions, fractures, lacerations, or avulsion of the renal pedicle (*i.e.*, vessels, ureter).

Diagnosis

The history may include a traumatic incident, or the owner may be unaware of any trauma.

Physical examination is often nonspecific. It may be impossible to identify a painful sublumbar mass or bruising. If hemorrhage occurs from vessels that communicate with the collecting system, there will be gross or microscopic hematuria. Hematuria can also occur with bladder, prostate, and urethral trauma. Uremia is unlikely unless both kidneys or the lower urinary tract are damaged.

Abdominocentesis may show intraperitoneal bleeding from damaged renal vessels with disruption of the peritoneum covering the kidney. Peritoneal urine is rarely detected with isolated kidney damage.

Survey radiographs may reveal fluid in the peritoneal cavity or a sublumbar mass displacing the colon ventrally. If the kidney is not visible on an excretory urogram, the renal artery may have been disrupted. With parenchymal damage, the contrast material will be retained within the capsule or within the retroperitoneal space. Renal injury is most commonly diagnosed during an abdominal exploration performed because of severe abdominal bleeding or trauma.

Treatment

The type of treatment depends on the severity of the injury. Contusions and intracapsular fractures require no treatment. When the kidney is surrounded by fat, it is difficult to identify active bleeding from the capsule or the parenchyma. Careful dissection of the fat may help determine the source of hemorrhage.

When there is laceration of the capsule and the renal parenchyma, the blood clots are removed from the wound, the edges are held together with digital pressure, and the capsule is sutured with synthetic absorbable 4-0 suture material. Temporary occlusion of the renal artery may improve visibility.

Preservation of part of a kidney with severe fragmentation or laceration of one pole may be possible with a partial nephrectomy. The renal artery is temporarily occluded. The damaged area is excised and bleeding vessels are ligated. The omentum is placed over the exposed area and tacked with fine sutures (Fig. 16-4). If bleeding occurs after release of the arterial occlusion, it may be necessary to ligate one or two interlobar vessels supplying the damaged area. The kidney should be tacked in its retroperitoneal position to prevent rotation. When more than half the kidney is damaged or the renal pedicle is avulsed, nephro-ureterectomy is performed. The other kidney must be functional.

Ureters

Ureteral Ectopia

Ureters are considered ectopic when they do not open into the trigone of the urinary bladder in the usual location. The ectopic ureter terminates most commonly in the urethra or vagina in dogs and the urethra in cats. The condition, which results from faulty differentiation of the mesonephric and metanephric ducts, may affect either ureter or may be bilateral.

Ureteral ectopia is sometimes associated with other urinary tract abnormalities (such as renal hypoplasia, ureterocele, ureteral dilatation, and hydronephrosis). Genetic involvement is suggested by familial aggregation in Labrador retrievers and Siberian huskies. High-risk breeds include Siberian huskies, West Highland terriers, fox terriers, and miniature and toy poodles.

Diagnosis

The presenting complaint is usually urinary incontinence, first noticed at the time of house training. The owner should be questioned about the dog's age at the onset of incontinence, reproductive status, and duration of incontinence. Examination of the neurologic system controlling micturition should reveal no abnormalities. The degree of voluntary control of voiding can be determined from the

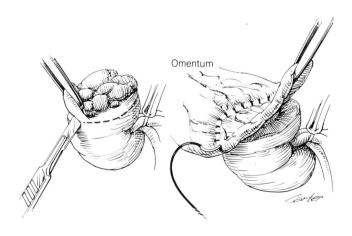

Omentum

Figure 16-4. Partial nephrectomy. *After the damaged portion of the kidney has been debrided, the cut surface is covered by tacking omentum to the capsule. (Bjorling DE. Traumatic injuries of the urogenital system. Vet Clin North Am [Small Anim Pract] 1984;14:70)*

history and from observation. Normal voiding has been observed in dogs with unilateral and bilateral ectopic ureters.

The abdominal wall is examined for moisture and abnormal openings as would occur with hypospadia or persistent urachus. For a thorough examination, it may be necessary to remove the hair from a long-haired dog. Concurrent urinary tract infection is diagnosed and treated before surgery if a urine sample can be obtained by cystocentesis. Otherwise, urine is collected during surgery.

Definitive diagnosis of ectopic ureters is usually based on the findings from an excretory urogram. The nephrogram phase of the excretory urogram should be examined for kidney abnormalities. A pneumocystogram combined with an excretory urogram will help identify the ureteral openings into the bladder. Fluoroscopic examination sometimes helps delineate the path of contrast medium and urine into the urethra or vagina.

A preoperative urethral pressure profile may give some indication of urethral function. At present, however, not enough data exists from preoperative urethral pressure profiles to aid surgical decision-making.

Four types of patent ectopic ureters have been recognized:

1. *Intramural.* The ureter enters the bladder wall and courses within the wall to open distal to the trigone.
2. *Extramural.* The ureter enters the urethra or vagina without entering and traversing the bladder.
3. *Intramural with troughs.* The ureter enters the bladder wall, courses within the wall, and opens into the bladder trigone in a normal location. The ureter then continues as a trough through the urethral sphincter area.
4. *Intramural with double openings.* The pathway of the ureter is the same as the intramural type. The ureter opens in a typical location in the trigone and then continues distally and has a second opening into the urethra or vagina.

Stenotic or nonpatent ectopic ureters have also been described, in which the intramural ectopic ureter passes beyond the trigone and then ends in a blind pouch. Dogs with this type of ectopic ureter will be continent if the urethra is functional. The initial clinical sign may be an abdominal mass from severe hydronephrosis and hydroureter.

Treatment

Surgical correction is the usual treatment. A ventral midline laparotomy is performed, and the kidneys and ureters are examined for abnormalities. If the kidney with the ectopic ureter is grossly diseased and the opposite kidney is normal, a nephro-ureterectomy is done. To determine the location of an ectopic ureter, a ventral cystotomy is done, and the bladder interior is inspected for ureteral openings and for intramural ureters. Identifying an intramural ureter may be facilitated by applying digital compression to the urethra, which will cause dilation of the ureter beneath the bladder mucosa. A proximal ureterotomy to catheterize the ureter is not recommended because of the risk of ureteral stricture.

The technique for establishing a new opening into the bladder depends on the type of ectopic ureter. If an intramural ureter is identified with no opening into the bladder, a new opening can be made directly into the trigone (Fig. 16-5). An incision is made through the bladder mucosa into the ureter in the area of the trigone. It may be necessary to excise the redundant portion of a greatly dilated ureter or ureterocele. The cut edges of the bladder mucosa are sutured to the cut edges of the ureter, creating a stoma. Four to six synthetic absorbable simple interrupted 4-0 sutures are used. The ureter distal to the neostoma is ligated by passing monofilament nonabsorbable sutures from outside the bladder around the ureter without penetrating the bladder lumen. If the ureter is small, the distal ectopic ureter can be incised longitudinally and sutured closed using synthetic absorbable suture material.

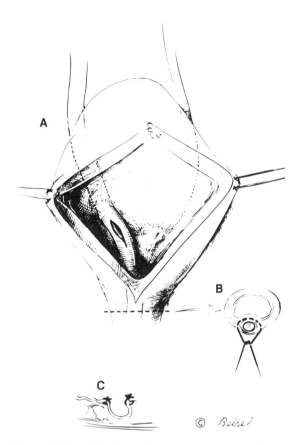

Figure 16-5. Creation of a neostoma in situ for an intramural ectopic ureter. *A, After a ventral cystotomy, the intramural ectopic ureter is identified. The bladder mucosa and ureter are incised longitudinally in a typical location for a ureteral opening. B, The ureter distal to the neostoma site is catheterized and sutures are placed from outside the bladder and urethra around the ureter beneath the mucosa. C, The ureter is sutured to the bladder mucosa to create the neostoma in situ.*

An extramural ureter is doubly ligated and transected as far distally as possible and reimplanted cranial to the trigone (Fig. 16-6). An incision is made in the bladder mucosa, and a straight hemostat is used to make a short submucosal tunnel. The tunnel exits through the serosa at an oblique angle from the mucosal opening. The hemostat is then used to grasp the ureter and draw it through the tunnel into the bladder lumen. The end of the ureter is sharply severed and then spatulated to increase its diameter. Four simple interrupted sutures are placed through the bladder mucosa and the ureter. If there are bilateral ectopic

ureters, both tunnels should be made before the ureters are passed into the bladder lumen. Care must be taken to avoid traumatizing the ureter or disrupting its blood supply.

When the ureteral orifice is at the normal location and the ureter then continues as a trough through the urethral sphincter, the ureteral orifice is not altered. The trough is closed with several simple interrupted sutures. If the opening into the trigone is more caudal than normal, the intramural ureter and bladder mucosa can be incised and then sutured open to create a more proximal neostoma before closing the trough.

The urinary bladder is closed routinely. Ureteral stents are not routinely used. When very small ureters have been reimplanted, ureteral stents may be inserted for 1 to 2 days to prevent occlusion of the ureteral openings by postoperative edema.

Most dogs show improvement after surgical repair of ectopic ureters. Some become incontinent during estrus or during pregnancy or have positional or rest incontinence. A few dogs may have persistent incontinence after surgery, requiring a thorough re-evaluation. Frequent voiding because of a hypoplastic bladder, cystitis, or renal failure must be distinguished from incontinence. Anatomic abnormalities contributing to incontinence should be ruled out. An excretory urogram may reveal that the distal ectopic ureter is still patent and needs to be religated. A vaginogram may show that an abnormally shaped vagina is allowing urine pooling and leakage. An ovariohysterectomy with excision of the proximal vagina may correct this cause of incontinence.

Urethral incompetence can be diagnosed by a urethral pressure profile at a referral center. Otherwise, empirical treatment with alpha-adrenergic drugs can be tried to increase urethral sphincter tone.

Ureteral Calculi

Ureteral calculi originate from a renolith that has fragmented or migrated. With ureteral obstruction, there may be proximal hydroureter and hydronephrosis (see "Hydronephrosis," p. 431).

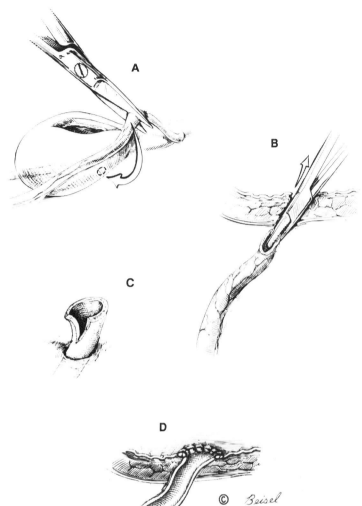

Figure 16-6. Reimplantation of an extramural ectopic ureter. *A, The extramural ectopic ureter is ligated as far distally as possible and reimplanted more cranially. A small piece of mucosa is excised at the location of the new opening. B, A mosquito forceps is passed from inside to outside the bladder and the ureter is grasped. C, The damaged end of the ureter is severed and the ureter is spatulated. D, The ureter is sutured to the bladder mucosa in a simple interrupted pattern using synthetic absorbable suture material.*

Diagnosis

Symptoms of ureteral calculi (such as flank pain) are usually not recognized. Ureteral calculus may be first diagnosed on abdominal radiographs taken for other reasons or by an excretory urograph. Renal function should be evaluated.

Treatment

The ureteral calculus is monitored by serial radiographs to determine if it is passing into the bladder. If it is stationary or if hydroureter and hydronephrosis are present, a ureterotomy is done (Fig. 16-7). Umbilical tape is placed as a tourniquet around the ureter prox-

imal and distal to the calculus. A transverse incision is made through the dilated ureter over the calculus. The calculus is gently removed. After removal of the umbilical tape, the distal ureter is flushed using a 3.5 French gauge soft catheter. The incision is closed with two to four simple interrupted sutures using 5-0 synthetic absorbable suture. Postoperative management is similar to that described earlier for nephrotomy.

Ureteral Neoplasia

The etiology and incidence of ureteral neoplasia in dogs and cats is unknown. Tumor types include papillomas, papillary carcinomas,

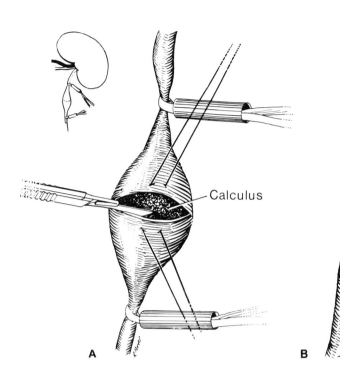

Calculus

Figure 16-7. Ureterotomy. *A,
The ureter is occluded and stabilized with umbilical tape. Retraction sutures are placed and a short
transverse incision is made over
the calculus. B, The ureteral edges
are approximated with interrupted
4-0 to 5-0 synthetic absorbable
sutures. (Stone EA. Surgical management of urolithiasis. Compend
Contin Ed 1981;3:627)*

transitional cell carcinomas, and mesenchymal
tumors.

Diagnosis

Clinical signs of ureteral tumors are similar to
those of renal tumors. Excretory urography
reveals a ureteral mass and possible ureteral
obstruction with proximal hydroureter and
hydronephrosis.

Treatment

Complete nephro-ureterectomy is recommended. The results of adjuvant therapy for
ureteral tumors have not been reported.

Ureteral Injury

Diagnosis

An animal with a damaged ureter may show no
abnormalities for several days after trauma.
Signs of pain, uremia, or abdominal fluid will
occur after the retroperitoneal space fills with
urine and/or the peritoneum ruptures, allowing urine to flow into the abdomen.

The diagnostic procedures are similar to
those described for renal injury. Significant
hemorrhage does not occur with isolated ureteral injury. The abdominocentesis and survey
radiographic findings depend on whether
urine is leaking into the retroperitoneal space
or into the abdomen.

An excretory urogram is usually diagnostic and will show contrast medium leaking
from the ureter. During an exploratory laparotomy, it is often difficult to determine the
location of ureteral damage, since the fat
around both ureters swells with urine and becomes discolored. The findings on the excretory urogram will help direct the exploration.

Treatment

An incomplete tear of the ureter (rare) is debrided and sutured with fine synthetic absorbable suture material. A transection near the
renal pelvis is usually best treated with a
nephro-ureterectomy, since it is difficult to
reattach the ureter to the pelvis. A transection
near the bladder is treated by first ligating and
severing the distal ureter at its entrance into

the bladder. After a ventral cystotomy, the proximal end is reimplanted into the bladder in the same manner as described for an extramural ectopic ureter (see Fig. 16-6).

In medium- to large-sized dogs, a midureter transection can be treated by careful debridement, spatulation, and anastomosis with 6-0 synthetic absorbable suture material (Fig. 16-8). In cats and small dogs, ureteral anastomosis requires microsurgical techniques, and usually a nephro-ureterectomy is performed if the opposite kidney is functional.

Bladder

Patent Urachus

The fetal urachus lies within the umbilicus and joins the urinary bladder to the allantoic cavity. After birth, the urachus should close and become the fibrotic midline (ventral) ligament of the bladder.

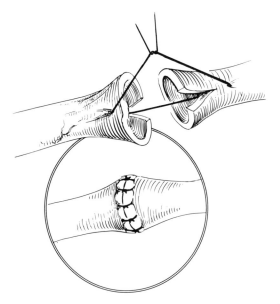

Figure 16-8. Ureteral anastomosis. *The debrided edges of a damaged ureter are spatulated by making a small longitudinal incision in each end of the ureter. The ureteral ends are reunited with 6-0 synthetic absorbable suture material. (Bjorling DE. Traumatic injuries of the urogenital system. Vet Clin North Am [Small Anim Pract] 1984;14:61)*

Diagnosis

If the urachus remains open, urine continues to dribble from the umbilicus. Urine scalds may occur on the ventral abdomen, and the dog may have a foul odor and recurrent urinary tract infections. Definitive diagnosis is by contrast cystography.

Treatment

Surgical excision is the treatment of choice. Following a ventral midline incision caudal to the umbilicus, an elliptical incision is made through the abdominal wall around the urachus. The urachus is traced to the bladder. The bladder around the urachus is excised, and the defect is closed as a routine cystotomy.

Vesicourachal Diverticulum

In this condition, the urachus remains partially open and forms a blind pouch on the bladder. It may predispose the animal to chronic bacterial cystitis. It is seen in some cats with feline urologic syndrome, but its contribution to that disease is not understood.

Diagnosis

Positive-contrast cystography will diagnose the diverticulum arising from the cranioventral surface of the bladder. A cystocentesis urine sample is cultured for aerobic bacteria.

Treatment

Treatment is by full-thickness excision of the defect with routine cystotomy closure. Associated cystitis is treated with appropriate antibiotics.

Cystourolithiasis

Uroliths are most commonly diagnosed in the urinary bladder. The most common type is struvite, composed of magnesium ammonium phosphate hexahydrate. Struvite uroliths can occur in any breed and are more common in female dogs. Urease-positive bacterial urinary tract infection (especially *Staphylococci* and

Proteus) and alkaline urine are common factors in the pathogenesis of struvite uroliths. Liberation of ammonia from urea by bacterial urease makes the urine more alkaline, decreasing the solubility of struvite.

Struvite cystouroliths in cats are less common than struvite urethral plugs. The uroliths are most commonly small, wafer-shaped stones and are not associated with urinary tract infection. Occasionally, large uroliths may be found in cats with *Staphylococci* or *Proteus* infection.

Urate uroliths are composed mainly of ammonium urate with small amounts of calcium oxalate or struvite. Urate uroliths occur most often in Dalmatians. All Dalmatians have a defect in uric acid metabolism in the metabolic pathway for degradation of purines. Uric acid is not converted to allantoin in the liver by the enzyme uricase, so more uric acid is excreted in the urine. Not all Dalmatians form calculi, so other unknown factors are also involved. Urate uroliths also occur in dogs with portovascular anomalies and high urine concentrations of ammonia and uric acid. Urinary tract infection may be a sequela to urate uroliths. Acid urine increases urinary ammonium output and ammonium urate supersaturation.

Cystinuria is an inherited disorder of renal tubular reabsorption involving cystine and three other amino acids. Cystine uroliths occur almost exclusively in male dogs, and not all dogs with cystinuria develop uroliths. Acidic urine increases the supersaturation of cystine.

Oxalate is a product of ascorbate and glyoxylate metabolism. The factors involved in the formation of oxalate uroliths are not well understood. Oxalate is not detected by qualitative mineral analysis; quantitative analysis suggests that oxalate may be more common than once reported.

Silicate calculi are rare in dogs in the United States. German shepherd dogs are most commonly affected.

Diagnosis

The signs associated with cystourolithiasis are typical of lower urinary tract disease (dysuria, hematuria, increased frequency of urination).

The uroliths may be diagnosed incidentally during routine physical examination and palpation of the bladder. Urinalysis may reveal hematuria, inflammation, or infection. Struvite crystals are a normal finding in urine, but cystine crystals are abnormal.

A quantitative urine culture with antibiotic sensitivity testing is performed, preferably from a sample collected by cystocentesis. If the bacterial count is greater than 10^3 bacteria/ml urine from a cystocentesis sample, a urinary tract infection is diagnosed. If a male dog is aseptically catheterized, a urine sample with a bacterial count greater than 10^5 is considered infected.

Occasionally, calculi are seen on survey abdominal radiographs. Contrast radiographs (retrograde urethrogram, double-contrast cystogram) are necessary to diagnose radiolucent calculi. With recurrent calculi, an excretory urogram is indicated to assess the size and shape of the kidneys.

Serum creatinine or urea nitrogen is measured before anesthesia. Other diagnostic tests may be indicated for dogs with abnormal history or physical examination findings.

Treatment

A special diet (Prescription Diet Canine S/D, Hill's Pet Products, Topeka, KS), in conjunction with control of the urinary tract infection, has dissolved struvite uroliths in dogs. The diet is low in phosphorus, magnesium, and protein and high in sodium chloride. Additional salt or acidifiers should not be added to the diet. The diet is continued for 1 month after uroliths are not seen on radiographs. The diet should not be fed to cats, young dogs, or pregnant or nursing female dogs. A precise protocol for medical dissolution of canine and feline struvite uroliths should be followed.

Surgical removal of cystouroliths is usually recommended unless other physiologic problems preclude anesthesia and surgery. A ventral cystotomy (Fig. 16-9) provides better access to the trigone, ureteral openings, and urethra. The risks of postoperative leakage and adhesions are similar for ventral and dorsal cystotomies.

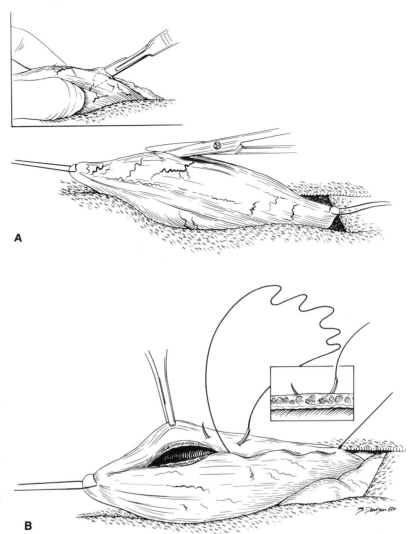

Figure 16-9. Cystotomy. **A,** A stab incision is made into the bladder. The incision is extended with scissors. **B,** The bladder is closed in one layer, using an inverting pattern. In a thickened bladder wall, a simple interrupted appositional pattern is used. (Stone EA, Barsanti JA. Small animal urologic surgery. Philadelphia: Lea & Febiger, in press)

After a laparotomy incision, the bladder is isolated from the abdomen with laparotomy sponges. Retention sutures are placed at each end of the planned incision. The bladder is emptied by cystocentesis, and a stab incision is made into the bladder with a scalpel. The incision is extended cranially and caudally with scissors. Calculi are removed with a bladder spoon, forceps, or saline flush. A catheter is passed into the urethra, and the urethra is flushed with saline to dislodge any calculi within the urethra.

The bladder is closed in one layer, using an inverting or simple interrupted pattern in a bladder wall of normal thickness and a simple interrupted pattern in a thickened bladder wall. The suture should not penetrate the mucosa. A monofilament nonabsorbable or a monofilament or braided synthetic absorbable suture material is used.

After surgery, the animal is allowed to urinate frequently. If this is impossible, the bladder should be decompressed by intermittent catheterization or by placing an indwelling urethral catheter connected to a sterile collection system.

Calculi are submitted for quantitative mineral analysis. Qualitative mineral analysis is not recommended because it may give false-positive results for urate and cystine and does not detect oxalate. Also, since many uroliths contain more than one mineral type, the layers of the stone must be quantitatively analyzed.

Prophylactic therapy should reduce the rate of recurrence, but clients should be warned that calculi can reoccur and that prolonged or even lifelong therapy may be required. Any concurrent urinary tract infection is treated, and food is salted to induce diuresis. Specific therapies for each urolith type have been reported. Special prescription diets are not recommended for the prevention of struvite cystouroliths since long-term use may cause hypoalbuminemia, increased calcium excretion, and hepatocyte changes.

Canine Polypoid Cystitis

Polypoid cystitis is an inflammatory condition of the bladder associated with chronic cystitis and characterized by a variable number of polypoid lesions protruding from the mucosa of the urinary bladder.

Diagnosis

The clinical and radiographic appearance is similar to tumors of the bladder. There may be lower urinary tract signs (hematuria, dysuria, stranguria). A space-occupying mass may be visible on contrast radiographs. The definitive diagnosis is based on a full-thickness biopsy of the bladder at the time of exploratory surgery. It must be differentiated from neoplasia by microscopic examination.

Treatment

The lesion is surgically excised. Chronic urinary tract infection is treated based on urine bacterial culture and antibiotic sensitivity results. Resolution may require a prolonged course of antibiotics, but remission and cure is possible.

Urinary Bladder Neoplasia

The bladder is the most common site for neoplasia of the urinary tract. Transitional cell carcinoma is the most common malignant tumor in dogs. Squamous cell carcinoma, adenocarcinoma, fibrosarcoma, leiomyosarcoma, rhabdomyosarcoma, and myxosarcoma have also been reported. Benign tumors of the bladder are rarely diagnosed. In cats, transitional cell carcinoma and squamous cell carcinoma are the most common bladder tumors.

Embryonal rhabdomyosarcoma (botryoid rhabdomyosarcoma, botryoid sarcoma) of the urinary bladder is a rare tumor that tends to occur in large-breed dogs younger than 2 years old. The tumor invades the bladder neck but does not metastasize.

Carcinomas may spread by direct invasion of the prostate gland, urethra, ureters, rectum, vagina, and/or uterus. The frequency of metastasis is unknown. Transitional cell carcinomas metastasize most commonly to the regional lymph nodes and lungs, but also may metastasize to the liver, long bones, and eyes.

The etiology of bladder neoplasia is unknown. Aromatic amine metabolites of tryptophan, which are excreted in high concentration in the urine of dogs, have been suggested as possible carcinogens. A significant positive correlation has been made between the proportional morbidity ratios for canine bladder cancer and the overall level of industrial activity in the host county of the veterinary hospital. Transitional cell carcinomas were found in three dogs after treatment with oral cyclophosphamide for other tumors, but a causal relationship was not proven.

Diagnosis

Clinical signs may include signs of lower urinary tract disease. There may be associated cystitis. Cytologic examination of urine may reveal tumor cells. Double-contrast cystography outlines bladder masses, and thoracic radiographs are examined for evidence of metastasis. Hypertrophic osteopathy can occur with bladder carcinoma and embryonal rhabdomyosarcoma. Definitive diagnosis of bladder neoplasia is based on microscopic examination of a biopsy, since pyogranulomatous masses and polypoid cystitis may have a similar gross appearance.

Treatment

Partial cystectomy is the most common treatment for localized canine and feline urinary bladder tumors. The bladder is opened at a point distant from the tumor. The tumor is excised with a 2-cm margin of healthy tissue. The remaining bladder is closed using a simple interrupted appositional pattern with synthetic absorbable suture material. A tube cystostomy or a urethral Foley catheter is placed to keep the bladder decompressed for 2 to 3 days after surgery. Frequent voiding occurs after surgery because of reduced bladder capacity. The bladder size will increase over several weeks, and further surgery to augment bladder size is seldom warranted.

For complete excision of extensive bladder neoplasia with urinary obstruction or severe hematuria, a cystectomy with trigone-colonic anastomosis (if the trigone is healthy) or ureterocolonic anastomosis is required. Dogs remain continent after these procedures, voiding watery feces several times a day, and most owners consider their animals to be acceptable pets. The main complications with the procedures are gastrointestinal and neurologic disturbances associated with metabolic acidosis, hyperammonemia, and/or uremia. These abnormalities can usually be controlled with sodium bicarbonate therapy and careful management of diet and fluid intake. Complete cystectomy is rarely curative, but may allow time for adjuvant therapy.

Bladder Injury

Rupture of the urinary bladder is the most common traumatic urinary tract injury in the dog and cat. Rupture occurs most commonly after external abdominal trauma and may have associated injuries, including pelvic fractures and visceral injuries. Rupture can also be caused by puncture wounds and by traumatic palpation and catheterization of the urinary bladder.

Diagnosis

The clinician should assume that any animal with abdominal or pelvic trauma could have a ruptured bladder. The clinical signs associated with a ruptured bladder are variable. Abdominal pain, vomition, and central nervous system depression may become apparent in less than 24 hours. The animal may still be able to urinate. Retrieving urine after urethral catheterization does not rule out bladder rupture. Any catheterization should be done using aseptic technique to prevent contaminating the peritoneal cavity. Diagnostic tests may reveal dehydration (elevated packed cell volume and total plasma protein) and elevations in serum creatinine, urea nitrogen, and inorganic phosphorus 24 to 48 hours after the rupture.

Abdominal paracentesis is done with a syringe and needle or with a peritoneal catheter. To determine if the fluid retrieved is urine, the urea and creatinine concentrations are measured in the fluid and peripheral blood and compared. Soon after urine leakage into the abdomen, the urea concentration of the fluid is higher than blood concentrations. After 24 hours, the urea concentration equilibrates between the abdominal fluid and the blood. Creatinine concentration, however, remains higher in the abdominal fluid than in the serum.

Survey radiographs are usually not diagnostic of a bladder rupture. Retrograde positive-contrast cystography using a water-soluble organic iodide preparation demonstrates the location of the rupture.

Treatment

Uremia, dehydration, and electrolyte abnormalities should be corrected before anesthesia and surgical repair of the ruptured bladder.

The surgical approach is through a midline incision extending from the umbilicus to the pubis. A complete exploration of the abdomen is done to check for other injuries. A sample of the abdominal fluid should be saved for microbiologic culture. The bladder tear is located. The edges are debrided back to bleeding tissue. The bladder is closed with a simple interrupted or a continuous Cushing suture pattern through the serosa and muscularis using absorbable or monofilament nonabsorbable suture.

If the tear is near the ureteral orifice, the ureter should be ligated near its entrance into the bladder and reimplanted more cranially. It may be necessary to enlarge the defect in the bladder to gain better access to the reimplantation site. After the ureter is reimplanted, the bladder edges are debrided and the bladder is closed.

If the tear is near the urethral junction, a urethral catheter should be passed from the bladder out the urethra to identify the urethral lumen. The lacerated edges are debrided to healthy tissue. The urethra is anastomosed to the bladder with simple interrupted appositional sutures using 4-0 synthetic absorbable suture material.

The abdomen is lavaged with copious amounts of warm saline, and the fluid is suctioned and removed. The bladder should be kept decompressed after repair by allowing the dog to urinate frequently, by urethral catheterization, or by a tube cystostomy; a tube cystostomy is preferable to a urethral catheter for ruptures occurring near the urethra. Fluid therapy should be continued after surgery until the animal is drinking on its own. Antibiotics are administered if the microbiologic culture is positive.

Urinary Bladder Herniation

The bladder may herniate through a traumatic rent in the abdominal wall or into a perineal hernia.

Diagnosis

There may be a history of trauma or an acute swelling. Catheterization of the urethra and reduction of the swelling is diagnostic. If a catheter cannot be placed, retrieval of urine by aspirating the swelling is diagnostic. A contrast cystogram also outlines a herniated bladder.

Treatment

The bladder can usually be reduced during the exploration of a traumatic hernia. Multiple cystocenteses may be needed. If the dog is a poor anesthesia risk, an indwelling catheter can be placed to drain the urine until the dog's condition can be stabilized.

Similarly, a bladder within a perineal hernia can usually be repositioned at the time of surgical repair of the hernia. If the bladder cannot be reduced, it may be necessary to perform a laparotomy to reposition the bladder. The bladder can be tacked to the abdominal wall (cystopexy) to prevent reherniation.

Urethra

Hypospadia

Hypospadia is a condition in male dogs in which the urethra opens on the ventral surface of the penis anywhere between the ischial arch and the normal urethral opening. It is a congenital defect resulting from a fusion failure of the urogenital folds and incomplete formation of the penile urethra. In humans, it is thought to be caused by inadequate androgen production by the fetal testis. The etiology in dogs is unknown.

Diagnosis

The dog may present with urine-soaked hair and skin around the urethral opening. The dog may lick excessively at the caudal abdominal area. The finding of an abnormal urethral opening and incomplete penis and prepuce on physical examination confirms the diagnosis.

Treatment

If the urethral opening is cranial to the scrotum, castration and scrotal urethrostomy are performed. If the urethral opening is in the perineal region, a perineal urethrostomy is done. The urethral groove and remnants of the prepuce and penis are excised.

After surgery, the patient is observed for signs of hemorrhage from the urethrostomy. Urine scalding may occur around the urethral opening and can be prevented by applying a water-insoluble ointment on the skin.

Urethrorectal Fistula

A urethrorectal fistula is a persistent communication between the urethra and the rectum. It is a developmental anomaly of the fetal cloaca.

Diagnosis

During voiding, urine passes simultaneously from the urethral opening and the anus. The signs usually are first observed after weaning. Rectal examination with a speculum may reveal the communication between the rectum and the urethra. A positive-contrast urethrogram demonstrates leakage of contrast medium from the urethra into the rectum. A cystocentesis urinalysis and urine bacterial culture often reveal concurrent cystitis.

Treatment

A caudal, ventral midline incision is made, and the pubic symphysis is separated in a young dog, or a pubic osteotomy is done in an adult dog. The fistula is identified, ligated, and excised. Concurrent cystitis is treated.

Prolapse of the Male Urethra

Prolapse of the male urethra is an eversion of the urethral mucosa through the urethral orifice. Sexual excitement and/or urethritis is thought to be contributory, but the exact cause is unknown. The results of urinalysis, urine culture, or contrast radiography have not been reported. An anatomic or hereditary predisposition may be present since young male English bulldogs and Boston terriers develop the condition.

Diagnosis

The dog may lick at the penis and preputial orifice. Urine and blood may dribble from the urethra. On physical examination, red, swollen, prolapsed tissue protrudes from the urethral orifice.

Treatment

Treatment requires general anesthesia. An attempt is made to reduce the prolapse gently with a soft urinary catheter. To prevent recurrence, four mattress sutures are inserted into the urethral lumen about 2 cm from the end of the penis. The sutures are tied outside the penis and are removed in 3 to 4 days.

If the prolapse cannot be reduced, or if the prolapsed portion is damaged or necrotic, the prolapsed portion is excised. After placing a urinary catheter, the urethra and penis are incised for one half of their circumference 2 to 3 mm proximal to the urethral orifice. The penile epithelium is sutured to the cut edges of the urethra. The remaining urethra and penis are incised and sutured to the penile epithelium.

After surgery, a side brace or Elizabethan collar is placed to prevent licking of the site. Tranquilization may be necessary. The dog should be kept separate from female dogs. If urethral prolapse recurs after reduction, resection of the prolapsed portion is recommended. Urinary tract infection should be treated if present.

Canine Urethroliths

Urethral uroliths originate from the bladder. Small, smooth calculi may pass through the urethra unnoticed, but clinical disease becomes apparent when the calculi become lodged within the urethra. Urethral obstruction occurs more often in male dogs than in females.

Diagnosis

Initially, the dog may have stranguria and dysuria. A dog with partial urethral obstruction may be incontinent, because the bladder distends until the intravesical pressure exceeds the urethral resistance from the urolith and urine dribbles out (paradoxical incontinence). With complete obstruction, the dog is anuric and the bladder may be greatly distended. The dog will begin to have the typical signs of postrenal uremia such as vomiting, anorexia, depression, and weakness. Evaluation of serum chemistries demonstrates azotemia and hyperkalemia.

Calculi within the pelvic urethra often can be palpated by digital rectal examination. Calculi may be palpable in the bladder. They often lodge in the urethra as it enters the proximal os penis. A urethral catheter may pass easily into the penile urethra and then meet resistance at the obstructing calculus.

Survey radiographs may reveal radiopaque uroliths within the urethra. Retrograde contrast urography is necessary to diagnose radiolucent calculi. Urine collected by cystocentesis should be submitted for urinalysis and bacteriologic culture and antibiotic sensitivity testing.

Treatment

Urethral obstruction requires immediate therapy since continuing postrenal uremia can be fatal. Permanent damage to the detrusor muscle, with subsequent bladder atony, can occur after prolonged distension. Intravenous fluid therapy is initiated and the bladder is decompressed by cystocentesis, unless there is a suspicion that the bladder is devitalized. Using a three-way stopcock, most of the urine is removed from the bladder during a single cystocentesis procedure. A small soft urethral catheter is used to try to bypass the urolith. A catheter should not be used to push the calculus into the bladder because of the risk of damaging the urethra.

Urohydropropulsion is used to dilate a portion of the urethra with fluid under pressure and wash the urolith into the bladder or out the urethra. A urethral catheter is passed aseptically to the level of the obstructing urolith. The distal urethra is occluded around the catheter with thumb and forefinger. An assistant places a gloved finger in the rectum and presses the urethra against the pubis. The urethra is dilated with sterile fluid from a 25-ml syringe attached to the catheter. Pressure on the urethra is quickly released, and the urolith

is flushed into the bladder. Alternately, the pressure around the distal urethra can be released so that the calculus can move out the urethra. If this procedure is unsuccessful, emergency surgical procedures should be considered.

Prescrotal urethrotomy, a temporary opening into the urethra, allows retrieval of uroliths from the prescrotal urethra (Fig. 16-10). Perineal urethral calculi can often be dislodged by catheterization and flushing of the urethra alternately through a cystotomy incision and the distal urethral opening. A skin incision is made from just caudal to the os penis to just cranial to the scrotum. If the incision extends onto the scrotum, the dog is more likely to excoriate the site, and there is the risk that the testes will prolapse through the incision.

Subcutaneous tissue is dissected to the level of the retractor penis muscle. The grayish corpus spongiosum and the paired white fibrous tissue covering the corpora cavernosa are located. If the corpora cavernosa fibrous covering is the most visible midline structure, the penis is rotated to bring the retractor penis muscle and corpus spongiosum to the midline.

The retractor penis muscle is retracted laterally, and a longitudinal incision is made in the corpus spongiosum and urethra. The shiny white urethra mucosal lining contrasts with the surrounding corpus spongiosum. The uroliths are removed, and a catheter is advanced.

The urethrotomy incision is closed with 4-0 synthetic absorbable sutures in a simple interrupted pattern, or it is allowed to heal by second intention, depending on the surgeon's preference and available materials. More postoperative hemorrhage may occur if the urethra is not sutured, but closing the urethra requires more time, gentle tissue handling, and delicate instruments to prevent stricture.

A *cystostomy catheter* is used to drain urine in a uremic animal with a urethral obstruction that cannot be easily corrected. A 1- to 2-cm skin incision is made in the caudal third of the abdomen (Fig. 16-11). In male dogs, the incision is made lateral to the prepuce. In

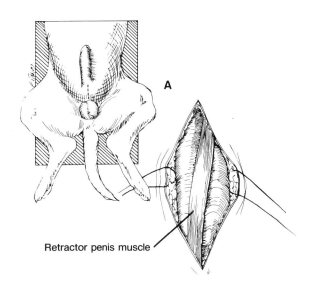

Figure 16-10. Prescrotal Urethrotomy—Canine. ***A,*** *The skin incision extends from just caudal to the os penis prepuce to just cranial to the scrotum (insert). Subcutaneous tissue is incised to the level of the retractor penis muscle.* ***B,*** *The retractor penis muscle is retracted laterally. A longitudinal incision is made in the corpus spongiosum muscle and the urethra, avoiding the corpus cavernosum.* ***C,*** *Retention sutures placed in the corpus spongiosum help identify the urethra. The urethrotomy can be left open or closed with 4-0 synthetic absorbable suture material in a simple interrupted pattern (insert). (Stone EA. Urologic surgery—An update. In: Breitschwerdt EB, ed. Nephrology and urology. New York: Churchill Livingstone, 1986;75)*

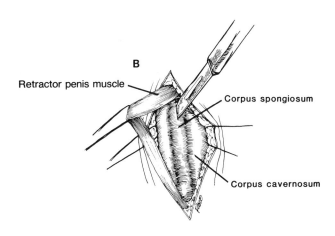

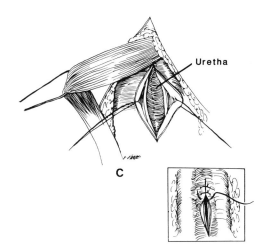

cats and female dogs, a midline incision is made.

The bladder is exteriorized, held in position with two retention sutures, and a purse-string suture, using absorbable suture material, is placed through the serosa and muscular layers of the cranial ventral wall. A stab incision is made within the purse-string, and an 8 French gauge or smaller Foley catheter is inserted into the bladder and inflated with sterile saline. Omentum can be incorporated into the purse-string as it is tied around the Foley

catheter. The retention sutures are passed through the linea alba or abdominal fascia and tied. The linea alba and skin incisions are closed, and the Foley catheter is secured to the skin. The catheter is connected to a closed drainage system and can be deflated and removed percutaneously after 3 days.

After urine flow is restored, fluid therapy is continued to correct the water, electrolyte, and acid-base disturbances. The kidneys may have an obligatory sodium and water diuresis for several days after the relief of urethral ob-

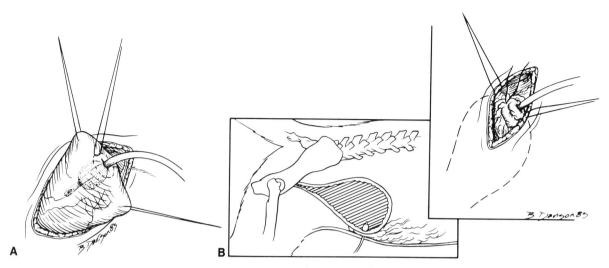

Figure 16-11. Cystostomy Catheter. **A,** *The Foley catheter is inserted into the bladder and inflated.* **B,** *Omentum can be incorporated into the purse-string suture as it is tied. The retention sutures are passed through the abdominal fascia and tied. After abdominal and skin incisions are closed, the Foley catheter is connected to a sterile closed drainage system. (Stone EA. Urologic surgery—An update. In: Breitschwerdt EB, ed. Nephrology and urology. New York: Churchill Livingstone, 1986;75)*

struction, so monitoring of hydration status, renal function, electrolyte levels, and urine output is necessary. When the dog's condition has stabilized, the dog can be anesthetized for a cystotomy to remove cystic calculi. Urethral calculi between the urethral opening and the bladder can usually be dislodged by flushing the urethra alternately from the bladder and from the urethral opening. A perineal urethrostomy (PU) is performed when calculi cannot be dislodged from the perineal urethra. The therapeutic plan to prevent recurrence of uroliths is based on quantitative mineral analysis of the calculi and urine bacterial culture and antibiotic sensitivity results.

Scrotal urethrostomy, a permanent opening in the urethra, is indicated for dogs that are recurrent stone-formers or for dogs with urethral strictures distal to the scrotum (Fig. 16-12). The procedure requires castration. The skin is incised around the scrotum at the junction of the scrotal and inguinal skin. The scrotal skin is excised, and the dog is castrated.

The subcutaneous tissue is incised to the retractor penis muscle. The retractor penis muscle is retracted laterally, and the urethra is incised directly on the ventral midline through the corpus spongiosum. The urethral incision extends caudally to where the urethra turns dorsally. A catheter can be passed to help determine the extent of the incision. The fascia of the corpora cavernosa is sutured to the subcutaneous fascia with absorbable suture material to help prevent tension on the urethra-to-skin sutures. The urethral mucosa is sutured to the skin with 4-0 nonabsorbable monofilament synthetic suture material. The caudal sutures are placed first to help align the urethral opening with the skin. The urethra-to-skin sutures are continued cranially for about 2 cm. The remaining skin is apposed.

A perineal urethrostomy is done only in dogs with irreparable damage or neoplasia of the distal perineal urethra. It is less cosmetically attractive and is more likely to cause urine scalding than a scrotal urethrostomy.

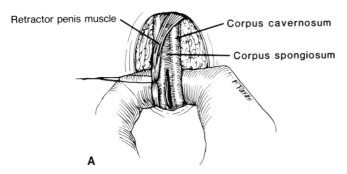

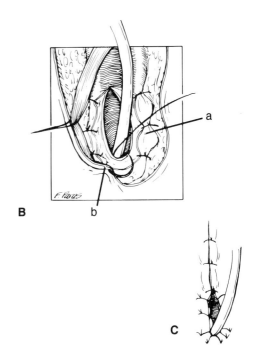

Figure 16-12. Scrotal Urethrostomy—Canine. **A,** *After the scrotal skin and testes have been excised, the subcutaneous tissue is incised to the retractor penis muscle. The muscle is retracted laterally and an incision is made through the corpus spongiosum and urethra. **B,** The fascia of the corpora cavernosa is sutured to the subcutaneous fascia with absorbable suture material (a). The urethral mucosa is sutured to the skin with 4-0 nonabsorbable monofilament suture material (b). **C,** The most caudal sutures are placed first. The urethra to skin sutures are continued cranially for 2 cm. The remaining skin is apposed. (Stone EA. Urologic surgery—An update. In: Breitschwerdt EB, ed. Nephrology and urology. New York: Churchill Livingstone, 1986;75)*

Feline Urethral Obstruction

Feline urologic syndrome (FUS) is a condition in cats of unknown etiology characterized by dysuria, hematuria, and sometimes urethral obstruction. It occurs in young adult male and female cats. Routine aerobic bacterial cultures are negative. Urethral obstruction occurs in male cats because of the narrow diameter of the penile urethra. The obstructing material is a plug of unorganized material formed of struvite (magnesium ammonium phosphate) crystals, mucus, and debris. The plug is not organized into a urolith.

Diagnosis

Nonobstructive urethritis and cystitis produce signs of hematuria, dysuria, increased frequency of urination, and urination in unusual locations. A urinalysis from a cat with uncomplicated FUS shows hematuria, proteinuria, and struvite crystals. There may be neutrophils, but no bacteria.

The signs of early obstruction are licking of the penis, straining, and anuria. On physical examination, a distended bladder is palpated. Cats may remain normal for about 48 hours following obstruction, but their condition will then rapidly worsen. About 10% of obstructed cats are critically ill at the time of presentation (*i.e.,* moderate to severe depression, azotemia, hypothermia, and acidosis).

Treatment

For a critically ill cat with urethral obstruction, an indwelling intravenous catheter is placed and blood is obtained to determine pretreatment laboratory values. Warm normal saline solution with 50 mEq Na bicarbonate is administered to correct fluid deficits. The total amount of fluid is based on the degree of hydration: for example, a 5-kg cat that is 8% dehydrated would require 400 ml of fluid. If the cat is hypothermic, it should be placed on a heating pad.

Catheterization is attempted to unplug the urethra. If unsuccessful, the bladder is drained by cystocentesis, then catheterization is reattempted. If a urethral catheter cannot be placed, multiple cystocenteses or a cystostomy catheter may be necessary.

Once urine production is re-established, fluid solutions are changed to a balanced electrolyte solution for 24 hours. The bladder is flushed with warm sterile saline. Force-feeding or tube-feeding should be started if the cat is not eating within 24 hours after relief of the obstruction. An obligatory postobstruction diuresis may occur after the relief of the obstruction. Fluid replacement (intravenous or subcutaneous) with a balanced electrolyte solution may be necessary for 2 to 3 days.

Infrequently, the urethra cannot be unblocked by backflushing and catheterization because of the obstructing material or urethral stenosis. In a healthy cat, a perineal urethrostomy (PU) can be done to unblock the urethra and create a wider urethral opening. If the cat is not a good anesthesia risk, or if the clinician is unfamiliar with the PU technique, a cystostomy catheter can be placed into the bladder using a local anesthetic. After the bladder distension is relieved, urine is drained while the cat is diuresed to decrease the uremia and hyperkalemia. A PU is done after the cat's condition has improved.

Bacterial urinary tract infection develops in about half of dogs and cats after 4 days of catheterization, even with closed drainage systems. Catheter-associated infections occur despite antibiotic therapy. Since animals given antibiotics tend to develop persistent infections with antibiotic-resistant bacteria, prophylactic antibiotics should *not* be used during urethral catheterization. When an infection develops, antibiotic administration is initiated based on culture and sensitivity results.

To prevent urethral reobstruction, a PU is recommended after two urethral obstructions within 6 to 12 months. Without surgery, obstruction recurs in at least 35% of cats within 6 months.

To perform a PU (Fig. 16-13), the cat is positioned in ventral recumbency with its tail taped cranially and its rear quarters elevated. A purse-string suture is placed in the anus. An elliptic skin incision is made dorsoventrally around the scrotum and prepuce, which are excised. An intact cat is castrated. The dissection is continued to the body of the penis. Five small blood vessels may need ligation. While the penis is retracted laterally, the ischiocavernosus muscle and penile crus on the opposite side is severed near their insertions on the ischium. The ventral ligament of the penis is palpated and severed between the penis and the floor of the pubis. Care is taken to keep the scissors flat on the pubis so that the pelvic urethra is not cut. The crus and ischiocavernosus muscle can be crushed and/or ligated to control hemorrhage. The procedure is repeated on the opposite side. Loose tissue surrounding the penis is cut. If the dissection extends too far dorsally, the rectum may be damaged. Finger dissection is used ventrally and laterally to free the penis. The retractor penis muscle is removed from the dorsal aspect of the penis. A transverse cut is made through the urethra 2 cm from the cranial edge of the bulbourethral glands. A catheter is inserted into the urethra. A dorsal longitudinal incision is made in the urethra with a #15 scalpel blade or with sharp iris scissors. The incision extends to the cranial edge of the bulbourethral glands. The incision extends into the pelvic urethra, which has a larger diameter. The dorsal end of the skin incision is sutured ventrally to the cranial end of the urethral incision. Skin sutures of 4-0 nonabsorbable monofilament material are placed between the urethra and the skin starting at the dorsal midline. If there is seeping hemorrhage, drains may be placed to help prevent blood clots from accumulating around the urethra, possibly forming a urethral stricture. Simple interrupted sutures are continued on both sides of the urethra 3 mm apart for 1.5 cm. The penis is ligated with a 3-0 surgical gut suture placed around the corpora cavernosa. The penis is amputated distal to this ligature. The lower end of the incision is closed with simple interrupted sutures. After the mucosa-to-skin flap is completed, the remaining skin wound is closed.

After surgery, an Elizabethan collar is put on the cat to prevent mutilation of the surgical site. Litter is removed from the litter box. Sutures are removed in 2 weeks using tran-

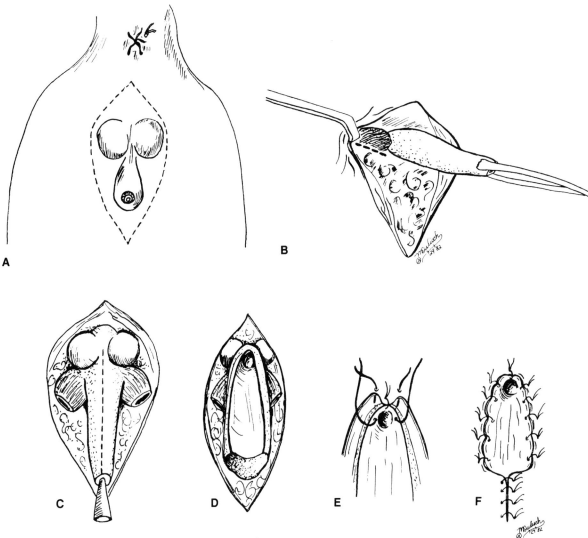

Figure 16-13. Perineal Urethrostomy (PU)—Feline.

A,   *An elliptical skin incision is made dorsoventrally around the scrotum and prepuce, which are excised. The cat is castrated, if intact.*

B,   *The penis is retracted laterally and the ischiocavernosus muscle and penile crus are severed near their insertions on the ischium.*

C-D, *A transverse cut is made through the urethra 2 cm from the cranial edge of the bulbourethral glands. A catheter is inserted into the urethra, and a dorsal longitudinal incision is made in the urethra to the cranial edge of the bulbourethral glands. This can be done with a #15 scalpel blade or with sharp iris scissors.*

E,   *Skin sutures of 4-0 nonabsorbable monofilament suture material are placed between the urethra and the skin starting at the dorsal midline.*

F,   *Simple interrupted sutures are continued on both sides of the urethra 3 mm apart for 1.5 cm. The penis is ligated and amputated distal to the ligation. After the mucosa-to-skin flap is completed, the remaining skin wound is closed.*

(Courtesy of Drs. ML Dulisch and PC Gambardella)

quilization or anesthesia if necessary. Synthetic absorbable sutures are not recommended because suture granulomas form at the junction of the mucosa and the skin.

Postoperative hemorrhage can be prevented by including the corpus cavernosum in each suture bite. If hemorrhage does occur after surgery, pressure on the incision site may control it. The mucous membrane color and packed cell volume should be monitored. Usually, the hemorrhage is not life-threatening and will stop without reoperation.

Anuria after a PU may be caused by a hypotonic bladder, obstruction of the urethra with blood clots, renal failure, or previous neurologic injury.

The owner should be warned that the PU procedure only prevents urethral obstruction. Cats may continue to have FUS with associated stranguria, dysuria, and hematuria. Prophylaxis for FUS is difficult since the etiology is unknown. One year after PU procedures, about 25% of cats have bacterial cystitis, possibly caused by a change in urethral sphincter function, anatomy, or both. If a cat with a PU has signs of lower urinary tract disease, a bacteriologic culture and antibiotic sensitivity test are indicated.

Stricture formation is prevented by careful attention to surgical technique and gentle tissue handling. Other causes of stricture include lacerations of the urethra during attempts to unblock the urethra, self-mutilation by the cat, and a suture left intact when the other sutures are removed. Occasionally, a minor stricture involving the most distal part of the urethra can be corrected by dilating the urethra with small forceps. Usually, however, additional surgery to make a new stoma is necessary. An elliptical incision is made around the urethrostomy site. It is helpful, if possible, to place a catheter to identify the urethral lumen. The penis is freed from any attachments in the pelvis (e.g., fibrous tissue, ischiocavernosus muscles). The dorsal aspect of the urethra is incised further cranially and the urethral mucosa is sutured to the skin.

If there has been extensive damage to most of the urethra, an antepubic urethrostomy is done by exiting the proximal urethra through the body wall. Alternately, a permanent cystostomy can be fashioned, but the cat will dribble urine continuously.

Minor wound dehiscence following a PU occurs most often when the sutures are pulled too tightly and lacerate the urethral mucosa. Major wound dehiscence may result from urine leakage in the subcutaneous space. This can be caused by urethral lacerations or improper apposition of mucosa to skin. The wound is managed as an open wound, debrided, lavaged, and allowed to heal by granulation. A Foley catheter is placed to prevent further urine contamination of the wound. Stricture is likely to occur and is managed as previously described.

Urethral Neoplasia

Neoplasms of the urethra are rare in dogs and extremely rare in cats. Older female dogs have the greatest incidence. Transitional cell carcinoma and squamous cell carcinoma are the most frequent tumor types. The etiology is unknown.

Diagnosis

Stranguria, ranging from mild straining to complete obstruction, hematuria, and urinary incontinence are common signs. Rectal and vaginal digital palpation may reveal an intrapelvic mass. A tumor at the distal end of the urethra may be seen by retracting the prepuce in a male or with vaginoscopy in a female. Urethral catheterization may be difficult or impossible. Tumor cells may be seen on urinalysis. A positive-contrast urethrogram reveals a space-occupying mass within the urethral lumen. Contrast cystography may help delineate the cranial extent of the tumor. Definitive diagnosis is by biopsy and microscopic examination. Local lymph nodes should be palpated and aspirated if enlarged. Thoracic and abdominal radiographs should be evaluated for metastatic disease.

Treatment

Complete surgical excision is often difficult because of the proximity of the surrounding tissues. The length of the required excision usually precludes direct anastomosis of the urethral edges. A urinary diversion procedure may be necessary. The effectiveness of chemotherapy or radiation therapy is unknown.

Urethral Trauma

Trauma is more common in male dogs. The urethra can be lacerated by pelvic fracture fragments, avulsed when the bladder is forced cranially, or crushed by external trauma. The penile urethra may be lacerated by fractures of the os penis or external lacerations.

Diagnosis

A history of trauma may be present. Physical examination findings depend on the location of the damage. If the urethra is avulsed from the bladder, urine may leak into the abdomen. Within the pelvic canal, there may be no external signs until the tissues swell and necrose. Alternately, a fistulous tract may develop, or damage to the urethra may not be recognized until scarring has obstructed the urine outflow.

A retrograde urethrogram, using water-soluble contrast material, is indicated if there is a suspicion of urethral trauma. An abdominocentesis will be positive only if urine is leaking into the peritoneal cavity. The serum creatinine and urea nitrogen may be elevated.

Treatment

For sharp penetrating injuries, surgical reapposition is not necessary. The urine is diverted from the site with a cystostomy catheter and/or a small urethral catheter. If there are lacerations with separation of urethral ends and/or urine leakage, surgical exploration is necessary.

To expose the pelvic urethra, a transsymphyseal approach is required. If the urethra is avulsed, a combined abdominal and transsymphyseal approach is necessary. Prostatic urethral damage may require partial or total prostatectomy. For perineal urethral in-

jury, a midline incision over the urethra is used. The ends of the damaged urethra are exposed and debrided. If possible, an end-to-end anastomosis is performed using 3-0 or 4-0 absorbable suture in a simple interrupted pattern. Urine should be diverted via a cystostomy (preferably) or a urethral catheter during urethral healing. Damage to the scrotal urethra may require castration and a scrotal urethrostomy.

Suggested Readings

Barsanti JA, Blue J, Edmunds J. Urinary tract infection due to indwelling bladder catheters in dogs and cats. J Am Vet Med Assoc 1985; 187:384.

Bovee KC, Reif JS, Maguire TG, et al. Recurrence of feline urologic syndrome. J Am Vet Med Assoc 1979;174:93.

Burrows CF, Bovee KC. Metabolic changes due to experimentally induced rupture of the canine urinary bladder. Am J Vet Res 1974;35:1083.

Finco DR, Barsanti JA. Bacterial pyelonephritis. Vet Clin North Am [Small Anim Pract] 1979; 9:645.

Goldschmidt MH. Renal neoplasia. In: Bovee KC, ed. Canine nephrology. Media, PA: Harwal, 1984;687.

Gregory CR, Vasseur PB. Long-term examination of cats with perineal urethrostomy. Vet Surg 1983;12:210.

Osborne CA, Polzin DJ, Kruger JM, Abdullahi SU. Medical dissolution and prevention of canine struvite uroliths. In: Kirk RW, ed. Current veterinary therapy IX. Philadelphia: WB Saunders, 1987;1177.

Patnaik AK, Schwarz PD, Greene RW. A histopathologic study of 20 urinary bladder neoplasms in the cat. J Sm Anim Pract 1986;27:433.

Stone EA, Barsanti JA. Small animal urologic surgery. Philadelphia: Lea & Febiger, in press.

Stone EA, Goldschmidt MH, Walter MC. Urinary diversion. Vet Clin North Am [Small Anim Pract] 1984;12:123.

Stone EA, Mason K. Surgery of ectopic ureters: Types, method of correction and postoperative results. J Am Anim Hosp Assoc, in press.

Stone EA, Withrow SJ, Page R. Ureterocolonic anastomosis in 10 dogs with transitional cell carcinoma. Vet Surg 1988;17:147.

17

Elizabeth A. Stone

The Genital System

The Ovary

Ovarian Cysts

Diagnosis

Follicular cysts, which develop from the Graafian follicle, may cause prolonged estrus with bloody vaginal discharge, nymphomania, cystic endometrial hyperplasia, cystic mammary hyperplasia, and genital fibroleiomyomas (fibroids). Cats may have prolonged estrus and behavioral changes such as aggressiveness and viciousness. Lutein cysts form from the corpus luteum following ovulation and may produce cystic endometrial hyperplasia or pyometra. The diagnosis of follicular and lutein cysts is based on clinical signs and is confirmed during exploratory celiotomy. Parovarian cysts arise from the remnants of either mesonephric (Wolffian) or paramesonephric tubules and ducts and do not cause clinical signs. They are usually found incidentally during ovariohysterectomy and are located between the ovary and uterine horn.

Treatment

Ovariohysterectomy is the treatment of choice for ovarian cysts.

Ovarian Neoplasia

Diagnosis

Any of the ovarian tumor types (granulosa cell tumor, papillary cystadenoma, and cystadenocarcinoma) may stimulate the theca to produce progesterone with associated signs of cystic endometrial hypoplasia and pyometra. Larger tumors may present as a cranial abdominal mass on palpation and abdominal radiographs. Granulosa cell tumors are the most common ovarian tumor in bitches and may

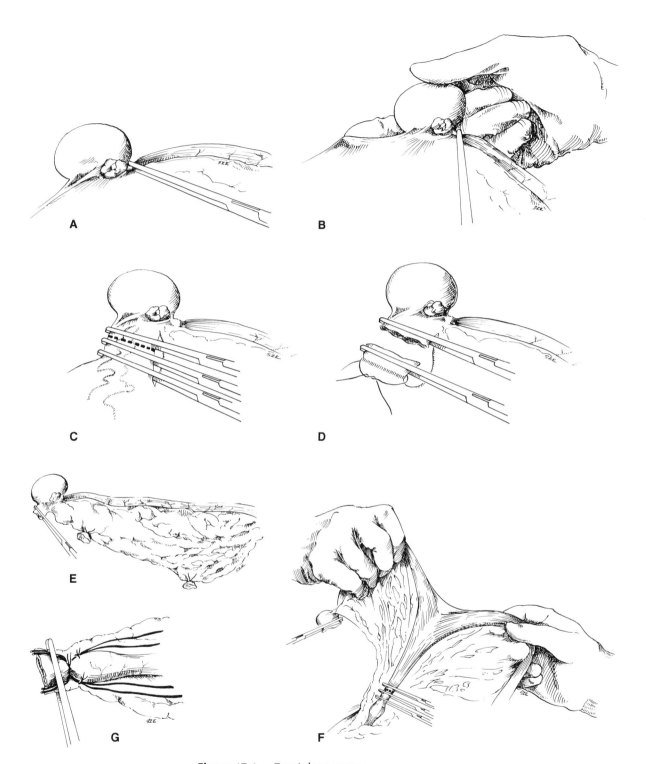

Figure 17-1. Ovariohysterectomy.

A, After the ovary is located, a clamp is placed on the proper ligament of the ovary.

B, The suspensory ligament is stretched or broken.

C, A window is made in the meso-ovarium caudal to the ovarian vessels. The ovarian pedicle is triple-clamped. The ovarian pedicle is severed between the clamp closest to the ovary and the middle clamp.

D, A ligature is placed in the groove left by the most proximal clamp.

produce prolonged estrus. Papillary cystadenomas and cystadenocarcinomas have also been reported in the bitch. Signs may include irregular estrous cycles, cystic endometrial hyperplasia, or ascites.

Treatment

In the early stages of ovarian neoplasia, surgical excision may be curative. Granulosa cell tumors may invade the body wall and kidney, requiring nephrectomy. Papillary cystadenocarcinomas often have peritoneal implants and lung metastasis. The success of adjunctive therapy has not been reported.

The Uterus

Sterilization

Elective sterilization is most often done by ovariohysterectomy. The incidence of mammary gland tumors in bitches spayed before the first estrous cycle is less than 0.5%. After the first estrous cycle, the risk increases to 8%; after two cycles, the risk increases to 26%. There is no preventive effect on mammary gland tumors if the ovariohysterectomy is done after 2.5 years. Sterilization by ovariohysterectomy is also indicated for animals with diabetes or epilepsy to prevent hormonal influences on therapy.

In young healthy animals, the minimum data base for an ovariohysterectomy is a packed cell volume, a total plasma protein concentration determination, and a urine specific gravity. In an older dog, a biochemistry panel and other tests, depending on the case

history and physical examination, may be indicated.

Treatment

There are many variations of the ovariohysterectomy technique. The following technique is useful for dogs and cats of any size and can be used on an enlarged uterus (Fig. 17-1). In a dog, a midline abdominal incision starts at the umbilicus and extends caudally for one third the distance between the umbilicus and the pubis. In a cat, the incision is started 2 cm caudal to the umbilicus and extended about 4 cm caudally. The abdominal incision should be longer if the uterus is enlarged or distended. The right uterine horn is located with a spay hook or an index finger. To use the spay hook, it is first turned so that the hook faces caudally, and then it is placed into the abdomen along the right body wall. It is advanced to the dorsal body wall, turned one quarter-turn toward the midline, then gently retracted. If this is unsuccessful after several attempts, the uterus is located by using a forefinger to palpate between the urinary bladder and the colon. The finger is hooked around the uterine horn, and the horn is lifted from the abdomen. A Carmalt clamp is placed on the proper ligament of the ovary (formerly named the utero-ovarian ligament). An index finger is placed in the hammock formed by the suspensory ligament and the meso-ovarium and slid cranially toward the kidney. The suspensory ligament is then torn or stretched by applying traction to the ligament in a craniolateral direction toward the abdominal wall. Care must be taken to avoid tearing more than the suspensory ligament.

E, *The broad ligament is ligated in one or two places and then severed.*
F, *The uterus is exteriorized and three clamps are placed on the uterine body just cranial to the cervix. The uterine body is severed between the proximal and middle clamps.*
G, *The uterine vessels are ligated on each side of the uterine body. The uterine body is ligated in the groove left by the most distal clamp.*
(Stone EA. The Uterus. In: Slatter DH, ed. Textbook of small animal surgery. Philadelphia: WB Saunders, 1985;1667–1669)

After a window is made in the meso-ovarium, a second Carmalt clamp is placed on the ovarian pedicle proximal to the ovary. A third Carmalt clamp is placed through the fenestration and clamped across the ovarian pedicle proximal to the ovary and proximal to the first clamp. The first Carmalt clamp is removed from the proper ligament of the ovary and placed on the ovarian pedicle between the second clamp and the ovary, if there is enough room, or through the fenestration and across the proper ligament of the ovary. The pedicle is severed proximal to the ovary between the first and second clamps. The index finger is used to protect adjacent structures. A ligature of 0 surgical gut (2-0 in cats) is passed around the most proximal clamp and the first throw of a surgeon's knot is loosely made. As the throw is tightened, the most proximal clamp is removed. The ligature is tightened into the crushed groove left after removal of the proximal Carmalt clamp. In large dogs and in fat dogs and cats, a second ligature may be placed just distal to the first ligature. The procedure is repeated on the opposite ovarian pedicle. The broad ligament is severed or torn. If it is vascular, it is ligated with one or two ligatures before it is cut.

The uterine body is ligated and severed using a three-clamp technique as described above. In small dogs and cats, the clamps may not be necessary before ligating. The uterine vessels are transfixed separately by passing a suture needle and 2-0 surgical gut into the edge of the uterine wall. The vessel ligatures should be placed just cranial to the cervix. The uterine body ligature is placed cranial to the vessel ligatures.

Ovariohysterectomy complications can be related to anesthesia, the laparotomy incision, or the ovariohysterectomy. Hemorrhage during surgery may be caused by improper clamping or ligation of the ovarian or uterine pedicles. To determine the source of bleeding, it may be necessary to extend the incision to accommodate the surgeon's hand in the abdominal cavity. The hand is advanced along the right abdominal wall until the right lateral lobe of the liver is palpated. The hand is moved slightly caudally and then medially to grasp the duodenum and bring it out of the incision. The mesentery of the duodenum is used as a retractor to locate the right ovarian pedicle. The left ovarian pedicle is located by first reaching down into the middle of the incision and grasping the descending colon. The mesentery of the descending colon is used as a retractor to identify the left ovarian pedicle. The urinary bladder is retracted ventrally and caudally to reveal the uterine pedicle between the neck of the urinary bladder and the rectum. The broad ligament is also examined for bleeding vessels. Intermittent vaginal bleeding can occur 4 to 16 days after ovariohysterectomy because of erosion of the uterine vessels or infection around the uterine vessel ligatures. An exploratory laparotomy is necessary to find and ligate the bleeding vessel.

Estrus following ovariohysterectomy is caused by residual ovarian tissue and requires excision of the remaining tissue to prevent further estrous cycles. Uterine stump pyometra can occur when residual uterine horns or body remain. The progesterone stimulus may come from remaining ovarian tissue or from medications, and complete excision of the uterus is curative. Fistulous tracts in the groin or flank may develop from tissue reaction to braided nonabsorbable suture material.

Delayed complications include urinary incontinence and weight gain. Incontinence can occur in older spayed bitches and is usually responsive to low-dose estrogen therapy.

Dystocia

Diagnosis

The owner of a dog with suspected dystocia should be questioned about the breeding date, gestation length, and previous whelpings and dystocias. A thorough physical examination is performed. Vaginal examination may reveal a fetus lodged in the pelvis or abnormalities in the vagina or vulva. Rectal examination is used to evaluate pelvic shape and size. Survey radiographs demonstrate the number of remaining feti, but are not diagnostic of fetal death until the puppies have been dead for several hours. Dystocia should be considered if there are signs of toxicity in a bitch in late pregnancy, strong contractions without delivering a puppy within 20 minutes, weak contractions for 2 to 3 hours without delivering a puppy, or prolonged gestation (>68 days from last mating).

Treatment

If medical management of dystocia is unsuccessful, cesarean section is indicated (Fig. 17-2). It is also indicated as the initial treatment when the fetus is obviously oversized or the pelvic canal is narrowed. Fluid therapy, antibiotics, and corticosteroids are administered as necessary to treat dehydration and toxic shock. The choice of anesthesia should minimize the anesthetic exposure of the fetuses with consideration of the available equipment, supplies, and personnel. As much surgical preparation as possible is done before induction of anesthesia.

The animal is placed in dorsal recumbency and rotated 15° to the right to shift the weight of the uterus from the caudal vena cava. A midline abdominal incision is made long enough to exteriorize the uterus easily. The uterus is gently lifted from the abdomen, and warm moistened laparotomy sponges are used to isolate it from the abdomen. The uterus is carefully examined. If it is devitalized from torsion or rupture, ovariohysterectomy may be necessary. For a cesarean section, a longitudinal incision is made in the uterine body. A fetus is manipulated into the incision by gentle pressure on the uterus. The amniotic sac is opened and the puppy is removed. The umbilicus is left attached to the placenta for a few minutes after uterine separation to allow the placental blood to flow into the puppy. The umbilical cord is clamped or ligated and sev-

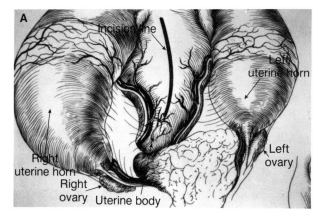

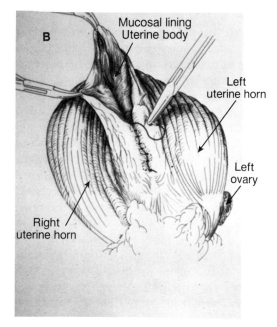

Figure 17-2. Cesarean Section. **A,** *A longitudinal dorsal incision is made in the body of the uterus.* **B,** *After the puppies have been removed, the uterine incision is closed with an inverting pattern. (Chambers JN. Caesarean section. In: Wingfield WE, Rawlings CA, eds. Small animal surgery. Philadelphia: WB Saunders, 1979;138)*

ered. Following delivery, the assistant dries the puppy and removes oronasal secretions. The uterine incision is closed in a one- or two-layer closure using synthetic absorbable suture material. If uterine leakage has occurred, the abdomen is lavaged with copious amounts of warm saline. Abdominal closure is routine. The puppies are united with the bitch as soon as she has recovered from anesthesia.

Pyometra

Pyometra is a disease of the diestral phase of the estrous cycle when the corpus luteum is actively secreting progesterone. Progesterone levels are not abnormally elevated, but there may be changes in the progesterone receptor cells in the endometrium and a corresponding increase in secretory activity of the uterine glands and inhibition of myometrial contractions. Bacterial invasion is not the initiating factor, but most dogs with pyometra have a secondary infection.

Diagnosis

The history of dogs with pyometra can be quite variable. It can occur in any intact bitch after the first heat, but appears to be more common in the middle-aged to older animal. A history of irregular estrous cycles, abnormal estrus, or false pregnancies does not predispose the dog to pyometra. Pyometra is uncommon in cats.

The signs most commonly seen in dogs with pyometra are vaginal discharge, anorexia, polydipsia/polyuria, and depression. Other signs are vomiting and diarrhea. On physical examination, vaginal discharge is present if the cervix is open. The vagina should be examined to rule out primary vaginitis or vaginal tumors as a cause of vaginal discharge. Abdominal palpation may reveal an enlarged uterus. Body temperature is usually within normal range, but toxemic dogs may be hypothermic. Vaginal cytology reveals large numbers of bacteria and neutrophils.

The minimum data base for a dog with pyometra should include a packed cell volume, total protein concentration, serum creati-nine or serum urea nitrogen, urine specific gravity from a midstream sample before fluid therapy, and a urine culture from a sample taken at the time of surgery. Other tests may be indicated based on the case history and physical examination findings.

Dogs with pyometra usually are leukocytic and hyperglobulinemic; some may be hypoalbuminemic. Older dogs may have chronic renal failure concurrent with the acute functional changes in the kidneys commonly associated with pyometra. Elevations in serum urea nitrogen and serum creatinine are caused by renal failure and prerenal dehydration and hypovolemia. A low urine specific gravity value in a dehydrated dog is diagnostic of renal failure, but cannot be used to determine chronicity or prognosis. On survey abdominal radiographs, homologous tubular structures of fluid density may be seen, but cannot be differentiated from early pregnancy or an immediate postpartum uterus.

Treatment

Ovariohysterectomy is the recommended treatment in most instances. Medical therapy using prostaglandin F_2-alpha has been generally restricted to the treatment of valuable breeding bitches with mild clinical disease. Therapy for dehydration, acidosis, and shock are started before surgery. Since these dogs may have compromised renal function, fluid therapy (balanced electrolyte solution) is continued (10 ml/kg/hr) during surgery.

The ovariohysterectomy procedure is similar to that described previously, with extra care taken to avoid rupturing the enlarged uterus. The uterus is isolated with laparotomy sponges to minimize contamination of the abdomen. The three-clamp technique is used on the uterine body in almost all dogs. If the cervix is greatly distended, an oversew technique can be used. Urine is taken by cystocentesis for bacterial culture, since urinary tract infection is commonly associated with pyometra. The abdomen is copiously lavaged with warm physiologic solution before closure. Antibiotics are administered if there has been spillage. Fluid therapy is continued after surgery until the dog can maintain hydration by drinking.

Uterine Torsion

In uterine torsion, the uterine body or one of the horns can twist along the long axis, or one or both uterine horns can twist around the opposite horn. A gravid uterus is more likely to twist than a nongravid uterus.

Diagnosis

Animals with uterine torsion develop acute abdominal pain. An owner may think that the animal is straining to defecate. The torsion may occur after delivery of a puppy or kitten. Physical examination may be unrevealing, with possible vaginal discharge and a tense and distended abdomen. Rarely, the rotated uterine body is felt by vaginal examination. Radiographic findings may include a large tubular structure filled with air or fluid.

Treatment

Appropriate fluid and shock therapy is initiated before surgery. A long midline abdominal incision is made, and the uterus is exteriorized. A cesarean section is done to remove any live feti, and an ovariohysterectomy is performed.

Uterine Prolapse

Prolapse of a uterine horn or the entire uterus through a dilated cervix occurs during or after parturition.

Diagnosis

The animal will either be in labor or in the early postpartum period. A tubular mass may protrude from the vulva or may be found within the vagina. The uterus may be ulcerated, hemorrhagic, and soiled. The animal's overall condition should be assessed.

Treatment

Manual reduction can be attempted in a healthy animal if the uterus is not damaged. After the animal is anesthetized, the uterus is cleansed with warm physiologic solution and lubricated with sterile, water-soluble jelly. The uterus is gently reduced with gloved fingers and a sterile syringe plunger. It may be necessary to do a celiotomy to complete the repositioning of the uterus. The risk of recurrence is unknown. If the reduced uterus has questionable viability, an ovariohysterectomy is done.

If manual reduction is impossible, the uterus is amputated. An incision is made into the cranial part of the uterine body near the vulva. The ovaries may be exposed by gentle traction on the cranial ends of the uterine horns. If the ovarian pedicle can be located, it is double-ligated and severed; otherwise, the uterine horns and uterine arteries are double-ligated and severed. The uterus is severed, and the stump is closed with absorbable suture material. The stump is repositioned through the vagina. If necessary, the ovaries can be removed later through a celiotomy incision.

Uterine Neoplasia

Uterine tumors are rare, with a reported incidence of 0.3% of all canine tumors. Leiomyomas are much more common than malignant tumors.

Diagnosis

Uterine tumors are often found incidentally during an elective ovariohysterectomy. Large uterine tumors may cause abdominal distension and signs associated with an abdominal mass. Hydrometra or mucometra can develop if the tumor occludes the uterine lumen.

Treatment

Surgical treatment is ovariohysterectomy.

The Vagina and Vulva

Congenital Anomalies

Segmental vaginal hypoplasia or aplasia, uncommon in dogs, is caused by abnormal development of the Müllerian duct system or urogenital sinus. Hypoplasia interferes with breeding and parturition. Aplasia (complete occlusion) causes retention of uterine fluids during estrus. A persistent hymen may cause annular fibrous strictures or vertical septae, which can cause breeding or whelping problems or vaginitis.

Diagnosis

Examining the vagina digitally and via a vaginoscope should identify vaginal hypoplasia, strictures, or septae.

Treatment

For segmental vaginal hypoplasia in a nonbreeding, nonsymptomatic animal, no treatment is needed. An ovariohysterectomy is recommended to prevent breeding and pregnancy. It is unknown whether the condition is hereditary in dogs.

Resection of vaginal strictures and septae usually requires an episiotomy. An episiotomy incision is made dorsally to extend the dorsal commissure of the vulva and enlarge the vulvar cleft. The animal is placed in ventral recumbency and a purse-string suture is placed around the anus. A straight incision is made through the vestibular wall. The incision should extend far enough dorsally to allow complete exposure of the vagina without entering the external anal sphincter. Hemorrhage can be controlled with ligatures, pressure, or electrocoagulation. If excessive hemorrhage occurs, straight Doyen intestinal forceps (not Carmalts) can be clamped along the edges of the incision. A urethral catheter is placed to identify the urethral orifice.

Once the episiotomy incision is made, an annular stricture is approached by first incising through the vaginal mucosa over the stricture and then dissecting out the fibrous band

forming the stricture. The mucosa is closed in a simple interrupted pattern with fine absorbable suture material. If the band cannot be removed, it is severed in several places and the circumference is stretched. Septae can be severed at each base and removed. The mucosa can be closed over the base for better hemostasis.

Closure of the episiotomy is with three or four layers in a simple interrupted pattern. In a large dog, the mucosa, muscle, and subcutaneous layers are closed separately. In small dogs, the muscle and subcutaneous layers can be closed together. Skin closure is routine.

When the vulva is hypoplastic, the episiotomy can be converted to an episiostomy by suturing the mucosa to the skin on each side of the incision to permanently enlarge the opening.

Vaginal Hyperplasia and Prolapse

Vaginal hyperplasia is an edematous swelling of the ventral vagina that occurs during periods of elevated estrogen levels (estrus, cystic ovaries). It may progress to vaginal prolapse, where the entire vaginal circumference everts. Vaginal prolapse may also occur after parturition.

Diagnosis

The dog will present with a fleshy mass obscuring the vagina. The everted tissue may be discolored, ulcerated, and soiled. With vaginal hyperplasia, the vaginal opening is dorsal to the mass. With vaginal prolapse, access to the vaginal canal is through a doughnut-shaped eversion. The urethra is usually caudal to the prolapsed tissue.

Treatment

No treatment is necessary for a small prolapse. It will regress during diestrus, but may recur during the next estrus. A large prolapse with healthy tissue can be cleansed, lubricated, and manually reduced. Temporary retention sutures are placed across the lips of the vulva. Ovariohysterectomy is performed in a nonbreeding animal to reduce the tissue edema during the current episode and to prevent recurrence. In a breeding bitch, it may be possible to use artificial insemination, but the condition may recur during the next estrus.

Surgical resection may be necessary if the tissue is necrotic or too large to be replaced. An episiotomy incision is made, and the urethra is catheterized and protected. Redundant vaginal tissue is amputated by making a transverse, elliptical incision around the base. The mucosa is closed with simple interrupted absorbable sutures, and the episiotomy is closed.

Vulvovaginitis

Diagnosis

Vulvovaginitis is most common in obese dogs. The dog may lick excessively at the area, and the hair may be matted. Generalized skin disease and pyoderma should be ruled out.

Treatment

Initially, the pyoderma is treated with cleansing and drying agents. If the infection is severe, skin culture and sensitivity testing should be followed by appropriate antibiotic therapy. Episioplasty (removal of redundant skin folds that predispose the area to moisture, irritation, and infection) is used to correct resistant vulvovaginitis.

For an episioplasty, the patient is placed in ventral recumbency and a purse-string suture is placed around the anus. To remove the redundant skin. a crescent-shaped, bilaterally symmetrical incision is made dorsal and lateral to the vulva. The skin and subcutaneous fat are removed. Temporary sutures are placed at 9 o'clock, 12 o'clock, and 3 o'clock to ascertain whether sufficient tissue has been removed. Once sufficient skin has been excised, interrupted subcutaneous sutures of 4-0 absorbable material are placed. Skin sutures are placed routinely.

Vaginal and Vulvar Neoplasia

Vaginal and vulvar tumors make up about 3% of tumors in dogs and are very rare in cats. Benign tumors are much more common than malignant tumors. The benign tumors are most often leiomyomas, fibromas, and polyps in older, intact female dogs. Lipomas may also occur in the vaginal area. The more common malignant tumors are leiomyosarcoma and squamous-cell carcinoma. Urinary tract carcinomas may originate from the urethra and extend to the urethral papilla, and then into the vagina or vestibule.

Diagnosis

The most common sign of vaginal and vulvar tumors is the sudden protrusion of a pedunculated mass. Vulvar bleeding or discharge may occur. Tumors are differentiated from vaginal hyperplasia and prolapse by their location, chronicity, and if necessary by cytology. During vaginoscopic examination, the urethral opening and papilla should be evaluated for tumor involvement. Transmissible venereal tumor (TVT) is usually a cauliflowerlike mass or multiple nodules. The surface may be friable and hemorrhagic. The gross appearance may be similar to a papilloma or squamous-cell carcinoma. The definitive diagnosis is based on histopathologic examination.

Treatment

The recommended treatment for benign, non-lipomatous tumors is surgical resection and ovariohysterectomy. The malignant tumors tend to be more diffuse and more difficult to excise completely. The efficacy of chemotherapy or radiation therapy is unknown.

Surgical excision of TVT is rarely complete and regrowth is common. TVT can be successfully managed using vincristine or radiation therapy.

Intersexuality

Intersexual dogs are usually male pseudohermaphrodites (female or ambiguous genitalia with internal or scrotal testes). These animals have an XX karyotype, but may have the H-Y gene located on an autosome or on the X chromosome. A specific type of male pseudohermaphroditism in the miniature schnauzer is characterized by persistence of Müllerian duct derivatives in male dogs with unilateral or bilateral cryptorchidism. The karyotype is XY, and the persistence of the Müllerian ducts is thought to be caused by a failure of Müllerian inhibitory activity.

Female pseudohermaphrodites have male or ambiguous genitalia, internal ovaries, and an XX karyotype. In addition to hereditary defects, female pseudohermaphroditism has been associated with the administration of progesterone, testosterone, or mibolerone during pregnancy.

True hermaphrodites are less common (25% of reported intersex cases in the dog). These dogs may have unilateral hermaphroditism, where one gonad is an ovotestis and the other is a testis or ovary; bilateral hermaphroditism, where both gonads are ovotestes; or lateral hermaphroditism, where one gonad is a testis and the other is an ovary. The karyotype may be XX or a mosaic (XX/XY and XX/XXY).

Diagnosis

The case history for dogs with female phenotypes may include irregular estrous cycles, reproduction problems, and vaginitis. On physical examination, an enlarged clitoris may be visible. Urinary incontinence can occur in both male and female phenotypes. Miniature schnauzers with Müllerian duct syndrome are unilaterally or bilaterally cryptorchid and can have signs referable to Sertoli cell tumors or pyometra, or both.

Treatment

In the female phenotype dog, the clitoris is excised and the dog is neutered. The dog is placed in ventral recumbency and an episiotomy incision is made. A urethral catheter is placed. The vaginal mucosa around the clitoris is incised, and the clitoris is dissected free. The mucosa is apposed with absorbable suture material. The dog is then repositioned and an abdominal incision is made. The neutering pro-

cedure is similar to an ovariohysterectomy. Treatment for pyometra in a male miniature schnauzer is the same as described previously for pyometra in a female. Removal of an abdominal testis is described below (see "Cryptorchidism," p. 472).

The Prostate

Benign Hyperplasia

Benign prostatic hyperplasia occurs in middle-aged and old dogs. Its development requires the presence of functioning testes. It may be caused by the prostate's altered sensitivity to serum androgens or in response to the relative decrease in the serum androgens compared to estrogens that occur with age. Squamous metaplasia of the prostate is caused by prolonged hyperestrogenism from Sertoli cell tumors or seminomas, or from exogenous estrogen administration.

Diagnosis

The dog may present for tenesmus or hematuria or it may be asymptomatic. The main clinical finding is a moderate, symmetrical, nonpainful prostatic enlargement. Ultrasound evaluation of the prostate has been quite useful in differentiating a homogenous enlargement of the prostate, as in benign hyperplasia, from cysts and abscessation.

Treatment

The treatment of choice is castration to decrease prostatic size. Persistent enlargement of the prostate suggests additional prostatic pathology, which should be diagnosed via biopsy.

Acute Bacterial Prostatitis
Diagnosis

Acute onset of hemorrhagic or purulent urethral discharge, caudal abdominal tenderness, fever, and lethargy in a dog suggests acute bacterial prostatitis. The prostate is painful on digital rectal palpation and may be slightly enlarged or normal in size. Blood may drip constantly or intermittently from the penis. The scrotal sac is carefully examined to rule out a primary orchitis.

Urinalysis reveals hematuria, bacteriuria, and pyuria. A positive urine culture from a cystocentesis sample is diagnostic of a urinary tract infection. In association with the aforementioned signs, urinary tract infection is indicative of acute bacterial prostatitis. A hemogram may be normal or may show leukocytosis.

Treatment

The dog is started on broad-spectrum antibiotics until the bacteriologic culture results are known. The type of antibiotic can be changed, if necessary, based on the antibiotic sensitivity results. Castration is recommended after the dog has been on antibiotic therapy for 1 week. Antibiotic therapy is continued for 2 weeks, and the dog is re-examined after 3 weeks. The urinalysis and urine culture are repeated. If the urine culture is negative, an ejaculate or prostatic massage sample is collected for cytology and quantitative culture. Persistent infection is indicative of chronic bacterial prostatitis.

Chronic Bacterial Prostatitis

Diagnosis

The dog usually presents with a history of recurrent urinary tract infection with or without urethral discharge. The prostate is usually not painful and may be small, normal, or enlarged. There are no signs of systemic illness with uncomplicated chronic bacterial prostatitis, but the prostate may be predisposed to abscessation and rupture.

A urinalysis and urine culture from a cystocentesis sample are performed. If the urine shows no evidence of urinary tract infection, an ejaculate or prostatic massage sample is collected for cytology and culture. Cytology from prostatic massage fluid or aspirate

correlates with the diagnosis from microscopic, radiologic, or microbiologic examination or clinical signs in most dogs.

Treatment

An antibiotic is selected based on sensitivity and ability to cross the blood-prostate barrier (*e.g.*, trimethoprim-sulfadiazine, erythromycin, oleandromycin, or chloramphenicol). The antibiotic is administered for 1 month. The dog is castrated after 1 to 2 weeks of antibiotic therapy. The cultures are repeated 1 week after cessation of antibiotic therapy. If the cultures are positive, the antibiotic therapy is continued for another month and the cultures are repeated as before.

Monthly cultures are repeated for several months after the initial negative culture. It may be impossible to eliminate the infection completely, and continual antibiotic therapy or prostatectomy may be required.

Prostatic Abscessation

Prostatic abscessation is a type of chronic bacterial prostatitis in which pockets of pus develop within the prostatic parenchyma.

Diagnosis

The signs may reflect systemic septicemia (fever, depression, anorexia, vomiting), lower urinary tract infection, and hemorrhagic or purulent urethral discharge. Digital rectal palpation may reveal the abscesses as soft, fluctuant swellings within the prostatic parenchyma or as an irregular surface on the prostate gland. Leukocytosis may be present, and the prostatic cytology will be inflammatory. Definitive diagnosis may require an exploratory laparotomy and biopsy.

Treatment

Surgical drainage of the abscess or prostatectomy is recommended, together with castration. The dog is started on antibiotic therapy before surgery. A urethral catheter is placed to identify the urethra.

For surgical drainage, the prostate is isolated from the abdomen with laparotomy sponges. A stab incision is made into the prostate with a hemostat. To minimize the spread of infection into the surrounding tissues, the periprostatic fat is not disrupted. The surgeon's finger is inserted into the abscess pocket to break down loculations. A single 5-mm Penrose drain is passed from ventral to dorsal on either side of the prostate. As the drain exits the dorsal surface, it is retrieved and passed lateral to the gland to exit through the same opening in the abdominal wall. No internal tacking sutures are used. The drains are secured to the skin and left in place 2 to 4 weeks. Antibiotic therapy is continued for 4 weeks, and then cultures are repeated 1 week later as described for chronic prostatitis.

The major long-term complications with the drainage technique are persistent or recurrent urinary tract infection and recurrent prostatic disease. Progression to pyelonephritis could cause irreversible renal failure.

For a prostatectomy, it may be necessary to osteotomize and reflect the cranial pubis to gain enough exposure. The periprostatic fat is removed from the ventral and lateral prostate, with care taken to avoid the neurovascular supply to the bladder and urethra dorsal to the prostate. The short vessels to the prostate and the vas deferens are ligated and severed. The prostate is dissected free from the bladder neck cranially and from the membranous urethra caudally. The urethra is severed as close as possible to the cranial and caudal surfaces of the prostate. The membranous urethra is anastomosed using 4-0 synthetic absorbable suture material in a simple interrupted pattern. A cystostomy catheter is placed in the bladder and exited lateral to the prepuce. A urethral catheter is placed through the external urethral meatus into the bladder. The abdomen is lavaged with copious amounts of warm physiologic solution and the abdomen is closed routinely.

Both the cystostomy and the urethral catheters are connected to closed drainage systems. The urethral catheter is left in place for 2 to 3 days, and the cystostomy catheter is retained for 1 week. Antibiotic therapy is continued for 1 month. One week later, urine cultures are repeated as described for chronic prostatitis.

The major perioperative problem with prostatectomy for dogs with prostatic abscesses is the prolonged anesthesia and surgical time and the excessive tissue manipulation required compared to the drainage technique. In a septic dog, it may be prudent to perform a castration and prostatic drainage initially, and then consider prostatectomy when the dog is in better condition and the prostatic size has diminished.

The major long-term complication with prostatectomy is urinary incontinence in 85% of dogs. Some dogs with prostatic disease may be incontinent before surgery. Approximately 25% of incontinent dogs have been reported to respond to alpha-adrenergic stimulants (*e.g.,* phenylpropanolamine) and/or detrusor muscle stabilizers (*e.g.,* oxybutynin).

Prostatic Cysts

Prostatic cysts may arise from the prostate gland itself or may be remnants of the Müllerian ducts. The cysts, which may extend into the perineal area, can become very large and may become infected.

Diagnosis

The diagnosis is based on abdominal or rectal palpation of a fluctuant mass and abdominal exploratory and prostatic biopsy.

Treatment

The dog is castrated. After an abdominal incision, the cyst is examined and a sample of cyst fluid is taken for culture and antibiotic sensitivity. If the cyst arises from a stalk, it may be completely excised. Otherwise, the cyst is marsupialized. A circle of skin (0.5 cm in diameter) is removed from the skin lateral to the prepuce. The cyst is sutured to the cut edges of the external rectus fascia with synthetic absorbable suture material. The cyst is incised and drained with suction. The cut edges of the cyst are sutured to the cut edges of the skin with monofilament nonabsorbable suture material.

The marsupialized cyst may drain for several weeks and then close over. If the drainage site closes before the cyst fibroses, the cyst will reform. If the cyst is infected, the stoma may never seal over and the cyst will continue to drain. In either of these instances, it may be necessary to reoperate and excise the cyst or prostate or both.

Prostatic Neoplasia

Prostatic neoplasia is most common in older dogs. Most primary prostatic neoplasms are adenocarcinomas. Other tumors (such as transitional cell carcinoma, rectal and colonic adenocarcinoma, and rectal and colonic squamous-cell carcinoma) can locally invade the prostate. Lymphosarcoma and perianal adenocarcinoma can metastasize to the prostate.

Diagnosis

The presenting signs are not specific for prostatic neoplasia (rear limb lameness, lumbar pain, dysuria, dyschezia, hematuria). Digital rectal examination reveals an enlarged, firm, irregular prostate gland. Radiographic changes also are not specific for prostatic neoplasia. The lumbar spine, pelvis, and lungs should be examined radiographically for metastasis. Examination of the urine sediment, ejaculate, or fluid obtained by prostatic massage occasionally reveals neoplastic cells. The definitive diagnosis is based on histopathologic findings from a biopsy.

Treatment

If diagnosed before metastasis has occurred, surgical excision (prostatectomy) may be curative. Unfortunately, early diagnosis is rare. Palliative therapy may include castration, estrogen therapy, and a cystostomy to divert urine from an obstructed urethra. The results of chemotherapeutic protocols have not been reported.

Testes and Vas Deferens

Sterilization

Castration is the primary method of sterilizing male dogs and cats. Castration may prevent or eliminate roaming, aggression toward other males, and urine marking or spraying in the house. Removing the testes will prevent prostatic hyperplasia and prostatitis. It might lessen the incidence of prostatic adenocarcinoma; however, prostatic neoplasia does occur in castrated dogs. Castration is combined with scrotal ablation when the scrotum is pendulous. Vasectomy (sterilization with maintenance of male hormones) is performed rarely.

Canine Castration

Castration can be performed using a closed or open technique. In the closed technique (Fig. 17-3), the testicular tunics are not incised. A skin incision is made through the median raphe just cranial to the scrotum. The testis is forced into the incision site and held with thumb and index finger. The subcutaneous tissue over the tunics is incised sharply with a scalpel blade. The spermatic fascia and scrotal ligaments are severed or broken with traction, and the tunics are stripped free of fat with a sponge. In a large dog, the spermatic ligament can be clamped and ligated before transection to prevent bleeding from the small vessel within the spermatic ligament. The tunic-enclosed spermatic cord is isolated. Three clamps are placed around the spermatic cord and it is severed between the two distal clamps. The most proximal clamp is removed and a ligature is placed in the groove. The pedicle is grasped with thumb forceps and the last clamp is removed. As tension is relaxed on the pedicle, the pedicle is carefully checked for hemorrhage. The procedure is repeated on the opposite testicle through the same incision.

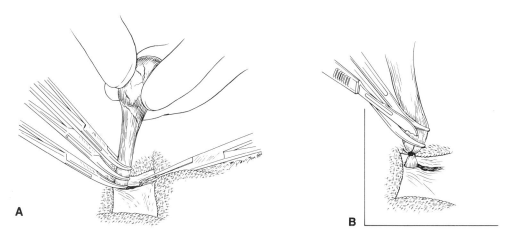

Figure 17-3. Canine Castration. **A,** *Three clamps are placed on the spermatic cord. **B,** The cord is transfixed and ligated in the crushed area of the most proximal clamp. The cord is transected between the most distal clamps. (Crane SW. Canine castration. In: Bojrab MJ, ed. Current techniques in small animal surgery. 3rd ed. Philadelphia: Lea & Febiger, in press)*

The advantages of the closed technique are decreased seroma formation at the incision site and less scrotal swelling. The major complication is postoperative hemorrhage from the pedicle because of improper placement or loosening of the ligature around the tunics and spermatic cord. If the surgeon is concerned about this possibility, the tunics can be carefully incised directly over the area to be ligated. Then the testicular vessels and vas deferens can be individually ligated and transected in the same position.

Postcastration hemorrhage manifests as scrotal swelling or abdominal bleeding or both. If the packed cell volume begins to decline or the dog begins to show signs of hemorrhagic shock, the dog should be anesthetized and prepared for an abdominal incision. The castration site can be initially examined for the bleeding pedicle. Usually the pedicle has retracted into the abdomen and can be found medial to the inguinal ring. The vessels are religated and the abdomen is closed routinely.

Feline Castration (Fig. 17-4)

The hair is plucked or shaved from the scrotum. A dorsoventral incision is made over each testicle. The testicle is partially extruded through the incision within the tunics (closed castration) or the common vaginal tunic is incised (open castration). In a closed castration, the spermatic cord and the tunics are excised together as described previously for the dog. In an open castration, the common vaginal tunic is retracted proximally, the ductus deferens and testicular vessels are ligated or occluded with a hemostatic clip, and transected. The scrotal incision is not sutured.

Cryptorchidism

The reported incidence of cryptorchidism in dogs is approximately 10%; it is occasionally seen in cats. The condition is inheritable by either a single autosomal sex-linked recessive gene or by multiple-gene inheritance. Intraabdominal testicles are more susceptible to spermatic cord torsion and to testicular neoplasia.

Diagnosis

A diagnosis of cryptorchidism is not made until the animal is at least 6 months old. The testicle may be palpable within the inguinal ring or may be completely within the abdomen. Bilaterally cryptorchid animals are usually

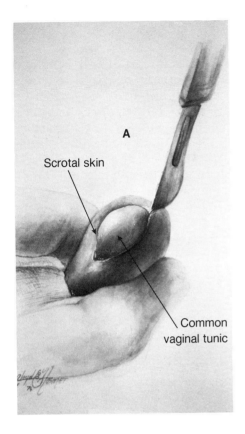

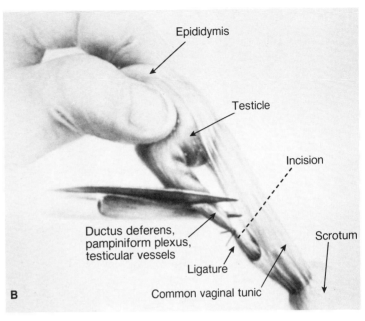

Figure 17-4.   Feline Castration. **A,** *A dorsal ventral incision is made in the scrotum over the testicle.* **B,** *For an open castration, the common vaginal tunic is retracted proximally and the ductus deferens and testicular vessels are ligated or occluded with a hemostatic clip and transected. (Rawlings CA. Feline castration. In: Wingfield WE, Rawlings CA, eds. Small animal surgery. Philadelphia: WB Saunders, 1979;148–150)*

sterile, but have normal secondary sex characteristics.

Acute abdominal pain in a cryptorchid animal should suggest possible torsion of the abdominal testicle. Radiographic examination reveals a soft tissue mass in the caudal abdomen. The diagnosis is confirmed by exploratory laparotomy.

A dog with a neoplastic abdominal testicle may have signs of an abdominal mass or excess estrogen or both.

Treatment

Castration is the only recommended treatment. If the owners elect not to have the cryptorchid testicle(s) removed, the dog should be regularly examined for testicular enlargement.

For castration, the animal should be prepared for prescrotal and abdominal incisions. The procedure for removing an inguinal testicle is the same as for a scrotal testicle. The spermatic cord and epididymis should be identified to distinguish the testicle from an inguinal lymph node. If the normal testicle is removed first in a unilateral cryptorchid, the surgeon can easily determine the side of the retained testicle.

A caudal abdominal incision is made to locate an abdominal testicle. The testicle is found between the inguinal ring and the kidney. The vas deferens can be traced from its insertion into the prostate back to the testicle. If the testicular vessels and the vas deferens exit through the inguinal ring, the testicle is outside the abdominal cavity. It may be necessary to enlarge the inguinal ring to retract the testicle back into the abdomen. After the testicle is located, the testicular vessels are ligated and severed. The vas deferens is ligated and severed. If the inguinal ring has been enlarged, it is partially closed with nonabsorbable sutures through the ventral fascia. Abdominal closure is routine.

Testicular Neoplasia

Testicular tumors are common in older, intact male dogs. The most common tumor types are Sertoli cell tumors, seminomas, and interstitial cell tumors. Metastasis is rare. Testicular tumors occur more often in cryptorchid testicles.

Diagnosis

Enlargement of the testis or a discrete nodule within the testicle may be palpable. A testicular tumor may be an incidental finding during an elective castration.

Dogs with Sertoli cell tumors, and less commonly with seminomas, may present with signs of hyperestrogenism such as bilaterally symmetric alopecia, epidermal hyperpigmentation, gynecomastia, and squamous metaplasia of the prostate. These signs may be caused by relative changes in the quantity of estrogen, conversion of testosterone or its precursors to estrogen, or *de novo* synthesis of estrogen. Bone marrow hypoplasia with pancytopenia may also occur.

Treatment

Bilateral castration is recommended since testicular tumors are frequently bilateral (50% in one report), and the tumor in the opposite testicle may not be clinically visible. As much spermatic cord as possible should be removed.

The Scrotum

The scrotal skin is very sensitive to clipper abrasions and antiseptic soaps. Chlorhexidine soaps are less likely to cause skin reactions than iodine soaps.

Scrotal Injury

Scrotal injuries include abrasions, contusions, and lacerations.

Diagnosis

Diagnosis is based on careful examination of the scrotum. Determining the extent of injury may be impossible until the animal is anesthetized and the area is surgically explored.

Treatment

Superficial abrasions and contusions can be treated with cleansing and topical antiseptic ointments. The dog must be restrained from licking and causing further damage. Lacerations through the scrotal skin are cleansed, lavaged, and sutured with subcuticular sutures (*i.e.*, within the dermis) using 4-0 monofilament absorbable or nonabsorbable suture material on a cutting needle. If the wound extends through the vaginal tunic, the vaginal cavity is lavaged and the vaginal tunic wound edges are debrided and closed with absorbable suture material before the scrotum is sutured.

When the wound is severely contaminated or involves most of the scrotum, or when the testicle is damaged, scrotal ablation and castration are recommended. In a valuable breeding animal, unilateral castration and scrotal closure with drainage can be attempted.

To start the scrotal ablation procedure, an incision is made around the base of the scrotum (Fig. 17-5). The area incised includes all of the scrotal skin. If the incision extends too far laterally from the scrotum, a tension-free closure will be difficult. The scrotum is elevated, and the scrotal ligament and fibrous connective tissue is incised. Care is taken not to dissect dorsally into the urethra or penis. The spermatic cord for each testicle is isolated, clamped, ligated, and severed as in a routine castration. Any remaining tissue holding the scrotum is dissected free, and the scrotum and testicles are removed. The subcutaneous tissue is apposed in a craniocaudal plane. The subcutaneous fascia and skin are closed routinely.

Scrotal Neoplasia

Mast cell tumors are the most common scrotal neoplasm. Other tumors include melanomas, papillomas, fibromas, fibrosarcomas, squamous-cell carcinomas, and adenocarcinomas.

Diagnosis and Treatment

Mast cell tumors may be diagnosed by aspiration cytology. Since most scrotal tumors are

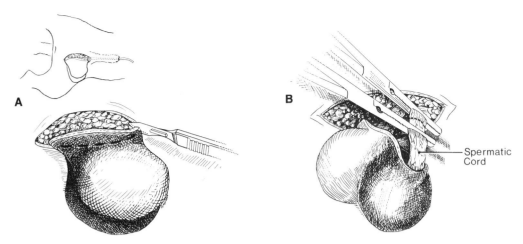

Figure 17-5.   Scrotal Ablation. ***A,*** *An incision is made around the base of the scrotum. The area incised should include all the scrotal skin, but does not extend laterally so that there is enough skin for a tension-free closure.* ***B,*** *The spermatic cord for each testicle is isolated, clamped, ligated, and severed. Any remaining tissue holding the scrotum is dissected free and the scrotum and testicles are removed. The subcutaneous tissue and skin are closed in a cranial-caudal direction. (Stone EA. Surgical management of urolithiasis. Compend Contin Ed 1981;3:627)*

malignant, scrotal ablation and castration usually is recommended.

The Penis and Prepuce

Persistent Penile Frenulum

The frenulum is located on the ventral surface of the penis and attaches the penis to the prepuce. In most dogs, it separates or ruptures on its own.

Diagnosis

If the frenulum persists, it may cause pain during sexual arousal or when the penis is extruded. The penis will bend ventrally when it is extruded.

Treatment

The frenulum is transected; no sutures are required.

Phimosis

Phimosis is the inability to extrude the penis through a small preputial opening.

Diagnosis

Retention of urine within the prepuce can cause balanoposthitis, ulceration, and necrosis.

Treatment

If the necrotic tissue sloughs, the preputial orifice is usually sufficiently enlarged. Surgical enlargement of the orifice can be performed to prevent ulceration and necrosis (Fig. 17-6). A longitudinal incision is made in the dorsal prepuce. If necessary for a larger opening, a wedge-shaped piece of prepuce is excised. The mucosal edges are sutured to the skin edges on each side of the incision to form a triangular opening.

Paraphimosis

Paraphimosis is the inability to retract a protruded penis into the prepuce after an erection.

Diagnosis

The exposed penis may become desiccated and traumatized. As the paraphimosis persists, the

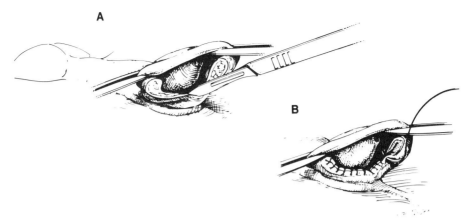

Figure 17-6. Enlargement of Preputial Opening. *A, A longitudinal incision is made in the dorsal prepuce. B, The mucosal edges are sutured to the skin edges on each side of the incision. (Rawlings CA. Correction of congenital defects of the urogenital system. Vet Clin North Am [Small Anim Pract] 1984;14:52)*

penis swells from tissue edema and venous stasis and can become strangulated.

Treatment

Preputial hairs are removed from around the penis. After the penis is cleansed and lubricated, an attempt is made to replace it in the prepuce. If it is replaced, a loose purse-string suture is placed in the prepuce orifice. If replacement is impossible, a longitudinal incision is made dorsally at the preputial orifice. After replacement, the incision can be closed as described for phimosis to enlarge the preputial opening. Severe necrosis of the penis or damage to the penile urethra or both requires amputation.

Fractured Os Penis

Diagnosis

The presenting signs are related to the severity of damage to the preputial tissue and urethra. The preputial area may be bruised and swollen; blood may drip from the penis. Urinary obstruction from soft tissue swelling or urethral damage may present as stranguria and, if the obstruction is complete, anuria; eventually, signs of uremia (anorexia, vomiting, dehydration) develop. Radiographs reveal the fractured os penis.

Treatment

If there is no apparent urinary obstruction, the dog is monitored for development of stranguria or anuria as the fracture heals. If there is urethral obstruction, a prescrotal urethrotomy is performed and is allowed to heal by second intention. Alternately, an attempt can be made to pass a urethral catheter. If successful, the catheter can be left in place and connected to a closed urine collection system for 7 days while the soft tissue swelling resolves. An unstable fracture can be exposed, reduced, and immobilized with a fingerplate. Persistent urethral obstruction requires a permanent prescrotal or scrotal urethrostomy (see Fig. 16-12 in Chap. 16, The Urinary System).

Penile and Preputial Neoplasia

Primary penile tumors are rare. Transmissible venereal tumors can occur on the penis. The preputial skin can develop the same tumors as the skin elsewhere on the body.

Diagnosis

The dog may be presented for excessive licking at the prepuce. A bloody discharge may be seen. If the tumor is not visible, retraction of the prepuce allows examination of the entire penis including the glans penis. Definitive

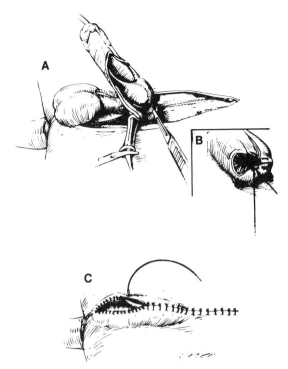

Figure 17-7. Penile amputation and preputial abla-tion. **A,** *After an elliptical skin incision is made around the prepuce and scrotum, the distal penis and prepuce are dissected from the body wall and the dorsal vessels of the penis and the superficial veins of the glands are ligated. A tourniquet is placed caudal to the bulbus glandis and the penis is severed.* **B,** *The tunica albuginea is sutured over the severed end of the penis.* **C,** *The scrotal urethrostomy is completed and the cranial extent of the incision is closed over the stump of the penis. (Hardie EM. Selected surgeries of the male and female reproductive tracts. Vet Clin North Am [Small Anim Pract] 1984;14:115)*

diagnosis is based on microscopic examination of cytologic and histopathologic samples.

Treatment

If a transmissible venereal tumor is small, it can be excised completely. Larger or recurrent transmissible venereal tumors should be treated with chemotherapy or radiation therapy.

Excising extensive tumors of the penis and prepuce requires complete amputation of the penis with scrotal urethrostomy (Fig. 17-7). An elliptical incision is made around the prepuce and extended around the scrotum. The dorsal vessels of the penis and the superficial veins of the glands are located and ligated. The cranial penis and prepuce are dissected from the body wall to the level of the bulbus glandis. A penile tourniquet is placed caudal to the bulbus glandis and the os penis. The penis is amputated just cranial to the tourniquet and the penis and prepuce are removed.

The tunica albuginea is sutured over the severed end of the penis. The tourniquet is removed and any bleeding is controlled with mattress sutures placed through the tunica albuginea into the cavernous tissue. The dog is castrated, and a scrotal urethrotomy is performed as previously described. The cranial extent of the incision used to excise the prepuce is closed in a routine manner over the remaining penis.

Suggested Readings

Barsanti JA, Finco DR. Treatment of bacterial pros-tatitis. In: Kirk RW, ed. Current veterinary ther-apy VIII. Philadelphia: WB Saunders, 1983; 1101.

Brodey RS, Roszel JF. Neoplasms of the canine uterus, vagina and vulva: A clinicopathologic survey of 90 cases. J Am Vet Med Assoc 1967;151:1294.

DeSchepper J, Van Der Stock J, Capiau E. Anaemia and leukocytosis in one hundred and twelve dogs with pyometra. J Sm Anim Pract 1987;28:137.

Hargiss AM, Miller LM. Prostatic carcinoma in dogs. Compend Cont Ed 1983;5:647.

Hardie EM, Barsanti JA, Rawlings CA. Complica-tions of prostatic surgery. J Am Anim Hosp Assoc 1984;20:50.

Lipowitz AJ, Schwartz A, Wilson GP, et al. Testicu-lar neoplasms and concomitant clinical changes in the dog. J Am Vet Med Assoc 1973;163:1364.

Reif JS, Maguire TG, Kenney RM, et al. A cohort study of canine testicular neoplasia. J Am Vet Med Assoc 1979;175:719.

Schneider R, Dorn CR, Taylor DON. Factors in-fluencing canine mammary cancer development and postsurgical survival. J Natl Cancer Inst 1969;43:1249.

18

J. E. Oliver, Jr.
Marc R. Raffe

The Nervous System

The Brain and Cranial Nerves

J. E. Oliver, Jr.

The central nervous system (CNS) is the most complex system of the body. The nerves emanating from it influence all physiologic processes and modify an animal's response to its environment. CNS abnormalities produce a variety of clinical signs; to interpret them, the veterinarian must be familiar with neuroanatomy and neurophysiology and must have a variety of diagnostic aids.

Axons of CNS tissue can regenerate, but seldom do because of the interference of fibrous tissue. Mature neurons do not replicate.

Brain surgery is uncommon in veterinary medicine. Intracranial tumors may be removed, and focal inflammatory lesions, including migrating parasites, may be resectable. Prefrontal lobotomy and olfactory tractotomy have been used to change behavior. Ventriculoatrial and ventriculoperitoneal shunts are used to treat hydrocephalus. Brain biopsies are useful adjuncts to diagnosis of generalized brain disease. Decompression of hematomas or fractures following head trauma is the most common indication for intracranial surgery and can be performed by most surgeons.

Surgical Anatomy

Cerebral Cortex

The cerebral cortex may be divided into four regions: frontal, parietal, occipital, and temporal. Functional areas do not exactly coincide

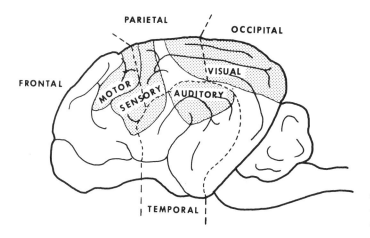

Figure 18-1. *Functional and anatomical areas of the cerebral cortex of the dog. (Archibald J, ed. Canine surgery. 2nd ed. Santa Barbara: American Veterinary Pub, 1974:843.)*

with these divisions (Fig. 18-1). The surgeon should be able to recognize landmarks, the gyri and sulci, so that major functional areas can be avoided when excising lesions or incising the cortex. The suprasylvian gyrus, for example, is a relatively "silent" area through which the cortex can be incised to explore the lateral ventricles.

Basal Nuclei

Deep to the cortex and ventral and lateral to the lateral ventricles are the large masses of basal nuclei. The caudate nucleus, putamen, and globus pallidus usually are included in the basal nuclei, which make up a significant part of the extrapyramidal system. The amygdala is sometimes included. These structures are rarely involved in surgical procedures, but portions of them may be exposed through the lateral ventricles.

Thalamus and Hypothalamus (Diencephalon)

The diencephalon is the most rostral part of the brain stem (Fig. 18-2). The pituitary gland is attached to the ventral surface of the hypothalamus. Extirpation of the pituitary gland may be accomplished from a lateral or ventral approach.

Midbrain (Mesencephalon)

The third and fourth cranial nerves originate in the midbrain, and the mesencephalic aqueduct traverses its length. The midbrain is especially vulnerable to compression lesions because of its position beneath the tentorium cerebelli separating the rostral and caudal compartments of the cranium. Transtentorial herniation of cerebrum caused by masses or brain swelling compresses the midbrain.

Pons

The pons is a major relay center for cortico-cerebellar pathways and is the origin of the

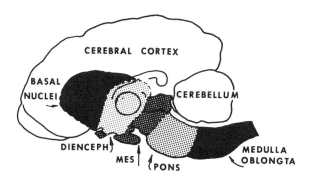

Figure 18-2. *The major divisions of the canine brain. Dienceph = diencephalon, Mes = Mesencephalon. (Archibald J, ed. Canine surgery. 2nd ed. Santa Barbara: American Veterinary Pub, 1974:844.)*

fifth cranial nerve. The blood supply to the tegmentum of the pons and midbrain is often damaged in accidents that produce brain hemorrhage.

Cerebellum

The cerebellum occupies most of the space in the caudal part of the calvarium. It is characterized by a median, prominent vermis and two small hemispheres. The flocculonodular lobe, which is intimately associated with vestibular function, is on the ventral aspect of the cerebellum. The caudal parts of the vermis are most easily reached surgically. Solid lesions that cause a shift of the brain may cause herniation of the caudal parts of the vermis into the foramen magnum (transforaminal herniation) and compress the medulla oblongata.

Medulla Oblongata

This is the most caudal part of the brain stem; it is continuous with the spinal cord. Numerous important areas, including the cardiovascular and respiratory centers and the nuclei of the fifth through twelfth cranial nerves are located in this area. Injury to the medulla causes alterations in cardiac and respiratory function; apnea is the most serious problem.

Ventricular System

The ventricles of the brain include two lateral ventricles in the cerebrum and a small, median third ventricle that communicates with the fourth ventricle by the mesencephalic aqueduct. The roof of the lateral ventricles is the cerebral cortex and its white matter; the floor includes the caudate nucleus and hippocampus. The third ventricle surrounds the interthalamic adhesion. The fourth ventricle is ventral to the cerebellum and dorsal to the pons and medulla oblongata. Two lateral apertures allow cerebrospinal fluid (CSF) to enter the subarachnoid space from the fourth ventricle.

Meninges

The fibrous membranes surrounding the CNS consist of the dura mater, arachnoid mater, and pia mater. Intracranially, the dura mater fuses with the endosteum that lines the cranial cavity. In the vertebral canal, there is a fat-filled epidural space between the dura and the endosteum.

Three formations of the dura mater are significant to the surgeon. The falx cerebri, which contains the dorsal sagittal sinus in its base, is a median fold extending between the cerebral hemispheres. Masses in one cerebral hemisphere may cause herniation under the falx cerebri (transfalcical herniation).

The membranous tentorium cerebelli is a transverse fold of dura mater arising from the osseous tentorium and extending rostroventrally between the cerebrum and cerebellum. Ventrolaterally, the membranous tentorium attaches to the petrous temporal bone, and its free border surrounds the midbrain. Masses in the cerebrum can cause portions of it to herniate under the tentorium cerebelli, compressing the midbrain (transtentorial herniation).

The diaphragma sellae is a fold of dura mater surrounding the stalk of the pituitary gland. Extirpating the pituitary gland from a dorsal approach may require incision of the diaphragma sellae.

The arachnoid is a delicate membrane lying against the internal surface of the dura; it is loosely connected to the pia mater by fine trabeculae. In the normal animal, there is only a potential subdural space between the dura mater and arachnoid. The CSF occupies the subarachnoid space between the arachnoid and pia mater. The pia mater adheres closely to the brain and extends deeply into the sulci.

Skull

The cranial cavity is formed by the frontal, parietal, occipital, temporal, sphenoid, and ethmoid bones. The surgeon must be able to recognize the different shapes of these bones in the extreme brachycephalic and dolichocephalic dogs as well as the range in size from the Chihuahua to the Saint Bernard.

The nuchal and sagittal crests, the temporal line, and the zygomatic process of the frontal bone are readily palpable in most dogs. These structures and the zygomatic arch form the boundaries of the temporal fossa, the usual site for craniotomy. To approach the frontal lobe of the brain, the frontal sinus must be opened in most dogs. Palpable fractures are most easily detected where they cross one of these prominences.

Suture lines between the bones of the calvaria may be separated if intracranial pressure was above normal before closure.

Muscles

Surgical exposure of the calvaria requires reflection of the auricular muscles from the midline. They should be resutured in their exact positions for normal functioning of the external ear.

The temporalis muscle occupies the temporal fossa. In smaller dogs, this muscle can be split for the placement of bur holes, but in larger dogs it is best to reflect the muscle subperiosteally from the fossa.

Arteries

Extracranial

The paired vertebral and internal carotid arteries provide the major blood supply to the brain. Of these four vessels, three may usually be ligated without causing significant neurologic deficit.

Lateral craniotomy exposes two important arteries. The caudal deep temporal artery may be encountered near the junction of the nuchal crest and the zygomatic process of the temporal bone. Incising the origin of the temporalis muscle along the nuchal crest too far ventrally may sever this vessel. The palpebral branches of the superficial temporal artery may be cut when the temporalis muscle is reflected along its attachment to the zygomatic

process of the frontal bone and orbital ligament. Both areas have an adequate collateral circulation.

Intracranial

The two vertebral arteries and ventral spinal artery unite to form the basilar artery. This vessel passes forward on the ventral surface of the brain stem to contribute to the arterial circle of the brain. The internal carotid arteries enter the skull and contribute caudal communicating and rostral cerebral arteries to complete the arterial circle (Fig. 18-3).

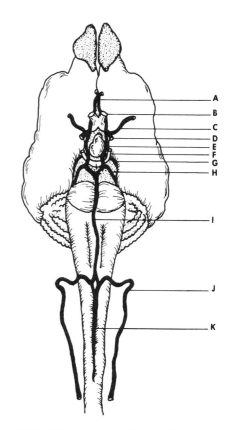

Figure 18-3. *The major arteries on the ventral surface of the canine brain: rostral cerebral—A; optic nerve—B; middle cerebral—C; internal carotid—D; caudal communicating—E; oculomotor nerve—F; caudal cerebral —G; rostral cerebellar—H; basilar—I; vertebral—J; ventral spinal—K. (Archibald J, ed. Canine surgery. 2nd ed. Santa Barbara: American Veterinary Pub, 1974:846.)*

The rostral, middle, and caudal cerebral arteries make up the major blood supply to the cerebrum. Occlusion of the rostral and caudal arteries does not cause any abnormality. Occlusion of the middle cerebral artery results in infarction of a large portion of the cerebral hemisphere.

Veins

Extracranial

The external jugular vein provides the main venous drainage from the head, and the maxillary vein furnishes the most direct drainage from the cranium to the external jugular. The angular vein of the eye, a branch of the facial vein, provides a direct route into the cavernous sinus (Fig. 18-4). This is a useful pathway for contrast media, and it also enables intracranial extension of infection.

Intracranial

Within the cranium, large venous sinuses constitute the major venous pathways. The dorsal sagittal sinus in the attached edge of the falx cerebri is of major importance because occluding it caudal to the point of entry of the dorsal cerebral veins causes severe cerebral congestion, edema, and usually severe neurologic impairment or death. The surgical approaches are designed to avoid the major venous sinuses.

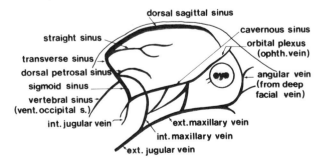

Figure 18-4. *Major venous channels of the dog's cranium. (Archibald J, ed. Canine surgery. 2nd ed. Santa Barbara: American Veterinary Pub, 1974:847.)*

The cavernous sinus on the floor of the skull may be involved in fractures of the base. The internal carotid artery has a short course within the cavernous sinus.

Physiology

The following selective discussion of physiology attempts to emphasize important concepts for the surgeon.

Metabolism

Neural tissue has a high metabolic rate; the brain uses 20% to 30% of the oxygen carried by the blood. Respiratory quotients indicate that glucose is the principal source of metabolic energy for the brain. Decreased levels of glucose or oxygen quickly result in abnormal brain function. Hypoxia or hypercarbia significantly increase the chance of cerebral edema. Hyperventilation of the surgical patient is recommended to reduce the likelihood of edema.

Brain Barrier Systems

The blood-brain barrier prevents some materials from passing from the circulating blood into neural tissues. Other tissues have similar, though less important, barriers. The barriers become important clinically when they break down or when systemic drugs are administered. Antibacterial agents that achieve high concentrations in the CNS include chloramphenicol, sulfonamides, and trimethoprim. Agents that achieve adequate levels when inflammation is present (*e.g.*, meningitis) include penicillin (and its synthetic analogues) and tetracyclines. Agents that do not achieve adequate concentrations include cephalosporins and aminoglycosides.

Cerebrospinal Fluid (CSF)

This fluid is produced by choroid plexuses in the brain's ventricles and by other vascular beds in the pia mater, brain, and spinal cord.

Although absorption occurs throughout the ventricular system, maximum absorption of proteins occurs in the subarachnoid space over the convexity of the cerebrum. Obstruction to the flow of CSF (lateral ventricle—third ventricle—mesencephalic aqueduct—fourth ventricle—subarachnoid space), results in increased pressure, enlarged ventricles, and hydrocephalus.

The metabolic functions of CSF in relation to brain tissue include excretion, nutrition, transport, and control of environment. The brain and spinal cord are suspended by the arachnoid trabeculae and are cushioned by the CSF that fills the subarachnoid space. Analyzing CSF protein and cells is a useful diagnostic tool.

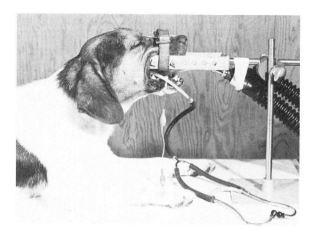

Figure 18-5. *A head holder for neurosurgery or radiography. It permits unrestricted exposure of the cranium, good venous drainage, and open air passages, and the anesthetist has access to the oral cavity. (Archibald J, ed. Canine surgery. 2nd ed. Santa Barbara: American Veterinary Pub, 1974:853.)*

Surgical Technique

Principles of Neurosurgery

Positioning the Patient

The animal should be securely positioned with its head immobilized for ease of observation by the anesthetist, for maintenance of patent air passages, for the comfort of the patient and surgeons, for adequate venous drainage without loss of CSF, and for drainage of the field (Fig. 18-5).

Anesthesia

Adequate anesthesia for neurosurgery requires provision for clear air passages, adequate ventilation with minimal expiratory resistance, and a rapid return of consciousness at the end of the operation. Only atropine should be used as a preanesthetic. Phenothiazine tranquilizers should not be used in animals with brain disease because they reduce the threshold for seizures. To avoid struggling, minimal doses of an ultrashort-acting barbiturate should be used for induction of anesthesia. Depressed animals may be induced with an inhalation agent, preferably halothane or halothane combined with nitrous oxide. Uncon-

scious animals must be intubated and maintained on controlled respiration. The anesthetist must be alert for any evidence of return of consciousness. Even a comatose animal must often have some anesthesia to abolish reflex responses that interfere with surgical procedures.

All neurosurgical patients should be intubated and provided with at least 50% oxygen. It is important to prevent coughing during endotracheal intubation because elevated intrathoracic pressures lead to cerebral venous stasis and further brain swelling. Topical analgesia of the larynx and, possibly, the use of muscle relaxants are indicated.

An inhalation agent should be used to maintain anesthesia. Halothane is preferred, although barbiturates have the advantage of reducing intracranial pressure.

Several techniques have been used to alleviate cerebral edema, including controlled hypotension, hypothermia, and hyperventilation. Hyperventilation is the only one that can be safely used without sophisticated monitoring equipment, and it should be applied on all neurosurgical patients. Lowering the arterial carbon dioxide tension lessens blood flow to the brain, reduces brain bulk, and helps prevent cerebral edema. Elevating the head encourages venous drainage during surgery, but there is some risk of air embolism and the heart should be monitored by auscultation throughout surgery. Corticosteroids in antiedema doses (30 mg/kg of prednisolone sodium succinate or 2 to 4 mg/kg of dexamethasone) should be given preoperatively to help prevent edema. An intravenous mannitol drip should be started at the onset of surgery if it is likely that edema is already present (*e.g.*, brain tumor, trauma).

Hemostasis

Controlling hemorrhage within the cranial cavity is imperative. If hemorrhage continues postoperatively, the escaping blood forms an expanding mass.

Hemostatic forceps and ligatures are of little value in neurosurgery. Hemorrhage usually is controlled with crushed muscle, electrocoagulation, absorbable gelatin sponge, cotton flannel pads, bone wax, arterial clips, and suction. Bleeding from the diploe can be stopped by rubbing bone wax into the cut edge.

Craniotomy and Craniectomy

The bone flap should be replaced in the rostrotentorial approach for craniotomy. The calvarial defect that remains following craniectomy may not cause serious problems if the temporal muscle mass is large, but some cerebral compression results.

The bone flap should not be replaced if the dura is not closed or if there is brain swelling. A bone flap cannot be preserved in the ventral or caudotentorial approaches.

Because the dura mater protects the brain from infection and trauma, it should always be sutured or replaced with a fascial graft. The temporal fascia is convenient and makes an acceptable graft. Although the dura mater cannot be closed if significant cerebral edema is present, a large graft can be used.

If the dura mater is to be closed, it must be stretched and kept moist throughout the surgical procedure. It is reflected as a rectangular flap with 5-0 stay sutures in each free corner, and the flap is compressed between strips of moist cotton flannel. Irrigation with physiologic saline solution will keep the flap, the brain, and surrounding structures moist.

Complications Encountered in Neurosurgery
Incisions

Skin incisions should be designed to provide optimal exposure. Midline incisions for a lateral craniotomy give a better cosmetic effect, but restrict the exposure.

Hemorrhage

Postoperative bleeding can be fatal. If the blood pressure drops low enough during surgery, hemorrhage from smaller vessels may be arrested, only to recur when the pressure returns to normal. Arterial spasm during manipulation may have the same effect. The surgeon must be alert to signs of increasing intracranial pressure. Blood in the subarachnoid space may produce a mild meningeal reaction.

Wound Problems

Subcutaneous hematomas and seromas are common problems following brain surgery. To prevent them, the subcutaneous tissues should be effectively united and a bandage applied.

Infection may be introduced if the frontal sinus is invaded during craniotomy, or when the pituitary gland is approached perorally. When the surgeon knows that contaminated areas will be encountered, antibiotics should be given pre- and postoperatively.

Hyperthermia

Serious elevations in temperature usually are associated with hypothalamic disturbances. Cranial trauma or pituitary gland surgery may also precipitate hyperthermia. Heat loss usually is impaired as a result of circulatory deficiencies. Ice-water enemas, corticosteroids, and fluids are beneficial.

Surgical Approaches to the Brain

The approaches to the brain are lateral (rostrotentorial), bilateral (rostrotentorial), suboccipital (caudotentorial), and ventral. Because the principles of operative technique are the same for all approaches, the lateral approach will be described in detail. Only modifications of this procedure are described for the other approaches. In the procedures to be described, hand instruments may be used, although air-powered drills and craniotomes are preferred.

Lateral (Rostrotentorial) Craniotomy

The lateral approach is through the temporal fossa, providing exposure of the cerebral hemisphere, pituitary gland, lateral ventricle, and rostral parts of the cerebellum. Bur holes to detect hemorrhage are made through this approach.

A large, curved (horseshoe) skin incision is made from caudal to the lateral palpebral commissure to the dorsal midline extended caudally to curve ventrally behind the ear. The auricular muscles are reflected from the midline. The temporal muscle is incised near its attachment, leaving enough fascia and tendon to allow closure. The temporal muscle is elevated from the skull subperiosteally and reflected laterally and ventrally. Four bur holes are placed at the corners of the bone to outline a flap and the flap is cut with a small bur in an air drill, or (preferably) one bur hole is made and the entire flap is cut with a craniotome. The craniotome's guard separates the dura from the skull. The flap can be cut in less time and with less trauma to the brain by this method. The cut should be angled to produce a beveled edge so that the flap will seat firmly

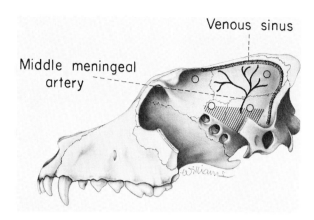

Figure 18-6. *Bur holes are joined by grooving and carefully penetrating the bone with a small pointed bur or a craniotome. The ventral side of the flap is broken to avoid the risk of cutting the middle meningeal artery. The craniotomy can be enlarged ventrally with rongeurs (hatched). (Oliver JE. Craniotomy, craniectomy and skull fractures. In: Bojrab MJ, ed. Current techniques in small animal surgery. Philadelphia: Lea & Febiger, 1975:361.)*

when replaced. Three sides of the flap are cut and the ventral side is broken by reflecting it (Fig. 18-6). If additional exposure or decompression is needed, rongeurs are used to enlarge the opening ventrally. Hemorrhage from the diploe is controlled with bone wax.

An arterial clip is placed on the middle meningeal artery. The dura mater is lifted away from the brain with a hook and incised on three sides to form a flap, which is reflected ventrally. A 5-0 suture is placed in each corner of the flap, which is kept stretched between two pieces of moist cotton flannel.

If the dog has been hyperventilated, gentle retraction of the brain and aspiration of CSF will decrease brain bulk. Retracting the brain with a spatula exposes the ventral median plane, including the pituitary gland; the first, second, and third cranial nerves; and the tentorium cerebelli. By incising through the suprasylvian gyrus with an electrosurgical instrument and a spatula, the lateral ventricle is exposed.

The brain must be kept moist by frequent irrigation with physiologic saline solution. All

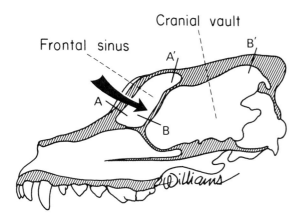

Figure 18-7. *In transfrontal craniotomy (lateral view), access to the frontal lobe of the brain is made through the frontal sinus. An initial bone flap is made over the frontal sinus (A to A'). The craniotomy flap is made between B and B'. (Oliver JE. Craniotomy, craniectomy and skull fractures. In: Bojrab MJ, ed. Current techniques in small animal surgery. Philadelphia: Lea & Febiger, 1975:361.)*

bleeding should be controlled and clotted blood flushed from the cavity before closure.

The dura mater is closed with interrupted 5-0 nonabsorbable sutures; a fascial graft should be used if necessary. Small holes are drilled in the skull and bone flap to wire the latter in place. The temporal and auricular muscles are then sutured to their attachments, and the fascia and skin are closed.

To expose the frontal lobe of the cortex, the frontal sinus must be opened in most dogs. A two-stage flap is necessary, as illustrated in Figures 18-7 and 18-8. The flap over the frontal sinus is removed first, the sinus is irrigated with antibacterial solution, and the second flap is made.

Depressed fragments of skull fractures must be elevated cautiously to avoid further damage to the brain. Bur holes may be placed adjacent to the fracture and a small elevator inserted beneath the fragments to lift them from below. Direct traction on a fracture fragment may result in a seesawing action, with laceration of the underlying brain (Fig. 18-9).

Bilateral (Rostrotentorial) Craniotomy

The bilateral approach should be used only to explore the dorsal median structures. If both cerebral hemispheres must be inspected, two separate lateral approaches are preferred. The difficulties and dangers involved in elevating the bone flap from the dorsal sagittal sinus limits the usefulness of this approach.

An H-shaped skin incision, with the cross bar on the midline, is preferred. After the muscles are reflected bilaterally, four bur holes are drilled, as in the lateral approach, with the dorsal pair made 0.5 cm from the midline. Another pair of dorsal holes is made

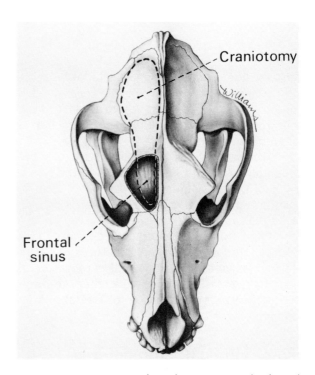

Figure 18-8. *In a transfrontal craniotomy, the frontal sinus bone flap is removed first. The large flap is then made, including the area inside the frontal sinus. Notice the increased area of the flap rostrally, as compared with that in Fig. 18-6. (Oliver JE. Craniotomy, craniectomy and skull fractures. In: Bojrab MJ, ed. Current techniques in small animal surgery. Philadelphia: Lea & Febiger, 1975:361.)*

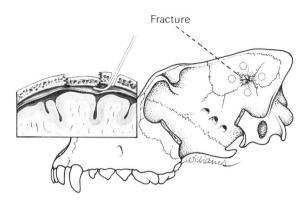

Fracture

Figure 18-9. *Placement of bur holes adjacent to fracture fragments and elevation of fragments. (Oliver JE. Craniotomy, craniectomy and skull fractures. In: Bojrab MJ, ed. Current techniques in small animal surgery. Philadelphia: Lea & Febiger, 1975:362.)*

on the other side near the midline. Cuts are made to connect the rostral and caudal pairs on one side and the rostral to caudal holes on the other side. The narrow bridge crossing the midline of bone between the two dorsal holes is cut rostrally and caudally. The large flap is then broken ventrally.

Emissary veins between the dorsal sagittal sinus and skull will bleed when the flap is elevated. The hemorrhage can be controlled by applying gelatin sponge and compressing it with cotton flannel.

The dura mater is reflected dorsally to the midline. If deeper midline structures are to be inspected, one or more dorsal cerebral veins may have to be severed as they enter the sinus.

Closure is the same as for the lateral approach.

Suboccipital (Caudotentorial) Craniectomy

The suboccipital approach is used to expose the part of the cranial cavity caudal to the tentorium cerebelli. The exposure is limited by the transverse sinuses to the central portions of the caudal aspect of the cerebellum. The rostral portions of the cerebellum must be ex-

posed through the tentorium by the lateral approach.

A dorsal midline or cross-bow skin incision is made. The dorsal cervical muscles are severed near their attachments to the nuchal crest and are reflected from the occipital bone to the foramen magnum. A self-retaining retractor is inserted for maximum exposure of the occipital bone and dorsal arch of the atlas. A bur hole is made just lateral to the median plane and the craniectomy is completed with rongeurs. Because of the extreme irregularity of the occipital bone, a bone flap is not made. The dura mater should be preserved, but this may be difficult in older dogs as it often is impossible to separate the dura from the bone.

A dural graft may be used or the muscles may be sutured directly over the cerebellum.

Ventral Craniectomy

The approach to the ventral surface of the brain is limited to a strip approximately 1 to 1.5 cm wide; consequently, the approach has limited application. The pituitary gland can be approached through the mouth or through the ventral midline. Large tumors of the pituitary gland cannot be removed through this approach, but microadenomas have been successfully removed. The approach through the mouth has been most frequently reported, but the approach through the neck offers the advantage of asepsis. The basilar artery, some of the cranial nerves, and the ventral surface of the pons and medulla can also be exposed through the ventral neck approach. A surgical microscope and air drill greatly assist this procedure.

The dog is placed on its back with the head extended and an endotracheal tube in place. The ventral midline skin incision extends from the intermandibular space to the level of the third cervical vertebra. By blunt dissection, the trachea, sternohyoideus, and sternothyroideus muscles are separated laterally; this dissection is continued between the carotid sheaths. The basioccipital bone is exposed by subperiosteal reflection of the longus capitis and rectus capitis ventralis muscles. An air drill is used for the craniectomy. The hamulus of the pterygoid bone serves as a convenient landmark. The opening is made just caudal to the intersphenoid suture. Frequent applications of bone wax are necessary to control diploic hemorrhage. The cavernous sinus forms a circle around the pituitary gland, with the rostral portion being incomplete. Careful removal of the bone will reveal the margins of the sinus so it can be avoided. The pituitary gland can be teased from the cavity with gentle dissection and moderate suction. Because vital parts of the brain and its blood supply may be injured, this procedure must be performed carefully.

Neurologic Diagnosis

The diagnosis of brain disease requires a history, physical examination, neurologic examination, and one or more special diagnostic tests. Accurate localization of the lesion is imperative if intracranial surgery is to be successful. The newer techniques of computerized axial tomography (CAT) and magnetic resonance imaging (MRI) provide more precise information on structural lesions of the brain than was possible previously. Details of neurologic diagnosis are covered in detail in several textbooks (see the "Suggested Readings" list at the end of this chapter).

Surgical Diseases of the Brain

Hydrocephalus

Hydrocephalus can be either congenital or acquired, but the most common form in the dog is congenital. Hydrocephalus is the accumulation of CSF within the skull, usually within the ventricular system. Communicating hydrocephalus is caused by decreased absorption of CSF in the subarachnoid space, usually secondary to inflammation and fibrosis of the me-

ninges and vessels, including the arachnoid granulations. Noncommunicating or obstructive hydrocephalus is caused by a blockage of the normal pathway of CSF flow. The most common site of obstruction is the mesencephalic aqueduct between the third and fourth ventricles. The obstruction causes an enlargement of the lateral and third ventricles. Rarely, hydrocephalus is caused by increased CSF production.

Congenital hydrocephalus is seen most commonly in toy and brachycephalic breeds.

Clinical signs are related to age of onset, degree of imbalance between production and absorption of CSF, and location of the defect. Details are available in the "Suggested Readings" listed at the end of this chapter.

The diagnosis can be confirmed by electroencephalogram (EEG) or ventricular puncture. Skull radiographs reveal thinning of the calvaria and open suture lines. A ventricular puncture may be performed in congenital hydrocephalus by inserting the needle through the open fontanelle at its lateral margin to avoid the dorsal sagittal sinus. An estimate of the thickness of the cortex is easily obtained in this manner. If there is doubt about the size of the ventricles, 1 to 3 ml of air is injected after fluid has been allowed to escape to atmospheric pressure. Lateral and frontal radiographs using a horizontal beam confirm the size of the ventricles. Positive-contrast ventriculography may be necessary to ascertain the site of obstruction.

Many cases of congenital hydrocephalus can be managed medically. The grossly malformed animal with severe brain destruction will not be normal. Acute progressive signs indicate a poor prognosis and the need for vigorous treatment.

Surgical treatment is reserved for cases unresponsive to medical treatment. Surgical treatment consists of a shunt from the lateral ventricle through a one-way valve to the right atrium or peritoneal cavity (Fig. 18-10). Complications include the need to replace the distal tubing as the animal grows, occlusion of the tubes by clots or fibrosis, and sepsis. Although

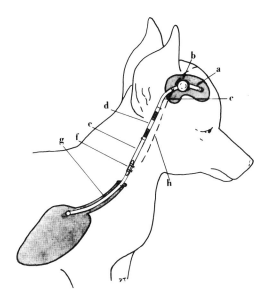

Figure 18-10. *Ventriculoatrial shunt system in a dog: ventricular catheter—a; reservoir—b; connecting tube —c; one-way valve—d; connecting tube—e; connector —f; atrial catheter—g; location of skin incision—h. (Archibald J, ed. Canine surgery. 2nd ed. Santa Barbara: American Veterinary Pub, 1974:860.)*

such shunts have functioned well in some dogs for years, the procedure is rarely performed.

Cerebral Edema

Cerebral edema is a major factor in the management of intracranial disease. Principally intracellular in the gray matter and extracellular in the white matter, it may result from trauma, inflammation, venous stasis, hypoxia, or intoxication.

The result of cerebral edema is increased volume within a closed compartment. After displacing the CSF (approximately 7 ml), the expanding brain tends to herniate through larger openings in the cranial cavity. If the swelling is confined to one cerebral hemisphere, the herniation may be under the falx cerebri (transfalcical) or tentorium cerebelli (transtentorial). Bilateral cerebral swelling usually results in transtentorial herniation. Massive cerebral edema or masses in the cau-

dal compartment will cause herniation of the cerebellum into the foramen magnum (transforaminal) with compression of the medulla.

The earliest sign of transtentorial herniation may be an ipsilateral dilated pupil. As the swelling continues to compress the third nerve and midbrain, lateral strabismus and signs of decerebrate rigidity will result. Decompression must be performed rapidly if the patient's life and CNS function are to be preserved.

Every effort should be made to prevent brain swelling. Adequate ventilation and unobstructed venous drainage are essential. The preoperative administration of corticosteroids may prevent edema during surgical exploration. Hyperventilation during anesthesia reduces brain bulk. Hypertonic solutions such as mannitol are indicated if swelling is already present and may be helpful when administered preoperatively. Mannitol is the safest of the osmotic diuretics, but it should not be administered to an animal in hypovolemic shock. It is given slowly at 1 to 2 gm/kg IV in a 10% to 20% solution. The dose is given at one hour intervals for a maximum of four doses. Corticosteroids (30 mg/kg prednisolone sodium succinate or 2 to 4 mg/kg dexamethasone) started at the same time will ideally be exerting their maximal effect by the fourth dose of mannitol. Continued administration of mannitol is not recommended because the gradient across the blood-brain barrier is reduced and fluid and electrolyte balance is difficult to maintain.

Intracranial Masses

Space-occupying masses in the cranium produce signs that are dependent on their location and rate of growth rather than their nature. Identifying their locations is based on a neurologic examination, EEG, ventriculography, angiography, nuclear scans, CAT scans, or MRI. The last two techniques are considerably more accurate than the others. The likely cause may be suggested by the history and CSF examination, but specific diagnosis may require surgery for confirmation.

Abscesses

Brain abscesses are diagnosed infrequently in small animals. Although they usually develop as an extension of infection from the ear, eye, nose, or sinuses, hematogenous metastasis may occur. Neutrophils may be present in the CSF but will be absent if the abscess is encapsulated. The source of infection should be identified and treated whenever possible by surgical drainage and administration of appropriate antibacterials.

Parasites

Parasitic larvae are occasionally found in the brain. If a parasitic lesion can be localized, resection may be possible. Surgical resection of Coenurus larvae in sheep has been reported.

Neoplasms

Brain tumors are reported in about 1% of necropsied dogs. Primary tumors, especially gliomas, are found more commonly in brachycephalic dogs, including boxers, Boston terriers, and English bulldogs. Meningiomas are slightly more common in German shepherds, collies, poodles, and cats. Plexus papillomas are more common in nonbrachycephalic breeds. Risk increases with age.

Primary brain tumors rarely metastasize. Metastatic tumors account for about one third of all intracranial tumors.

Clinical signs depend on the tumor's location. Convulsions or syncope are often the earliest signs. As the tumor enlarges, a persistent neurologic deficiency becomes noticeable. A diagnosis of brain tumor should be considered in any dog over 5 years of age that develops seizures. The occurrence of seizures in a brachycephalic dog and progression of signs increase the probability of neoplasia.

Successful excision of brain tumors in dogs and cats is being reported more often. Radiotherapy with or without excision has also been successful in prolonging life. Successful excision depends on an early and accurate diagnosis of a mass localized in an accessible area.

Cerebrovascular Disease

Primary vascular disease causing CNS disorders is rarely diagnosed. Cerebrovascular lesions have been described, but their relationship to CNS disease has not been clarified.

Cerebral vasospasm, thrombosis, and embolism may occur more often than is realized. More widespread application of angiography and the newer imaging techniques increase the probability of diagnosis.

The arteries supplying the basal nuclei and internal capsule appear to be more susceptible to occlusion than those of other areas. Dogs with congestive heart failure were found to have infarcts in these areas. These vessels are comparable to the human "stroke" arteries, and their occlusion may account for cases of hemiparesis seen in dogs. An occlusive cerebrovascular disease of unknown etiology is seen in cats. Infarction of a large area of the cerebral hemisphere from occlusion of the middle cerebral artery has been reported.

At this time, gross hemorrhage in the subdural space is the only cerebrovascular disorder likely to benefit from surgery. The use of a surgical microscope may enable treatment of more discrete vascular lesions.

Seizure Disorders

Seizures can result from a variety of lesions. Neoplasms, circulatory disturbances, and post-traumatic scarring may be treated surgically. Surgical excision of an epileptogenic lesion may provide at least temporary relief.

Brain Biopsy

Diagnosing many degenerative and inflammatory diseases may be impossible with the usual diagnostic methods. Brain biopsy may be useful in making a positive diagnosis in some of these cases. It is usually reserved for the animal with a diffuse, progressive brain syndrome such as storage or demyelinating diseases. Although there is no treatment for these disorders, they are important models of human disease and are genetically transmitted. Antemortem diagnosis may be important for development of breeding studies. This also provides an alternative for the owner who does not want to elect euthanasia without a definitive diagnosis.

Behavior Modification

Prefrontal lobotomy to modify aggressive behavior has been reported in dogs. Results have been variable, so the procedure should be considered a last resort. Olfactory tractotomy can alter micturition habits such as spraying in cats and marking in dogs and cats. Cats unresponsive to progestin therapy may respond to olfactory tractotomy; approximately half of male cats and almost all female cats are improved.

The Peripheral Nerves

Marc R. Raffe

General Surgical Principles

Successful results in peripheral nerve surgery depend on the surgeon's familiarity with surgical concepts, an understanding of tissue biology, appropriate surgical instruments, practice, and patience. Paying attention to detail and spending a few extra moments to obtain technical perfection are rewarded by a higher success rate and less time lost in repeat exploratory procedures.

The two most important decisions to the surgeon and the patient are whether surgery should be performed and when it should be done. Exploratory surgery is justified:

1. To establish an accurate diagnosis in cases where diagnostic methods have been inconclusive or contradictory,
2. To inspect the extent and severity of the lesion,
3. In cases where incomplete loss of function has occurred, but no clinical improvement is evident,
4. Where injury has occurred more than 3 weeks before surgery and no function has returned,
5. To improve function of the nerve in question by surgical means, and
6. To establish a prognosis.

The timing of surgical repair depends on the type of injury encountered and facilities available for repair at the time of initial presentation. Two times of surgical repair have been advocated in the literature; immediate (primary) repair 8 to 12 hours after injury, and early delayed (secondary) repair 2 to 6 weeks after initial injury. Immediate repair is indicated in cases of nerve trunk transection related to a clean sharp wound. Advantages of immediate suture repair include earlier return to function, better visualization for more accurate realignment of nerve tissue, and decreased tension on the suture line.

Delayed (secondary) repair is preferred in cases when major trauma and contamination are associated with nerve damage. Advantages of delaying repair for 2 to 6 weeks after injury include hypertrophy of epineurium for easier suturing and greater tensile strength, demarcation of injured nerve elements at the site of injury for easier resection of neuroma, and changes in cell physiology related to regrowth.

Disadvantages include stump retraction and neuroma debridement, increased tissue fibrosis and hemorrhage in the surgical field, and later return of function. Delaying definitive repair beyond 6 to 8 weeks can result in poor clinical results.

Peripheral nerve surgery instruments can be purchased from manufacturers of ophthalmic and microsurgical instruments. Generally, ophthalmic instruments are adequate for all but the most sophisticated repair procedures and are generally less expensive. Standard surgical instruments are appropriate for the surgical approach. Suggested instruments for peripheral nerve surgery should include a small ophthalmic needle holder, two pair of jeweler's forceps, a 10-cm strabismus scissor, a 10-cm iris scissor, a mouse-tooth Adson forceps, and a razor-blade holder. Disposable supplies should include lint-free sponges made from Gelfoam (Upjohn Co., Kalamazoo, MI) or Weck-Cel (Edward Weck Co., New York, NY), wooden tongue depressors, double-edged razor blades or scalpel blades, silicone nerve cuffs, and suture material. The type and selection of suture material is optional; I prefer monofilament suture material that has low tissue friction, such as polypropylene or nylon in 5-0 to 7-0 sizes with a swaged taper-point needle.

Preparation of surgical instruments is critical. Cleansing in a detergent-free soap solution is recommended. Instruments should be placed on a tray lined with a lint-free towel material; disposable dental napkins may be used. The instruments should be sterilized by dry heat or ethylene oxide. Repeated use of moist heat may corrode instruments and dull working edges. Sharp edges of razor or scalpel blades may also be dulled by moist heat.

Optical magnification and supplemental lighting help the surgeon achieve optimum results. A binocular magnifying loupe similar to one used in ophthalmic surgery is helpful. Interchangeable eyepieces allow 2.5 to 5.0 times magnification. Supplemental lighting may be provided by spot-type surgical lamps, fiber-optic headlamp sources, or flexible neck light sources.

The surgical approach to the injury site is important. Hemostasis and minimal tissue damage are critical because the presence of blood and tissue debris promotes excess scar formation. Tissue dissection should occur along anatomic lines. If exposure requires separation of muscle tissue, the muscle should be split in the direction of its fibers. If this is impossible, transecting the muscle at its ligamentous attachment is recommended. Lavage of the surgical site to remove tissue debris is helpful. Hemostasis can be achieved by low-voltage electrocoagulation of transected vessels.

After exposing the nerve, it is mobilized. Each nerve is surrounded by an adventitial tissue (mesoneurium) that contains collateral vessels. Some mesoneurium must be incised and stripped from the nerve trunk. While the amount of tissue that can be safely removed is controversial, it appears that 6 to 8 cm can be stripped without adverse effects. This is usually enough to permit adequate mobilization of the nerve trunk.

The nerve trunk should be manipulated with great care. Nerve tissue can be safely handled by several methods. The epineurium may be handled gently with jeweler's forceps, taking care to avoid incorporating nerve fascicles with the forceps. Manipulation of the nerve stump using mesoneurium may also be used. Most commonly, traction sutures are placed and manipulated through the epineurium. In addition to providing traction, these sutures can serve as landmarks for alignment if resection and anastomosis of the nerve trunk is required.

The nerve is then examined. The injured area often includes firm, swollen tissue (a neuroma). Presence of a neuroma indicates axontomesis or neurotomesis. The shape and location of the neuroma may give an estimate of prognosis. If the neuroma is firm, fibrosis has occurred at the point of injury, and there is little chance of spontaneous recannulation of neurotubules by regenerating nerve. Spontaneous functional healing is more likely if the neuroma is of soft consistency.

The neuroma's location within the nerve trunk may also aid in judging the lesion's severity (Fig. 18-11). Lateral neuromas indicate partial injury, with some functional tissue remaining. If the injury is less than half the width of the nerve trunk, spontaneous recovery may occur without surgical intervention. However, if more than 50% involvement is present, resection and reanastomosis of the nerve is indicated. Bulbous and dumbbell-shaped neuromas suggest widespread injury with poor prognosis for spontaneous recovery. Excision of the neuroma and neurorrhaphy is indicated in these cases.

If a neuroma is encountered at the time of exploration, it should be classified as described above and a decision should be made for or against surgical resection. If resection is elected, the neuroma is transected back to normal nerve tissue. Serial transverse sections 1 mm thick are removed from the incised edge of the neuroma until normal tissue is seen. This procedure is done on both the proximal and distal stumps. Constant inspection of the excised tissue and maintenance of adequate length are necessary. Wide and extensive tissue excision must be avoided so that anastomosis without undue tension can be accomplished.

Hemostasis is imperative following resection because excessive fibrosis and distortion of nerve architecture may occur. Lint-free ophthalmic sponges or absorbable gelatin sponges should be used. The degree of intraneural vasculature is surprising. If excessive hemorrhage is encountered, it may be controlled by using sponges dipped in 1:100,000 epinephrine solution, or bipolar electrocoagulation.

Surgical Techniques

Epineural Suture Repair

The most common technique of nerve repair (neurorrhaphy) involves placing simple interrupted sutures through the epineurium. Low-power magnification from a five-power binocular loupe is helpful in distinguishing structures and ensuring that sutures pass through only the epineurium. The epineurium is grasped and tensed with jeweler's forceps. Because the tissue has elastic fibers, the epineurium may be stretched slightly to facilitate suture placement. Before suture placement, the surgeon should be confident that peripheral nerve stumps have been realigned correctly.

Sutures should be placed approximately 0.5 to 1.0 mm from the incised edge. The suture material is placed from the surface of the nerve and emerges subepineurally. It is brought out to the free edge, and the process is continued in the opposing nerve stump. The second passage begins subepineurally and emerges on the surface. This completes one simple interrupted suture (Fig. 18-12). The number of sutures

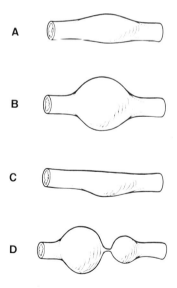

Figure 18-11. *Neuroma classification.* **A,** *Fusiform neuroma,* **B,** *Spherical neuroma,* **C,** *Lateral neuroma,* **D,** *Dumbbell neuroma. Neuroma appearance in* **A** *and* **C** *will not absolutely require resection and anastomosis. Neuroma appearance in* **B** *and* **D** *will require surgical resection. (Raffe MR. Peripheral nerve injuries in the dog. Part II. Compend Contin Ed Sm Anim Pract 1979;1:207)*

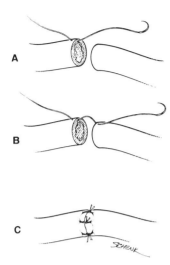

Figure 18-12. *Epineural suture repair of a transected peripheral nerve. Simple interrupted sutures are placed just below the fibrous sheath (epineurium) approximately 0.5 mm from the transected edge (**A** and **B**). All sutures are tied at the same time to maintain even tension at the repair site (**C**). (Raffe MR. Peripheral nerve injuries in the dog. Part II. Compend Contin Ed Sm Anim Pract 1979;1:207)*

needed to align the stumps adequately varies depending on the nerve's diameter. Using as few sutures as possible minimizes the inflammatory reaction to the suture material; however, aligning the nerve stumps is critical to the procedure's success. It is advisable to preplace sutures and then tie them all at the same time. This minimizes the chance of applying excess traction at one point and having the suture tear tissue.

To begin, two sutures are placed in the nerve trunk 180° apart. These sutures maintain the alignment of the nerve stumps. An additional suture or sutures is placed in the upper portion of the nerve. Several or all of these sutures may be tied to obtain adequate alignment. The suture ends may then be carefully grasped and the nerve trunk rotated to expose the underside of the nerve. An additional suture or sutures are then placed and tied to complete apposition of the nerve trunk. All sutures should be tied with equal tension,

and that tension should be just enough for alignment and contact of the neural bundles. Excessive tension may result in crushing and misalignment of the nerve bundles, which may lead to poor recannulation of distal nerve tubules and neuroma formation at the surgical site. All knots should be inspected for equal tension.

An alternate anastomosis technique involves placing a single suture along the nerve trunk's longitudinal axis. The two ends of the suture are secured with small buttons on the outside of the nerve trunk. Sutures may be placed in one of two ways. In the first method, the suture is begun 7 to 8 mm from the transection site. It is directed perpendicular to the longitudinal axis in the center of the nerve trunk. The suture is then redirected to follow the central axis of the nerve trunk and emerge at the center of the transection site. It is then carried to the opposing stump and the needle is inserted in the central axis, advanced for 7 to 8 mm, and then redirected to emerge 180° opposite the initial suture placement. The result resembles the letter Z.

The second method involves double-armed suture material. Each needle is centrally inserted into one of the nerve stumps, then directed down the longitudinal axis and redirected so that it emerges 180° from its counterpart. This modification increases the likelihood of central suture placement, which is critical for proper alignment (Fig. 18-13).

Fascial or silicone buttons approximately 3 mm square are prepared. Each end of the suture is attached to a button, which acts as an anchor. One end is secured with a square knot on top of the button. The other button is affixed with a slip knot, which acts to apply tension for alignment and apposition of the nerve trunks. The slip knot involves a triple suture passage, and use of a loop and suture strand to tie a square knot to provide good alignment and knot security.

The main advantage of the one-suture technique is that less postsurgical neuroma formation and ingrowth of scar tissue are seen. However, the technique is more technically

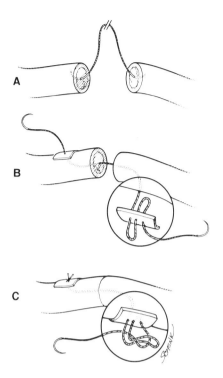

Figure 18-13. *Intraneural suture repair of a transected peripheral nerve. The suture is placed in the axial center of the nerve and advanced for 6 or 7 mm (**A** and **B**). Emergence is on opposite sides of the nerve trunk. Fascial of silicone buttons are attached (**B**). A slip knot is tied to provide appropriate suture tension (**C**). (Raffe MR. Peripheral nerve injuries in the dog. Part II. Compend Contin Ed Sm Anim Pract 1979;1:207)*

difficult and may result in severe complications. The most common complication is stump rotation and instability, resulting from a suture that was not carefully centered in the nerve trunk.

Nerve Cuffs

Nerve cuffs are used to inhibit ingrowth of connective tissue from the area surrounding the site of nerve repair. Inhibiting ingrowth encourages axons to regenerate in a rapid, orderly manner.

Silicone rubber compounds (Silastic) are commonly used as a shielding implant after nerve repair. Silicone rubber is relatively inert, flexible, thin-walled, and uniform in diameter. Assorted diameters and lengths are available. The material is provided in sterile glass vials and is ready for use.

The cross-sectional area of the cuff should be two to three times that of the nerve trunk. A smaller cuff may constrict the anastomotic site as nerve swelling occurs and may predispose to neuroma formation. A larger cuff may invaginate and constrict the nerve trunk. The cuff should be no longer than 8 to 10 mm. A longer cuff may inhibit collateral circulation to the nerve trunk, and a shorter cuff may not provide sufficient shielding at the surgical site (Fig. 18-14). Complications of cuff use result from improper sizing of the cuff.

The cuff is placed on the nerve stump before anastomosis. The epineurium is gently grasped and the cuff is slipped onto the nerve stump, using a jeweler's forceps or small hemostat. After anastomosis, the cuff is centered over the anastomotic site and fixed in position with epineural sutures. One suture at each end of the cuff will provide sufficient anchorage and will prevent cuff distortion.

Nerve Grafts

In extensive injuries, nerve tissue loss may result in an irreducible gap. Nerve stumps may be stretched to a limited extent to attain apposition, depending on the direction of the nerve, vascular supply, and species involved. However, any degree of stretching decreases the

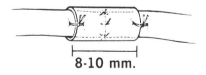

8-10 mm.

Figure 18-14. *Proper nerve cuff sizing for enshielding the anastomotic site. The cuff should be two to three times the diameter of the nerve trunk and at least 8 to 10 mm long. (Raffe MR. Peripheral nerve injuries in the dog. Part II. Compend Contin Ed Sm Anim Pract 1979;1:207)*

possibility of nerve healing. Generally, enough length is available in most nerves to overcome a 2- to 3-cm gap, but stretching or mobilizing any more than this endangers the vascular supply to the nerve and predisposes the repair to failure by increased suture-line tension. In experimental studies, the regeneration rate through a suture line under tension was no greater than that through a properly used nerve graft.

A free graft may be used to overcome irreducible gaps. Free graft donor sites in the dog are the lateral cutaneous nerve of the thigh and the median nerve of the forearm. The decision to use a nerve graft should be based on the diagnosis of irreducible gap at the time of surgery. Anatomical mapping experiments show that nerve bundles are not distinct subunits, but undergo a continuous process of division and integration with neighboring units. The pattern of change is approximately every 0.5 cm along the course of a peripheral nerve. Unless grafts are united to individual bundles by microsurgical techniques (cable grafting), interposition of a nerve graft segment does not guarantee perfect axonal migration in the distal stump.

The graft diameter should be close to the diameter of the nerve trunk to be grafted. An inadequate graft diameter may predispose to incomplete axonal regrowth due to the insufficient number of Schwann tubes provided by the graft. The graft length should be 15% to 25% longer than the gap to be spanned, to allow for graft shrinkage and to release tension on suture lines at anastomotic sites (Fig. 18-15).

Nerve grafts may fail for several reasons, including inadequate training and instrumentation, failure to match graft diameter and length to the injured nerve, improper matching of donor and host bundles, and tension at either suture line. Biologic aspects of nerve grafting are also important. Nerve grafts are similar to other devascularized tissue. Regeneration of blood supply must be provided by surrounding tissues to provide nutrition for neural elements. It is important to remember

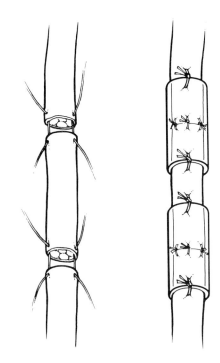

Figure 18-15.   *An example of an interposed nerve graft. Note that two suture lines and shielded areas are present. Matching of individual nerve fibers between the graft and nerve is critical for optimal results. (Newton CD, Nunamaker DM, eds. Textbook of small animal orthopaedics. Philadelphia: JB Lippincott, 1985:810)*

that a race is always ongoing between regeneration of axons across a free graft and destruction of patent Schwann tubes.

Nerve Gaps

Occasionally, an irreducible gap may be encountered without immediate provision for graft repair. In these cases, an alternate approach is to bring the nerve stumps together as close as possible and suture the stumps with epineural sutures to a dry tissue bed, creating a nerve gap without continuity. This technique may be used for defects no longer than 1 to 2 cm. Successful regeneration across nerve gaps has been reported in the dog and in children. Bioabsorbable tubes to bridge nerve gaps may be used, although increased time of regeneration should be expected.

Postoperative Care

Routine surgical closure is performed after nerve repair. If tension at the suture line is evident at the time of surgery, the limb should be splinted or cast in a flexed position to relieve suture line tension for no less than 2 weeks. After this time, passive motion of the limb may be started; the goal should be to achieve full range of motion by the sixth postoperative week.

The denervated limb must be protected from mutilation until evidence of reinnervation is apparent. Protection may be provided by padded bandages, splints, or moldable cast material. In some cases, the animal may attempt self-mutilation of the denervated area; this may be correlated with early stages of axon growth and reinnervation of sensory-deprived areas. Conservative management—a protective bandage, side brace, bucket collar, or muzzling—usually is sufficient to prevent further damage.

Periodic examination and electrodiagnostic evaluation are used to assess progress. Although 100% function will not be regained, the goal is to restore enough function to allow adequate locomotion and activity.

Qualitative measurement of sensory function by dermatome examination and evoked nerve potentials (motor nerve conduction velocity) can be used as early indicators of functional recovery. Somatosensory evoked cortical potentials can be used as the sole or adjunctive diagnostic assessment of reinnervation.

Factors Influencing Success of Surgical Repair

Surgical repair of peripheral nerve injuries only sets the stage for healing. Unfortunately, it is not uncommon that complications arise and failure in operative repair occurs. Although most failures can be attributed to technical error during surgical repair or postoperative management, biologic considerations also are important.

Injury to a pure motor or sensory nerve is usually accompanied by a more uncomplicated recovery course. Axons in mixed-function nerves may become transposed during regeneration, causing end organ reinnervation. This can result in patient disorientation and a lower level of functional recovery. Younger patients recover more completely and more quickly. Proximal injuries require greater metabolic biosynthesis for healing, which may exceed the capabilities of the nerve cell body and result in cell death. If this occurs on a widespread basis in the nerve, regeneration failure will occur.

The extent of the injury is also important. Lesions in continuity, those with focal neuroma formation, or small gaps will respond better than injuries with irreducible gaps or large defects. This is related to factors such as vascular supply, suture line tension, and biologic considerations in nerve grafting. In addition, large defects interrupt nerve architecture and increase the potential for cross-functional innervation. Clean tissue beds decrease the potential for neuroma formation. Rerouting of the nerve may be necessary to achieve the best site for regeneration. Tension at the suture site may result in regeneration failure; minimal tension increases the potential for nerve healing. Also, as time increases from injury to surgical repair, progressive changes occur in the anatomy of the nerve trunk.

Suggested Readings

The Brain and Cranial Nerves

Evans HE, Christensen GC. Miller's anatomy of the dog. Philadelphia: WB Saunders, 1979.
Hart BL. Olfactory tractotomy for control of objectionable urine spraying and urine marking in cats. J Am Vet Med Assoc 1981;179:231.
Oliver JE Jr., Lorenz M. Handbook of veterinary neurologic diagnosis. Philadelphia: WB Saunders, 1983.

Oliver JE, Hoerlein BF, Mayhew IG. Veterinary neurology. Philadelphia: WB Saunders, 1987.

Skerritt G, Stallbaumer M. Diagnosis and treatment of coenuriasis (gid) in sheep. Vet Rec 1984; 115:399.

The Peripheral Nerves

Gourley LM, Synder CC. Peripheral nerve repair. J Am Anim Hosp Assoc 1976;12:613.

Peacock EE, VanWinkle W. Wound repair. Philadelphia: WB Saunders, 1972.

Raffe MR. Peripheral nerve injuries, Parts I and II. Compend Contin Educ [Sm Anim Pract] 1979;1:207, 269.

Swaim SF. Peripheral nerve surgery in the dog. J Am Vet Med Assoc 1972;161:905.

Swaim SF. Peripheral nerve surgery. In: Hoerlein BF, ed. Canine neurology. Philadelphia: WB Saunders, 1978.

19

Jonathan N. Chambers
Tommy L. Walker

The Spine

The Cervical Spine

Jonathan N. Chambers

Introduction

Surgical diseases of the cervical spine fall into two general categories: unstable lesions and compressive lesions. Some diseases involve both instability and compression at some stage. Compressive lesions require decompression, unstable lesions require stabilization, and when both are present the surgical procedure must handle each.

Two elements related to the diagnosis, prognosis, and treatment of cervical spine lesions deserve preliminary mention. The first is the relative sizes of the epidural and subarachnoid spaces. Although the spinal cord diameter is large in the cranial cervical region and

again at the brachial intumescence (C5—T2), the spinal canal diameter is correspondingly large. The ratio of spinal canal to spinal cord diameter is actually higher than in lower parts of the spine. Compared to the thoracolumbar region, a space-occupying mass (e.g., a herniated intervertebral disk) in the cervical region may be much larger before causing clinical signs, and a surprising accommodation for cervical vertebral displacement is possible before signs of spinal cord compression develop.

Of course, these facts must be considered in the light of acceptable tolerances. Although serious, an animal can live with a severe displacement of the spinal cord in the thoracolumbar region. A similar displacement in the midcervical region would probably be instantly fatal due to the proximity of the vital cardiorespiratory pathways.

The second important factor to remember when treating cervical lesions is that external supports (bandages, splints, braces, or casts) are relatively ineffective and impractical. Many human neck problems (for which there are counterparts in the dog) are treated entirely or partially with external support. But even under ideal circumstances, support with external skeletal traction is only moderately effective in neutralizing forces on the upper neck in humans. External support alone is not sufficient for the treatment of very unstable lesions, even if the conditions could be reproduced for animals. Therefore, veterinary surgeons must often rely on the most secure means of internal fixation that can be devised, even though it may seem radical.

Atlantoaxial Subluxation

Introduction

Atlantoaxial subluxation is a specific diagnosis in the dog, but instability of this joint may be either slowly progressive (typical) or may be due to traumatic fracture-luxation of an otherwise normal joint (less common). The two problems often have differing histories and physical findings, but the biomechanical considerations are the same.

Anatomic Considerations

The atlantoaxial articulation is a fairly simple smooth ball (axial facets) in a shallow socket (caudal atlantal ring). The joint capsule is thickened dorsally and laterally (atlantoaxial membrane), but restricts motion very little. The dens and its complex of ligaments limit the joint's motion predominantly to rotation around the axis of the spinal canal. The transverse atlantal ligament tethers the dens to the floor of the atlas and is the most important stabilizing structure for the joint. This ligament, in conjunction with the apical ligament, limits flexion to a few millimeters.

Absence or disruption of the dens or the transverse atlantal ligament allows serious subluxation of the joint in flexion. The caudal atlas is displaced ventrally and the cranial axis dorsally. Traumatic rupture of the transverse atlantal ligament is the most dangerous situation because of severe encroachment on the spinal cord by the dens. If the dens is fractured but remains secured to the floor of the atlas, less spinal cord encroachment is expected. Agenesis or hypoplasia of the dens and its ligaments, the most common problem, causes slowly progressive instability with intermittent pinching of the spinal cord. Surgical stabilization is almost always indicated.

Examination

Atlantoaxial subluxation is characteristically a disease of toy breeds, particularly the Chihuahua. It is also common in Yorkshire terriers and toy poodles. The dog is most often younger than 1 year. The history usually shows a slowly developing myelopathy with intermittent episodes of severe spinal cord compression. An uncoordinated gait is usually present and postural reaction deficits may be noted in all limbs. Occasionally, a dog will present with severe weakness or tetraplegia. Even if the dog is still ambulatory, the owner will usually report past episodes of transient tetraplegia lasting for short periods. Neck pain or guarding is an inconsistent finding. Great care should be taken in examining any dog suspected of having atlantoaxial instability, and flexion of the craniocervical junction should be avoided.

Diagnosis

Survey film radiographs are usually sufficient to establish the diagnosis. The initial study should be done with the dog fully awake and able to guard the neck against undue stress. The lateral film is most valuable and the malalignment is usually so gross that making the diagnosis is easy. The tip of the axial spinous process is widely displaced caudodorsally from the atlas. The atlas is tipped forward with the dorsal arch close to the occipital bone. The body of the axis rides dorsally, encroaching on the spinal canal at the atlantoaxial junction. In the rare instance that the initial survey film is insufficient for diagnosis, the dog should be anesthetized under close supervision by the surgeon and the neck should be very gently flexed for a repeat study. Special radiographic techniques are rarely required, but myelography and tomography have been advocated when the diagnosis is still uncertain.

Surgical Techniques

Dorsal stabilization is the time-honored approach to surgical correction. This procedure has been used successfully in humans for many years, and the technique used in the dog is an adaptation. The human procedure often involves multiple interarcuate wires and incorporates autogenous cortical bone grafts to induce a fusion. Fusion has not been found necessary in many cases in dogs, but could be considered.

The dog is positioned in sternal recumbency with a small sandbag supporting the chin. The muzzle or ears are taped to the table to maintain symmetry.

The approach is made through the dorsal midline. The paraspinal muscles are bluntly separated and elevated from the dorsal arch of C1 and the dorsal spinous process of C2. Entrance to the epidural space is gained through incisions in the dorsal atlanto-occipital and atlantoaxial membranes. These should be made directly adjacent to the atlantal arch. The underlying dura often adheres to the membranes, and care must be taken not to penetrate it.

A loop of 22- to 24-gauge stainless steel wire is gently passed under the arch of the atlas from caudal to cranial through the epidural space. It is grasped as it appears at the atlanto-occipital joint and is pulled back to the axis. Two holes are drilled in the spinous process of the axis. One of the wire strands protruding from the atlantoaxial joint is passed through the caudal hole and twisted with its mate. The wire loop protruding from the atlanto-occipital joint is cut and one end is

passed through the cranial hole. The wire is pulled tight as the luxation is reduced by gently forcing the axis in a ventral and caudal direction. Final stabilization is achieved when the wire through the cranial hole is twisted to its mate (Fig. 19-1). Decompressing the spinal cord beyond the act of reducing the luxation is unnecessary and only weakens the stabilization.

A variation of the technique has been developed for very small dogs to avoid passing heavy orthopedic wire through the epidural space. A loop of wire suture (32 to 36 gauge) is used as a passer for a strand of nonabsorbable suture material such as polyethylene-impregnated Dacron (size 0 to 2). The luxation is reduced and the suture is secured to the spinous process of the axis as with the wire technique. An additional advantage of this technique over traditional repair is that it avoids fatigue failure of wire.

The surgeon must be prepared for anatomic variations that may require further modification of the dorsal fixation technique. An alternate technique of ventral pin fixation ap-

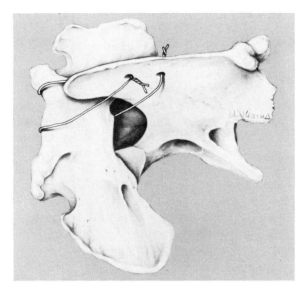

Figure 19-1. *Final positioning of a wire used for stabilizing atlantoaxial subluxation (Cook JR, Oliver JE. Atlantoaxial luxation in the dog. Compend Contin Ed Pract Vet 1981;3:247)*

pears to be indicated in the rare case when the dorsal anatomy is deficient.

Postoperative Care and Prognosis

The dog's activity should be strictly limited and supervised for several weeks. A padded bandage or fiberglass splint should be used to support the neck for 4 to 6 weeks after surgery.

Excellent results can be expected in patients presenting with intermittent symptoms intermixed with periods of relative normalcy. Patients with well-established neural signs may show moderate improvement after surgery; those with advanced symptoms are unlikely to show improvement, but the surgery will prevent further deterioration.

Cervical Intervertebral Disk Herniation

Introduction

Cervical intervertebral disk disease is primarily a problem in small breeds, with dachshunds, beagles, and toy poodles accounting for over 80% of the cases. More than 50% of cervical disk herniations occur at C2-3, with the frequency decreasing sequentially from C3-4 through C6-7.

The primary, and often the only, symptom of cervical disk herniation in the dog is pain, although some dogs will have a compressive myelopathy that produces postural reaction deficits and motor deficits varying from paresis to paralysis. The pain of disk herniation can originate from one or a combination of three sources. The annulus fibrosus is supplied with sensory nerve endings and discogenic pain is caused by the abnormal pressures within the disk and disruption of the annular fibers. Nerve root or radicular pain is caused by direct irritation or ischemia of the root by herniated disk material and the intense spasm of the cervical muscles supplied by the root. The meninges contain sensory endings and pressure or inflammation around her-

niated disk material can produce meningeal pain.

These multiple sources of pain are probably why treatment failures have been encountered. In theory, fenestration (partial removal of the disk) could relieve discogenic pain, but it will do nothing for (and may aggravate) radicular or meningeal pain if either is the source. In fenestration, a slit or window is created in the ventral annulus and the nuclear material still contained by the annulus is removed. This procedure will not affect disk material that has escaped the annulus into the spinal canal, or around nerve roots. Disk material within the spinal canal or compressing nerve roots can only be removed by creating a ventral slot through the vertebral bodies, or by dorsal laminectomy.

Examination

The pain of cervical disk disease is excruciating and will rarely be mistaken for another problem. The dog will hold the neck rigid, usually with the head lowered. Intermittent and sudden bouts of loud crying are usually present and are easily elicited by manipulating the neck. Careful palpation will often allow localization of the pain to within one or two vertebral segments. Rhythmic spasms of the neck muscles are common and can often be induced by palpation. The spasm may radiate to muscles of the ear or shoulder.

Significant spinal cord compression from herniated disk material is first manifested by loss of proprioception in the limbs. Weakness or paralysis may be acute or slowly progressive in onset. The postural reaction or motor deficits may be severe or quite subtle. The spinal reflexes usually localize the compression to spinal cord segments C2-6, but a massive herniation at C5-6 or C6-7 could produce lower motor neuron signs in the forelimbs.

Diagnosis

A presumptive diagnosis of cervical disk herniation can be made from the history and physical examination. Further diagnostic tests serve mainly to confirm and localize the lesion.

Survey radiographs should always be taken if surgery is contemplated. Anesthesia is necessary to obtain meaningful radiographs. Marked narrowing or wedging or complete collapse of a disk space are significant localizing signs (Fig. 19-2), but these signs are often subtle, or multiple spaces may be suspect. A mineralized density within the spinal canal is highly significant, but this is not a consistent finding, even in patients with obvious clinical signs of spinal cord compression. It is important to accurately define the extent of the radiographic lesion and to correlate it with the severity of clinical signs to choose the proper surgical technique.

Figure 19-3 is an algorithm that helps the surgeon select the logical therapy based on combined clinical and radiographic findings. Using this system, a concerted attempt is made to confirm the presence or absence of disk material within the spinal canal or intervertebral foramina, and to remove it if found. A myelogram can be very helpful in many cases. Oblique views highlight the intervertebral foramina and should be obtained whenever prior studies have proved fruitless and the suspicion of a lateralized disk extrusion remains high. The second most common problem causing these symptoms is infectious meningitis; therefore, cerebrospinal fluid collection

and analysis is always prudent before myelography.

Treatment

Conservative therapy, including rest and analgesic-antiinflammatory drugs, can be recommended only with the full understanding that the symptoms can be protracted and often recur. If a protrusive mass is left in the spinal canal, organization of the mass into a fibrotic, calcific, or osseous lesion can cause irreversible spinal cord damage.

Surgical Techniques

Ventral Approach for Cervical Disk Fenestration

Fenestration is indicated when pain is the only clinical sign and intervertebral disk disease remains the most likely diagnosis, even though no disk material is demonstrated in the spinal canal on either survey radiographs or a myelogram. (In my experience, this is a rare set of circumstances.) The more common indication is as prophylaxis at other commonly offending sites, in combination with a decompressive procedure at the primary site.

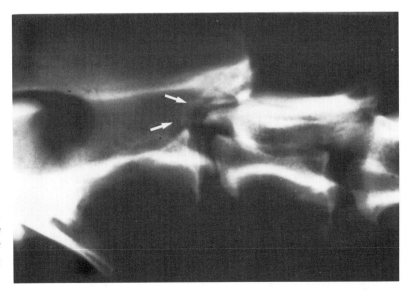

Figure 19-2. *Lateral survey radiograph of a dog with cervical disk disease. The C2-3 disk space is wedged and a mass of calcified disk material can be seen in the canal over the disk space (arrows).*

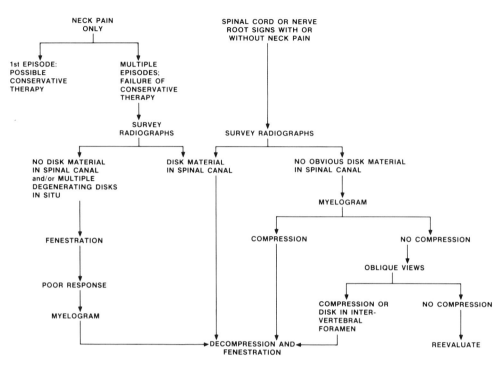

Figure 19-3. *An algorithm to guide the surgeon in selecting the proper therapy for cervical intervertebral disk disease.*

General anesthesia with endotracheal intubation is used. The end of the endotracheal tube must be near or below the thoracic inlet to prevent tracheal collapse from manipulation and retraction. Tube placement should be checked occasionally during the procedure.

The dog is placed in dorsal recumbency, with a sandbag under the neck to produce moderate extension. The forelimbs are pulled caudally and tied in place. The clipped and scrubbed area should include at least the rectangle formed by the bases of the ears and points of the shoulders.

The skin incision is on the ventral midline and extends from the mid-laryngeal region to the manubrium. The deep dissection is by blunt muscle separation between the paired sternohyoideus muscle bellies (midline) or the sternothyroideus and sternocephalicus (sternomastoideus) muscle bellies on the right side. (Advocates of the latter approach claim that it is less traumatic and affords more protection for the trachea, right recurrent laryngeal nerve, right vagosympathetic trunk, and right carotid artery.) Dissection should proceed

gently, and the aforementioned structures and the esophagus should be identified and protected. The Frazier or Rigby self-retaining retractors are relatively atraumatic and are well suited to this procedure. The ventral paraspinous muscles are exposed by blunt dissection of the overlying loose areolar connective tissue. The paired longus colli muscles lie on the midline, with the longus capitus muscles lying lateral to them. The ventral tubercles of the vertebral bodies should be palpated on the midline deep to the longus colli tendons and should be differentiated from the transverse processes, which lie 1 to 2 cm laterally.

The ventral tubercles are protuberances from the caudal vertebral bodies at the intervertebral disk space, and each should be identified. The C1-2 space can be identified by placing the thumb and middle finger against the caudal borders of the wings of the atlas. The index finger is positioned on the midline and the pointed ventral tubercle of C1 is palpated (there is no disk at C1-2). The C2-3 through C6-7 spaces can be identified by sliding the index finger caudally on the midline.

Another way to identify the spaces is to place the thumb and middle finger on the cranial aspect of the large transverse processes of C6. The C5 ventral tubercle (C5-6 space) is palpated with the index finger on the adjacent midline, and the other spaces are identified by counting cranially or caudally.

The confluence of the ventral longitudinal ligament and ventral annulus is exposed by forcing the closed tips of a small hemostat between the paired tendons of the longus colli muscle just caudal to their attachment on the ventral tubercle. As the hemostat is opened, the ventral longitudinal ligament and annulus are seen as white opalescent tissue that can be differentiated from the dull white of the bony endplates of the vertebra. More exposure is gained by incising the tendons, but this causes hemorrhage and is rarely needed for routine fenestration. The slit or window in the annulus is made with a #11 Bard-Parker scalpel blade. The ventral annulus will be 3 to 5 mm thick depending on the dog's size. The blade tip should not be inserted into the disk space more than one-half the measured height of the disk as determined from the lateral radiograph. The proper angle of insertion is slightly caudoventral to craniodorsal, and the slit or window is developed with a sawing motion. The plug of annulus is removed with a small toothed tissue forceps. The nucleus pulposus is gently removed from the disk space. A variety of small, blunt instruments can be used to accomplish this. The most popular is a thin-bladed dental scaler, but I prefer a size 0000 bone or ear curette. The C2-3 through C6-7 spaces are fenestrated.

Closure is by simple reapproximation of the separated sternohyoideus (or right sternothyroideus and sternomastoideus) muscle bellies with 2-0 or 3-0 suture material in an interrupted or continuous pattern. Closure of dead space created by loose areolar dissection is difficult, and drainage can be considered, although clinically apparent seroma formation is uncommon.

Postoperative care includes very limited activity for 2 to 3 weeks after surgery. The use of a padded support bandage is optional.

When fenestration alone is used, immediate relief of pain is a good indication that the pain was primarily discogenic and that the surgery has been both therapeutic and prophylactic. Continuing pain after surgery suggests that fenestration alone was insufficient, and a protracted course of pain can be predicted.

Ventral Decompression (Slotting) for Cervical Intervertebral Disk Herniation

Ventral slotting is indicated when the presenting clinical signs, survey radiographs, or myelogram indicate that disk material is present within the ventral aspect of the spinal canal. Intervertebral body screws, plates, bone grafts, and other forms of vertebral body fixation can also be applied through this approach.

The approach to the spine and localization of the offending disk are the same as for fenestration. The longus colli tendons are incised at their attachment on the ventral tubercle of the cranial vertebral body, and the muscles are reflected laterally with a periosteal elevator. Hemorrhage is controlled by hemostats and electrocautery. Stubborn seepage usually comes under control as Gelpi retractors are placed at the mid-vertebral body region on both sides of the disk space.

The ventral annulus and nucleus pulposus are removed as described for routine fenestration. The intervertebral body slot is created using a power bur (see "Thoracolumbar Hemilaminectomy," below, for specifics of pneumatic bur technique). The length of the slot should include approximately one-third of the vertebral body on each side of the disk space; the width should include approximately the central half. This leaves a shelf of bone and lateral annulus intact bilaterally. The proper-sized bur depends on the dog's size, and the shape of the bur is the surgeon's preference. Progressively smaller burs are used as the depth of the slot approaches the spinal canal. The tendency to create a funnel-shaped defect should be avoided, because this greatly limits exposure at the level of the spinal canal. The surgeon also should recognize that the disk space at the level of the spinal canal is more directly dorsal to the ventral tubercle of the cranial vertebra than the ventral annulus. The final thin layer of cortical bone is delicately removed with fine rongeurs or a small bone curette. Tags of the dorsal annulus and dorsal longitudinal ligament are grasped with a fine thumb forceps or hemostat and excised with a #11 scalpel blade or similar fine cutting instrument. Herniated disk material is removed with a nerve root retractor, fine blunt probe, thumb forceps, or small curette.

The fragile vertebral sinuses are allied with the dorsal annulus, dorsal longitudinal ligament, and periosteum lining the floor of the canal. They can be best avoided by limiting manipulations to the exact midline and the region of the disk space. Unfortunately, the sinuses are often obscured and displaced by the herniated disk, and laceration is common. Bleeding can be profuse and difficult to control. Judicious suctioning and light direct pressure will often allow completion of the canal exploration. Blood pressure should be monitored closely and volume replacement used as necessary to prevent hypotension.

Short, wide slots, as described above, resolve by spontaneous fusion within a few months, and routine intervertebral fixation or bone grafting is unnecessary. The longus colli muscle bellies are apposed over the slot, and light direct pressure over the closed muscle will usually control any residual vertebral sinus hemorrhage. The rest of the disk spaces should be fenestrated before or after the slotting procedure. Closure of the wound is as described for fenestration.

The dog's activity should be severely restricted for several days. Some surgeons routinely use a padded neck bandage, and analgesic-antiinflammatory drugs might also be used. The prognosis is good.

Indications for Dorsal Approach and Laminectomy

Dorsal decompression (laminectomy) is indicated when a mass lesion is lateral or dorsolateral to the spinal cord. The dorsal approach is also indicated when liberal decompression and exposure are needed, as in cases of suspected tumors. Ventral or ventrolateral lesions, especially herniated disks, are best managed through a ventral slot.

The dog is placed in sternal recumbency with forearms crossed to separate the scapulae. Sandbags support the chin and neck, allowing gentle ventroflexion. Additional sandbags support the thorax laterally and help maintain axial symmetry. Endotracheal intubation is mandatory, with the end of the tube at or beyond the thoracic inlet. Positional compression of the jugular veins should be avoided.

The prominent C2 and T1 dorsal spinous processes should be palpated. They are significantly longer than the relatively rudimentary C3-6 processes and can be used as landmarks for localizing the involved segment(s). The skin incision is on the dorsal midline from the occiput to between the scapulae. Deep dissection should be confined precisely to the midline to minimize trauma and hemorrhage. The median raphe is sharply incised, releasing the paired bellies of the platysma, trapezius, rhomboideus, cleidocervicalis, serratus dorsalis cranialis, splenius, and semispinalis capitus muscles. The nuchal ligament is now evident and is held with self-retaining retractors for isolation of the tips of the dorsal spinous processes. The remaining epaxial muscles (spinalis cervicis and multifidus) are elevated from both sides of the dorsal spinous processes.

The dorsal spinous process(es) is removed at its base with a bone-cutting forceps. The canal is entered by incising or excising the interarcuate ligament. The laminectomy can be completed with a rongeur, or a power bur followed by a rongeur. If possible, the facets and their capsules are maintained, as they are the only remaining dorsally stabilizing structures. Articular facet arthrodesis and other fixation techniques can also be accomplished through this same approach. Wound closure is routine, but special care should be taken to obliterate dead space to prevent seroma formation.

Caudal Cervical Spondylopathy
(Cervical Vertebral Instability; Cervical Vertebral Malformation; Canine Wobbler Syndrome)

Introduction

This affliction is common to Doberman pinschers and Great Danes but has also been reported in other large and giant breeds. The consensus is that the primary problem is an inherited, probably congenital weakness of the structures supporting the spine. The weakness leads to intervertebral instability, and the spinal cord becomes damaged either from primary subluxation or, more commonly, from compression by a variety of secondary degenerative lesions that develop in response to the instability. Immature dogs, often only several months old, present with primarily subluxation; this is more common in the Great Dane. Mature dogs often do not show signs until middle age, and then the secondary lesions are more prominent; this is the more common presentation for Doberman pinschers. Affected males outnumber females by as much as 4:1.

The C6-7 segment is most commonly involved; C5-6 is the other common site. Involvement at other sites (including C7-T1) has been reported but is uncommon. Multiple site involvement has also been reported.

The lesions are:

Intervertebral Disk Herniation—The combined mass of dorsal annulus fibrosus and dorsal longitudinal ligament is displaced into the spinal canal. The lesion most closely resembles a Hanson's type II disk herniation, with protrusion of degenerated nuclear material into the spinal canal but still contained by a thin layer of degenerated annulus (Fig. 19-4). The resultant cord compression can be either static (constant) or dynamic (relieved by traction). This is the most common lesion.

Subluxation—The cranial end of the vertebra is displaced dorsally. The spinal cord is compressed between the craniodorsal margin of the vertebral body and the arch of the vertebra in front of it.

Misshapen Vertebral Bodies—This can be considered either malformation in the skeletally immature dog or a process of remodeling in the adult. Instability probably precedes the change, in either instance. The disk space becomes malformed or obliterated.

Sagittal Stenosis of the Vertebral Canal—The spinal canal within a vertebral segment is funnel-shaped as viewed from the side, with the cranial end abnormally narrowed to the point of spinal cord compression. This can also be a consequence of dysplasia or remodeling, depending on the dog's age.

Transverse Stenosis of the Vertebral Canal—The canal is narrowed on the sides by large, malformed articular processes and/or their supporting pedicles.

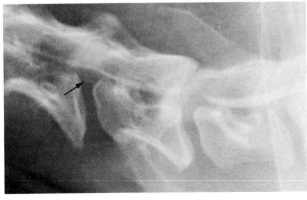

Figure 19-4. *Myelogram of a dog with cervical spondylopathy. Note the severe ventral spinal cord compression at C6-7 and the dense soft tissue mass ventral to the spinal cord at C5-6 (arrow). (Chambers JN, Betts CW. Caudal cervical spondylopathy in the dog: A review of 20 clinical cases and the literature. J Am Anim Hosp Assoc 1977;13:571)*

Interarcuate Ligament Hypertrophy—The inter-arcuate ligament is enlarged and/or folded into the dorsal spinal canal to the point of spinal cord compression.

Examination

Progressive ataxia in the hind limbs is the first sign. In puppies, the owner might initially mistake this for the normal clumsiness of a rapidly growing dog. In the older dog, it might be mistaken for other degenerative skeletal problems (*e.g.*, hip dysplasia). The ataxia may progress slowly or rapidly or may wax and wane, depending on the dog's activity. The ataxia may progress to the forelimbs, but this is rarely as obvious to the owner.

A complete neurologic examination can localize the source of the ataxia to the cervical spinal cord. The postural reactions will be abnormal in all limbs, but typically the rear-limb deficits are obvious and those in the forelimbs are more subtle. The hindlimb spinal reflexes will be exaggerated (upper motor neuron). Neck pain or stiffness is an inconsistent finding.

Diagnosis

A presumptive diagnosis can be made based on the breed predilection, history, and physical examination. Survey radiographs are usually sufficient to confirm it.

If surgery is contemplated, the complexity and multiplicity of the lesions make high-quality survey radiographs (with the dog anesthetized) and a myelogram mandatory. Radiographs taken with the neck flexed, extended, and with traction have been recommended. Care should be taken when performing these manipulations, because normal mobility might be interpreted as instability, or a dog with an extreme instability could be harmed. Emphasis should be placed on identifying areas of static or dynamic spinal cord compression rather than mere subarachnoid space deviation.

Therapy and Surgical Techniques

Conservative therapy, including confinement and forced rest, affords inconsistent long-term benefit. Commonly, an initial improvement is followed by deterioration when normal activity is resumed. Older dogs with static compressive lesions are unlikely to improve without surgical decompression.

Proper selection of a decompressive procedure for disk herniation begins by determining whether the compression can be relieved by traction. This is done by stretching the neck during myelography. If the compression is static, the protruding mass must be excised through a ventral slot or dorsal laminectomy. If the lesion is reduced by traction, this force can be reproduced and maintained surgically. An abbreviated ventral slot is formed to the level of the cortex lining the spinal canal (see "Ventral Decompression [Slotting] for Cervical Intervertebral Disk Herniation" above). Accessible dorsal annulus and dorsal longitudinal ligaments are excised, and an autogenous or allogenous bone graft is wedged into the slot, placing the intervertebral space under permanent tension. Some surgeons use plate or pin-methylmethacrylate fixation to help maintain the tension and retain the graft. Instability alone should be managed by arthrodesis of either the vertebral bodies or articular facets.

Spinal cord compression from sagittal stenosis, transverse stenosis, or interarcuate ligament encroachment is best relieved by dorsal laminectomy. Concomitant instability can be managed by articular facet arthrodesis through the approach described for dorsal decompression. The joint capsules are incised and the articular cartilage removed with a bur or curette. The facets are fixed with a screw directed slightly caudolaterally through their centers. Care must be taken not to damage the vertebral vessels or cervical nerves when drilling the hole and inserting the screw.

Postoperative Care and Prognosis

Many of these patients require arduous nursing and physiotherapy. Paralyzed patients need constant attention to prevent bladder distention, pressure sores, and atrophy. The prognosis is guarded, and some degree of permanent impairment can be expected if the symptoms were long-standing before surgery.

Cervical Spine Fractures and Luxations

Introduction

Some cervical spine injuries are immediately fatal because they disrupt the vital pathways controlling respiration. However, a surprising number of animals not only survive the initial injury, but may present as ambulatory patients. Most injuries appear to follow an all-or-nothing pattern: either they are fatal due to surpassed tolerances, or they produce transient quadriplegia followed by a high potential for recovery, provided that the spinal cord can be protected from further damage.

Skull traction combined with casts or braces is minimally effective and impractical for use as the only treatment for the unstable cervical spine in the dog. Primary internal fixation and planned fusion is the best treatment in most cases, even when the instability initially appears minor. Without surgery, gradually increasing instability with a worsening neurologic status is the rule rather than the exception.

Achieving a highly stable internal fixation of the cervical spine is difficult and involves technical problems not encountered in the thoracolumbar region. The dorsal spinous processes of C3-7 are too small for dependable plate fixation, and the location of the vertebral artery prevents the use of lateral body plates. This limits fixation sites to the dorsal lamina and facets, or the ventral aspect of the vertebral bodies.

It was once thought that most traumatic spinal cord lesions required decompression, but this philosophy has changed over the last few years. The original theory was that it could do no harm and might improve the chances of recovery, but this has proved false. Routine laminectomy offers minimal (if any) benefits and may in fact increase morbidity and mortality due to additional spinal cord trauma and spinal instability. The current recommendations are to effect decompression by reducing the displacement and to reserve laminectomy for cases with irreducible displacement, bone or disk fragments in the spinal canal, or an otherwise unexplained subarachnoid block as shown by myelography.

Diagnosis

Any dog presenting with acute quadriparesis or quadriplegia (or a history thereof) should be suspected of having sustained cervical spine trauma, especially if it belongs to a breed rarely afflicted by spontaneous disk herniation. Neck pain is a consistent physical finding, but the motor, spinal reflex, or postural reaction changes may be subtle and mild. Severe head injuries are often accompanied by neck injuries, and comatose trauma victims should be evaluated for cervical spine injury before proceeding with therapy or diagnostic tests requiring excessive manipulation. If cervical trauma is suspected, the neck should be protected and further diagnostic tests carried out under the direct and constant supervision of a veterinarian. A bulky support bandage or brace should be applied immediately if the spine is palpably unstable.

Lateral and ventrodorsal radiographs should be taken. Extreme caution should be exercised in positioning the patient, as outlined for atlantoaxial subluxation above. Because most cervical fractures occur through the base of the dens, body, or body-laminar junction of the axis, radiographs of this area should be studied carefully.

Although less common, the character of a caudal cervical fracture (C3-7) should be studied to ascertain the extent of instability, as this will determine the surgical approach and method of repair. If stressed-view radiographs are needed, they should be done gently and judiciously, with the veterinarian doing the positioning. Ideally, image intensification should be used.

Fractures caused by overflexion will be either the classic compression or wedge fracture, characterized by a collapsed, shortened vertebral body, or a more severe injury causing ventral subluxation of the cranial vertebra with tearing of the supporting soft tissues dorsally and luxation of the facets. The intervertebral disk may be ruptured. Fractures caused by overextension are usually transverse vertebral body fractures. They are often self-reducing, but the intervertebral disk may also be disrupted with this type of injury. Rotational forces combined with flexion, extension, or traction will produce fractures or luxations of the facets or pedicles. Myelography is indicated whenever soft-tissue compression is suspected, such as traumatic intervertebral disk herniation.

Techniques for Specific Fractures and Luxations

Atlanto-Occipital Dislocation

Dislocation of the atlanto-occipital joint has been reported in two dogs. Both cases were managed by closed reduction followed by plaster casting, with excellent results.

Fractures of the Atlas

Fractures of the atlantal wing rarely require treatment other than rest and short-term pain relief. Fractures of the atlantal arches usually split the vertebra in roughly equilateral halves. This rare injury is caused by a blow on the head. Both the dorsal and ventral arches must be repaired using interfragmentary wires, or screws and wires, and the ligamentous support for the dens must be assessed.

Axial Fractures and Luxations

Traumatic disruption of the ligamentous support of the dens may be managed like congenital atlantoaxial instability (*i.e.*, by dorsal wiring or ventral pinning). Fractures of the dens often go to nonunion, and achieving stable internal fixation may prove difficult. Although successful odontoidectomy without additional stabilization has been reported, the importance of the dens-ligament complex should not be underestimated, and additional internal fixation is recommended to prevent latent or chronic atlantoaxial instability.

Probably the most common cervical spine fracture in the dog is through the junction of the axial body and the cranial articular facets. Reducing the overriding fragments is difficult from a dorsal approach; even if it is accomplished, dorsal wiring (as if for atlantoaxial luxation) may prove insufficient for stability. A ventral approach is thus recommended, because more direct traction or leverage of the fragments is possible, and the cranial fragment can be partially removed if necessary to effect reduction. The fracture can be fixed with a small plate(s) or pins incorporated in methylmethacrylate (Fig. 19-5). More fixation may be added dorsally in the form of wires and autogenous grafts if the fracture is still unstable.

Fracture of the Caudal Cervical Spine (C3-7)

The surgical approach and method of stabilization for fractures in the C3-7 region depends entirely on the nature of the fracture. Fractures that produce primarily a disruption of the ventral structures (vertebral body, intervertebral disk) may be approached ventrally (see "Ventral Decompression [Slotting] for Cervical Intervertebral Disk Herniation," above). The ventral approach allows direct examination and manipulation of fragments. The fracture can be stabilized with a small interbody plate (contoured metal or plastic) or pin-methylmethacrylate combination. Autogenous bone grafts should be used to encourage rapid healing.

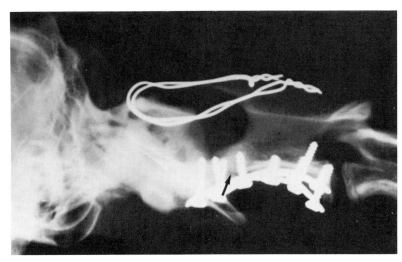

Figure 19-5. *Repair of an axial fracture through the body-laminar junction with two plates and an augmenting dorsal wire. The fracture site is indicated by the arrow.*

Fractures or luxations involving disruption of the dorsal complex (interarcuate, intraspinous, and supraspinous ligaments, dorsal spinous processes, facets and capsules, pedicles) may be managed through a dorsal approach initially (see "Indications for Dorsal Approach and Laminectomy," p. 508). This allows direct inspection and repair of the damage. A good method of stabilization is small pins (Kirschner wires) laid along the bases of the spinous processes bilaterally and secured with wires around the laminar arches or to the facets and spinous processes (Fig. 19-6). This can be augmented with interfacet screw or wire fixation (this might be used as the sole method of fixation for cases of simple facet luxation).

External support with bulky bandages, braces, or splints should be provided after surgery to augment internal fixation. The prognosis depends entirely on the degree of pre-existing spinal cord damage and the ability to attain and maintain spinal stability.

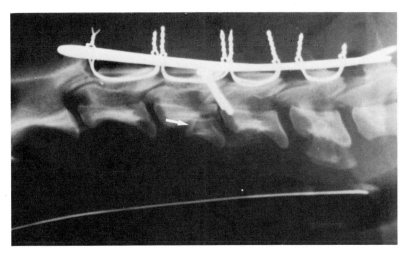

Figure 19-6. *Repair of a C4 fracture with a dorsal pin affixed to the vertebra by sublaminar wires. The fracture is indicated by the arrow.*

The Thoracolumbar Spine

Tommy L. Walker

Thoracolumbar Disk Syndrome

Indications

The most common thoracolumbar spinal disorder in the dog is the intervertebral disk syndrome. Disks of chondrodystrophoid breeds (dachshund, Pekingese, American spaniel, beagle) undergo an inherent chondroid degeneration of the nucleus pulposus that predisposes them to disk extrusions at an early age (Hansen Type I disk disease). Some 80 other breeds have been recognized as having disk disease, but usually at an older age after undergoing a fibrinoid change in the nucleus pulposus (Hansen Type II disk disease). Spontaneous and traumatic intervertebral disk extrusions occur in cats and must be differentiated from thromboembolism of the iliac arteries or abdominal aorta, trauma, tumors, or inflammatory cord disease.

In one report, 73% of dogs 3 to 6 years of age had signs of disk disease; about 65% of these lesions occurred between T11-12 and L1-2, with T12-13 the most commonly affected space. The protrusion (thrusting dorsal or lateral) or extrusion (expulsion) of the disk from its normal position toward the spinal canal or nerve roots is responsible for the clinical syndrome.

The basic lesion resulting from thoracolumbar disk protrusion or extrusion is a compressive myelopathy (a nonspecific, functional disturbance of the spinal cord) or a compressive radiculopathy (disturbance of nerve roots). The first sign of disk disease is pain over the specific area of involvement. The animal will be reluctant to move and may have the back arched in an attempt to relieve the painful pressure of a dorsal protrusion or extrusion. The variety and severity of clinical signs that follow depend predominantly on four factors:

1. The rate at which a disk extrudes.
2. The amount of disk material extruded.
3. The location of the extrusion.
4. The length of time a severe extrusion compresses the cord.

Generally, the more acute an extrusion or protrusion, the more severe the spinal cord damage. The dynamic changes involving edema, hemorrhage, and inflammation complicate the mechanical pressure caused by the disk itself. When a vicious cycle of edema and anoxia begins, the acute focal compression may spread to a localized necrotic myelopathy (myelomalacia). This can become diffuse and lead to an ascending and descending progressive, hemorrhagic necrosis of the spinal cord (hematomyelia or hemorrhagic myelomalacia). Conversely, a large mass of disk material that ruptures slowly (over days) is usually not accompanied by edematous or hemorrhagic changes and may not be as clinically severe.

The location of the disk extrusion is important when considering the resulting clinical effects. An extrusion in the lower lumbar spinal canal (L6,7), which contains only nerve roots, is much less dangerous than an extrusion in an area where the epidural space is narrow (e.g., the area filled by the lumbosacral intumescence L4-5). The location of neurologic involvement also determines whether the neurologic status is one of upper or lower motor neuron signs. Lower motor neuron involvement via extrusions at L4-5 and L5-6 can damage neurons that give rise to the femoral, sciatic, perineal, and pelvic nerves and affect weightbearing and reflex defecation and micturition. An acute, severe extrusion in the thoracolumbar area can also produce a Schiff-Sherington syndrome, the only neurologic syndrome in which clinical signs are manifested cranial to the site of the lesion.

The surgeon must be able to localize the lesion and confirm its etiology before surgery. The clinical application of the neurologic examination, especially the spinal cord reflexes, must be correlated with radiographic findings before the etiology, treatment plan, and prognosis can be established. When the neurologic examination does not correlate with the radiographic changes, further work-up or myelography is indicated.

Surgery should be considered whenever neurologic deficits are present or when repeated attacks of intervertebral disk disease occur. The more dramatic the clinical signs and dynamic their severity, the more important surgery becomes for a good clinical recovery. Cases with first attacks commonly recover with medical therapy but must be carefully monitored to ascertain whether return of function is continuing.

Prognosis

The rate of onset and duration of significant neurologic deficits are critical in the functional neurologic status and assessing and establishing a prognosis. The all-important prognostic component of the neurologic examination is the conscious perception of pain when a noxious (painful) stimuli is applied to the tail and digits of the pelvic limb. When conscious pain perception is intact and the factors of rate of extrusion and duration of compression are favorable, the case generally has a good prognosis. When pain perception has been lost, the prognosis deteriorates rapidly. The duration of time in which an animal without conscious pain perception from the limbs can still recover with surgery is often related to the pathophysiologic changes associated with acute and extensive disk extrusions.

I argue that paralyzed dogs that have lost this sensory capability from the pelvic limbs for 1 to 12 hours should receive immediate decompressive surgery and intensive medical therapy to combat cord edema. These cases will not, as a general rule, recover with the high success rate of good surgical candidates but will respond in sufficient numbers, and with a quality of recovery high enough, to warrant surgery. Dogs presented without pain perception for over 24 hours will occasionally recover with sufficient quality of motor ability to sustain eliminations and prevent decubiti, but will continue to need intensive nursing care.

For an animal to recover to a state of "spinal walking," with reflex control of bladder and bowel function, cord segments L4 through S3 must remain intact and viable. These cases should not be considered functional recoveries or surgical successes.

Surgical Technique

The most common techniques involve hemilaminectomy, with concurrent dorsolateral fenestration, and modified dorsal laminectomy. The involved vertebrae can be identified by radiographically documenting and maintaining the position of a small hypodermic needle, placed adjacent to a dorsal spine, or by injecting a small amount of methylene blue into the identified area after noting the needle's position. This marks the spot for the surgeon when the dorsal spines are approached. The dog is placed in ventral recumbency, with a sandbag or towel under the abdomen to elevate the site of the lesion. If compression of the caudal vena cava leads to excessive hemorrhage via congestion of the vertebral venous sinuses, or if respiration is hampered during surgery, the towel or sandbag should be removed. Dexamethasone is given presurgically (2 mg/kg).

Hemilaminectomy

A right-handed surgeon should work from the animal's left side. When radiographic evidence suggests that a mass is located primarily in the right side of the spinal canal, the surgeon should consider an approach from the right, even though dissection will be awkward and more traumatic.

Centering on the location of the disk extrusion, a dorsal incision is made over a length of four to five vertebrae. The dorsolumbar fascia is incised adjacent to the spinous processes on the surgeon's side. The following dissection should proceed in phases. Preparing the spinous processes, articular processes, and the involved accessory process is achieved systematically. Starting at the caudal most exposed dorsal spinous process and working in a cranial direction, subperiosteal elevation of the musculature and removal of tendinous attachments as close as possible to the spinous processes minimizes tissue trauma (Fig. 19-7). A periosteal elevator is introduced at the caudal ventral aspect of the cranial articular facet of L4 and used to elevate the muscular attachment until only its tendinous insertion is visible (Fig. 19-8). The tendon is cut adjacent to the bone, leaving the cortical surface free of all soft tissue. A surgical sponge can be placed into this area to complete hemostasis while the next articular facet is exposed in a similar manner from L4 to T11. Only the accessory process at the hemilaminectomy site requires exposure by careful division of the thin tendinous muscle attachment. Gelpi retractors may be placed near the involved disk, with one point positioned deep into the paravertebral musculature and the other placed between the spinous processes to afford better exposure. Spinal nerves and blood vessels are easily located cranial and ventral to the accessory process where they are protected by the intact muscular attachments.

If the location of the thoracolumbar junction has thus far been estimated by palpating the last rib through the incision and not by marking the vertebral processes at initial radiography, it is important to identify the landmark by dissecting along the vertebral bodies and identifying the transverse process of L1 and the rib attached to T13. A preoperative ventrodorsal radiograph will confirm that 13 paired ribs exist and may prevent the confusion caused by an anomaly.

A decompressive hemilaminectomy is initiated by removing the articular facet dorsal to the involved disk space with a pair of large rongeurs. For small dogs or cats with thin cortices, the spinal canal is most easily entered with a Lempert rongeur. A towel clamp placed in the cranial spinous process can be used to separate the remaining articular base, using a forward and upward motion. One blade of the rongeur is wedged into the space to begin the

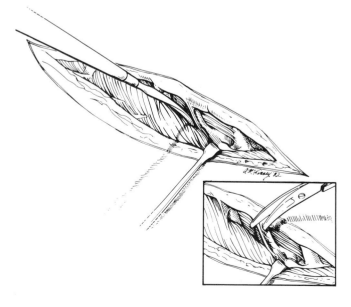

Figure 19-7. *Working in a caudal to cranial direction, the spinous processes of L4 through T11 are exposed with subperiosteal elevation over the body of the process and incision of the tendinous insertions of the multifidus lumborum and multifidus thoracis muscles.*

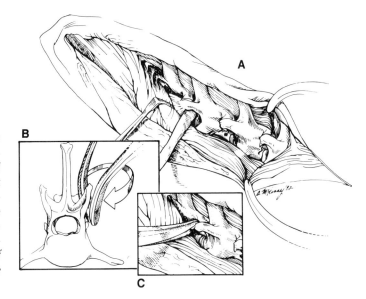

Figure 19-8. *Caudal to cranial isolation of the facets is initiated by inserting a periosteal elevator or scalpel handle at their caudal ventral border (**A**). With the instrument kept against the bone, the muscle can be elevated by advancing and rotating the elevator along the facet's ventral surface (**B**) until only the tendinous insertions of the multifidus and longissimus muscles remain attached. Incision of these tendons as close to the bone as possible will minimize hemorrhage (**C**).*

hemilaminectomy (Fig. 19-9). An alternate entry is a modified lateral decompressive technique that allows the surgeon to rongeur only the lateral intervertebral foramen below the articular facets. This allows for a more stable vertebral architecture when only small amounts of disk material and cord swelling are involved.

In dogs with thicker cortices or any large-breed dog, a high-speed surgical drill (A200 Air Drill, 3M, St. Paul, MN; Moto-Flex Tool, Dremel, Racine, WI) can be used to facilitate entry into the canal (Fig. 19-10). Sharp spherical burs are used in a paintbrush fashion to remove a thin layer of bone with each sweep of the bur.

Landmarks for determining the burr's depth are critical. First encountered is the dense outer cortical layer, followed by the trabecular cancellous layer and a thin inner crust of cortical bone adjacent to the spinal canal.

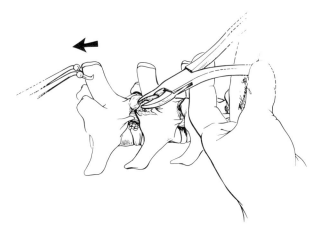

Figure 19-9. *In small and thin-boned dogs, the articular facets can be opened by traction on the rostral vertebrae to get a "toe hold" with a small ronguer (Lempert) to initiate the hemilaminectomy.*

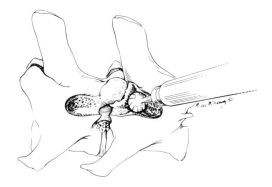

Figure 19-10. *An air drill can be used to facilitate entry into the spinal canal.*

Final entry into the canal is made with a blunt dental scaler and rongeur. A bur should never be used to enter the canal due to the potential for iatrogenic cord damage. Whichever drill is used, the importance of sharp burs cannot be overemphasized. A dull bur will fill with bone more quickly and lose its effectiveness in cutting. Burning of bone results, which obliterates the contrast of dense outer cortical bone and inner trabecular cancellous bone. When the depth perception is obscured, premature entry into the spinal canal with the drill is more likely.

The initial burring should extend from the base of the next cranial articular facet to the base of the articular facet caudal to the site of disk extrusion. The length of the decompressive hemilaminectomy should be extended until epidural fat is reached at both its cranial and caudal extent, because the loss of epidural fat around the spinal cord is representative of cord compression. The extruded disk material and blood clots that may have resulted from rupture of the venous sinus are gently removed with a dental scaler or similar instrument. Care must be taken to tease the material from around the cord without trauma. Often, material in the right spinal canal can be removed from the left-sided hemilaminectomy opening. Normothermic saline irrigation is used to bathe the area frequently. A syringe and blunt needle can be used to flush remnants of nucleus from beneath the cord with a gentle "water jet" action. If hemorrhage should occur from the venous sinuses, packing the area with a gelatin pad (Gelfoam, Upjohn Kalamazoo, MI), a small wedge of muscle, or a surgical sponge will facilitate clotting. Suction should be used with caution to prevent traumatic injury to the cord by the suction tip.

In cases of suspected focal myelomalacia where exploratory surgery is being performed or when a swollen spinal cord protrudes from the decompression site, a durotomy is indicated for both prognostic and decompressive reasons. A #12 scalpel blade, a 20-gauge needle with a 90° bend in the sharp tip, or Potts-Smith cardiovascular scissors with a 60° angle can be used to make the durotomy incision. Durotomies are most safely performed from a dorsal approach, but can be done from the lateral dural surface via a hemilaminectomy. The site is covered with an absorbable gelatin sheet (Gelfoam, Upjohn, Kalamazoo, MI) or an autogenous fat graft from the dorsolumbar area.

Fenestration

Disk fenestration can be performed after the decompression is complete or while controlling hemorrhage from a venous sinus. In chondrodystrophic breeds or other breeds showing radiographic signs of disk degeneration adjacent to extruded disks, fenestration is a standard prophylactic practice in many clinics. Although fenestration's role in preventing future extrusions is controversial, when performed properly it is a viable means of transforming a potentially degenerative disk into a stabilized fibrotic space.

After identifying the articular facet, the accessory process is identified with its muscular attachments intact. The spinal nerves and vessels are located cranial and ventral to the process while the disk is located caudal and ventral. A periosteal elevator or scalpel handle and sponge can be used to elevate the soft tissue from the vertebral body and lateral annulus of the disk (Fig. 19-11). In the lumbar area, these disks are just cranial to the junction of the transverse process and vertebral body; in the thoracic area, they are just cranial to the rib head. The muscular attachments to the accessory processes are used to protect the spinal nerves, acting as a pad between delicate bundles and the instrument.

Once the disk is located, a House curette or fenestration knife is introduced into its central point and directed horizontally until its tip is buried in the nuclear area. The disk is removed by a downward and outward rotation of the instrument, forming a window (fenestration) in the lateral annulus. The motion is repeated until little or no disk material can be removed. A 12- to 14-gauge intravenous needle can also be used to fenestrate the disk. It is

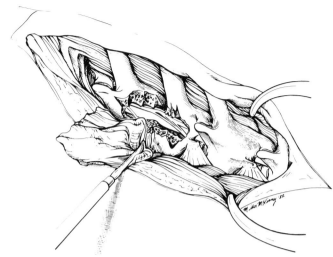

Figure 19-11. *The disk space is exposed by using a gauze sponge and periosteal elevator to elevate the soft tissue from the vertebral body and lateral annulus and is always approached from a caudal to cranial direction to protect the nerve roots with the muscles and tendons inserting on the accessory process.*

placed in a similar manner but is used in a boring action to remove cores of nuclear material.

The important steps in fenestration are adequate visualization of the disk, hemostasis, and removal of the entire nucleus pulposus. Curettage of the dorsal or ventral annulus is of little value. The nuclear material should be removed from radiographically degenerative disks in the surgical area. Some surgeons routinely fenestrate T11-12 through L1-2 to eliminate the disks at highest risk. The most difficulty is encountered at T11-12, where the disk is narrow and more vertical than in the lumbar area. If L4-5 and L5-6 are fenestrated, extra care must be taken to protect the nerve roots. The nerves exiting L4, L5, and L6 form the femoral nerve, and damage to any part of the nerve root could result in a permanent motor deficit to the involved limb.

Fenestration is widely used alone for prophylaxis in dogs with several episodes of nonparalytic disk disease. The intent is to remove the disks via fenestration before a dorsal protrusion can occur that results in paralysis.

Dorsal Laminectomy

Several types of dorsal laminectomies have been described to treat intervertebral disk disease and to explore the spinal canal (Fig. 19-12). The most important is the modified dorsal laminectomy, which allows greater decompression than other techniques.

The preparation and basic approach to the dorsal spine is identical to that for hemilaminectomy, except that the dorsal exposure extends ventral to the articular facets on both sides of the dorsal spines. At least two vertebrae are exposed cranial and caudal to the involved disk. The dorsal spinous processes of the two vertebrae involved are removed with rongeurs and the dorsal lamina burred away using a high-speed drill (A200 Air Drill, 3M, St. Paul, MN). In the original technique, a 4-mm egg-shaped bur with notched flutes (Amsco/Hall, Santa Barbara, CA) is used to drill laterally, leaving the cranial articular process intact and removing the caudal (more medial) articular processes to gain width in the decompression. It allows accurate undercutting of the laminectomy edges for improved decompression, but requires extreme caution in the vertebral interspaces where only dense cortical bone and intra-articular ligaments are present. With only a thin inner cortical layer of dorsal lamina left intact, a 2.3- or 1.6-mm round carbide-tip bur is used to remove the thin dorsal plate of bone by drilling around the edge of the laminectomy site, holding the drill at a 45° angle away from the spinal cord (Fig.

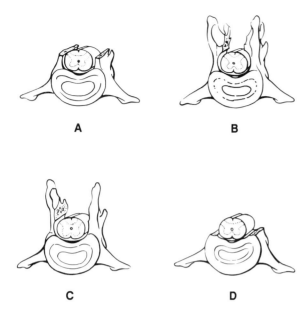

Figure 19-12. *Types of dorsal laminectomies.* ***A,*** *Funkquist A, which is subject to secondary cicatricial compression.* ***B,*** *Funkquist B, the standard dorsal laminectomy procedure. The dorsal lateral arches remain above the cord so that cicatricial compression is not a problem.* ***C,*** *Modified dorsal laminectomy (Trotter), which provides a more spacious decompression.* ***D,*** *Modified deep dorsal laminectomy (total dorsal laminectomy), which may be used for severe cord trauma in spinal fractures.*

19-13). The inner cortical shelf is elevated and removed. Further decompression depends on the amount and location of fat in the epidural space.

The modified dorsal laminectomy allows the surgeon to inspect the spinal canal and remove lateralized disk material or other compressive masses. When peracute disk extrusions result in bulging of the dural tube, a dorsal midline durotomy or, in some cases, myelotomy can be performed to evaluate the cord for myelomalacia or hematomyelia and to aid in the treatment of severe traumatic spinal injuries.

Closure

Regardless of which technique is used, complete hemostasis and repeated normothermic saline flushing to remove bone chips are nec-

essary during surgery. The elevated periosteum and musculature is returned to its proper position and the dorsolumbar fascia is sutured with absorbable material in a simple interrupted pattern. Redundant subcutaneous fat is apposed with a continuous pattern of absorbable material. Subcutaneous tissues are approximated and closed, as is the skin. Bandaging is unnecessary if good hemostasis and adequate closure of tissue dead spaces have been achieved.

Postoperative Care

Although recommendations for their postsurgical use differ, adrenocorticoids should not be used in paraplegic animals any longer than 72 hours after surgery. The relationship between prolonged steroid use and colonic or duodenal ulcers is convincing, limiting their once-indiscriminant use. Currently, several clinics give one or two doses of dexamethasone (1 to 2 mg/kg IV) after surgery at 12-hour intervals. A broad-spectrum antibiotic is given for at least three days after steroid therapy is discontinued; therapy should be prolonged if a urinary infection exists.

Urinary bladder tone must be maintained if a prompt return to reflex emptying is to be expected. The patient's bladder should be expressed twice daily or catheterized if necessary to ensure emptying. The patient must remain in the hospital until conscious urinary control returns or until the owner understands the techniques and importance of expressing and maintaining the bladder in a healthy state.

Foam pads, elevated cage liners, and water pads markedly reduce the incidence of decubiti in paralyzed dogs. Whirlpool baths after suture removal or after coating the incision with collodion not only improve circulation and prevent muscle atrophy, but also clean the animal and aid in recovery. Walking exercises with the aid of an abdominal sling and manual physical therapy of the pelvic limbs also greatly facilitate motor recovery. Between periods of physical therapy, the patient should be confined to a playpen or cage to

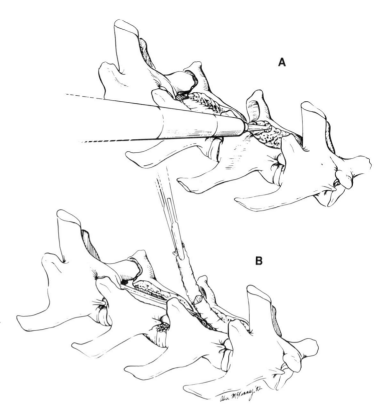

Figure 19-13. *Angled drilling into the cancellous bone around the periphery of the thin plate of inner cortical bone avoids working directly over the spinal cord (**A**). The deeply undercut edge allows easy removal of the dorsal arch and increased spinal cord exposure (**B**).*

prevent self-mutilation or further aggravation of the condition.

Thoracolumbar—Sacral Spinal Trauma

Indications

The thoracolumbar and lumbosacral areas may be the most common areas of vertebral derangement from trauma. Regardless of the type of fracture or combination of fractures, the mode of treatment and necessity of decompression and/or fixation depend on five factors:

1. A serial neurologic examination
2. The stability of the fracture and the assessed compression of the cord
3. The animal's size
4. The integrity of the vertebral spinous processes and vertebral body
5. The fracture's location.

The radiographic diagnosis establishes the type of fracture or subluxation and the specific location of involvement, but it provides only a skeletal picture of what existed when the image was taken. In any vertebral fracture, profound motor deficits and radiographic findings of severe vertebral displacement do not necessarily mean a poor prognosis. Regardless of the degree of displacement, the conscious response to pain remains the only viable prognostic indicator. Patients having stable, mildly displaced fractures or subluxations with minimal neurologic deficits often are best handled conservatively. Most surgeons still consider the most consistent medical treatment to be corticosteroids used during the initial stages of injury.

In these cases, the fragments are not likely to move or cause neural damage during healing. Strict confinement to a cage for 4 to 8 weeks and good nursing care will often allow satisfactory recovery. Excessive movement during this critical period may cause the healing callus to enlarge, resulting in secondary cord compression after an initial clinical improvement. In an animal with an unstable or grossly displaced fracture, the animal's size and the radiographic examination of the spinous process and vertebral bodies will determine the mode of fixation. Many unstable fractures require decompression to assess cord damage not visualized on plain radiographs. Because a laminectomy will further destabilize the area of trauma, it should be used only when needed to evaluate cord integrity.

Surgical Technique

Decompressive hemilaminectomy or modified lateral hemilaminectomy should be used in conjunction with most forms of spinal stabilization. Hemilaminectomy allows removal of depressed bone fragments, redirection of the spinal cord around an abnormal contour of the vertebral canal, durotomy for decompression or prognostic exploration of a swollen cord, and removal of epidural hemorrhage or foreign bodies. The number of vertebrae exposed and the dissection ventral to the articular processes are minimized. Dorsal laminectomy provides decompression but requires the removal of the vertebral spinous processes, which may be needed for fixation and provide postsurgical protection. When a unilateral hemilaminectomy provides inadequate spinal decompression, a bilateral modified lateral hemilaminectomy may be indicated.

The thoracolumbar spine can be stabilized by plating or pinning either the vertebral spinous processes or vertebral bodies. Reducing the fracture may be unnecessary and should be performed only after decompression to help prevent iatrogenic trauma. When the vertebral spinous processes are used for fixation, each one used must be intact. The dorsal approach is modified to reflect a broad band of thoracolumbar fascia to cover the plates. When the vertebral body is used for immobilization, the standard dorsolateral approach allows adequate exposure for decompression and implant application. A combination of both spinous process and vertebral body fixa-

tions provides the most secure means of fixation.

Spinous Process Stabilization

Metal Plates

Metal plates (Auburn Spinal Plates, Richards Mfg. Co., Memphis, TN) are best fitted for transverse and compression vertebral body fractures, as well as luxations and subluxations of the lower thoracic and the entire lumbar spine in dogs over 12 kg. The spinous processes of these vertebrae are wide enough to support a bolt placed through their base. The plates range in length from 3.5 to 12.4 cm and should be long enough to include two spinous processes cranial and two caudal to the fracture. They should be positioned as low on the spinous processes as possible to gain maximum purchase of bone when the holes are drilled. Adjusting the plate along the long axis of the spine will align most holes with the center of the process; rongeurs can be used to create a grove in the ridge of laminar bone between the articular and spinous processes (Fig. 19-14) for more ventral seating.

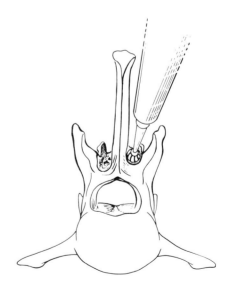

Figure 19-14. *Removal of the ridge of laminar bone between the articular and spinous process with a bur or ronguer allows the plate to fit more ventrally against the spinous process.*

With one plate held in place, a hole is drilled with a drill bit to allow easy movement of the bolt through the plate and spinous processes. After each hole is drilled, a bolt is placed to engage a plate, the spinous process, and a second plate. When all bolts are in place, they are secured with a washer and nut and firmly tightened without crushing or breaking the spinous process (Fig. 19-15). Excess bolt material is cut off adjacent to the nut.

Plastic Plates

The indications and basic approach for applying plastic plates (Lubra Plates, Lubra Co., Ft. Collins, CO) to the thoracic and lumbar spinous processes are identical to those for metal plates. These plates are made of a vinylidine fluoride resin and have one smooth and one roughened friction grip surface. Four plate sizes (ranging from small to extra-large) allow the incorporation of two or three spinous processes on each side of the fracture. The plastic can be contoured to some degree with rongeurs, high-speed burs, or a scalpel to maintain better plate contact with the base of the spinous processes. Vitallium nuts and bolts (Vitallium, Howmedica, Rutherford, NJ) en-

gage both plates between the spinous processes rather than through them. Stainless-steel bolts similar to those described for metal plates can be used, but they may loosen if not applied with a nut and washer on each side of the plate. Tightening the bolts apposes the plates and holds them to the spinous process by friction and compression (Fig. 19-16).

These plates are more useful in the thoracic area than the stainless-steel plates because no holes are drilled through the base of the narrow thoracic spinous processes. Plastic plates are available in longer lengths for use in giant breeds and may be more practical than stainless-steel plates in these animals. Their disadvantage lies in how they establish fixation. The pressure required for the plate to hold or "sandwich" the spinous processes can cause remodeling of bone where the plate touches the bone. As the fracture stabilizes and the dog becomes more active, more active spinal flexion and extension may cause the grip on the cranial and caudal spinous processes to loosen. The resulting movement instigates a seromatous response that often requires plate removal for resolution.

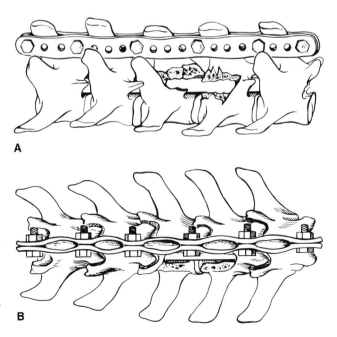

Figure 19-15. *Lateral (**A**) and dorsal ventral view (**B**) of metal spinal plates in place with at least two spinous processes cranial and two caudal to the site of instability. The plates are placed as low as possible on the spinous processes to provide a greater purchase of cortical bone by the bolts.*

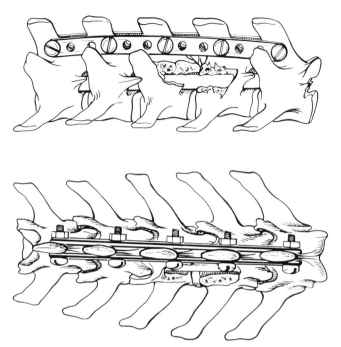

Figure 19-16. *Plastic plates hold the spinous processes between their friction grip surfaces. The bolts and nuts are placed between the spinous process.*

Stainless-Steel Pins and Wires

Spinal staples are an excellent means of fixation in the thoracic, lumbar, and sacral spine in cats and in dogs weighing less than 12 kg. Small holes are drilled at the base of the spinous process of the fractured vertebra and two spines on both sides of the fracture. The diameter of the end holes should be the same as the pin used for fixation. The fixation pin is selected (0.15 to 0.11 mm in diameter) according to the animal's size. The pin is bent at a 90° angle at exactly the length between the most cranial and caudal holes. The ends of the pin are left long and inserted through the holes until the pin lies against the base of the spinous processes. The long ends are then bent back toward the fracture and can be cut off 2 to 3 cm from the bend (Fig. 19-17) or may be left long to allow double strength (Fig. 19-18). Final crimping secures both sides of the fixation pin against the most cranial and caudal spinous processes. Orthopedic wire (22 to 24 gauge) is then passed through the holes and around the pin to secure the intervening spines. In cases of compression fracture, the pin may be bent at a length 1 to 2 mm longer than the distance between the most cranial and caudal holes to allow for distraction of the fracture. Allowing too much distraction or using a shorter length to compress the fracture can lend to disastrous results.

Transilial Pinning

When a fracture subluxation of the lumbosacral joint occurs, the sacral component usually travels cranial and ventral to the main portion or remnants of L7. The pathophysiologic changes occurring at the lumbosacral junction differ from those at the thoracic and lumbar spine because only nerve roots are compressed, and a decompression must occur through a limited dorsal laminectomy. The integrity of these nerve roots—vital for proper function of the micturition and defecation reflex—cannot be overemphasized. Also, although exact reduction after decompression is not always necessary in other parts of the spine, it is important in the lumbosacral area for immobilization. Once the nerve roots are decompressed and the fracture-subluxation

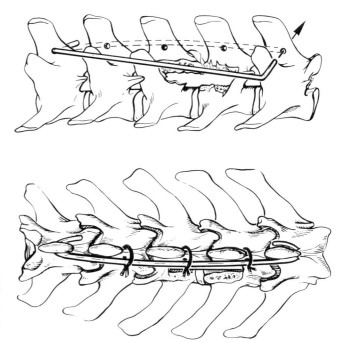

Figure 19-17. *Spinal stapling using a 1.6-cm stainless steel intramedullary pin bent at right angles to span the distance between the predrilled cranial and caudal spinous processes. The ends are cut 2 to 3 cm from the bend, inserted into the holes, and crimped as shown.*

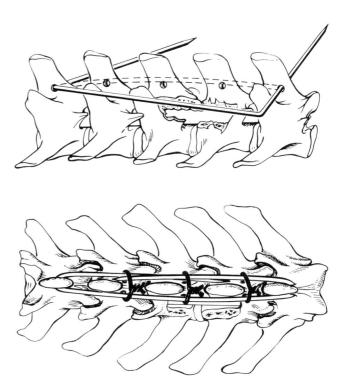

Figure 19-18. *Spinal stapling modification. Doubling the pin provides additional strength.*

reduced, dorsal spinal plates (metal or plastic) may be placed from the lower lumbar spines to the sacral spinous processes. In small dogs and cats, the sacral processes are too small to accept a bolt and often will not hold when a plastic plate is applied. In large-breed dogs, a plate large enough to immobilize the lumbosacral junction may be too large to secure the sacrum.

Using a transilial pin either by itself (Fig. 19-19) or with a plate provides the necessary extra fixation (Fig. 19-20). The pin (or pin and plate) touches the dorsal surface of L7 to prevent the ilium-sacral unit from subluxating ventral to it and prevents further displacement. The transilial pin can be secured by bending the ends of the pins flush with the ilium or using a threaded pin and nut to secure one end of the pin and a 90° bend at the other end.

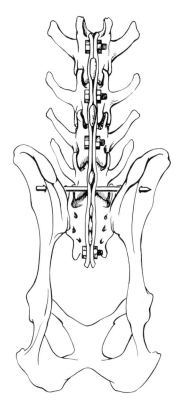

Figure 19-20. *Transilial pin used in conjunction with dorsal plates provides additional support for lumbar or lumbosacral fractures.*

Vertebral Body Stabilization

Vertebral Body Plating

Vertebral fractures in a medium to large dog in which a majority of the vertebral body remains intact may be repaired by applying small bone plates (Vertebral Body Plates, Richards Mfg. Co., Memphis, TN) to the dorsolateral vertebral body surfaces. Exposure and vertebral size limit the technique to the caudal thoracic area and the cranial lumbar region (T12—L4). The approach is less extensive but otherwise identical to that for the dorsolateral hemilaminectomy, which may be used for decompression before plate fixation. It may also be helpful to position the animal with the left side slightly elevated, placing the vertebral body at an elevated 30° angle and facilitating screw-hole placement.

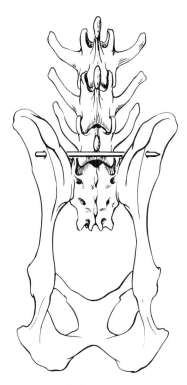

Figure 19-19. *Transilial pin used to stabilize a fracture of the body or a lumbosacral subluxation.*

The plate is positioned so that it rests at the transverse process—vertebral body junction just ventral to the hemilaminectomy defect (Fig. 19-21). The spinal nerve exiting the involved interspace is located and severed to prevent entrapment by the plate or future osteophyte formation; therefore, plates cannot be applied where roots of the lumbosacral plexus are present (L4-5 through L7-S1). The plate size is selected so that two holes are located cranial and two holes caudal to the fracture or subluxation. Comminuted and transverse fractures that do not allow adequate purchase of bone with the screws are not candidates for this type of fixation.

A hole is drilled through the cranial or caudal plate holes in a ventral lateral direction to allow threads to engage in the maximum amount of bone possible. It is important to cover the hemilaminectomy defect with a finger to prevent the screwdriver from slipping off the screw and injuring the cord.

Applying the plates to the caudal thoracic area requires temporary dislocation of

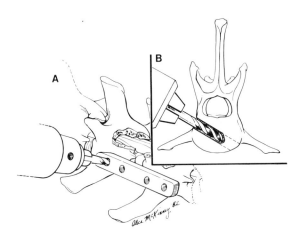

Figure 19-21. *The vertebral body plate is placed at the junction of the transverse process and the vertebral body in the lumbar area (**A**). The spinal nerves are severed at the site of placement, which prevents placement of a plate at the L4 through L7 interspace. Proper path of the drill through the vertebral body to supply maximum purchase of cortical bone (**B**).*

the rib heads from their costovertebral articulation. A small Kirschner wire is used to drill a dorsoventral hole in the head of each rib to be separated from its vertebrae. The rib heads are separated with bone cutters and retracted ventrally, allowing plate application as previously described. A pneumothorax is sometimes unavoidable when rib disarticulation is performed; this should be considered in the anesthetic management of the case before surgery. In a severely traumatized area, tissues must be dissected and handled carefully to facilitate closure of the thoracic wall defect.

When decompression and plating are complete, approximating the ribs to their original position allows a more cosmetic closure. Stainless-steel orthopedic wire is used to elevate the rib by passing from the predrilled rib head to the corresponding spinous process. Closure is identical to that for hemilaminectomy.

Vertebral Body Pinning

Cross-Pinning

This method of fixation is useful in repairing subluxations, particularly in the lumbar area. It is frequently used after other methods have been exhausted due to fractured spinous processes, vertebrae that are too small for bone plating, or immature bone too soft for traditional fixation. It is not used in the thoracic area due to limited exposure and rib location.

The standard hemilaminectomy approach and decompression is used. Pins from 0.15 to 0.11 mm in diameter are used most often; larger pins have been suggested in larger breeds. In most cases, the subluxation is immobilized by cross-pinning the involved vertebral bodies. One pin is introduced into the vertebral body cranial to the lesion to a point midway along the vertebral area or the ribs in the caudal thoracic area. The pin is aimed in a caudal ventral direction to cross the involved disc space and seat with a good purchase of bone in the next caudal vertebral body. A second pin in introduced into the caudal vertebra

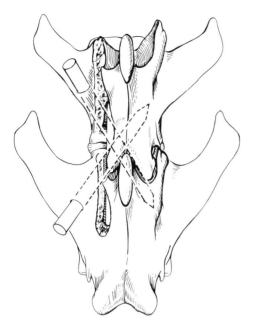

Figure 19-22. *A cross-pin technique is used to span a single intervertebral space or fracture.*

and directed to assume a similar diagonal course, resulting in the cross-pinning configuration (Fig. 19-22). It may be necessary to introduce the pins through the paravertebral musculature and direct them into the vertebral body to achieve the proper angle of insertion.

Vertebral body pinning has been used in cases of transverse vertebral fractures by anchoring each pin in adjacent normal vertebral bodies. This type of fixation is difficult and

would probably require a form of spinous process immobilization.

Methylmethacrylate
Small intramedullary pins or Kirschner wires can be inserted into the vertebral bodies (Fig. 19-23) cranial and caudal to the fracture or subluxation. The pins are placed from a dorsolateral point on the vertebral body and directed ventrally and medially. The pins are cut at the level of the dorsal spinous processes and crimped with a pin-cutter to allow a better cement interface.

The laminectomy is covered with gelatin foam sponge. The mixed methylmethacrylate is placed around the pons, avoiding the spinal cord due to the excessive temperatures generated during polymerization. Sterile styrofoam, as well as copious lavage with cool saline during polymerization, can be used to protect the cord when a hemilaminectomy is used.

Postoperative Care

The postoperative medical therapy discussed for severe thoracolumbar disk cases applies equally to trauma patients. Immature or large-breed dogs with internal fixation may fracture the spinous processes if the fixation is not supplemented with external support for 3 to 4 weeks after surgery.

The splint should be applied under profound sedation or anesthesia. Appropriate

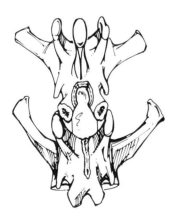
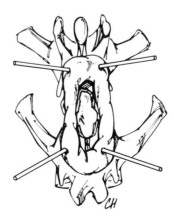

Figure 19-23. *Before and after pin placement and application of methyl methacrylate.*

support material of thin plywood, yucca board, or aluminum splint rod should be cut to the correct length, the material should be heavily padded on each end to prevent pressure on the incision, the entire area of the body to be splinted should be wrapped with case padding and roll gauze, and finally the entire area should be covered with casting material or heavy tape.

The material should fit snugly in the flank area and may require anchoring to the hair cranially. A wedge or triangle is cut to free the prepuce when necessary. Many splints are found to be excessively loose soon after application due to emptying of gas from the stomach or poor coaptation to the caudal abdomen. Heavy taping, therefore, provides a more secure fixation that is more amenable to modification. A body cast or splint applied securely over the thoracic area must not impair respiration.

Cauda Equine Syndrome

Indications

The cauda equina syndrome is a neurologic problem resulting from any compression, destruction, or displacement of the nerve roots that form the cauda equina.

Developmental abnormalities such as stenosis of the lumbar and/or sacral canal, stenosis of the intervertebral foramen, and abnormal articulation at the lumbosacral joint may not cause clinical signs until old age. Long-term biomechanical stress results in bony changes or hypertrophy of the ligamentum flavum from trauma, neoplasia, intervertebral disk protrusions, hypertrophic spondylosis, or diskospondylitis. Many of these degenerative-type diseases are characterized by pronounced spondylosis ventral to the lumbosacral joint, subluxation, and spondylolisthesis (vertebral displacement). The result of the stenosis, regardless of etiology, is cauda equina compression and nerve-root entrapment.

The most common clinical sign is pain in the lumbosacral spinal area and tail. Other common signs include pelvic limb lameness, difficulty in rising, paresis of the tail, urinary and/or fecal incontinence, perineal hyperalgesia or analgesia, paresthesia, and occasionally self-mutilation of the tail and perineal areas. Lumbosacral spinal reflexes may be decreased or absent. Clinical signs vary greatly, owing to multiple etiologies and different degrees of nerve-root compression. Although no age, breed, or sex predilection has been established, reportedly there is a higher incidence in older dogs and, particularly, breeds with a higher incidence of hip dysplasia. Unless motor signs are apparent, the early clinical signs of this syndrome can be easily confused with hip dysplasia. Other differential diagnoses include degenerative myelopathy, type II disk protrusion, diskospondylitis, and spinal neoplasia.

Radiographic findings for cauda equina syndrome include stenosis of the lumbar and/or sacral canals, stenosis of the intervertebral foramina, malformation and/or angulation of the lumbosacral joint, spondylosis deformans of the lumbosacral space, and diskospondylitis. Survey radiographs alone do not usually provide enough evidence to confirm the diagnosis, but can show compatible changes. Diagnosis is based on history, clinical signs, physical and neurologic examinations, and radiographic findings consistent with the diagnosis. Because the subarachnoid space is usually absent at the cauda equina, myelography is often inconclusive. Transosseous vertebral sinus venography, epidurograms, and electromyography are valuable in confirming the diagnosis.

Surgical Techniques

L7-S1 can be decompressed by a deep dorsal or conventional dorsal laminectomy. The etiology and the extent of the compression determine the type of surgery required. Once the dorsal spines of L7 and the sacrum are exposed, the dorsal-ventral manipulation of these structures will demonstrate any instability. When vertebral stabilization is indicated, the articular facets and spinous processes should be retained for fixation identical to that for fractures of the lumbosacral joint.

The dorsal approach to the lumbosacral spine is a modification of the thoracolumbar dorsal approach. A midline skin incision from L6 to S3 is followed by reflection of the hypaxial musculature from the spinous processes and dorsal lamina of the sacrum and of L6 and L7 vertebrae. Gelpi retractors are placed in the musculature. Using an air drill or small rongeur, the dorsal lamina is removed between the articular facets (Fig. 19-24). A hypertrophied ligamentum flavum may be present and should be removed with caution due to its close association to the cauda equina. When the L7 nerve root is entrapped, a foraminotomy is indicated. Generally, only a small part of the

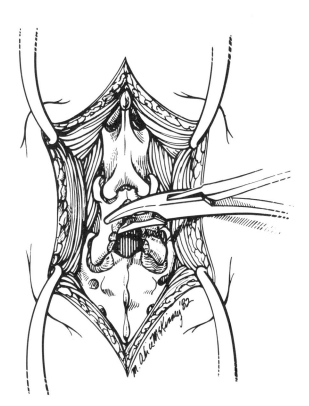

Figure 19-24. *Removal of the dorsal lamina with air drill or ronguers allows decompression of the cauda equina.*

cranial aspect of the foramen is removed. Bilateral foraminotomies, which can extend to include facetotomies (excision of the articular facets), may be required in cases of massive root compression. Placing a gelatin sponge over the laminectomy site may help prevent cicatrix formation.

The spinal cord ends at L6 or L7 in the dog and terminates as nerve roots and a dural sac through the lumbosacral area. A durotomy performed through the laminectomy will allow examination of S1, S2, and S3 nerve roots. Further examination or fenestration of the lumbosacral joint can be accomplished by gently elevating the roots and dura over the disk space. Because the roots traversing the area are required for reflex urination and anal tone, gentle decompression is of utmost importance.

Before closure, the lumbosacral joint should be checked for stability. A towel clamp placed in the dorsal spinous process of L7 is used to elevate the vertebral body. If more than 1 mm of subluxation occurs at the L7 sacral articular processes, a transilial pin is indicated for stabilization. Failure to recognize and stabilize an instability can lead to prolonged recovery and deterioration of clinical signs.

Closure and Postoperative Care

The dorsal fascia, subcutaneous tissues, and skin are closed routinely. Bladder function should be monitored closely and appropriate treatment instituted for urine retention cystitis, as needed. When instability is evident, exercise should be restricted for 6 to 8 weeks. Analgesics or sedatives may be indicated immediately after surgery when paresthesia or lumbosacral hyperesthesia are present.

Spinal Neoplasia

Vertebral tumors, whether malignant or benign, metastatic or primary, generally gain clinical significance when the mass compresses nervous tissue or the invasive growth pattern of the tumor debilitates the vertebral architecture, resulting in pathologic fracture. Decompression and vertebral fixation are usually palliative and of limited long-term clinical value due to the tumor types often involved (*e.g.*, osteosarcoma). The exception to this rule is multiple cartilaginous exostoses. These benign proliferations affect vertebrae and all other bones formed by endochondral ossification. Growth of the tumor ceases at maturity, making cord decompression a more permanent form of treatment. Advances in chemotherapy may render other tumors (such as multiple myeloma and lymphosarcoma) more amenable to decompressive treatment by managing tumor size and possible metastasis.

Myelography is required for all tumors that involve the spinal canal or spinal cord but do not destroy normal bone. These tumors may be classified as extradural (hemangiosarcoma, lymphosarcoma), intradural-extramedullary (neurofibroma, meningioma), or intramedullary (astrocytoma). Meningiomas can be removed with a favorable prognosis if discovered early in their clinical course.

Surgery for all suspected intramedullary and most metastatic extradural tumors is of an exploratory and diagnostic nature and should not be considered a viable form of treatment. The modified dorsal laminectomy provides the best exposure for most exploratory decompressions in the thoracolumbar region.

Suggested Readings

The Cervical Spine

Basinger RR, Bjorling DE. Cervical spinal luxation in two dogs with entrapment of the cranial articular process of C6 over the caudal articular process of C5. J Am Vet Med Assoc 1986;188:865.

Chambers JN, Betts CW. Caudal cervical spondylopathy in the dog: a review of 20 clinical cases and the literature. J Am Anim Hosp Assoc 1977;13:571.

Cook JR, Oliver JE. Atlantoaxial luxation in the dog. Compend Contin Ed Pract Vet 1981;3:242.

Felts JF, Prata RG. Cervical disk disease in the dog: intraforaminal and lateral extrusions. J Am Anim Hosp Assoc 1987;19:755.

Raffe MR, Knecht CD. Cervical vertebral malformation—a review of 36 cases. J Am Anim Hosp Assoc 1980;16:881.

Seim HB, Prata RG. Ventral decompression for the treatment of cervical disk disease in the dog: a review of 54 cases. J Am Anim Hosp Assoc 1982;18:233.

Seim HB, Withrow SJ. Pathophysiology and diagnosis of caudal cervical spondylopathy with emphasis on the Doberman pinscher. J Am Anim Hosp Assoc 1982;18:241.

Sorjonen DC, Shires PK. Atlantoaxial instability: a ventral surgical technique for decompression, fixation, and fusion. Vet Surg 1981;10:22.

Stone EA, Betts CW, et al. Cervical fractures in the dog: a literature and case review. J Am Anim Hosp Assoc 1979;15:463.

Withrow SJ, Seim HB. Caudal cervical spondylopathy and myelopathy in large-breed dogs. In Bojrab MJ, ed. Current techniques in small animal surgery. Philadelphia: Lea & Febiger, 1983:541.

The Thoracolumbar Spine

Bitetto WV, Thacher C. A modified lateral decompressive technique for treatment of canine intervertebral disc disease. J Am Anim Hosp Assoc 1987;23:409.

Griffiths IR. Trauma of the spinal cord. Vet Clin North Am 1980;10:131.

Oliver JE, Lorenz MD. Handbook of veterinary neurologic diagnosis. Philadelphia: WB Saunders, 1983;159.

Smith GK, Walter MC. Fractures and luxations of the spine. In: Newton CD, Nunamaker DM, eds. Textbook of small animal orthopedics. Philadelphia: JB Lippincott, 1985;307.

Trotter EJ. Thoracolumbar intervertebral disc disease. In: Current techniques in small animal surgery. 2nd ed. Philadelphia: Lea & Febiger, 1982;475.

Turner WD. Fractures and fracture-luxations of the lumbar spine: A retrospective study in the dog. J Am Anim Hosp Assoc 1987;23:459.

Walker TL, Tomlinson J, Sorjonen DC, Kornegay JN. Diseases of the spinal column. In: Slatter DH, ed. Textbook of small animal surgery. Philadelphia: WB Saunders, 1985;1385.

Walter MC, Smith GK, Newton CD. Canine lumbar spinal internal fixation techniques—a comparative biomechanical study. Vet Surg 1986;15:191.

20

Charles D. Newton

Orthopedic Basic Sciences

Structure and Function of Bone

Cellular Components and Bone Formation

Bone is a dynamic tissue composed of three cell types (osteoblasts, osteocytes, and osteoclasts), matrix, and mineral (hydroxyapatite). The organic matrix, which is about 35% of the weight of a bone, is composed of 95% collagen, and 5% proteoglycans and other low molecular weight proteins. The remaining 65% of the weight of bone is contributed by the hydroxyapatite.

Osteoblasts, the chief cells responsible for new bone formation, contain abundant amounts of endoplasmic reticulum, numerous ribosomes (which produce collagen), golgi fields (which produce protein polysaccharides), and mitochondria (Fig. 20-1). Specific membrane-bound matrix vesicles found within the osteoblast probably are responsible for the initiation of bone mineralization.

To form new bone, osteoblasts produce an organic matrix (osteoid), which is primarily collagen; then the osteoid is mineralized by the deposition of hydroxyapatite crystals. Ribosomes produce procollagen, which is extruded into the extracellular space and polymerized to form collagen fibrils. Proteoglycans are produced by the golgi field. The combination of proteoglycans and collagen fibrils forms a mineralizable matrix. This product is also called osteoid. The area around an osteoblast which contains osteoid is called an osteoid seam.

As collagen fibrils package themselves more tightly, a 640 Å-banding pattern is evident. The impregnation (somehow initiated by matrix vesicles) of the fibrils and the intrafibrillar and interfibrillar spaces with mineral (hydroxyapatite) results in mineralized new bone. This process is capable of producing appositional new bone at a rate of 1.5 μm per day in the dog and cat.

Osteocytes are mature osteoblasts which are entirely surrounded by bone. The cells are smaller than osteoblasts and lie within lacunae, connecting with other osteocytes only by means of cytoplasmic processes that touch through canaliculi (Fig. 20-2). Because osteo-

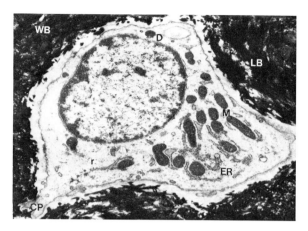

Figure 20-2. *Mature osteocyte surrounded by woven bone (WB) and lamellar bone (LB). Individual profiles of endoplasmic reticulum (ER), mitochondria (M), ribosomes (r), and dense bodies (D) are present. A cytoplasmic process (CP) extends into a canaliculus. (Glutaraldehyde × 11,575—Fetter AW. Ultrastructural evaluation of bone cells in pigs with experimental turbinate osteoporosis [atrophic rhinitis]. Lab Invest 1971;24:392. Copyright © 1971, US–Canada Division of the IAP)*

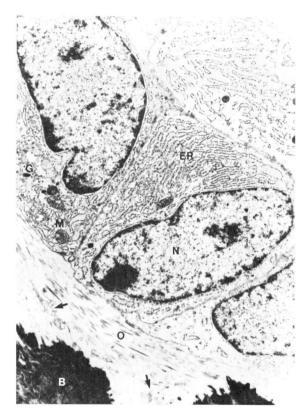

Figure 20-1. *Osteoblasts lining a trabeculum of cancellous bone. The cytoplasm contains rough endoplasmic reticulum (ER) and scattered mitochondria (M). Golgi complexes (G) are well developed and have cisternae distended with fibrillar material. Cytoplasmic processes of osteoblasts (arrows) extend into adjacent osteoid (O), which is interposed between the osteoblasts and underlying mineralized matrix of woven bone (B). Osteoblast nuclei are shown (N). (Original magnification × 6420—Fetter AW. Electron microscopic evaluation of bone cells in pigs with experimentally induced Bordetella rhinitis [turbinate osteoporosis]. Am J Vet Res 1975;36:15.)*

cytes are buried within bone, they cannot be farther than 150 μm from blood supply, or they die. The main function of osteocytes is calcium exchange between bone and body fluids. Osteocytes can destroy the bone around themselves and release calcium by osteocytic osteoclasis, thereby forming a source of calcium in the body fluid, as needed by the animal.

The osteoclast is a very large, multinucleated cell responsible for bone destruction as well as bone remodeling (Fig 20-3). Osteoclasts isolate bone underlying themselves from surrounding bone by their peripheral projections that seal the canaliculi. The isolated bone is removed by acidification, which breaks down the hydroxyapatite, and by the release of enzymes that destroy the organic matrix. The resulting depression on a bone surface is called a Howship's lacunae. Bone destruction can be very rapid, a single osteoclast can remove bone at a rate of 50 to 60 μm per day.

In the mature animal, bone remodeling of cortical (lamellar) bone is constantly taking place. This remodeling is carried out by a re-

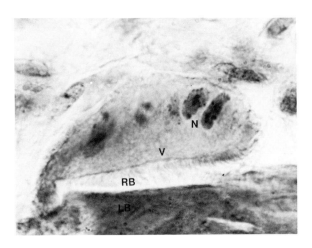

Figure 20-3. *Osteoclast adjacent to lamellar bone (LB). Note the multiple nuclei (N) and vacuolated cytoplasm (V) in the vicinity of the ruffled border (RB). The mineralized section of bone is stained with Goldner's modified trichrome stain. (Newton CD, Nunamaker DM, eds. Textbook of small animal orthopaedics. Philadelphia: JB Lippincott 1985:11.)*

sorptive unit (cutting cone) composed of one or more osteoclasts that destroy bone as they advance through it. The resulting space (resorptive cavity) left behind the advancing osteoclasts will be filled by an advancing capillary loop. Osteoblasts migrate from the capillary to the outer surface of the cavity to form new bone, and they become osteocytes as they are incorporated in new bone. In this fashion, mature bone can be remodeled and replaced with new osteons (haversian systems). This type of bone remodeling will go on throughout the entire life of the animal.

General Anatomy of a Long Bone

The idealized long bone is shown in Figure 20-4. The epiphysis ceases to exist when skeletal maturity has been reached. The entire expanded end of the bone is called the metaphysis. It is composed of trabecular (cancellous or spongy) bone.

The diaphysis is a hollow tube of cortical (compact) bone. Compact bone is composed primarily of haversian systems (osteons). The central cavity contains the medullary arterial supply and is occupied chiefly by fatty marrow. A portion of the medullary cavity of some long bones contains hematopoietic elements, however these are found primarily in the cancellous bone of the metaphysis in the immature animal.

The surface of a long bone, except the ends which are covered by articular cartilage, is covered by periosteum. Periosteum comprises an inner osteogenic layer (cambium), which provides appositional growth before maturity, and an outer fibrous layer, which is purely supportive. Under normal conditions the periosteum is loosely attached to the undersurface of covering muscle bellies. Endosteum lines the inner surface of the medullary cavity.

Blood Supply to a Long Bone

The blood supply to a long bone typically is a centrifugal system. Arterial blood (the afferent arm of this system) enters the medullary cavity

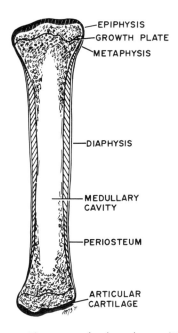

Figure 20-4. *The parts of a long bone. (Rhinelander FW. Circulation in bone. In: Bourne G, ed, The biochemistry and physiology of bone, Vol 2, 2nd ed. New York: Academic Press, 1972.)*

through the nutrient (medullary) artery, divides into ascending and descending medullary arteries, and then further breaks down into arterioles and capillaries supplying the cortex of the diaphysis. The smallest vessels in this afferent system are the central capillaries in each haversian system. The efferent arm of the system, the venous side, is peripheral to the bone (it does not return into the medullary cavity). Venous blood is collected in interfascicular venules and intramuscular veins, eventually returning to systemic veins.

The only exception to the above centrifugal system exists in immature animals. At surfaces with large muscular insertions (*e.g.*, the insertion of the adductor muscle on the femur), a periosteal blood supply may exist. This supply originates from periosteal arteries, breaks up into periosteal capillaries, and is recollected in periosteal veins. This system is very localized to the area of attachment and does not penetrate deeper than the outer one third of the cortex.

Bone Healing

Classical Fracture Healing

Classical bone healing is an inflammatory process, which proceeds through a continuum of cellular and vascular changes, ultimately resulting in the production of collagen and the deposition of mineral into the resulting matrix.

Bone usually is forced to heal in the face of some degree of motion, therefore the form of healing seen and documented on radiography is healing with motion. Healing with motion passes through inflammatory, reparative, and remodeling stages.

Inflammatory Phase

Following fracture the bone and surrounding soft tissues are damaged (Fig. 20-5). Because of torn blood vessels a hematoma forms within and around the fracture site. Osteocytes at the fracture end are deprived of normal nutrition (blood supply) and die. Periosteum and other

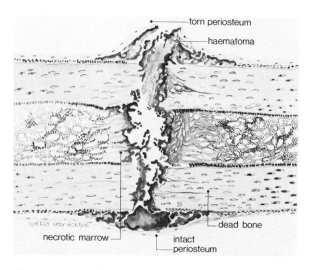

Figure 20-5. *The initial events involved in fracture healing of long bone. The periosteum is torn opposite the point of impact and, in many instances, is intact on the other side. There is an accumulation of hematoma beneath the periosteum and between the fracture line. (Cruess RL, Dumont J. Healing bone, tendon, and ligament. In: Rockwood CA, Green DP, eds. Fractures. Philadelphia: JB Lippincott, 1975:98.)*

surrounding soft tissues may also contain dead and necrotic material.

The presence of necrotic bone and soft tissue elicits a rapid and intense, acute inflammatory response. Acute inflammatory cells, such as polymorphonuclear leukocytes and macrophages, migrate to the region. Further events during this phase are identical to those described for general wound healing (see Chap. 3, The Surgical Wound).

Reparative Phase

The reparative phase begins with organization of the hematoma (Fig. 20-6). The hematoma serves principally as a fibrin scaffold, over which repair cells perform their function. Because of cell death and poor blood supply, the microenvironment at the fracture site is acid, which may be an additional stimulus to cell behavior during the early phases of repair. The pH gradually returns to neutral and then slightly alkaline as the repair process advances.

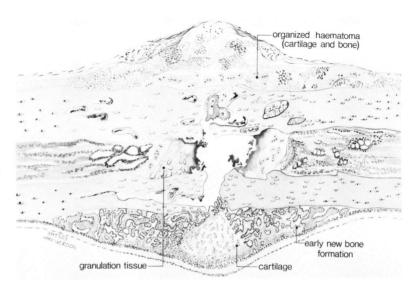

organized haematoma
(cartilage and bone)

early new bone
formation

granulation tissue

cartilage

Figure 20-6. *Early repair. There is organization of the hematoma, early primary new bone formation in subperiosteal regions, and cartilage formation in other areas. (Cruess RL, Dumont J. Healing of bone, tendon, and ligament. In: Rockwood CA, Green DP, eds. Fractures. Philadelphia: JB Lippincott, 1975:99.)*

Pluripotential cells of mesenchymal origin are responsible for the repair of fractures. These cells, probably of common origin, form collagen, cartilage, and bone. Variations in the microenvironment and the stresses they are subjected to probably determine the behavior of these cells. Some cells are derived from the cambium layer of the periosteum, other cells probably are derived from the endosteum.

Most of cells directly involved in fracture healing enter the fracture site with the granulation tissue that invades the region from the surrounding vessels. Repair is linked with the ingress of capillary buds. It appears that under ordinary circumstances following fracture of the bone and medullary artery, the periosteal vessels contribute most of the capillary buds early in the process; the medullary artery becomes important later in the process. Surgical interference with either the vessels of the periosteum (via stripping of the periosteum) or the intramedullary system will delay healing.

Cells invade the hematoma and begin rapidly producing callus, which is composed of fibrous tissue, cartilage, and immature bone. This callus rapidly envelops the bone ends and leads to a gradual increase in stability of the fracture fragments. Cartilage is eventually resorbed by a process indistinguishable from endochondral bone formation. Bone will be

formed by those cells that receive sufficient nutrients and appropriate mechanical stimulation (Fig. 20-7).

The initial appearance of mineral occurs as a result of an interaction between metastable solutions of calcium and phosphate and groups of specific amino acid side chains within the holes of the organized collagen fibrils to produce mineralized bone, as in the process of bone remodeling previously discussed.

As this phase of bone repair takes place, the bone ends gradually become enveloped in a fusiform mass of callus containing increasing amounts of bone. Immobilization of the fragments becomes more rigid because of this internal and external callus formation, and eventually a *clinical union* will occur. It should be stressed that union as an end point does not yet exist, because in the middle of the reparative phase, the remodeling phase begins with resorption of unneeded or inefficient portions of the callus and the laying down of trabecular bone along lines of stress.

Remodeling Phase

In 1892, Wolff recognized that the architecture of the skeletal system corresponded to the mechanical need of this system. He postulated his

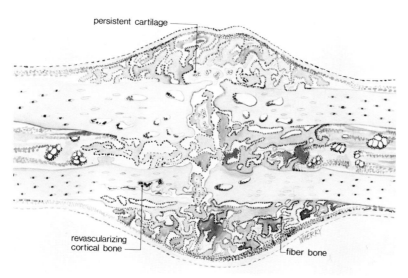

persistent cartilage

revascularizing
cortical bone

fiber bone

Figure 20-7. *At later stage in the repair, early immature fiber bone is bridging the fracture gap. Persistent cartilage is seen at points most distant from ingrowing capillary buds. In many instances these are surrounded by young new bone. (Cruess RL, Dumont J. Healing of bone, tendon, and ligament. In: Rockwood CA, Green DP, eds. Fractures. Philadelphia: JB Lippincott, 1975:100.)*

law: "The form of the bone being given, the bone elements place or displace themselves in the direction of the functional pressure and increase or decrease their mass to reflect the amount of functional pressure."*

The remodeling of a fracture takes a long time. Osteoclastic resorption of superfluous or poorly placed trabeculae occurs, and new struts of bone are laid down along lines of stress. The cell behavior control mechanism is piezoelectric; electropositivity occurs on the convex surface and electronegativity on the concave.

The cellular module that controls remodeling is the resorptive unit (cutting cone), which consists of osteoclasts that first remove bone, the ingrowth of a capillary loop, and then osteoblasts that produce new bone. The result of remodeling is the formation of new osteons across the fracture site which lend strength, much like the reinforcing rods in concrete. The end result of remodeling is a bone that, whether or not it has returned to its original form, has been altered so that it may best resist the stresses which are applied to it.

* Wolff J. Das gesetz der transformation. Transformation der knochen. Berlin: Hirschwald, 1892.

Primary Fracture Healing

The foregoing discussion of classical fracture healing described the method of healing if motion is present. Generally motion is minimized by internal or external fixation; however, micromovement may still be present. On occasion, rigid fixation can be accomplished (absolutely no motion or even micromovement at the fracture site); in this circumstance, primary fracture healing can occur.

Primary bone formation occurs under rigid fixation in areas where small gaps occur through *gap healing*. During the first stage of gap healing the fracture gap is filled via primary bone formation (neither connective tissue nor fibrocartilage has been present prior to new bone being laid down). The pattern of the newly formed bone does not correspond to the original structure of the cortex; the new bone lamella and their collagen fibrils are transverse to the long axis of the diaphysis.

Extensive necrotic areas are present on both sides of the fracture as a result of interruption of the vascular circulation in the haversian canals fracture site.

The second stage of gap healing is longitudinal reconstruction of the fracture site by haversian remodeling. This begins with the formation of resorption cavities that penetrate longitudinally through the necrotic fragment ends and approach the newly formed tissue within the fracture gap.

Groups of osteoclasts form a cutting cone that advances longitudinally through the new bone in the gap, producing this resorptive cavity (Fig. 20-8). The osteoclasts are followed by a thin-walled capillary loop, which runs in the center of the resorptive cavity and is accompanied by mesenchymal cells and osteoblast precursors. Newly formed osteoblasts eventually line the resorptive cavity and begin producing osteoid. Eventually the resorptive cavity will entirely fill with consecutive layers of new bone and become an osteon. The synchronized action of both bone-resorbing and bone-forming cells results in a regenerating osteon capable of advancing in a longitudinal direction parallel to the long axis of bone (Fig. 20-9). This is the identical remodeling process as described for classical fracture healing.

Primary bone formation, as it occurs under rigid fixation in areas where bone is tightly held in contact, is called *contact healing*. In contact healing, because there are no gaps present, haversian remodeling of the fracture site begins immediately, leading simultaneously to the union and reconstruction of the fracture ends (Fig. 20-10).

Complications of Bone Healing

Many factors can frustrate the process of normal union. The most common complications include osteomyelitis, delayed union, nonunion, and malunion.

Osteomyelitis

The most common cause of inflammation of the bone in dogs and cats is an infectious or suppurative inflammation of bone marrow and adjacent bone called osteomyelitis. Although osteomyelitis is usually caused by suppurative organisms, nonsuppurative osteomyelitis also occurs. Nonsuppurative osteomyelitis results from granulomatous organisms or from metalosis.

Suppurative Osteomyelitis

Pathogenesis
Suppurative osteomyelitis occurs when bacteria infect bone. Bacteria may reach bone by hematogenous routes, by extension of soft tissue infection into bone, or more commonly by direct contact with bone (*i.e.,* open fracture or prolonged surgery). Regardless of the source of

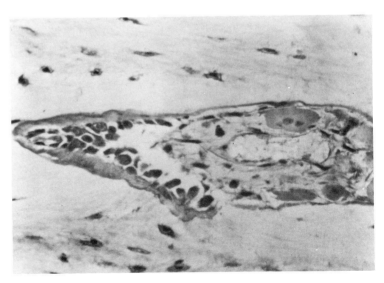

Figure 20-8. *A cutting cone which is creating a new osteon. Osteoclasts are advancing to the right, creating a resorptive cavity. A thin walled capillary is present in the center of the resorptive cavity. Osteoblasts (to the left) are beginning to form new bone on the peripheral surface of the resorptive cavity.*

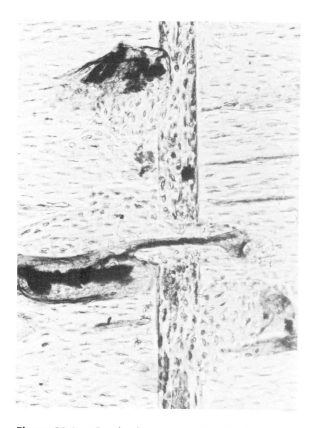

Figure 20-9. *Gap healing. In a rigidity fixed gap area, direct ossification takes place after ingrowth of blood vessels. The original structure of bone is later restored by secondary haversian remodeling in the long axis of the bone. (Rahn BA, Gallinary P, Baltensperger A, et al. Primary bone healing: an experimental study in the rabbit. J Bone Joint Surg 1971;53(A):783.)*

contamination, once bacteria are present, bone mounts an inflammatory response that is similar to that seen in soft tissues.

Bone inflammation results in the infiltration and localization of granulocytic leukocytes. Many of the infiltrating cells are destroyed by the bacteria and release proteolytic enzymes into the bone. Tissue necrosis ensues, and the bacteria and the lytic products of necrosis (the purulent debris) are mingled to form a focus of suppuration.

The severity of osteomyelitis depends on many factors: whether the process is in cortical or metaphyseal bone, the contribution of other disease to bone abnormality, and the animal's age and general health. If the inflammatory process is successful, the osteomyelitis may be contained. If, however, the infection proves overwhelming to the inflammatory process, osteomyelitis will disseminate within the bone.

Infection in metaphyseal bone may break through the thin cortex and spread subperiosteally to most of the diaphysis. Infection in diaphyseal cortical bone spreads through the haversian canals. As infection spreads, vascular thrombosis occurs, resulting in localized areas of cortical bone ischemia. If ischemia is incomplete, the bone may respond by producing new bone around the area of infection. If ischemia is severe, bone death may result. Complete bone death results in cell death, and

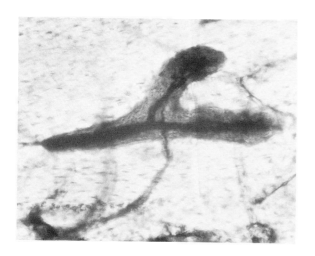

Figure 20-10. *Contact healing vascular supply. By means of India ink filling, the vascular supply of an osteon crossing the osteotomy can be traced directly to the endosteal circulation. (Rahn BA, Gallinaro P, Baltensperger A, et al. Primary bone healing: an experimental study in the rabbit. J Bone Joint Surg 1971;53(A):783.)*

the resulting area is thus composed only of collagen and mineral. Such dead bone may be slowly revascularized, undergo lysis and subsequent new bone formation, or be sloughed. Dead bone is called a sequestrum; it often sits within a granulation-tissue-filled bony depression (involucrum—Fig. 20-11).

Acute osteomyelitis describes these early changes, which, when recognized, require prompt treatment. Chronic osteomyelitis occurs when the process continues for an extended period of time, and the inflammation fails to contain the infection. Chronic infection will usually result in disseminated infection within the bone, bone death, and evidence of aborted attempts at containment (*i.e.,* involucrum and suppurating exudate, or pus that drains to the skin).

Diagnosis

Acute or chronic suppurative osteomyelitis usually presents with pain, local swelling, and pyrexia. With chronicity, obvious tracts and drainage also may be present. Most animals do not demonstrate significant hematologic alterations; moderate leukocytosis with a left shift is found occasionally.

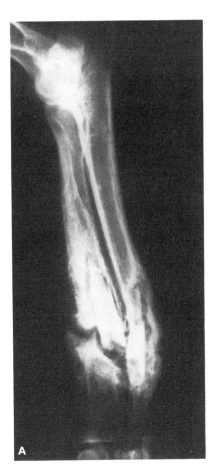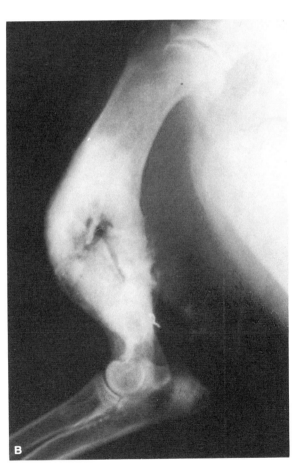

Figure 20-11. *Osteomyelitis with evidence of sequestration of bone within an involucrum. **A,** An infected nonunion of the radius and ulna. Note the two very dense bony sequestrae within the nonunion site. The cavity they lie within is termed the involucrum. **B,** Multiple bony sequestrae within an involucrum in the mid-diaphysis of a humerus.*

On radiography, bone change associated with suppurative infection is limited to bony lysis; areas of periosteal new bone (Fig. 20-12); or the presence of a sequestrum, a nonvascularized fragment of bone that is relatively more opaque than adjacent bone. Typical lytic and periosteal bone changes are not evident for 10 to 14 days following onset of infection. Soft tissue changes are visible within 24 hours; such changes include soft tissue swelling and loss of fascial planes, and sometimes a fistulous tract.

Bacteriologically, the most frequent organism isolated in the dog and cat with osteomyelitis is *Staphylococcus aureus*. Streptococcal infections follow *S. aureus* in frequency. About 50% of clinical osteomyelitis cases are mixed infections.

Treatment

The treatment method depends on the type of osteomyelitis—acute or chronic. In acute osteomyelitis, if fluid is present, the first step is to decompress and provide drainage from the area. The drain should be protected with a bandage against contamination from its surroundings. An alternative is to leave the wound open for complete drainage.

Systemic antibiotics are used at this time, and although many antibiotics may be considered, a bactericidal drug should be chosen. If fluid is available, it is submitted for culture, identification, and sensitivity. Systemic antibiotics are used in the interim before the results of the culture are known. The choice of antibiotic is important, because the first few days of treatment may determine the course of the infection. Most forms of gram-positive cocci and bacilli, and gram-negative cocci respond well to amoxicillin, oxacillin, or cephradine. The remaining gram-negative organisms usually respond to gentamycin or kanamycin. Dosage depends on circulation: higher concentrations of antibiotics are needed when blood perfusion is poor, such as in cases of sequestered bone fragments or soft tissue edema and stasis around the fracture.

Support of the limb by a bandage may be indicated to lessen soft tissue swelling, but if used, should be checked and changed daily. If internal fixation is used, rigid fixations should be left in place. Unstable internal fixation should be removed and replaced with a rigid form of fixation. Bone will heal, even if infected, if the fixation is *rigid*. Radiography at 10-day intervals is helpful to evaluate the extent and course of infection.

The treatment of chronic osteomyelitis may be similar to that of acute osteomyelitis; however, areas of dead bone or sequestra must be surgically removed. Following surgical removal, curettage of dead bone to uncover healthy bleeding bone is performed. Rigid in-

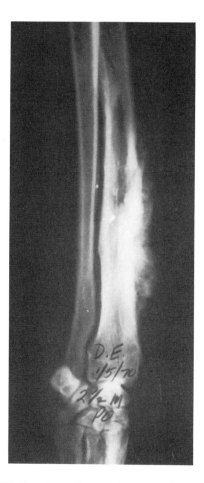

Figure 20-12.   *Acute bacterial osteomyelitis secondary to gun shot. Note the periosteal new bone.*

ternal fixation is imperative. The placement of drains is often necessary to remove blood or other postoperative debris, although open drainage is also appropriate. Culture of the deep wound or bone determines the organisms present and permits antibiotic sensitivity testing.

Chronic osteomyelitis is a difficult disease to cure and may persist despite extensive treatment.

Nonsuppurative Osteomyelitis

A noninfectious, nonsuppurative osteomyelitis (metalosis) often occurs around metal implants, which may result from metal corrosion, use of dissimilar metals, or animal allergy to an implant. Metalosis usually manifests itself clinically by lameness or draining tracts. The tract effluent will be serous and will not grow bacteria. Animals are not febrile and do not have marked hematologic abnormalities. Radiographic evidence of metalosis is bony lysis around the implant. A halo effect will be present around part or all of the implant. Treatment will be unsuccessful unless the implant is removed. Following removal, recovery is uneventful; antibiotics are unnecessary.

Delayed Union

Any fracture that is not healed in the time normally required for such a fracture is considered a delayed union. The period during which normal healing is expected to occur depends on the species of animal, age of the animal, site of the fracture (cortical vs. cancellous bone), or the shape of the fracture.

The usual causes of delayed union include inadequate immobilization, inadequate blood supply, malalignment of fracture fragments, interposition of soft tissues in the fracture site, bone loss, or infection. Systemic factors, such as high doses of corticosteroid drugs, starvation, age, or other metabolic diseases may also result in delayed bone union.

The diagnosis of delayed union is made when, based on your experience, radiographic

healing of a fracture is taking longer than it should. Treatment is prolonged immobilization. If the method of fixation appears adequate, restrict activity, wait, and re-radiograph in 4 weeks. With adequate time and immobilization, most fractures will unite. When immobilization is inadequate and continues over a prolonged period, a delayed union becomes a nonunion.

Nonunion

Nonunion occurs when fracture repair ceases, and union cannot occur without surgical intervention. The most common cause is inadequate immobilization of the fracture. Clinically, nonunions are usually associated with painful motion at the fracture site, muscle atrophy in the involved limb, progressive deformity of the involved limb, and limb disuse. Radiographic evidence includes sclerotic bone ends, a gap between the bony fragments, sealed medullary cavities, smooth fracture ends, and, perhaps, pseudarthrosis (a false joint).

Two types of nonunion exist: vascular (hypertrophic) nonunion and avascular nonunion. Vascular nonunion occurs in the face of adequate blood supply and numerous unsuccessful attempts at union (Fig. 20-13). As a result the nonunion evidences large volumes of proliferative new bone unsuccessfully attempting to bridge the fracture site. Of course, avascular nonunion displays no attempt at union, because without blood supply, bone cannot heal, and very little or no new bone is present (Fig. 20-14).

Treatment of nonunion relies on the surgeon's ability to identify and treat the etiology of the problem. If a fracture is unstable, provide adequate stability. If the nonunion also lacks osteogenic ability, add autogenous cancellous bone. If the nonunion is avascular, encourage vascularity by adding an autogenous cancellous graft.

Any form of rigid internal fixation will be successful if the nonunion site is debrided, stabilized, and an autogenous graft is added.

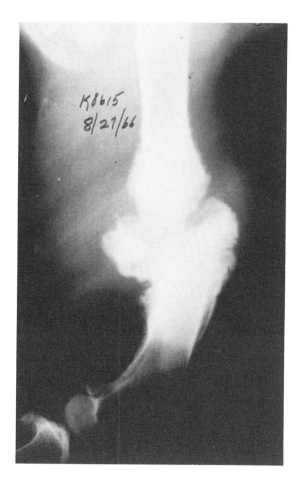

Figure 20-13. *A vascular (hypertrophic) nonunion of the femoral diaphysis.*

Although bone plates are usually used, they are not the only successful form of fixation. Plates do, however, offer one advantage; if the fibrous and cartilaginous tissue of the nonunion is compressed (best done with a plate), the tissue can convert directly to bone without the need for debridement and grafting.

Infected nonunion poses a very challenging problem for the surgeon; however, by combining the treatment plans of osteomyelitis and nonunion, the bone will heal. The nonunion site must be approached surgically. All dead and necrotic bone (sequestra) must be removed, then the bone is cultured for identification of organism and antibiotic sensitivity.

Rigid internal fixation is provided, and an autogenous cancellous graft is packed into the nonunion site. Normal bone will heal in the face of infection and so will a nonunion.

Malunion

Malunions occur when bones have been allowed to heal into malposition or nonfunctional anatomic position (Fig. 20-15). Malunion usually results from fractures that were never treated or in fractures where the internal or external method of fixation was removed prematurely, allowing the incompletely healed bone to deform.

If malunions are compromising the pelvic canal, they can result in severe problems with defecation or parturition. Malunions of long bones commonly result is degenerative arthritis of the joints above and below the malunion. Treatment of malunion requires osteotomy of the site and realignment, followed by rigid internal fixation.

Biology of Bone Grafts

Bone grafts used in veterinary medicine are either cancellous or cortical. Because the surface of cancellous bone is covered with osteoblasts, cancellous grafts can be used to transplant their osteogenic potential to another site. In this way cancellous bone can be used to fill defects (Fig. 20-16) or to help promote bone union in an arthrodesis, fresh fracture, or nonunion. Cortical grafts provide structural strength but do not transplant significant numbers of osteoblasts. Cortical grafts are used to provide strength in bridging bone gaps or can be used as a method of internal fixation similar to a bone plate. It must be stressed that a cortical bone graft becomes dead bone once it has been separated from its blood supply.

Bone grafts can be autogenous (from the same animal), homogenous (allograft, from another member of the same species), or heterogenous (xenograft, from a member of another

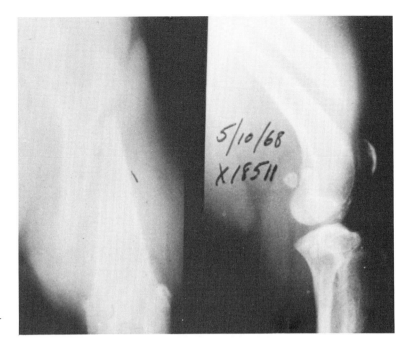

Figure 20-14. *An avascular non-union of the femoral diaphysis.*

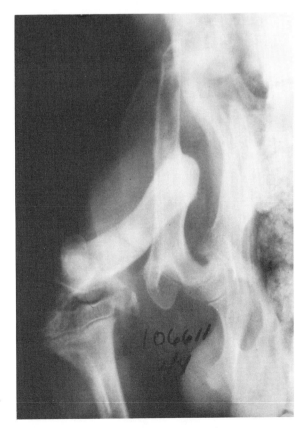

Figure 20-15. *Malunion of a femoral diaphyseal fracture. The distal fragment has united perpendicular to the center of the proximal fragment. Ambulation on this limb was very difficult.*

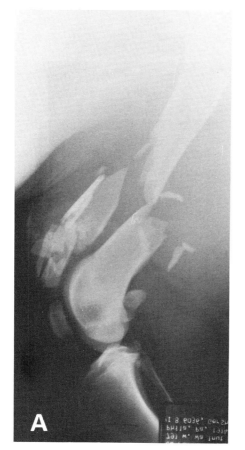
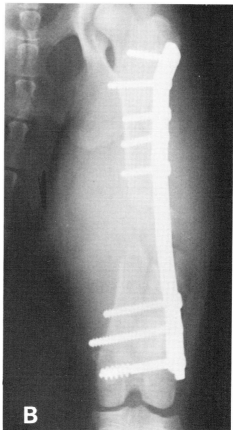
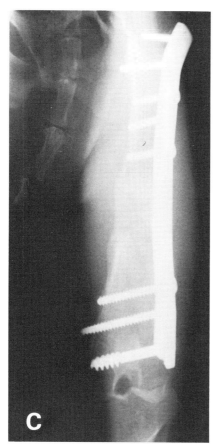

Figure 20-16. *A comminuted fracture in a large breed dog.* ***A,*** *Treatment using a cancellous autograft to fill the large gap after internal fixation.* ***B,*** *Internal fixation with a plate and screws.* ***C,*** *Radiographic consolidation of the fracture occurred in 8 weeks.*

species). Autogenous cancellous grafts are preferable, although cortical grafts are successful if either autogenous or homogenous in origin.

Cancellous bone has the ability to incorporate rapidly into the site of transplantation. The graft is readily revascularized, and the surface osteoblasts rapidly begin to form bone. Although the process of transplantation may actually result in cell death of as many as 90% of the surface osteoblasts, the remaining 10% are capable of contributing considerable new bone to the site. Cancellous bone can be harvested by opening the bone cortex with a drill or Steinmann pin over the appropriate sites. The best sites are the proximal humeral meta-

physis, the wing of the ilium, the greater trochanter, or the proximal tibial metaphysis. Bone is harvested using large bone curettes, and moved directly to the recipient site. Cancellous bone should never be allowed to dry on the surgical table.

Cortical bone must be incorporated into the recipient site by a process know as *creeping substitution*. The dead cortical bone is first broken down or removed by osteoclasts, then the bone is revascularized and ultimately undergoes formation of new bone and remodeling. During this process, the graft will be entirely removed and replaced by new bone (Fig. 20-17). This may take months or years depending on the size of the graft. Cortical bone

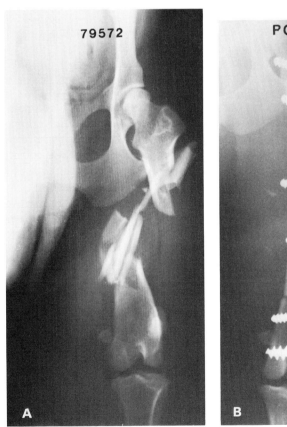
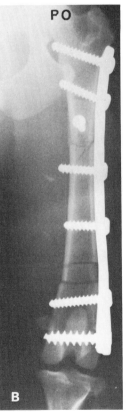
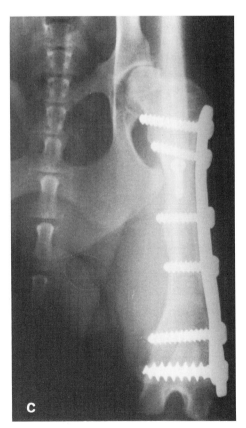

Figure 20-17. *A,* A 2-year-old dog presented for treatment of a comminuted femoral fracture. *B,* The fracture was repaired with a segmental cortical allograft and fixed using a plate and screws. *C,* Radiographic healing is seen at 8 months following surgery. (Courtesy of Dr. W. D. Hoefle)

grafts can be harvested from the diaphysis of another bone in the same animal, from the diaphysis of a fresh donor animal of the same species, or from an aseptically collected donor graft that was frozen at an earlier date.

Tendon Biology and Surgery

Tendons and Tendon Sheaths

Most skeletal muscles are attached to bone or cartilage by a tendon, aponeurosis, or by direct attachment. Tendon attachment is by far the most important and is present wherever the point of insertion is distant or the muscle must exert its forces of contracture across a joint.

A tendon is composed of collagenous tissue that is highly resistant to extension, but is relatively flexible and can therefore be sharply bent around bones or joints. A tendon is usually round, oval, or elongated in cross section and consists of fascicles of collagen fibers, imbedded in a ground substance, that generally run parallel to the long axis of the tendon.

In areas where there is marked change in the direction of a tendon, or where tendons pass under ligamentous structures, or through fascial slings, a tendon sheath or synovial sheath surrounds the tendon. The tendon invaginates into the sheath to form a closed double-walled cylinder. This anatomic device clearly reduces friction, but its most fundamental purpose is to produce a discontinuity between structures that must move in relation to each other.

Healing of Tendon

Following surgical coaptation of divided tendon ends, fibroblasts from surrounding connective tissue migrate into the wound, including the space between the tendon ends. The healing process follows the general pattern common to all tissues (see Chap. 3, The Surgical Wound), and the fibroblasts synthesize and discharge into the wound monomeric collagen and mucopolysaccharides needed for synthe-

sis of mature scar. Rapid polymerization of monomeric subunits converts the initial fine reticular network immersed in a viscous ground substance into discernible fibrils and finally into dense connective tissue scar.

Obviously there are two aspects of tendon healing that distinguish healing of this tissue from that of other tissues. The first is the tremendous tensile strength that must develop between the tendon ends. The second aspect is the development of a type of separation in the single scar so that the healed tendon can move or glide within the surrounding scar tissue.

Tendon Surgery

Tendon Laceration

In small animals the most frequently injured tendons are located in the lower limbs. These consist of the superficial and deep flexors and extensors of the forepaw and, not infrequently, the calcanean tendon. Most of these injuries, particularly the flexor injuries, are the result of lacerations caused by sharp objects; whereas extensor injuries appear to be most commonly associated with mechanical injury.

When repairing an injured or lacerated tendon, several general principles apply.

- The surgical procedure itself should cause as little additional injury to the tendon and surrounding soft tissues as possible.
- Damage to the surrounding tissues that make up the gliding mechanism must be avoided.
- At no time should the tendon or the surrounding soft tissues be allowed to dry.
- At no time should the tendon be grasped with forceps or wrapped in gauze.
- The traumatized portion of the end of the tendon can be removed with a sharp scalpel, exposing a fresh cross section of normal tendon prior to beginning suturing.

The ideal tendon suture should have high tensile strength, should tie in such a way that extra knots are not required, and should not create reaction within the tissue. A simple

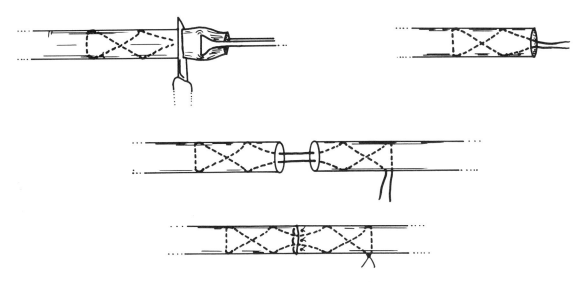

Figure 20-18. *The Bunnell–Meyer tendon suture pattern. (Newton CD, Nunamaker DM, eds. Textbook of small animal orthopaedics. Philadelphia: JB Lippincott, 1985:837.)*

pattern, containing a minimum of suture material, that will not tend to strangulate tissues is best. No one suture pattern is satisfactory for all tendons; therefore, a variety of patterns are employed, and the choice of patterns is based on the anatomic configuration of the tendon. Round or semiround tendons can accept the use of a Bunnell–Meyer suture pattern (Fig. 20-18) or locking-loop tendon suture (Fig. 20-19); whereas flat tendons require overlapping suture patterns. At the end of the repair, the tendon ends are aligned and slightly buckled with no suture material visible.

The fundamental principle in postoperative motion is to encourage secondary remodeling of the scar tissue, while simultaneously avoiding rupture of the adhesion. Following 3 weeks of absolute rest (a long leg cast may be needed), a sutured tendon is not sufficiently strong to endure active motion and full weight bearing. Increased collagen synthesis has been measured for as long as 35 days after tendon anastomosis. After 3 weeks of immobilization, the tendon should be supported by less rigid external fixation for at least an additional 3 weeks. Continuous absolute immobilization

beyond 3 weeks is probably not desirable; there is no significant increase in tensile strength at 5 weeks compared to 3 weeks. However, if limited active motion is allowed after 3 weeks of immobilization, the tensile strength at 5 weeks will be 3 times greater than at 3 weeks.

Lengthening Tendons

Tendon contracture commonly occurs, usually as the result of contraction of the muscular attachment to the proximal end of the tendon

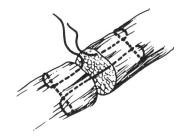

Figure 20-19. *The locking loop (Kessler–Mason–Allen) suture technique. (Tomlinson J, Moore R. Locking loop tendon suture use in repair of five calcanean tendons. Vet Surg 1982;3:105.)*

following trauma. If the contracture is severe, as is often seen in contracture of the flexor tendons of the paw, surgical intervention may be necessary.

The simplest procedure for lengthening the tendon is tenotomy, wherein the tendon is divided and allowed to retract. The resultant gap will fill with scar that will function as the tendon, provided the tendon retracts less than 3 cm. If, however, the tendon ends retract more than 3 cm, the resulting union will be weak owing to thinness of the scar, and the scar will lack the tensile strength of a normal tendon. In these cases another method of tendon lengthening must be used. (Note, teno-

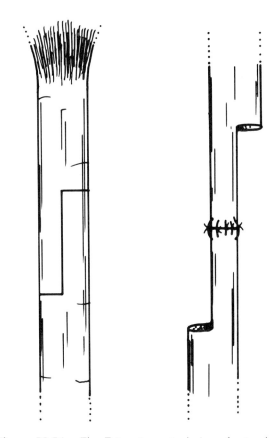

Figure 20-21. *The Z tenotomy technique for tendon lengthening. (Newton CD, Nunamaker DM, eds. Textbook of small animal orthopaedics. Philadelphia: JB Lippincott, 1985:838.)*

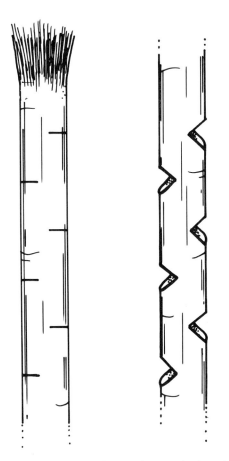

Figure 20-20. *The accordion technique for lengthening a tendon. (Newton CD, Nunamaker DM, eds. Textbook of small animal orthopaedics. Philadelphia: JB Lippincott, 1985:838.)*

tomy within a tendon sheath is contraindicated.)

An alternative is the accordion method of lengthening, which is simple to apply. In this technique, a series of cuts are made on opposite sides of the tendon (Fig. 20-20), allowing the tendon to stretch. The most common method of lengthening a tendon, when it is necessary to lengthen it more than 3 cm, is that of the Z tenotomy. In this procedure a longitudinal cut (equal to the length the tendon is to be lengthened) is made in the center of the tendon. A transverse cut is then made at each end of the incision on opposite sides of the tendon. This will make an elongated Z pattern (Fig. 20-21). The ends of the tendon can then be reunited by sutures.

Shortening Tendons

An abnormally long tendon generally results from a breakdown of supporting structures during the growth phase of the animal, which places strain on the tendon. It can also occur after severance when the joint is placed in hyperextension or flexion during the immobilization period. There are several methods for shortening tendons (Fig. 20-22).

Reattachment of Tendon to Bone

There are two basic methods by which a tendon can be reattached to bone. The first is by resecting a small piece of the periosteum from the area where the tendon is to be attached and placing the cut end of the tendon on the de-

nuded area of bone. The tendon can then be sutured to the bone by passing a needle through the margins of the tendon and the adjacent periosteum. A second method, which is somewhat simpler, is to drill a small hole in the bone and place a Bunnell-Meyer suture in the end of the tendon. The suture can then be pulled through the bone, drawing the tendon up against the periosteum. The suture is then fastened to the periosteum and other surrounding soft tissues.

Ligament Biology and Surgery

Ligament Anatomy and Sprain

Ligaments are composed of connective tissue in which fibers form a thick bundle. This connective tissue is predominantly collagenous, but some elastic components are present. Ligaments connect bones to other bones.

Ligaments are easily injured whenever a joint is forced beyond its normal range of motion. Minor injury is sprain. Classification schemes for sprain generally focus on the qualitative aspects of the ligamentous injury. First degree sprain injury involves minimal tearing of the ligament and associated fibers, as well as a varying degree of internal hemorrhage. Second degree sprain usually results in definite structural breakdown as a result of partial tearing. Hemorrhage is both internal and periligamentous, with inflammatory edema being moderately extensive. Third degree sprain is most severe and often involves complete rupture of the ligament body. Avulsion at the points of origin or insertion usually results in small bone fragments.

Healing of Ligament

The basic concepts of ligament healing resemble those of tendon healing; however, the process is simpler because gliding is not involved.

Under suitable conditions, injured ligaments have the ability to reform a structure that very closely approximates the original structure. Healing occurs via formation of col-

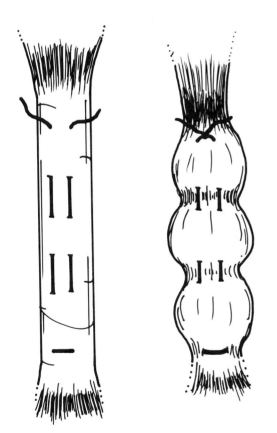

Figure 20-22. *Hoffa's method of shortening tendons. (Newton CD, Nunamaker DM, eds. Textbook of small animal orthopaedics. Philadelphia: JB Lippincott, 1985:839.)*

lagen and remodeling of this scar tissue. Fibroblastic activity comes from the ligament itself as well as from surrounding tissues. As in tendon healing, the *one wound concept* prevails: healing proceeds in the wounded ligament and in the wounds in surrounding structures, just as it would in a wound of a single structure.

If the ligament ends are separated, a gap or irregular fibrous tissue is formed between the ends. If the ends are sutured carefully, an organized scar develops in which collagen fibers are regularly oriented. The tensile strength of this organized scar exceeds that of the irregular fibrous tissue between separated ends of a ligament. In addition, if gapped ligament ends are allowed to heal, the resulting healed ligament is not only weaker than a sutured ligament, it is also longer. This leads to instability of the joint supported by the ligament.

Ligament Surgery

Repair of Collateral Ligaments

Collateral ligaments are found medial and lateral to all major appendicular joints except the shoulder. Often, in extremes of varus, valgus, rotation, or trauma, the structure will tear (third degree sprain). Collateral ligaments are short, relatively inelastic structures, which can be difficult to repair, but many methods have been devised.

Nonsurgical Management
External fixation of a joint in its midrange position may encourage healing but requires very rigid fixation for a minimum of 6 to 8 weeks. At best, this technique is 25% successful. Success requires healing and scarring of the torn ligament.

Surgical Management
Surgical reconstruction of collateral ligaments rarely involves primary suture of the torn ligaments, because most have been shredded beyond repair.

Collateral avulsions, which have torn with a bony fragment, may be reconstructed by interfragmentary screw fixation of the bone fragment. If the fragment is too small to accommodate a hole for the screw, then the ligament can be trapped into its normal location using a spiked washer. The reconstruction must be as anatomic as possible if normal joint function is to result.

Collateral ligament tears are usually reconstructed by supporting the joint with wire or nylon to mimic the collateral function; then, if possible, the torn ends are sutured. The most basic technique requires placing a cortical screw at each attachment point of the collateral ligament and then connecting the screws with orthopedic wire or nylon suture (Fig. 20-23). If screws are unavailable, orthopedic staples can be used or holes can be drilled through the attachment points.

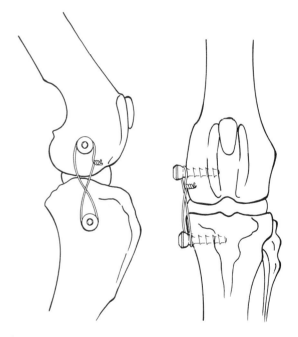

Figure 20-23. *Technique for a repair of a collateral ligament using two cortical screws and a figure-8 orthopedic wire. The screws must be placed as near as possible to the anatomical points of attachment of the ligament being reconstructed. This figure illustrates use of the technique to reconstruct the medial collateral ligament of the stifle. (Newton CD, Nunamaker DM, eds. Textbook of small animal orthopaedics. Philadelphia: JB Lippincott, 1985:849.)*

The wire should be sufficiently tightened to give a stable joint but not to crush the opposing cartilage surface. It is generally agreed that the wire or nylon prosthesis will break eventually and probably require removal. Prior to breakage, however, the collateral ligament scars, resulting in a stable repair.

A few anatomic variations may require alteration in these techniques. Specifically, the very prominent medial malleolus makes wire placement difficult at the hock; therefore, a technique using holes through the malleolus and nylon may prove more useful.

Aftercare

Prolonged postoperative external immobilization will lead to joint stiffness. It is recommended that a supportive external bandage may be helpful for 7 to 10 days but should not remain longer. Following removal, exercise should be restricted to leash walking for an additional 2 to 4 weeks.

Repair of the Patellar Ligament

The patellar ligament can be torn if the stifle is severely flexed while the quadriceps are contracted. This trauma may result in avulsion from the tibial tuberosity, or a tear through the ligament. Laceration may occur because of automobile trauma.

Repair requires removing tension from the ligament and primary suturing using nonabsorbable suture material. To remove tension from the patellar ligament, a tension band wire should be affixed between the patella and the tibial tuberosity by looping the wire over the top of the patella (Fig. 20-24). The distal attachment is through a transverse hole in the tibial tuberosity. The tension band wire should be tightened until the patellar ligament ends lie in apposition. The ligamentous repair is achieved by a large tension suture and simple interrupted pattern at the cut ends. In instances of severe ligamentous loss, strips of dense fascia lata may be sutured into the defect.

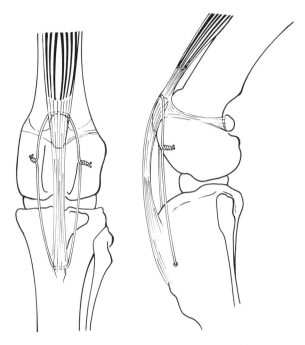

Figure 20-24. *Technique to remove tension from a severed patellar ligament to allow suture. The proximal point of purchase of the tension-band wire is the proximal pole of the patella. The wire is over the patella and through the quadriceps muscle insertion. (Newton CD, Nunamaker DM, eds. Textbook of small animal orthopaedics. Philadelphia: JB Lippincott, 1985:850)*

Postoperative care is similar to collateral ligament aftercare: soft supportive bandage for 7 to 10 days, followed by 2 to 4 weeks of restricted activity. The wire will break and probably necessitate removal at a later date.

Muscle Biology

Muscle Function and Form

Muscle is made up of bundles of fibers that can contract, and by so doing, move body parts. The fibers are arranged in bundles (fasciculi or myonemes) of various sizes and patterns. Connective tissue, (endomysium) fills the space between fibers in a fasciculus. Each fasciculus or bundle is surrounded by a strong connective tissue sheath (the perimysium).

Another strong connective tissue sheath (epimysium) surrounds the muscle body and is continuous internally with the other perimysial septa and externally with the connective tissue of surrounding structures.

Muscles can be grouped according to orientation of their fasciculi or bundles, which can be parallel, oblique, or spiral relative to the final direction of pull at their attachment.

Healing of Muscle

Wounds of skeletal muscle occur as a result of surgical dissection, laceration wounds, spontaneous ruptures, and contusions. Muscle tears and ruptures are particularly common in racing greyhounds.

Wounds of skeletal muscle can heal both by fibrosis and regeneration of myofibrils. If the muscle wound edges are displaced, healing is by the usual fibrous protein synthesis and formation of scar tissue, which has the ability to strangle the myofibrils and prevent regeneration. This scar tissue between muscle ends can remodel and elongate to such an extent that muscle function is reduced.

If the edges of a muscle wound are carefully debrided (either of dead and devitalized tissue in a fresh wound or of scar tissue in an old wound) and approximated by sutures, optimal healing can be obtained by fibrous tissue formation and regeneration of myofibrils. Muscle does not heal by cell division but by myofibril regeneration across the defect. Fibers on each side of the defect break up into nucleated cylinders of cytoplasm, then macrophages remove dead material but leave the basement membrane intact. The muscle fiber cylinders now fuse and grow back inside the original basement membrane to form a myotube, until eventually the two growing undamaged ends fuse and fill this gap. Surviving portions of the muscle begin to form these fine outgrowths in 6 to 7 days, and cross striations can develop in 8 to 14 days. The rate of muscle regeneration by this type of sarcoplasmic outgrowth appears to be about 1.5 mm/day.

Bursae

Bursae are connective-tissue sacs lined by secretory endothelium, the synovial membrane, and containing a viscous fluid, synovial fluid. They are interposed between moving parts and at points of unusual pressure. Thus, they are situated between many bony prominences and tendons, ligaments, or muscles; or occasionally between two tendons.

Joint Biology

Normal Synovial Tissue

Synovial tissue lines all diarthrodial joints and is composed of one to three layers of cells known as synovial lining cells. Synovium has different names to describe the tissue it overlays. In fibrous synovial membrane, lining cells tend to be few and lie directly on dense fibrous tissue; its surface tends to be flat. In areolar or fatty synovial membrane, small vessels are present immediately under the synovial lining cells and in connective tissue septa extending between fat cells. The surface of areolar synovium tends to be undulating.

The cells making up synovial membrane are active phagocytes (type A cells), cells responsible for secretion of hyaluronic acid (type B cells), and type C cells that mimic both type A and B cells.

Synovial Healing After Incision

Like all tissue healing, synovial healing is an inflammatory process. The initial response to incision, with or without suturing, is bleeding, hematoma formation, and fibrin organization of the hematoma. During the first 3 days the defects are filled with neutrophils, erythrocytes, and fibrin. By day 7, with the ingrowth of capillaries and the formation of granulation tissue, fibroblasts become prominent at the periphery and the base of the wounds. The fibroblasts cover the wounds by 10 days postincision, and the incision appears healed. Eventually, the ground substance and the collagen produced by the fibroblasts will heal and contract the wound. In the dog this process extends over a period of only 14 days.

The healing of large synovial membrane defects mimics the process of incisional healing in type of healing and time of healing.

Normal Articular Cartilage

The hyaline articular cartilages constitute a unique and extraordinary body tissue (or perhaps more appropriately, "organ"), the structural, biochemical, and metabolic characteristics of which endow the mammalian diarthrodial joint with a remarkable resiliency and almost frictionless movement.*

Hyaline cartilage is a connective tissue consisting of cells and fibers embedded in matrix. Hyaline cartilage can be described as a gel consisting of 70% water and a firm component, chondroitin sulfate, produced by chondrocytes. The matrix contains two macromolecular materials: collagen and a combination of a linear protein and polysaccharides, known as proteoglycan.

Chondrocytes are situated in lacunae, and are 30 to 40 μm in diameter. The cartilaginous surface is divided into four characteristic zones. The layer of chondrocytes most superficial toward the joint surface is termed the gliding or tangential zone. Both the elongated cells of this zone and the collagen run parallel to the surface of the cartilage. This zone is found to be rich in collagen but rather poor in proteoglycans, when compared to the deeper zones. The next deeper zone of rounded or oval-shaped cells is termed the transitional zone. The next deeper area is called the radial zone. Chondrocytes are lined up in short irregular columns of about five to seven cells. The deepest zone is termed the calcified zone; here the matrices of the cells are heavily encrusted with hydroxyapatite.

* Mankin HJ. The articular cartilages. In: Newton CD, Nunamaker DM, eds. Textbook of small animal orthopaedics. Philadelphia: JB Lippincott, 1985:90.

Because mature cartilage lacks vessels, survival of chondrocytes depends on diffusion of proteins and electrolytes; once total mineralization of the calcified zone has occurred, underlying bone can no longer nutritionally support the cartilage. The survival of chondrocytes depends on diffusion from the fluid in the joint. Mature cartilage also lacks lymphatics and nerve fibers.

Healing of Cartilage

Partial thickness (not extending to the level of subchondral bone) lacerations or injuries to articular cartilage are incapable of healing.

Full thickness hyaline cartilage injuries heal similarly to other more vascular connective tissues. The defect immediately fills with blood, and the resulting hematoma organizes with fibrin. White blood cells and undifferentiated cells from the bone marrow and endothelium modulate into primitive fibroblasts. As surrounding capillaries grow into the defect, the fibrin clot becomes a vascular fibroblastic repair tissue. With progressive fibrosis of the granulation tissue, the defect becomes filled with a loose fibrovascular network that gradually becomes more cellular and less vascular. The vascular fibrous tissue in the defect undergoes progressive hyalinization and subsequently becomes "chondrified," to produce a fibrocartilaginous mass.

Full thickness cartilage defects that heal while the joint is undergoing continuous passive motion heal more rapidly and with a tissue that more closely approximates hyaline cartilage than fibrocartilage.

Cartilage Surgery

Very little primary surgery of cartilage is performed. The usual procedure is to remove osteochondritic flaps and trim the margin of the resulting defect, or to trim the margins of osteochondral fragments that are encountered during intra-articular fracture repair. A few basic principles must be adhered to:

- Never allow the surface of articular cartilage to dry.
- Always trim cartilage edges perpendicular to the surface of the cartilage.
- Partial thickness defects will never heal.
- An obliquely cut edge will never heal smoothly with the surface.
- If you encounter a partial thickness defect, convert it to a full thickness defect, so that healing can occur.

Neoplastic Bone Disease

Malignant Bone Tumors

Osteosarcoma of the Dog

Osteosarcoma in dogs is a malignant primary tumor of bone consisting of malignant osteoid, bone, or cartilage formation. It is the most common bone tumor in the dog, accounting for 80% of all bone tumors. The average age of onset is about 7.5 years with a range of 1 to 15 years. Males and females are about equally affected.

The breed of dog is an important factor in the diagnosis of osteosarcoma. The German shepherd has the highest incidence, followed by the Great Dane, Saint Bernard, boxer, Irish setter, Labrador retriever, Doberman pinscher, and collie. If data are compared with the relative risk of a dog of any breed developing osteosarcoma, then the greatest risk is to the Saint Bernard, followed by the Great Dane, golden retriever, Irish setter, Doberman pinscher, and German shepherd dog.

Most osteosarcomas (75%) originate in long bones, and 25% arise in flat bones. The appendicular to axial ratio is 4:1. The forelimb to hindlimb ratio is 1.7:1. About 75% of the tumors will arise in the metaphysis of the affected bone. Limb osteosarcoma is most prevalent "away from the elbow" (*i.e.*, in the distal radius and proximal humerus) and "around the knee" (*i.e.*, in the distal femur and proximal tibia).

Clinical signs include rapid onset of lameness over 2 to 5 days, localized swelling around the lesion, and, occasionally, fever and anorexia. Pathologic fracture is not uncommon. Metastases to the lungs (the most common site—90%) occur in 80% of the cases by 6 months after the original diagnosis.

Radiographs reveal solitary lesions in the bones with either aggressive lytic or blastic areas or both (Fig. 20-25). A periosteal reaction is present in about 95% of the lesions, with 33% having a sunburst periosteal reaction. An eroded cortex and poorly demarcated lesion margins are common with neoplastic bone extending beyond the cortex. Growth rate of the tumor is rapid with a large amount of soft tis-

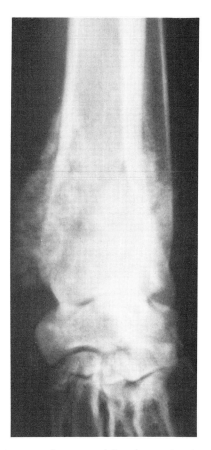

Figure 20-25. *Craniocaudal radiograph of the distal antebrachium of a dog with a radial osteosarcoma. Note that there is both lytic (bone loss) and blastic (bone proliferation) present within the same tumor. (Newton CD, Nunamaker DM, eds. Textbook of small animal orthopaedics. Philadelphia: JB Lippincott, 1985:878.)*

sue swelling usually present. Pathologic fracture may be present. Pulmonary metastases may not easily be recognized in the early stages of the tumor.

Histologically, osteosarcoma presents with a wide range of morphologic patterns. These include a broad range of matrix patterns aligned in a haphazard way with osteonecrosis or new bone production.

Diagnosis of osteosarcoma is confirmed by biopsy of the lesion. Care must be taken to sample several sites, specifically the margins of the tumor will be more likely to give an accurate diagnosis. Radiography following biopsy is helpful to confirm that the appropriate sites have been examined by biopsy. In lieu of biopsy, clinical signs, age, breed, location of the lesion, and radiography may be used to make a tentative diagnosis.

Treatment of osteosarcoma continues to be an area of ongoing research; the present reality is that only 10% to 15% of dogs survive longer than nine months following diagnosis or amputation. Amputation of the involved limb will alleviate pain, although clinical impression is that amputation does not necessarily prolong the life of the dog, unless it is coupled with an aggressive program of other modalities, such as chemotherapy, immunotherapy, and radiotherapy. The most promising information available today indicates that amputation coupled with the administration of Cisplatin has resulted in mean survival times of 47.5 weeks in a group of 12 dogs. This is encouraging, because amputation alone results in a mean survival time of only 18 weeks.

The prognosis for survival with osteosarcoma is very poor, although a few dogs do survive for years following diagnosis. Most dogs die within 9 months following the diagnosis regardless of the modality of treatment.

Osteosarcoma of the Cat

Malignant and benign bone tumors are less common in the cat than in the dog. The clinical, radiographic, and pathologic appearance of bone tumors in the cat is similar to that in the dog.

Osteosarcoma is the most common bone tumor seen in the cat and is most commonly associated with the appendicular bones (15 of 22 cats in 1 study). Axial tumors have been documented in the skull, vertebrae, and pelvis. Cats with osteosarcomas present at a mean age of 10 years (range 1–20 years).

Presenting signs are usually associated with lameness or neurologic dysfunction in the case of spinal involvement. Radiographically, 80% of the appendicular tumors appear primarily as aggressive lytic lesions with a marked absence of new bone and periosteal proliferations. Axial tumors are primarily characterized by proliferative new bone formation.

Treatment, using amputation of appendicular tumors without the addition of chemotherapy or immunotherapy, has had surprisingly good results. In one small study of 12 cats, 5 cats died with a mean survival time of 49 months, 6 cats were still alive at (mean 64 months), and 1 cat was lost to follow-up. Cats with axial tumors who were treated with various chemotherapeutic agents all died, with a mean survival time of only 5.5 months.

Metastasis is less common in cats than in dogs. When it does occur, it is by the hematogenous route, usually to the lungs or other internal organs. Although the prognosis for this tumor is still very guarded, the outcome appears to be better than for the same tumor in the dog.

Parosteal Osteosarcoma

Parosteal osteosarcoma is the second most common bone tumor in the cat. This tumor is found immediately adjacent to the bone and arises on the outer surface of the cortex. It arises from fusiform cells that produce chondroid and osseous foci. The tumor is seen affecting long bones (primarily the humerus and femur) and the frontal bones and ramus of the mandible. Affected animals range in age from 1 to 14 years old with a mean age of 6.6 years.

This is a very slow-growing tumor that usually results in lameness due to expansion into surrounding muscles. In very chronic cases the tumor may erode through the cortex and extend into the medullary cavity. Metastasis to the lungs is possible but is rare. As a rule, amputation of the affected limb or area of tumor will be curative.

Chondrosarcoma

Chondrosarcoma is a malignant tumor in which the cells produce a neoplastic chondroid and fibrillar matrix but never directly produce neoplastic osteoid or bone. If neoplastic osteoid or bone is produced, then the tumor is classified as an osteosarcoma. Canine chondrosarcoma is the second most common bone tumor, comprising 10% of all canine bone tumors. The median age of affected dogs is 6 years (range, 1–12 years); there is no sex predilection. Major sites of origin are the ribs, nasal bones, and the pelvis.

Clinical signs are related to the location of the lesion: rib involvement—large, hard, painless swelling at the costochondral junction; pelvis—lameness; and nasal cavity—sneezing, epistaxis, and nasal swelling.

Radiographically, chondrosarcoma can produce either ostcolysis, osteoblastic or reactive periosteum with mineralization of the chondrosarcoma, or all of these.

Although frequently difficult, treatment is best accomplished by surgical removal of the tumor. The prognosis is good to guarded if complete excision of the tumor is accomplished. Metastasis to the lungs via a hematogenous route occurs in 10% of all chondrosarcomas. Radiotherapy with or without surgery appears to be effective for treating nasal chondrosarcoma.

Fibrosarcoma

Fibrosarcoma arises from malignant fibrous connective tissue elements that produce a collagenous matrix but no neoplastic cartilage or bone.

Fibrosarcoma of bone is rare in the dog; fibrosarcomas and hemangiosarcomas account for 7% of all long bone tumors in the dog. These bony tumors mostly occur in medium to large sized, male dogs. The tumors arise primarily in the metaphyseal area of the long bones. In my experience this is very commonly the distal femoral metaphysis.

Clinical signs are often masked for a period of time when the tumor is growing under a sizable muscle mass. Lameness or obvious swelling usually brings the animal to the veterinarian's attention. Radiography can be helpful, but it is almost impossible to differentiate between the primary and metastatic tumors of bone. Periosteal proliferation is seen early and is followed by erosion of the bone adjacent to the tumor. Soft tissue swelling is more apparent early in the course of the disease.

Treatment requires surgical excision of the tumor mass. Local radiation therapy following the amputation is often helpful. It is my experience that fibrosarcomas, although slow growing, will recur and can result in pulmonary metastasis as long as 1 year following amputation.

Benign Bone Tumors

Osteoma

Osteomas are protruding tumor masses composed of abnormally dense, but otherwise normal, bone formed in the periosteum. These tumors are most commonly seen on the skull and face but are rare in both the dog and cat. Clinical signs are only referable to the structures upon which they may impinge. Surgical removal is recommended only if tumor growth compromises another structure or the tumor is cosmetically unacceptable.

Chondromas

Chondromas are benign tumors of cartilage origin. These rarely seen tumors usually occur on flat bones. Clinical signs are referable to the distortion of surrounding structures. Surgical excision is only necessary if the clinical signs suggest compromise of a vital system in the animal.

Mineralizing Hematoma

Mineralizing hematomas can occur at many sites but are commonly seen on the dorsum of the skull in rapidly growing giant breed pups. They result from the animal striking the top of its skull on the underside of a table or other piece of furniture. The trauma results in a hematoma on top of the skull; because the trauma also breaks the periosteum, the hematoma mineralizes as does a fracture hematoma. Although these masses can be very cosmetically displeasing to the owner, they are very difficult to remove, because the surgery commonly results in more trauma and the formation of another hematoma.

Metastatic Tumors of Bone

Metastatic tumors of bone occur in both the dog and cat. These tumors include carcinomas, melanomas, nephroblastomas, aortic body tumors, sarcomas, fibromas, lymphosarcomas, hemangiosarcomas, reticulum cell sarcomas, and meningiomas.

References

Basset CAL. Current concepts of bone formation. J Bone Joint Surg 1962;44A:1217.

Boyd HB. Delayed union and nonunion of fractures. In: Crenshaw AH, ed. Campbell's operative orthopedics, 5th ed. St Louis: CV Mosby, 1970.

Brodey RS, Sauer RM, Medway W. Canine bone neoplasms. J Am Vet Med Assoc 1963;143:471.

Butler HC. Surgery of tendinous injuries and muscle injuries. In: Newton CD, Nunamaker DM, eds. Textbook of small animal orthopaedics. Philadelphia: JB Lippincott, 1985:835.

Caywood DD, Wallace LJ, Braden TH. Osteomyelitis in the dog: A review of 67 cases. J Am Vet Med Assoc 1978;172:943.

Cruess RL, Dumont J. In: Rockwood CA, Green DP, eds. Healing of bone, tendon and ligament. Philadelphia: JB Lippincott, 1975:988.

Cruess RL, Dumont J. Basic fracture healing. In: Newton CD, Nunamaker DM, eds. Textbook of small animal orthopaedics. Philadelphia: JB Lippincott, 1985:35.

Farrow CS. Sprain, strain and contusion. Vet Clin North Am 1978;8:169.

Goldschmidt MH, Thrall DE. Malignant bone tumors in the dog. In: Newton CD, Nunamaker DM, eds. Textbook of small animal orthopaedics. Philadelphia: JB Lippincott, 1985:877.

Goldschmidt MH, Thrall DE. Primary and secondary bone tumors in the cat. In: Newton CD, Nunamaker DM, eds. Textbook of small animal orthopaedics. Philadelphia: JB Lippincott, 1985:911.

Mankin HJ. The articular cartilages. In: Newton CD, Nunamaker DM, eds. Textbook of small animal orthopaedics. Philadelphia: JB Lippincott, 1985:90.

Nunamaker DM. Management of infected fractures. Vet Clin North Am 1975;5:259.

Peacock EE, Van Winkle W. Wound repair. 2nd ed. Philadelphia: WB Saunders, 1976.

Rahn BA, Gallinaro P, Perren SM. Primary bone healing. J Bone Joint Surg 1971;4:783.

Rhinelander FW. Normal vascular anatomy. In: Newton CD, Nunamaker DM, eds. Textbook of small animal orthopaedics. Philadelphia: JB Lippincott, 1985:12.

Schenk RF. Histology of fracture repair and nonunion. Bern: A-O Bull, 1978:14.

Spjut HL, Dorfman HD, Fechner RF. Tumors of bone and cartilage. In: Atlas of tumor pathology. 2nd series, fascicle 5. Washington: Armed Forces Institute of Pathology, 1971.

Turrell JM, Pool RR. Primary bone tumors in the cat: A retrospective study of 15 cats and a literature review. Vet Radiol 1982;23:152.

Wolff J. Das gesetz der transformation. Transformation der knochen. Berlin: Hirschwald, 1892.

21

Marvin L. Olmstead
Charles D. Newton

Principles of Fracture Treatment

First Aid and Transportation

Owners of injured animals often fail to protect themselves while attempting to assist the injured animal, because the animal is a trusted pet. Therefore, it is important to caution owners about the need to protect themselves, by muzzling the animal if necessary, and to instruct them in administering first aid and transporting their injured animal to the veterinary office. Advise the owner of the following:

- If the animal is bleeding profusely, cover the area with a clean or sterile cloth and apply direct pressure to the site of hemorrhage.
- If an open fracture is present and bone ends are exposed, cover the bone ends and wound with a clean or sterile cloth to prevent further contamination.
- During transportation, do not allow the animal's injured limb to dangle freely or be further injured by the animal's movements.

- If the animal is unable or unwilling to right itself, slip a board under the animal.
- If it is necessary to roll the animal on the board, roll both the front and back legs at the same time in the same direction, and stabilize the head, moving it in unison with the rest of the body to minimize any potential trauma in the area of the spinal cord.
- Present the injured animal to the veterinarian as quickly as is reasonably possible so that a thorough medical evaluation can be performed.

Priorities of Polytrauma

Although a polytraumatized animal should always be evaluated for possible injuries to all its body systems, the order of evaluation should be as follows:

1. The number one priority is to be sure that the animal can breathe freely.

2. The next system to be evaluated is the cardiovascular system. Areas of profuse bleeding are controlled by placing a sterile bandage over the site of bleeding and applying direct pressure. Hemorrhage control is maintained until the injured area can be properly surgically explored.
3. Assessment of the central nervous system is next. The stage of consciousness should be evaluated. Any reluctance or inability of the animal to stand on either the front or back limbs should be evaluated neurologically. If a fracture in the spinal column is suspected, great care should be taken in moving the animal. Obvious neurologic signs require further neurologic evaluation.
4. The urinary system should be evaluated to ensure that the bladder or urethra is not ruptured. Damage to the kidneys may be more difficult to assess; therefore, in the severely traumatized patient it is prudent to place a catheter so that urinary output can be monitored.
5. Evaluation and initial treatment of a polytraumatized patient's musculoskeletal injuries usually are low in priority. If a patient with an open fracture presents with other life-threatening injuries, then a sterile gauze should be applied to the open wound, and the other emergencies attended to first. If the patient is stable, extensive evaluation of the musculoskeletal injury can be performed.

In the case of an open fracture, the wound should not be probed until the surgeon is ready to perform the initial wound debridement. Exposed bone ends and tissue can be covered with sterile lubricant jelly while the hair is being clipped from around the wound margin. The clipped area should be adequate to allow extensive debridement of the area, if necessary. Once the tissue has been debrided, the bone ends should be positioned under the skin, muscle, and fascia. Generally it is better to leave the wound margins open unless the wound has been so thoroughly cleaned that there is no chance of any contamination being trapped under the skin.

Principles of Fracture Management

The treatment goal in fracture management is to achieve normal, undisturbed bone healing and to have the patient return to normal function. Achieving this goal is dependent both upon factors that are completely under the control of the surgeon and factors that are outside that sphere of control. For every fracture, more than one method of acceptable fixation is possible. It is the surgeon's responsibility to choose the method of fixation that will provide the greatest opportunity for successful resolution of the problem with least risk to the patient.

The surgeon must decide between internal and external fracture stabilization and then must apply the chosen treatment method according to the guidelines established for the treatment selected. Following the fixation of a fracture, a controlled, monitored convalescence is critical to ultimate success. The surgeon must work in concert with the animal's owners to ensure a successful result.

Factors that influence the selection of a treatment plan include the location of the fracture, the degree of trauma involved, the age of the patient, the activity of the patient, the reliability of the owner, and the capabilities of the surgeon. The surgeon, while trying to reduce the fracture gap, must also remember to respect the soft tissue surrounding the fracture and to provide an environment that is conducive to fracture healing. When surgical stabilization of a fracture is undertaken, early limb motion or weight bearing is generally desirable. This means that the fracture stabilization must be adequate to negate the forces that will act at the fracture site, (e.g., compression, tension, shear, rotation, and bending movements —Fig. 21-1). The choice of a fixation method will depend on many factors (see "Methods of Fracture Management," p. 570).

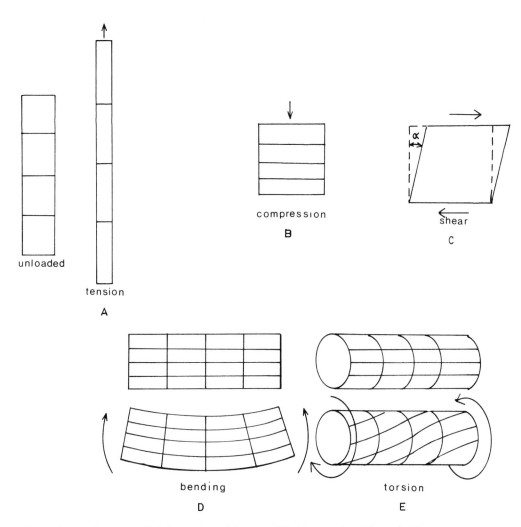

unloaded

tension

A

compression

B

shear

C

bending

D

torsion

E

Figure 21-1.   *Patterns of deformation. (Newton CD, Nunamaker DM, eds. Text-book of small animal orthopaedics. Philadelphia: JB Lippincott, 1985:199.)*

Principles of Joint Surgery

Because of the important role joints and articular cartilage play in locomotive function, fractures that involve articular surfaces or affect the normal mechanics of the joint must have anatomic reconstruction and rigid fixation. Without reconstruction and fixation the end result will be degenerative joint disease. Discrepancies in alignment that would not be a problem in shaft fractures because of the remodeling process cause disastrous results in joint fractures. Because of these demands fractures that involve the joint are almost never treated by nonsurgical methods.

The surgical approach must give adequate exposure to the joint, yet not be so extensive that it damages critical blood supply or creates excessive inflammation at the surgical site. The standard accepted approaches have been well documented. Fracture segments that contain cartilage surfaces must be aligned anatomically and rigidly fixed with either intramedullary pins or, more preferably, lag screws, whenever possible. Free fragments of cartilage should be removed from the joint, and cancellous bone grafts should be applied to areas of bone deficit. Following reconstruction and stabilization of the fracture, the joint should be inspected for ligamentous instabilities, and corrective surgery for these instabilities should be performed.

In most cases it is critical to the success of joint fracture repair to institute early motion in the joint following surgery. This may be passive or may occur through controlled active weight-bearing. Early motion helps eliminate or minimize the development of fracture disease. Fracture disease is defined as stiffness in joints, muscle atrophy, fibrosis, limb edema, and resultant disuse or impaired use of a limb. When repairing the joint, avoid unnecessary damage to muscles, tendons, and ligaments, and try to avoid destabilizing an already traumatized joint. Incisions in the joint capsule should be made in such manner that they minimally affect blood supply, joint stability, and joint function. There must always be enough joint capsule available on either side of the incision to allow closure at the end of the surgery. An absorbable, noninflammatory monofilament suture is best for closure of the joint capsule. A simple interrupted or cruciate pattern very effectively closes the joint capsule.

While fracture repair is being performed, care should be taken not to cause additional damage to the articular cartilage. Following fracture repair, the joint should be thoroughly lavaged and examined for other damage. The joint should always be passively manipulated through a normal range of motion after the fracture has been stabilized to ensure that a smooth gliding motion within the joint has been reestablished.

Etiology, Diagnosis, and Classification of Fractures

A fracture is a dissolution of bony continuity with or without displacement of the fragments. It is accompanied by torn vessels, bruised muscles, lacerated periosteum, and contused nerves. The trauma to soft tissue must be con-

sidered, because such trauma is often more important than the fracture itself.

Etiology of Fractures
Extrinsic Causes of Fracture

Trauma is the most common cause of fractures and usually results from automobile injury or falling from a height. Because direct trauma is rarely delivered in a calibrated amount to a specific place, the resultant fracture is rarely predictable. Most fractures resulting from marked direct trauma are either comminuted or multiple.

Fractures due to indirect trauma are more predictable than those from direct trauma. Generally a force is transmitted to a bone in a specific fashion, and a fracture occurs at a "weak link" within the bone.

Bending fractures occur when force is applied to a specific focal point on a bone. The fracture occurs when the traumatic force overcomes the elastic limit of the bone diaphysis. Bending fractures are generally oblique or transverse or may have a butterfly fragment.

Torsional fractures occur when a twisting force is applied to the long axis of a bone; one end of a bone is placed in a fixed position, while the other end of the bone is forced to rotate. The resulting fracture will be a spiral with sharp points and, often, sharp edges.

Compressive forces along the long axis of a bone may force the smaller diaphyseal or metaphyseal portion of a bone to impact into the larger epiphysis, which is crushed. Similarly a compressive force directed along the axis of the spine may result in collapse of a vertebral body.

A shearing fracture is caused by a force transmitted along the axis of a bone that is then transferred to either a portion of the same bone that lies peripheral to the axis or across a joint to other bones. The force shears off that bony portion unable to continue transmission of the force along the axis. The fracture line in a shear fracture will run parallel to the direction of the applied force. Shearing forces result in fracture of bony prominences.

Intrinsic Causes of Fractures

Fractures caused by contraction of a muscle are called avulsion fractures. They may occur because of strong isometric contraction, but more commonly are associated with trauma that results in forceful muscular shortening. These fractures commonly occur in immature animals with relatively weak open physeal plates.

Pathologic fractures occur because of underlying bony or systemic disease. In these cases, many, or all, bones of an animal's skeletal system are abnormal, thus more susceptible to fracture. Pathologic fracture may be due to any of the following types of bony pathology: neoplasia, bone cysts, osteoporotic bone, or localized osteomyelitis.

Diagnosis of Fractures

Clinical Signs of Fracture

Clinical signs associated with diagnosis of a fracture are uncomplicated in most instances; often the owner observes lameness. The practitioner needs a systematic, logical approach to isolate the fracture site and evaluate the fracture. Lameness is the most common indicator of fracture. Paralysis may indicate spinal fracture, unconsciousness can point to cranial fracture, and masticatory dysfunction may reflect mandibular fracture. Pain over the site of fracture is common and may be the only clinical indication present in cases of incomplete fracture. If the fracture is open, the surrounding area may demonstrate swelling, hematoma, contusion, or laceration. Acute onset of abnormal posture or limb positioning following trauma is a clear indication of fracture. Bony crepitus, the grinding sensation felt by palpation, which indicates contact of broken bone ends on each other, is a consistent sign of fracture. Abnormal motion of the limb at a point that should be rigid is a pathognomonic sign of a fracture. This abnormal motion occurs with a complete fracture of the shaft of a long bone but not with an incomplete or impacted fracture. Miscellaneous signs sometimes associated with fracture include: fever (seen rou-tinely 24–48 hours following a fracture), anemia, shock, nerve injury, necrosis or gangrene, and fat in synovial fluid.

Radiographic Signs of Fracture

Fracture, either diagnosed or suspected, should be documented through radiography. At least two views, including the joint above and below the fracture, are needed. Fracture of joints and fractures of special anatomic locations may require additional radiographs or special positioning.

The specific radiographic signs of fracture are: a break in the continuity of a bone, a line of radiolucency when the fragments are distracted, and a line of radiopacity when the fragments are compressed or superimposed.

Classification of Fractures

Fractures are classified into many types based on the severity of the fracture, whether it communicates through the skin, the shape of the fracture line, and the anatomic location of the fracture within an individual bone.

Classification of Fractures by Severity

Incomplete Fractures. If a bone has not completely lost continuity and some portion of the bone remains intact, the fracture is incomplete (Fig. 21-2). The following are specific types of incomplete fractures.

A greenstick fracture resembles the break caused when a supple green branch of a tree is bent and breaks incompletely. Usually the side opposite the bending force fractures completely, while the side under the force remains intact. Greenstick fractures occur primarily in immature animals.

Fissure fractures are cracks or fissure lines that occur when direct trauma is applied to any long or flat bone. Generally the fissures are formed in one cortex of the bone and are covered by an intact periosteum. Bones may have single or multiple fissure lines.

Depression fractures represent areas where multiple fissure fracture lines intersect. With sufficient force, the entire area will depress from the direction of force.

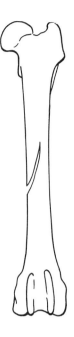

Figure 21-2. *Incomplete fracture of the femoral diaphysis. (Newton CD, Nunamaker DM, eds. Textbook of small animal orthopaedics. Philadelphia: JB Lippincott, 1985:187.)*

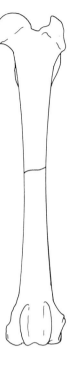

Figure 21-3. *Transverse fracture line. Drawing represents a reduced transverse fracture of the midshaft femoral diaphysis. (Newton CD, Nunamaker DM, eds. Textbook of small animal orthopaedics. Philadelphia: JB Lippincott, 1985:187.)*

Complete Fractures. These fractures are indicated by the entire loss of bony continuity allowing bone overriding and limb deformation. Complete fractures are far more common than incomplete fractures. Further classification of complete fractures is by the shape of the fracture line.

Classification of Fractures by Line Shape

Transverse fractures are transverse to the long axis of the bone (Fig. 21-3). Most are caused by bending forces.

Oblique fractures are oblique to the long axis of the bone (Fig. 21-4). The two cortices of each fragment are in the same plane without spiraling. These fractures generally result from bending with superimposed axial compression.

Spiral fractures spiral along the long axis of the bone and are caused by torsional twisting or rotational forces (Fig. 21-5). Spiral fractures tend to have extremely sharp points and edges.

Comminuted fractures have at least three fracture fragments with all the fracture lines interconnecting (Fig. 21-6). Comminuted frac-

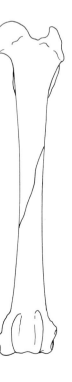

Figure 21-4. *Oblique fracture line. Drawing represents a reduced oblique fracture of the midshaft femoral diaphysis. (Newton CD, Nunamaker DM, eds. Textbook of small animal orthopaedics. Philadelphia: JB Lippincott, 1985:188.)*

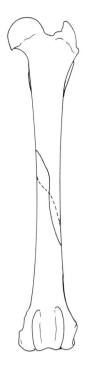

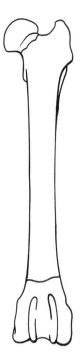

Figure 21-5. *Spiral fracture line. Drawing represents a reduced spiral fracture of the midshaft femoral diaphysis. (Newton CD, Nunamaker DM, eds. Textbook of small animal orthopaedics. Philadelphia: JB Lippincott, 1985:188.)*

Figure 21-7. *Multiple fractures. Drawing represents a reduced femoral neck fracture and a reduced transverse fracture of the distal femoral metaphysis. (Newton CD, Nunamaker DM, eds. Textbook of small animal orthopaedics. Philadelphia: JB Lippincott, 1985:188.)*

tures are generally caused by high energy trauma.

Multiple fractures have three or more fracture fragments in a single bone but the fracture lines do not interconnect (Fig. 21-7). Typically, multiple fractures present with two completely independent fractures affecting the same bone.

Compression fractures describe a fracture in which cancellous bone collapses and compresses on itself (Fig. 21-8). Most typically this occurs in vertebral bodies following trauma to the spine.

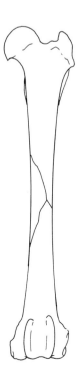

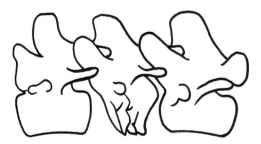

Figure 21-6. *Comminuted fracture lines. Drawing represents a reduced comminuted fracture of the midshaft femoral diaphysis. (Newton CD, Nunamaker DM, eds. Textbook of small animal orthopaedics. Philadelphia: JB Lippincott, 1985:188.)*

Figure 21-8. *Compression fracture. Drawing represents an unreduced compression fracture of a lumbar vertebral body. (Newton CM, Nunamaker DM, eds. Textbook of small animal orthopaedics. Philadelphia: JB Lippincott, 1985:189.)*

Classification of Fractures as Open or Closed

In a closed fracture, the skin remains intact. The fracture does not communicate with the outside environment. The open fracture does communicate with the outside environment (Fig. 21-9*A, B*). This may occur through a large soft tissue and skin wound or through a tiny puncture wound. The force or object creating the wound may come from inside or outside the leg.

Classification of Fracture by Location

This method clarifies fractures by their anatomic location with a specific bone. Identifying a fracture by location does not define if the fracture is open or closed or its type (*i.e.*, transverse, oblique, spiral).

Diaphyseal fractures are called midshaft if they occur near the axial center of diaphysis. All other fractures of the diaphysis are referred to by breaking the diaphysis into equal thirds (*i.e.*, proximal third, middle third, or distal third).

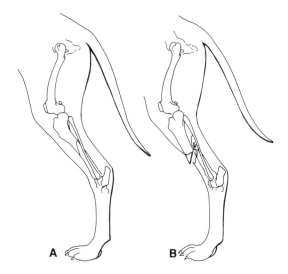

Figure 21-9. **A,** *Closed reduced oblique fracture of the midshaft tibial diaphysis.* **B,** *Open unreduced oblique fracture of the midshaft tibial diaphysis. (Newton CD, Nunamaker DM, eds. Textbook of small animal orthopaedics. Philadelphia: JB Lippincott, 1985:189.)*

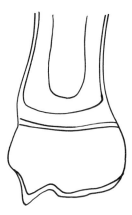

Figure 21-10. *Type I epiphyseal plate injury: separation of the epiphysis. (Redrawn after Salter RB, Harris WR. Injuries involving the epiphyseal plate. J Bone Joint Surg 1963;45(A):587.)*

Metaphyseal fractures are any fractures within the anatomic metaphysis of a long bone. For a clearer description, the terms proximal or distal should be added.

Fractures of the epiphyseal plate occur in immature animals during the time the epiphyseal plate (proximal or distal) remains open and cartilaginous. Epiphyseal plate fractures in immature animals are further classified to accurately describe their shape. The method of Salter–Harris is the standard classification for all species:

Type I—Epiphyseal separation is displacement of the epiphysis from the metaphysis at the growth plate through the zone of hypertrophied cartilage cells (Fig. 21-10).

Type II—A corner of metaphyseal bone fractures and displaces with the epiphysis (Fig. 21-11).

Type III—Fracture occurs through the epiphysis and part of the growth plate, but the metaphysis is unaffected (Fig. 21-12).

Type IV—Fracture exists through the epiphysis, growth plate and metaphysis (Fig. 21-13).

Type V—Impaction of the epiphyseal plate occurs with the metaphysis driven into the epiphysis (Fig. 21-14).

Fractures of the epiphysis in the mature animal with closed growth plates are called

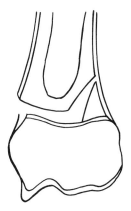

Figure 21-11. *Type II epiphyseal plate injury: fracture-separation of the epiphysis. (Redrawn after Salter RB, Harris WR. Injuries involving the epiphyseal plate. J Bone Joint Surg 1963;45(A):587.)*

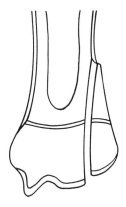

Figure 21-13. *Type IV epiphyseal plate injury: fracture of the epiphysis and epiphyseal plate. (Redrawn after Salter RB, Harris WR. Injuries involving the epiphyseal plate. J Bone Joint Surg 1963;45(A):587.)*

epiphyseal fractures and further classified by describing them as proximal or distal.

Condylar fractures affect the distal ends of the humerus or femur or the proximal tibia. Because a condyle is anatomically composed of metaphysis, physis, and epiphysis, a descriptive classification system is used (see Fig. 21-15). Condylar fractures are further defined as medial or lateral, depending on the location of the fracture. If both condyles fracture off the shaft as a unit, the fracture is called supracondylar. Both condyles may fracture from the shaft and from each other, leading to what is

termed an intercondylar or diacondylar fracture, and may be classified as "Y" or "T" fracture to better describe the shape of the fracture lines (Fig. 21–15).

The term articular fracture indicates that the subchondral bone and articular cartilage are involved in a fracture. Such a fracture may be further classified by indicating which end of the bone (proximal or distal) or which specific joint is fractured.

Avulsion fracture refers to a fracture of the bone under an insertion or origin site of a

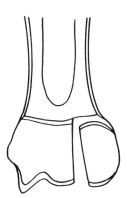

Figure 21-12. *Type III epiphyseal plate injury: fracture of part of the epiphysis. (Redrawn after Salter RB, Harris WR. Injuries involving the epiphyseal plate. J Bone Joint Surg 1963;45(A):587.)*

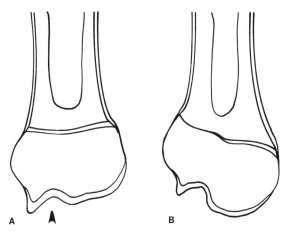

Figure 21-14. *Type V epiphyseal plate injury:* **A,** *Crushing of the epiphyseal plate;* **B,** *Premature closure. (Redrawn after Salter RB, Harris WR. Injuries involving the epiphyseal plate. J Bone Joint Surg 1963;45(A):587.)*

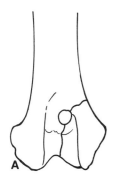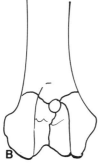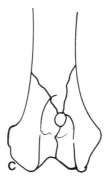

Figure 21-15. *Condylar fractures. **A,** Lateral humeral condyle fracture. **B,** Intercondylar and supracondylar fractures of the distal humerus (T fracture). **C,** Intercondylar and supracondylar fractures (Y fracture) of the distal humerus. (Newton CD, Nunamaker DM, eds. Textbook of small animal orthopaedics. Philadelphia: JB Lippincott, 1985:191.)*

muscle, tendon, or ligament. The prominences that fracture are usually separate centers of bone formation called apophyses. Avulsion fractures are classified by the prominence that has been avulsed.

Fracture dislocation describes fractures of joints which produce sufficient joint instability to result in a simultaneous subluxation or luxation of the affected joint.

Methods of Fracture Management

Because all fractures can be managed by more than one method, a number of factors must be evaluated when choosing a method of fixation. The age of the patient, the location of the fracture, the configuration of the fracture, the mechanical forces acting at the fracture site, equipment available, and the surgeon's capabilities and experience all play an important role in the decision-making process. The ultimate goal of fracture management, regardless of fracture type, should be undisturbed bone healing and return to normal limb function. Thus, surgeons must understand each of the methods of fixation available to them and the basic principles involved in their proper application. The standard methods of fixation include casts, splints, orthopedic wire, intramedullary pins, external fixators, bone screws alone, and bone plates with screws.

Closed Reduction and External Fixation

Most fractures encountered in small animal practice will be best repaired by open reduction and internal fixation (ORIF); however, there are those occasions when closed reduction and external stabilization of a fracture are indicated. In most cases where closed reduction is used, the animal will be young, and the fracture will be comprised of only two pieces or may even be an incomplete fracture. Casts or splints are usually used to maintain reduction of these fractures. On some occasions an intramedullary pin or an external fixator may be used in fracture repair without ever opening the fracture site. The advantage of closed reduction and external fixation is that the risk of infection is lowest, and further trauma to already damaged tissues from surgical exposure is avoided. Also, the cost of initial treatment using a closed reduction is generally less than that encountered with any open reduction procedure. The disadvantages of closed reduction and external fixation include a decreased ability to achieve anatomic realignment of the fracture site, prolonged anesthesia if the first reduction is unacceptable and the procedure must be repeated, and the development of fracture disease when casts and splints are used. With cast and splint application, follow-up reevaluation must be performed much more frequently than when other forms of fixation are applied.

The application of casts and splints for fracture repair should be limited to those fractures that occur below the stifle or elbow and are relatively nondisplaced or can be easily reduced.

Although plaster of paris has been the standard material used for casting, new water-activated resins are being used more and more in the place of plaster of Paris. These new resins are stronger and lighter in weight than plaster of Paris and achieve functional strength within minutes, as opposed to the many hours required of plaster of Paris. The new resins also allow better air circulation, which helps to keep the skin dry, thus decreasing the chance of a dermatitis developing under the cast.

Casts

For most fractures that are to be cast, it is best to lay the animal on its side with the fractured leg closest to the table. Traction can be applied to the limb by securing the axilla or groin area and pulling on the foot. Palpation of the bone fragments and the axial alignment of the bone will aid the surgeon in knowing when reduction has been achieved. It may be necessary to toggle the fragments into position. This maneuver is performed by creating an angle at the fracture site, so that the two fracture edges of one side of the bone can be engaged, and then straightening the limb using the engaged edges as a fulcrum (Fig 21-16). This procedure works with transverse or shorter oblique fractures but is little help in treating long oblique or spiral fractures.

Once the fracture is reduced, two anchor tapes or foot stirrups are applied to opposite sides of the limb (Fig. 21-17). These anchor tapes should extend 10–15 cm beyond the tip of the foot. A tongue depressor placed between the surfaces of the tape prevents them from sticking to each other. An assistant may use the anchor tapes as a handle to maintain traction and reduction of the fractured limb. The

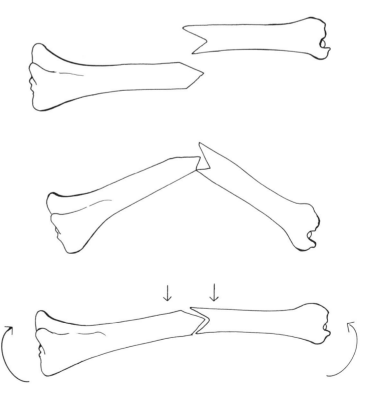

Figure 21-16. *Illustration of the method of "toggling" to achieve fracture reduction. Bone fragments must be placed in correct rotational orientation and angled to provide edge-to-edge cortical contact. Gradual straightening of the bone is accomplished by digital pressure applied away from sharp fracture ends. (Newton CD, Nunamaker DM, eds. Textbook of small animal orthopaedics. Philadelphia: JB Lippincott, 1985:208.)*

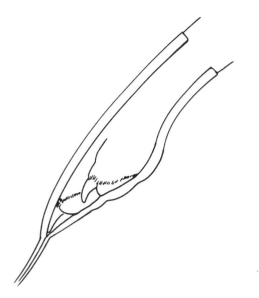

Figure 21-17. *Application of a foot stirrup is shown on the dorsal and volar surface of the paw. (Newton CD, Nunamaker DM, eds. Textbook of small animal orthopaedics. Philadelphia: JB Lippincott, 1985:250.)*

gauze stockinette is rolled up the leg until it fits high into the groin or axilla, depending upon which leg is being cast. Cast padding is started at the bottom of the foot at a level that will allow only the middle two toes to be exposed once the cast is complete; then the padding is wrapped towards the top of the leg. The cast padding should overlap at least 50% throughout the wrapping procedure. It should also be applied as snugly as possible, so that the conformation of the leg can be observed once the cast padding is applied. At potential pressure points, such as over the accessory carpal bone, at the point of the elbow or tuber calcanei, and at the cranial portion of the stifle, the cast padding should be wrapped in such a manner that a minimum of six layers of cast padding cover each of these areas. The casting material, be it plaster of Paris or resin, is then applied, starting at the bottom of the foot and working upward. When resin is used, one or two layers of cast material that overlap 50% are generally adequate. If plaster of Paris is the substance used, first, a layer of overlapping

plaster of Paris should be wrapped on the leg, followed by folded plaster of Paris splints, and then strips of plaster of Paris gauze applied to the front and back of the leg. These layers are then covered by a second and possibly third layer of plaster of Paris, depending on the size of the animal. No matter which cast material is used, the cast should be applied snugly to the leg, so that it will not be loose when the procedure is finished. To complete the cast, a 2- to 4-cm strip of the stockinette that was originally applied to the leg is rolled over the edge of the cast material at the top and bottom of the leg. The anchor tapes are folded back along the cast material as well. They may be cut off so that they are the same length as the folded back stockinette. A strip of casting material is used to secure the stockinette at the top of the cast and the stockinette and anchor tapes at the bottom of the cast.

Once the cast has been applied, radiographs are taken to ensure that the fracture reduction has been maintained. The owners should be instructed that they must check the cast daily for odor, slippage, drainage, chewing, and dryness. The owners should also examine the two exposed toes for swelling, perception of sensation, and evidence of inflammation. The veterinarian should evaluate the cast every 7 to 14 days.

The cast should be applied so that the joints of the limb are moderately flexed as they would be when the animal is standing on the leg. In areas where high humidity exists, it may be desirable to place cotton between the toes before the limb is covered with stockinette to help avoid a moisture-induced dermatitis.

Splints

Some veterinarians prefer to use a Schroeder–Thomas splint instead of a cast. This splint consists of an aluminum rod that is bent to accommodate the shape of the forelimb or hindlimb (Fig. 21-18). At the top of the splint, the rod has been bent in the shape of a ring, which is about the same width as the limb at that point. The part of the ring that fits either into

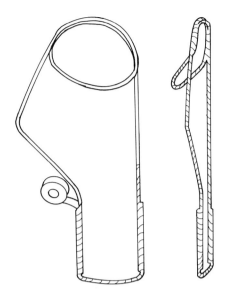

Figure 21-18. *A pelvic limb Schroeder–Thomas splint. The finished splint is shown with flattened tilted groin bar. Tape is applied to keep the traction members from slipping. (Newton CD, Nunamaker DM, eds. Textbook of small animal orthopaedics. Philadelphia: JB Lippincott, 1985:255.)*

the axilla or the groin is bent inward to accommodate the musculature of the limb. This portion of the ring is then padded with cotton and taped. The caudal bar for a hind leg and the cranial bar for a front leg is kept straight, while the natural bend of the elbow and carpus and the bend of the stifle and hock are followed by the bars that are adjacent to these areas. Once the leg length is determined, the front and back bars are bent square and taped together. The foot is anchored to the bottom bars with strategically placed tape. Tape and padding at various points on the limb are used to maintain the limb in the desired position (Fig. 21-19). Follow-up care for patients with this splint is the same as it would be for a cast.

A metasplint is sometimes used for fractures below the antebrachiocarpal joint and below the talocrural joint (Fig. 21-20). These fractures should be nondisplaced and generally involve the metatarsals and metacarpals or phalanges. The foot is wrapped with cast padding and anchor tapes, and the metasplint is incorporated in the final securing tape.

Internal Fixation of Fractures

Orthopedic Wire

Orthopedic wire is generally used as an adjunct to other methods of fracture repair. The most common function of orthopedic wire is to hold fragments in anatomic position. This can be achieved in several different ways. The wire may function as a full cerclage wire, which is passed completely around the circumference of the bone. Hemicerclage wire passes through holes that have been drilled in the bone. A figure-8 skewer pin is created by driving an intramedullary pin between two segments of bone and seating wire on the outside of the bone, using the two points of the exit of the intramedullary pin as anchors and crossing the wire between the pins. Orthopedic wire is also used as a tension band for avulsion fractures or osteotomies that were created in a surgical approach. A tension band counters the pull of a muscle or the force exerted on a ligament where these structures insert on to the bone fragment.

When applying a cerclage wire, several rules must be followed (Fig. 21-21). The wire should be at least 18 to 22 gauge, depending on the size of bone to be immobilized. This size will ensure that the wire has adequate strength to perform the required task. Wire should not be placed within a fracture line but should cross fracture lines. It should always be at least 1 cm away from the end of a bone spike and the nearest cerclage wire. When full cerclage wires are used, at least two should be applied, and, in the case of an oblique or spiral fracture, the length of the fracture should be at least two times the diameter of the bone to ensure that enough bone length will be present to accommodate the application of the cerclage wires. It is critical that the wires be placed tightly around the bone. Any motion of the wire on the bone surface will cause resorption of the bone and could disrupt the healing pro-

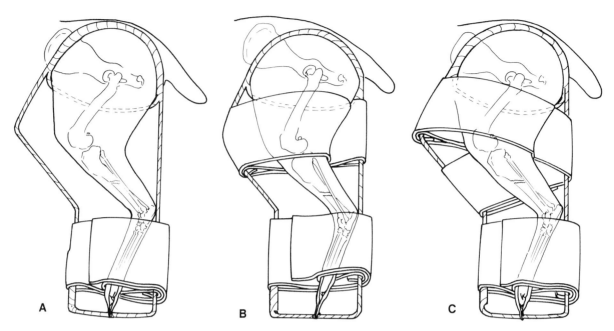

Figure 21-19. *Application of a Schroeder–Thomas splint.* **A,** *The bottom sling is placed first, as shown. Following completion, the combine roll material is taped in place.* **B,** *The process is reversed to apply the top combine roll to pull the femur forward, thereby applying traction to the tibia.* **C,** *Medial support is applied to the tibia by continuation of the bandage medial to the tibia. (Newton CD, Nunamaker DM, eds. Textbook of small animal orthopaedics. Philadelphia: JB Lippincott, 1985:256.)*

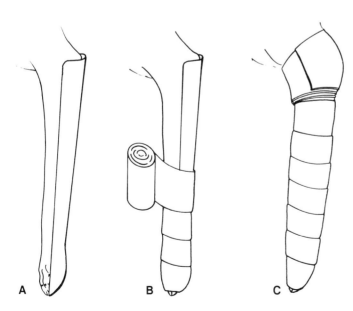

Figure 21-20. *Application of a metasplint.* **A,** *A ready-made metasplint is used to immobilize the forelimb. The device is often padded and may be used alone or with additional padding. The splint is usually attached with a foot stirrup, but some veterinarians attach it around the elbow with tape.* **B** *and* **C,** *Coaptation of the splint is done with gauze and tape. (Newton CD, Nunamaker DM, eds. Textbook of small animal orthopaedics. Philadelphia: JB Lippincott, 1985:259.)*

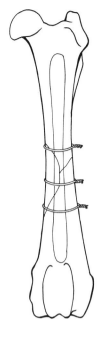

Figure 21-21. *Full cerclage wiring. Multiple cerclage wires are placed before the introduction of a Steinmann pin. (Newton CD, Nunamaker DM, eds. Textbook of small animal orthopaedics. Philadelphia: JB Lippincott, 1985:280.)*

ture line. The holes drilled for hemicerclage wires should be drilled toward the fracture line so that the wire does not have to make sharp turns as it enters and exits the bone. Hemicerclage wires may be passed in front of or around intramedullary pins (Fig. 21-23).

A figure-8 skewer pin is applied as described above. The intramedullary pin should protrude through the opposite cortex just enough so that a wire can be looped around the end of the pin. The two free strands of the wire are placed under tension and tightened until they rest snugly on the bone's surface. The continuous wire strand of the figure 8 should always be under the free ends, which have been twisted together. The intramedullary pin is then bent at 90° at the point where it first entered the bone and is cut off short. By bending the pin, migration is prevented. When using this technique, the pin is most ideally placed perpendicular to the long axis of the

cess. While the wire is being tightened, tension should be applied to the wire to ensure that a snug fit of the wire is achieved (Fig. 21-22). Full cerclage wires should be applied perpendicular to the long axis of the bone whenever possible. This helps ensure that the wire maintains its tight fit and does not rotate during the healing process. Hemicerclage wires may be placed perpendicular to the frac-

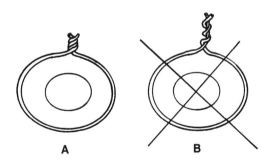

A   **B**

Figure 21-22. *Techniques of orthopedic wire tightening. **A,** Proper wire tightening allows the wire to twist around itself; and **B,** does not allow one wire to twist around the other. (Newton CD, Nunamaker DM, eds. Textbook of small animal orthopaedics. Philadelphia: JB Lippincott, 1985:280.)*

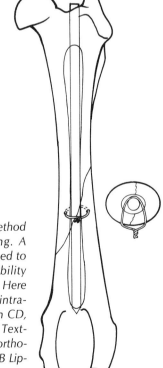

Figure 21-23. *One method of hemicerclage wiring. A hemicerclage wire is used to provide rotational stability and prevent overriding. Here it is used around the intramedullary pin. (Newton CD, Nunamaker DM, eds. Textbook of small animal orthopaedics. Philadelphia: JB Lippincott, 1985:281.)*

bone but may be placed perpendicular to the fracture line.

Cerclage, hemicerclage, and figure-8 skewer pin wires are always used as an adjunct to other methods of fracture repair. Their primary purpose is to aid in the anatomic reconstruction of the bone and to help stabilize the bone fragments during fracture healing.

Tension-band wiring can be used as the sole means of fixation of some fractures (Fig. 21-24). This technique is used to repair avulsion fractures or surgical osteotomies that have been performed in areas where tendons, ligaments, or muscle attach to bone. The wire used in this technique directly counters the tension forces on the free bone fragment created by muscle pull or weight bearing. Because of the presence of this wire, instead of displacement of the bone fragments, compression is created along the fracture line. Generally this technique is applied by first driving two intramedullary pins through the fragment into the main body of bone. These pins are bent at a 90° angle as they exit the bone. A hole is drilled in the main body of bone perpendicular to the long axis of the bone, and the wire to be used for the tension band is passed through this hole. This wire is wrapped in a figure 8 around the two pins that were placed to maintain rotational stability. The wire is then tight-

ened while tension is applied to the two free strands of wire, until it lies flush with the bone surface. This technique is commonly applied to the trochanter, olecranon, tibial tuberosity, malleolus, tuber calcis, and acromion process.

Intramedullary Pins

The Steinmann pin or the Kirschner drill wire are the most commonly used intramedullary pins in veterinary surgery. Depending on the type of fracture, these pins may be used by themselves or in combination with other fixation techniques to achieve fracture reduction. These pins are introduced in either an open or a closed fashion. When an open approach is used, the fracture is exposed through a surgical incision. In a closed approach the fracture site is not exposed, and reduction is achieved by manual manipulation of the fragments. Obviously, closed reduction is limited to those fractures that are simple in nature and reduce easily. This method of fixation is very limited in its application. It is generally better to open the fracture site and visually observe fracture reduction and the effectiveness of the intramedullary fixation. Intramedullary pins can be introduced retrograde (from the fracture site toward either end of the bone) or normograde (from the end of the bone toward the fracture

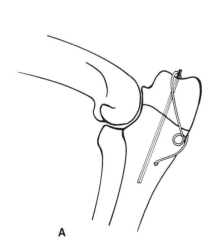
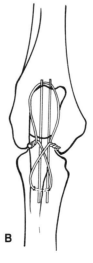

A   **B**

Figure 21-24. *The tension-band wire. **A,** The loop of the tension-band wire is shown prior to tightening. **B,** The tension-band wire is tightened by twisting the wire and cutting off the ends. (Newton CD, Nunamaker DM, eds. Textbook of small animal orthopaedics. Philadelphia: JB Lippincott, 1985:266.)*

site). Normograde fixation can be used in all of the long bones, whereas retrograde introduction of the pin is not recommended in all of the long bones (see Chap. 22, Management of Specific Fractures and Traumatic Dislocations).

The size of intramedullary pin chosen will depend upon the method of fracture repair used, the bone involved, and the type of fracture present. An intramedullary pin may be used singularly or in a stacked fashion with two or more pins placed in the medullary cavity. When used singularly, the intramedullary pin generally should fill at least two thirds of the medullary cavity, and, in some cases, it is desirable to completely fill the medullary cavity at its narrowest point. When a stacked pin technique is used, it is desirable to have the combined diameters of the two pins almost equal the narrowest diameter of the bone being pinned.

If a fracture interdigitates well, then an intramedullary pin, which provides axial alignment, may be adequate by itself. How-ever, if the fracture is found to be unstable after the intramedullary pin is introduced, then auxiliary orthopedic implants (orthopedic wire or external fixators) should be applied.

External Fixators

External skeletal fixation can be used as the sole means of fracture repair or as an adjunct to other methods of fixation. With this type of fixation, half pins are inserted through the skin and through the near and far portions of the cortical bone. In this fashion at least one pin is inserted in each segment of the fracture. The pins are connected outside the skin with the use of clamps and connecting bars. Three different types of configurations of external fixators have been identified. Multiple variations exist within each type (Fig. 21-25).

- The half pins in a Type I external fixator penetrate through the skin and the near

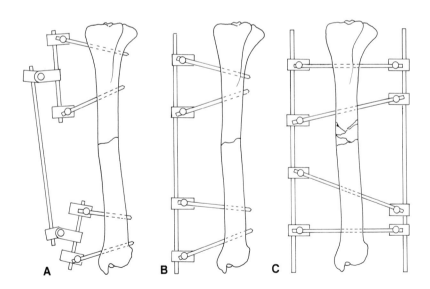
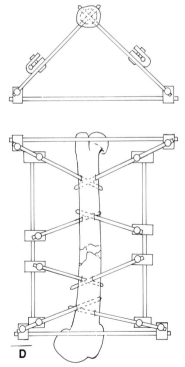

Figure 21-25. *Configurations of Kirschner-Ehmer apparatus commonly used in veterinary practice. **A,** Double-clamp (half-pin) [Type I] configuration. **B,** Single connecting-bar (half-pin) [Type I] configuration. **C,** Double connecting-bar (full-pin) [Type II] configuration. **D,** Triangular (half-pin) [Type III] configuration. (Newton CD, Nunamaker DM, eds. Textbook of small animal orthopaedics. Philadelphia: JB Lippincott, 1985:211.)*

and far cortex of bone but do not penetrate the skin on the opposite side.

- The half pins in a Type II external fixator penetrate the skin on both sides of the leg and both cortices, and bars are affixed to both sides of the limb.
- A Type III external fixator is three-dimensional and combines the aspects of Type I and Type II external fixator.

When a Type I external fixator is applied, the pins should be inserted with a hand chuck or a low-speed drill at an angle that is 30° to 45° from the midline. The first pins placed are near the proximal and distal end of the bone, thereby providing the best mechanical advantage against bending and torsional forces. This type of arrangement is used in combination with intramedullary pinning when the external fixator is used as an adjunct to increase the stability of fixation. By adding a second or third angled pin to each fracture segment, the stabilization provided by the external fixator is increased, and axial alignment of the segments is also maintained. These pins may all be secured to a common connecting rod. Double clamps and auxiliary connecting bars can also be used to connect the proximal to the distal pin block. The pins nearest the fracture site provide the greatest stability to the fracture. They should be placed relatively close to the fracture.

The Type II external fixator is most easily applied to the radius and tibia. Generally, if this type of fixation is the primary stabilizing apparatus, only the most proximal and distal pins need to pass entirely through the limb and bone; the pins nearest the fracture can be applied as they would be with a Type I fixation. This means that there would be a bar and two clamps on one side of the leg and a bar and four or more clamps on the opposite side.

The Type III fixation is generally not needed except in highly comminuted fractures in large dogs.

After the apparatus is applied, it may be desirable to wrap the clamps with gauze and then cover this with tape. The limb itself should not be wrapped. The bandaging of the splint is designed to minimize the possibility of the splint catching on objects and to cover the sharp edges of the pins. The exit holes where the pins leave the skin must be kept clean. Pin tract drainage is a common sequela to the application of an external fixator. This quickly resolves itself when the external fixator is removed. Those fixators that are used as adjuncts to other means of fixation can be removed when enough internal callus has been built up to take over the function of the external fixator. In most cases this buildup occurs in 4 to 6 weeks.

Bone Screws

In veterinary surgery two basic bone screws are used: the cancellous screw and the cortex screw. Cancellous screws have a wider thread and a steeper pitch than cortex screws. Thus, cancellous screws have fewer threads per unit of length than cortex screws. Cancellous screws are designed to hold in soft or loosely packed bone such as that found in the epiphysis and metaphysis. Cortex screws have better holding power in the dense compact bone found in the diaphysis.

Bone screws can have three functions: as plate screw, lag screw, or position screw. A cortex screw, because of its full threaded design, can have all three functions; but a cancellous screw only functions as either a lag screw or a plate screw.

Plate screws are those screws that pass through the screw hole in the plate and fix the plate into position.

A lag screw provides interfragmentary compression along a fracture line (Fig. 21-26). This compression occurs when the threads of the screw take hold only in the bone farthest away from the screw head. If this effect is to be achieved with a cancellous screw, then the shank of the cancellous screw that passes through the near fragment should be devoid of threads. Because cortex screws only come fully threaded, for this screw to function as a lag screw, the hole that is drilled in the bone

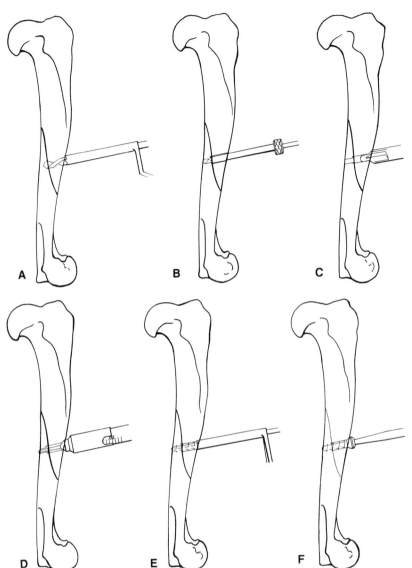

Figure 21-26. *Technique for placing an interfragmentary cortical bone screw. **A,** The large gliding hole is drilled using a drill guide. **B,** The smaller-threaded hole is drilled using the insert to center the hole precisely. **C,** The countersink is used to align the screw head to the hole in the shaft to prevent bending of the screw head. **D,** The hole is measured using the depth gauge. **E,** The hole is tapped. **F,** The screw is placed, producing interfragmentary compression. (Newton CD, Nunamaker DM, eds. Textbook of small animal orthopaedics. Philadelphia: JB Lippincott, 1985:272.)*

nearest the screw head must have the same or larger diameter as the threads of the screw used. The hole in the fragment opposite the screw head is always the same diameter as the inner shaft of the screw. The threads in the bone are cut with a tap, because self-tapping screws can cause microfractures and are thus not desirable as bone screws. Ideally, lag screws are placed at 90° to the fracture line. Lag screws should not be placed too close to the end of a fragment, because this placement

will cause the tip of the fragment to fracture. They also should not be placed in a line, because this placement may result in a linear split along the line of compression. Lag screws may be used to reconstruct the fracture segments before a plate is applied to the bone, or they may be placed through the plate and thus have a secondary function as a plate screw.

On rare occasions screws are used as position screws to hold bone fragments in a position, not to provide interfragmentary compression. When a screw is used as a position screw, threads are present on either side of the fracture line, resulting in some distraction of the fracture fragments. In situations where a lag screw will cause collapse of a bone segment into the medullary cavity, the screw should be used as a position screw, thus maintaining a more anatomic position of the bone fragment.

Bone Plates

Properly applied bone plates provide rigid internal fixation of a fractured bone, thus allowing the limb to return to normal function more quickly. To accommodate animals and bones of many different sizes, bone plates are available in a large selection of sizes and shapes. It is desirable to maintain the anatomic contours of the bone by molding the plate in special bending presses to a shape that follows the desired contour. Twisting irons are used to torque the plate when necessary.

Bone plates will have one or more of the following functions depending on the type of fracture they are applied to: dynamic compression, static compression, neutralization, and buttressing.

Plates have dynamic or static compression function when they are applied to the surface of the bone most frequently exposed to tensile forces, and the fracture involved is transverse or short oblique. Static compression is provided by one of three methods. A tension device may be hooked to the end of the plate after the plate has been secured with a bone screw to the segment farthest away from the tension device (Fig. 21-27). As the tension device is tightened, compression is achieved at the fracture line. The tension is maintained by inserting the screws in the fragment closest to the tension device. Once both fragments of bone have been secured to the plate with bone screws, the tension device is removed, and all holes in the plate are filled with screws. Compression may also be achieved by prestressing the plate, which means that rather than bending the plate flush to the bone, a 1- to 2-mm gap is left between the plate and bone at the frac-

ture site (Fig. 21-28). As the screws are inserted on either side of the fracture line, the bone is drawn towards the plate, thereby providing compression along the fracture line. The third method of providing static compression along the fracture line is achieved with screw hole geometry. If oblong holes are present in the plate, a special load guide may be used to drill a hole that is eccentric in its location (Fig. 21-29). As the screw is tightened, the head of the screw will engage the edge of the plate at the screw hole due to the eccentric position of the screw hole. Further tightening of the screw pushes the plate away from the fracture line. Because the plate has already been secured to the bone by placement of a screw through the plate into the opposite fragment, that portion of bone will be pulled towards the segment where the eccentrically placed screw is being inserted. This method provides compression along the fracture line. This process can be repeated twice on either side of the thick central part of the plate. The amount of compression provided will depend on the size of the plate used.

Dynamic compressive function is achieved when a plate is placed on the tension side of the bone and the bone is loaded with force provided by either weight bearing or the pull of muscles. Dynamic compressive function tends to be cyclic in nature. When no load is present, there will be no compression at the fracture line.

A plate has neutralization function when the shaft of bone has been fully reconstructed with the use of lag screws and the plate is used to protect these screws from all of those forces that act at the fracture line. The lag screws may be placed either through the plate or outside the plate as the fragments are reconstructed. Neutralization plates are applied to long oblique spiral fractures or comminuted fractures.

Buttress function is achieved when plates are used to support bone fragments, thereby maintaining length and axial alignment. Therefore, plates that prevent the collapse of a joint surface, whether or not there is a deficit in the

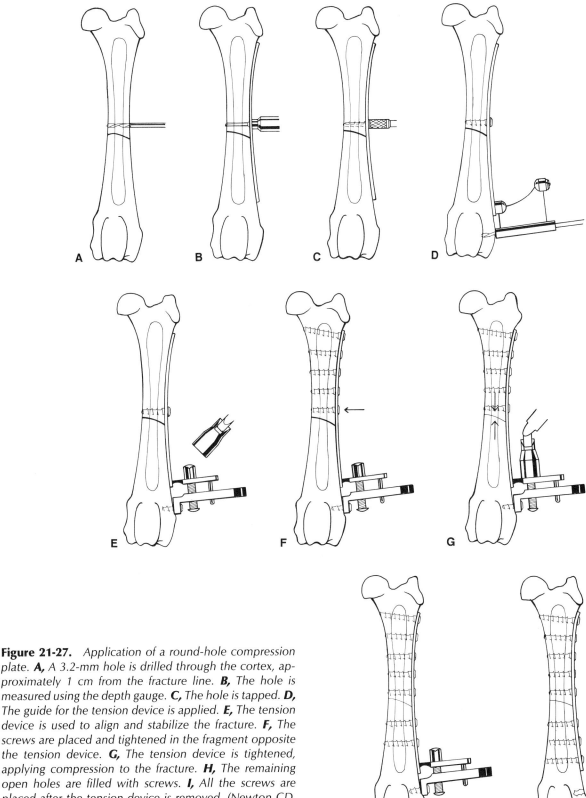

Figure 21-27. *Application of a round-hole compression plate. **A,** A 3.2-mm hole is drilled through the cortex, approximately 1 cm from the fracture line. **B,** The hole is measured using the depth gauge. **C,** The hole is tapped. **D,** The guide for the tension device is applied. **E,** The tension device is used to align and stabilize the fracture. **F,** The screws are placed and tightened in the fragment opposite the tension device. **G,** The tension device is tightened, applying compression to the fracture. **H,** The remaining open holes are filled with screws. **I,** All the screws are placed after the tension device is removed. (Newton CD, Nunamaker DM, eds. Textbook of small animal orthopaedics. Philadelphia: JB Lippincott, 1985:274.)*

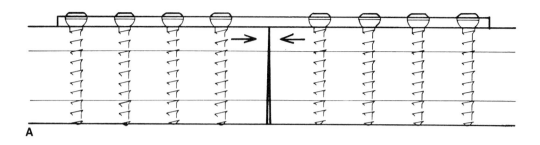

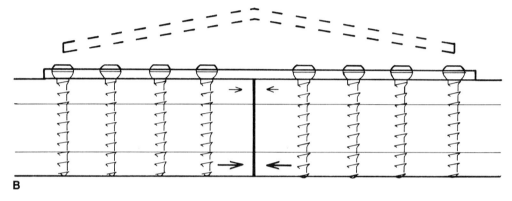

Figure 21-28. *Effects of prebending compression plates.* **A,** *Compression applied to a straight bone using a straight plate will give compression under the plate and a gap opposite the plate.* **B,** *A prebent plate will provide compression on the cortex opposite the plate as well as underneath it. (Newton CD, Nunamaker DM, eds. Textbook of small animal orthopaedics. Philadelphia: JB Lippincott, 1985:278.)*

fracture reconstruction, have buttress function. When a plate is used as a buttress plate in the shaft, however, there is either loss of bone or such severe comminution that the shaft cannot be totally reconstructed with the use of lag screws. Because buttress plates will be exposed to the greatest amount of strain, they should be the thickest or longest plates applied to a fracture repair.

No matter what the function of the plate, a minimum of two screws or four cortices should be engaged on either side of a fracture line. If at all possible, particularly in fractures involving the diaphysis of the bone, three screws should be inserted on either side of the fracture line. Screws should not be placed any closer than 5 mm from the edge of a fracture line.

Pediatric Fractures

The bone in young animals is usually soft; therefore, implant devices are not as secure as they would be in a more mature animal. The fact that immature bones are growing in length and width must be taken into consideration when the method of fixation is chosen. Because young bone is more elastic than older bone, there is a greater tendency for the bone to bend rather than break. Fractures seen in young patients often are far less comminuted than those encountered in the older animal. Bone in young animals generally heals much more rapidly than that in older animals. In the very young animal, the healing process may take only a few weeks. Because the young animal is

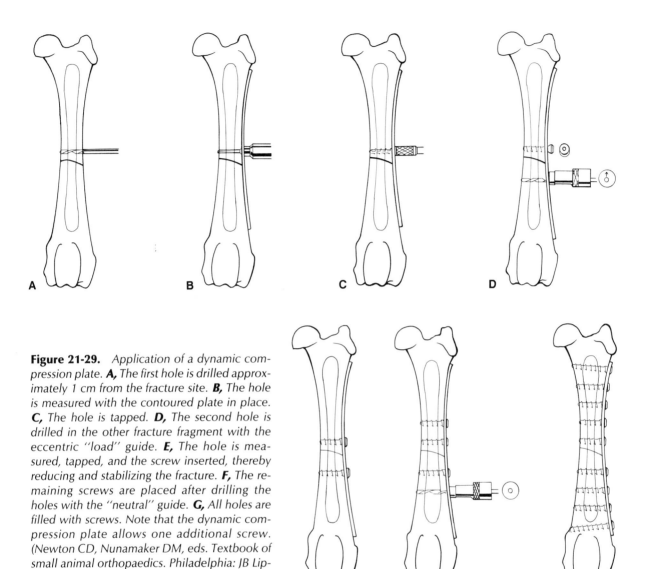

Figure 21-29. *Application of a dynamic compression plate.* ***A,*** *The first hole is drilled approximately 1 cm from the fracture site.* ***B,*** *The hole is measured with the contoured plate in place.* ***C,*** *The hole is tapped.* ***D,*** *The second hole is drilled in the other fracture fragment with the eccentric "load" guide.* ***E,*** *The hole is measured, tapped, and the screw inserted, thereby reducing and stabilizing the fracture.* ***F,*** *The remaining screws are placed after drilling the holes with the "neutral" guide.* ***G,*** *All holes are filled with screws. Note that the dynamic compression plate allows one additional screw.* *(Newton CD, Nunamaker DM, eds. Textbook of small animal orthopaedics. Philadelphia: JB Lippincott, 1985:276.)*

actively making new bone, the callus formed in the pediatric patient may be relatively greater than that observed in a more mature animal. This active state, however, also means that the remodeling process will occur much more quickly.

The Salter–Harris classification of fractures has been previously described (see "Classification of Fractures by Location"). Fractures occur frequently in young animals at or near the physis, because the cartilage pres-

ent in the physis is the weakest part of the bone. Implants that cause compression across the growth plate or have a bridging effect on the growth plate will result in premature closure of the physis. For this reason, bone plates should not be positioned such that the physis is bridged, and the pins for external fixators should be placed only in metaphyseal and diaphyseal bones. Straight intramedullary pins can pass through the epiphysis, the physis, and into the metaphysis without resulting in premature closure of the growth plate, if the pins are less than 20% of the overall surface area of the physis and pass parallel with the longitudinal alignment of the cartilage columns within the physis. Generally speaking, intramedullary pins are used to stabilize fractures that involve the physis. If the epiphysis is fractured along with the physis, as is observed in Salter–Harris III and IV types of fracture, then the bone is reconstructed, whenever possible, with a lag screw. It may be necessary, when a traction apophysis has avulsed, to replace that structure with the use of two pins and a tension-band wire. Because the tension-band wire provides compression across the fracture line, it is imperative that this wire be removed in 2 to 4 weeks (depending on the age of the animal). If the two pins alone provide adequate stabilization of the apophysis, then their use alone is the preferred method of stabilization. It is very important to achieve stable fixation and anatomic reduction of fractures that occur near or within a joint surface.

Fractures of the diaphysis that are not complete (greenstick fractures), are only minimally displaced, or can be reduced with good interlocking of the pieces, may be placed in either a Schroeder–Thomas splint or a cast, as long as these fractures occur in bones below the stifle and elbow.

Intramedullary pinning is often the method of choice when dealing with fractures in young animals. Generally a relatively small pin can be used to stabilize a fracture in a pediatric patient. Young bone has more cancellous bone in the medullary cavity, thus reducing the size of pin necessary for fracture stabilization. External fixators may be used in young animals as they are in adults, except that the anchoring pin should never be placed in the epiphysis.

It is usually not necessary to use bone plates on young bone. If a bone plate is used, it should be the smallest size possible that will still lend adequate support to the bone. Plate removal as soon as the fracture is radiographically healed is recommended in young animals to assure that the plate does not interfere with expansion of the bone or the development of blood supply within the bone. With the exceptions already noted, fracture repair in young animals is performed as described in each of the individual long bones (see Chap. 22, Management of Specific Fractures and Traumatic Dislocations).

Management of Open Fractures and Gunshot Wounds

When open fractures or gunshot fractures are present, the patient's entire system must be assessed, because these types of injuries often are accompanied by severe trauma to other organs of the body. With a gunshot fracture, the entrance wound and, if present, the exit wound will provide a clue as to the path of the missile. It should be remembered, however, that bullets can tumble in tissue rather than pass from one point to another in a straight line. It is up to the surgeon to determine the severity of the open fracture, which will dictate to some extent the urgency of fracture repair and the aggressiveness of the treatment needed. Proper wound management is always of paramount importance when handling these cases. Hair should be clipped from the edge of the open wound outward providing a wide hair-free margin around the wound site. Care must be taken to see that no small hair particles fall into the wound during the clipping process. Liberally covering the wound with sterile, water-soluble jelly will help trap any small hair particles in the jelly, and these can later be flushed out with liberal amounts of sterile lactated Ringer's solution. All animals with an open fracture should be started on broad-spectrum antibiotic therapy. If the wound is small (less than 1 cm), and there is no indication of severe trauma to the soft tissues, the fracture can be handled as any closed fracture would be handled. However, if the wound is large, and there is severe trauma to the soft tissues, then the soft tissues should be cleaned and debrided thoroughly at the time the animal is presented. It may also be necessary at that time to effect primary repair of the fractured bone. If the animal is not stable or the tissues are very badly damaged, then temporary stabilization should be provided until such time as either the animal or the tissues are in a better state of health. An external fixator or reinforced splint can be used for temporary stabilization.

When a wound is caused by a gunshot injury, the damage can be quite extensive to the soft tissues. This is particularly true if the bullet was fired from a high-muzzle-velocity rifle (over 700 m/sec). The tissue damage will be very extensive because of the massive wound cavitation that results from the energy released as the bullet passes through the tissue. Fortunately, most civilian rifles are low velocity and do not cause the extensive damage that a high-velocity rifle does. If the wound is extensive or massive contamination is present, then it is best to leave the wound open following debridement. Closing the wound will merely trap any infection within the body, whereas leaving the wound open allows for constant drainage and wound care. It may be necessary to debride a wound more than once depending on the body's response to the trauma. In cases with severe contamination and a high probability of extensive damage to the regional blood supply, the more rigid forms of an external fixator (Type II or Type III) may be the best choice of fixation. Because a rigidly stabilized fracture will heal even in the face of infection, it is of paramount importance that no matter what fixation method is chosen for repair of an open fracture, the main fracture segments must be rigidly fixed. Tiny fragments of comminution that are too small to incorporate in the shaft reconstruction should be removed

if active infection is known to be present. If the fracture site is only considered contaminated and not infected, then the small fragments may be left in place, because excessive tissue damage may result from trying to find all of the tiny fragments. Fragments of metal from a bullet may also be left in the soft tissues. They, however, should not be left in a joint space, because the fragments will act as a mechanical irritant to the joint space. Lead, which dissolves into the joint fluid, will poison the chondrocytes of the joint.

In a severe open wound, it is oftentimes necessary to allow the wound to heal by second intention, so that the infection can be controlled. All of the major implants used for fracture stabilization of an open fracture should be removed after the fracture has healed. If these implants are not removed and infection is present, the infection may remain in the bone at a subclinical level for years. Disastrous results may occur if this is allowed to happen. There is some evidence that fracture-related sarcomas have been caused by these subclinical infections.

Suggested Readings

Bojrab MJ. Current techniques in small animal surgery. Philadelphia: Lea & Febiger, 1983.

Brinker WO, Hohn RB, Prieur WD. Manual of internal fixation in small animals. Berlin: Springer-Verlag, 1984.

Brinker WO, Piermattei DL, Flo GL. Handbook of small animal orthopedics and fracture treatment. Philadelphia: WB Saunders, 1983.

Newton CD, Nunamaker DM, eds. Textbook of small animal orthopaedics. Philadelphia: JB Lippincott, 1985.

Piermattei DL, Greely RC. Atlas of surgical approaches to the bones of the dog and cat. 2nd ed. Philadelphia: WB Saunders, 1979.

Slatter DH, ed. Textbook of small animal surgery. Philadelphia: WB Saunders, 1985.

22

Marvin L. Olmstead
Charles D. Newton

Management of Specific Fractures and Traumatic Dislocations

Repair of Common Fractures

The fracture treatment methods previously described (see Chap. 21, Principles of Fracture Treatment) will be employed in the stabilization of the fractures described below. As each bone is discussed, the special aspects related to care of fractures in a specific region of the bone will be emphasized. Different methods of repair will be described where applicable. Remember that each fracture can be repaired in more than one fashion. The surgeon must choose a method of repair that is most appropriate for the situation presented.

Management of fractures of the mandible is described in Chapter 6, The Oral Cavity. Management of vertebral fractures is described in Chapter 19, The Spine.

Fractures of the Scapula

Fractures of the scapula are uncommon for several reasons, the primary one of which is that the scapula is well protected by sur-

rounding musculature. Primarily a flat bone, it tends to undergo elastic deformation rather than fracturing. If the fracture is relatively nondisplaced and does not either directly or indirectly affect the scapulohumeral joint, then a nonoperative approach can be taken. Generally, a non-weight-bearing flexion sling, a Velpeau sling, (Fig. 22-1) applied for a period of 10 days to 4 weeks, depending on the animal's age and the nature of the fracture, is adequate stabilization in most nonoperatively-treated cases. If the above criteria are not met, then surgical treatment should be considered. Muscle spreading approaches should be used in lieu of approaches that require osteotomies, when exposing the scapula surgically.

Displaced fractures of the blade of the scapula can be effectively treated with either wiring techniques or application of bone plates and screws. The objective of wiring techniques is to bring the bone fragments into approximate alignment. The wire is passed through holes drilled in the bone, and the wires are

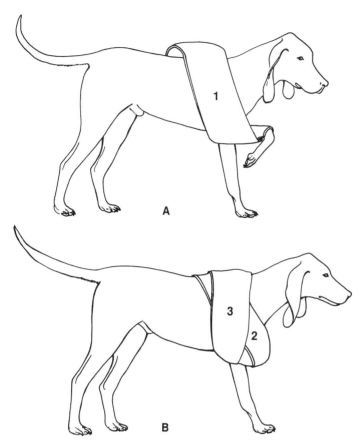

Figure 22-1. *Application of a Velpeau sling. **A,** The Velpeau sling is shown with the first revolution in place. **B,** The finished Velpeau sling, with the second and third wrap shown. (Newton CD, Nunamaker DM, eds. Textbook of small animal orthopaedics. Philadelphia: JB Lippincott, 1985:251.)*

tightened, forming a simple interrupted suture. More than one of these simple interrupted wire sutures should be placed. More stable fixation can be achieved by using a bone plate. The plate should be placed where the bone is the thickest, (*i.e.,* along the caudal ridge of the scapula or at the junction between the spine and the blade of the scapula). A one-third or one-half tubular plate turned upside down and placed along the scapula at the spine–body junction is an effective method of treatment of blade fractures. In this instance the screws can be easily angled through the thickest part of the bone.

Fractures involving the neck of the scapula should be reduced, because fractures in this area result in abnormal alignment of the scapulohumeral joint (Fig. 22-2). Other cross-pin techniques (Steinmann or lag screw fixation) or small bone plates can be used to stabi-

lize this fracture. Care must be taken to protect the suprascapular nerve where it crosses this area. Bone plates used in this area will generally have buttress function. A T-shaped or L-shaped plate with the short segment in the distal fragment and the long segment placed along the spine–body junction in the infraspinatus fossa is generally an effective method of stabilizing this fracture.

Any fracture that involves the glenoid fossa should be anatomically reduced, because this area is an articular surface (Fig. 22-3). Placement of lag screws, minifragment bone plates, or intramedullary pins are all effective methods of treating fractures in this area. The suprascapular nerves should be protected. When intramedullary pins are used, an attempt should be made to carefully bend the pins over before they are cut off, thus helping to prevent pin migration. Placement of intra-

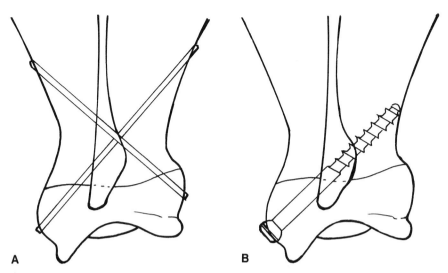

Figure 22-2. *Internal fixation for a scapular neck fracture: **A,** Crossed Steinmann fixation, **B,** Lag screw fixation. (Newton CD, Nunamaker DM, eds. Textbook of small animal orthopaedics. Philadelphia: JB Lippincott, 1985:339.)*

medullary pins in the scapula is difficult, because the bone is thin. It is, therefore, imperative that pin placement be accurate so that effective fracture stabilization can be achieved.

Fractures involving the supraglenoid tubercle can be repaired with the use of either a lag screw or two pins and a tension band wire (Fig. 22-4). The tension band wiring technique is biomechanically more correct, because this

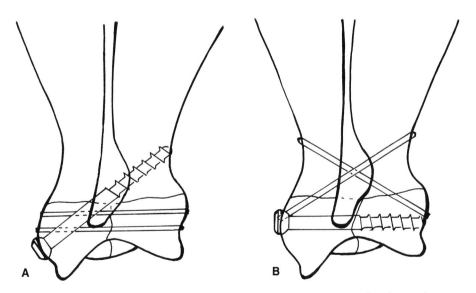

Figure 22-3. *Methods of internal fixation for a combination glenoid and scapular neck fracture: **A,** Two pins and one lag screw; **B,** One lag screw and crossed Steinmann pins. (Newton CD, Nunamaker DM, eds. Textbook of small animal orthopaedics. Philadelphia: JB Lippincott, 1985:340.)*

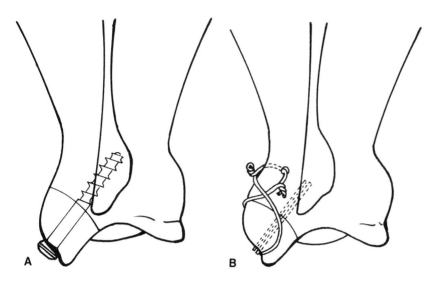

Figure 22-4. *Methods of internal fixation for a supraglenoid tubercle fracture: **A,** Lag screw fixation; **B,** Tension-band wire fixation. (Newton CD, Nunamaker DM, eds. Textbook of small animal orthopaedics. Philadelphia: JB Lippincott, 1985:339.)*

technique will effectively counter the pull of the biceps brachii muscle, which attaches to the supraglenoid tubercle.

Fractures involving the spine of the scapula can be repaired by wiring the spine to the body. If the acromion process is fractured, the tension band principle is the most effective means of dealing with this problem, because it will counter the distraction forces created by the pull of the deltoid muscle (Fig. 22-5). Either

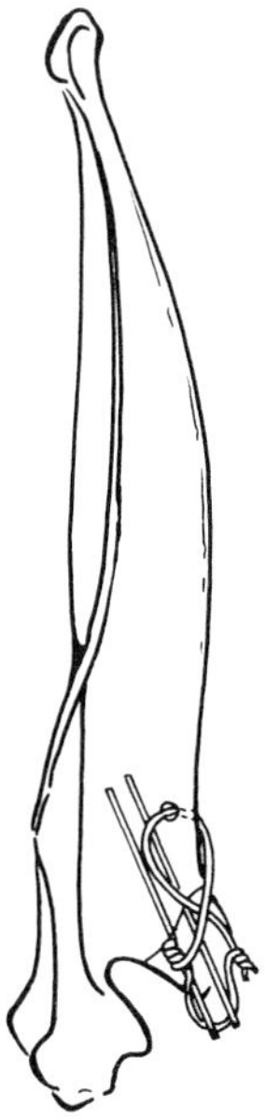

Figure 22-5. *Placement of a tension band wire for fixation of an acromial fracture. (Newton CD, Nunamaker DM, eds. Textbook for small animal orthopaedics. Philadelphia: JB Lippincott, 1985:338.)*

two simple interrupted orthopedic wire sutures or two carefully placed intramedullary pins and a tension band wire are effective.

If the stabilization of scapular fractures is rigid, then limited activity during the convalescent period should be adequate to allow proper fracture healing. If, however, there is any question as to whether the stabilization employed can withstand weight bearing, then the affected limb should be placed in a Velpeau sling for a period of 7 to 14 days. This sling will provide adequate time for fibrosis to develop. Controlled weight bearing can be allowed beyond this point.

The prognosis for scapular body fractures is excellent; conversely, fractures of the glenoid are more likely to result in some degenerative joint disease and limited range of motion.

Fractures of the Humerus

Proximal humeral fractures are relatively uncommon. When they do occur, however, the function of the nerves of the brachial plexus should be critically evaluated, because this plexus lies directly medial to the humerus. Salter–Harris Type I and II fractures may involve the proximal humeral physis. These fractures should be reduced and, in most instances, can be stabilized with the use of two or three small intramedullary pins that pass from the greater tubercle into the shaft of the bone. If the animal still has growth potential left, then extreme care should be taken to avoid damaging the germinal cells of the growth plate. If the animal has no growth potential left, then it may be possible to reduce the fracture with the use of a lag screw either through the greater tubercle or from the cranial–proximal portion of the humerus, just below the greater tubercle, angled into the humeral head, but not penetrating the articular cartilage. In some instances, it may be desirable to place a buttress plate along the cranial shaft of the humerus to stabilize the fracture segment. If only the greater tubercle has fractured off, then two pins and a tension band wire are generally very effective in reconstructing normal anatomy and stabilizing the fracture segments.

If the fracture involves the area from the proximal metaphysis to the distal diaphysis, any number of methods of fixation may be used. Although fractures of the proximal metaphysis are uncommon, two-piece fractures can be repaired with the use of an intramedullary pin that enters the bone at the greater tubercle and is seated distally in the metaphysis just above the supracondylar fossa. This pin may be driven either normograde or retrograde. If the fracture is oblique or spiral, then either full cerclage or hemicerclage wires can be used as axillary stabilization for the fracture. If there is comminution that prevents the fracture from being stabilized, then in addition to intramedullary pins, a Type I external fixator using two to six intramedullary stabilizing pins may be applied from the lateral to the medial side of the bone. In many instances, the external fixator can be removed in 4 to 6 weeks, when enough callus has been produced to take over the function of the external fixator.

Bone plates are applied cranially, medially, or laterally for fractures of the shaft of the humerus. Care must be taken when applying a bone plate laterally or cranially to protect the radial nerve where it crosses the bone with the brachialis muscle. When using a bone plate, use lag screws for fragments that can be

reduced anatomically. If deficits exist, then a cancellous bone graft should be used to fill the fracture gap. The plate should be contoured to match the normal anatomy of the humerus. When a plate is applied to the lateral side, it must be bent in a concave fashion, as well as twisted, to match the contours of the bone.

Most humeral shaft fractures will heal uneventfully. The prognosis for full return to function is excellent.

Supracondylar fractures of the humerus occur just proximal to the supratrochlear fossa. Open reduction of this fracture will provide the best results. If the fracture is a two-piece fracture, intramedullary pinning can provide satisfactory results. The fracture may be approached either medially or laterally or with a combination of the two approaches. A pin is driven retrograde from medial to lateral up the proximal medullary canal until it exits through the greater tubercle. By placing the chuck on the segment that has exited at the greater tubercle, the pin is withdrawn until the point is below the fracture surface. The fracture is reduced and the pin is seated in the medial condyle. By itself, this approach will not provide adequate rotational stability for repair of this fracture. To resolve this problem, a second pin is driven, starting just caudal to the lateral epicondyle towards the medial cortex. This pin crosses the fracture line at the level of the lateral condyle. Should comminution prevent stable fracture fixation from being achieved, then a Type I external fixator may be applied to the humerus to provide additional stability. It is also possible to repair these fractures with the use of a bone plate, which is placed on the caudal medial condylar ridge. Screws in this plate are positioned from caudal to cranial. The fracture line must be high enough to allow at least two screws to be placed in the distal fragment.

One of the most common fractures involving the distal humerus is that of the lateral condyle. Medial condylar fractures occur, but much less frequently than lateral condylar fractures. The radial head articulates directly with the lateral condyle, and the lateral condyle is relatively weakly attached to the humeral shaft as compared to the medial condyle. When repairing lateral condylar fractures, a craniolateral approach allows inspection of the joint surface thus aiding in fracture reduction. The most effective method of stabilization of the condylar fractures is with a transcondylar lag screw. The size of screw chosen will depend on the size of the humerus involved. The screw should be placed so that it lies just distal and cranial to the lateral epicondyle. This will place the screw below the physis, so that if the fracture has occurred in a young animal, growth will not be compromised. In a young dog, care must be taken when inserting the lag screw so that the head of the screw does not bury too deeply into the bone. In the soft bone that allows the screw head to bury deeply, a washer may be used with this screw to prevent burying from occurring. Once the fracture is stabilized with a lag screw, an antirotational pin should be placed from just behind the lateral epicondyle through the medial cortex in the opposite fragment. Fractures of the medial epicondyle may be approached in a similar fashion except that the surgeon is working from medial to lateral.

Diacondylar fractures ("T" or "Y" fractures) involve both the medial and lateral condyle. These fractures are best repaired with open reduction and internal fixation. Usually these fractures are approached through a transolecranon approach. In some instances, however, the fractures may be approached by combining a medial and a lateral approach. As with any joint fracture, it is of paramount importance to reduce the articular surfaces anatomically. A transcondylar lag screw is used to stabilize the intercondylar (articular) portion of the fracture. This fracture can now be stabilized like a supracondylar fracture with intramedullary pins or a plate placed on the caudal aspect of the medial condylar ridge. The best results are achieved with bone-plate fixation. The fixation must be stable so that early, controlled active or passive joint motion can be instituted. This will help preserve the integrity of the elbow joint, because the elbow can become stiff relatively quickly if it cannot move.

Most fractures of the distal humerus (supracondylar or intercondylar) will result in loss of range of motion. Articular fractures are likely to cause degenerative joint disease as the animal ages. Excellent results are not common.

Fractures of the Radius and Ulna

Two-piece fractures involving the proximal ulna are generally repaired via the tension-band principle so that the pull of the triceps muscle, which attaches to the olecranon and distracts the proximal bone fragment, is countered. Two intramedullary pins, starting at the most proximal point of the olecranon are driven distally. A figure-8 wire is passed through a hole that has been drilled transversely in the distal segment and is passed around the ends of the pins in the proximal segment. This is the most effective method of repairing a transverse or short oblique fracture of the proximal ulna. In large dogs or where the comminution is severe, a bone plate may be placed along the caudal edge of the ulna. This bone plate also acts as a tension band. Fractures in the shaft of the ulna may be repaired with the use of single intramedullary pins driven either retrograde or normograde, or, if the animal is large enough, a bone plate may be applied to the shaft of the ulna. Fractures of the styloid of the ulna can be repaired with the use of a single intramedullary pin or a pin and tension-band wire. If the ulnar fracture is stabilized through its ligamentous attachment to the radius, and the radius is stabilized internally, it may not be necessary to fix the ulna. Splints or casts may suffice in nondisplaced fractures, particularly in young animals.

Fractures of the proximal radius are relatively uncommon. A Salter–Harris Type I fracture of the proximal radius may be repaired with the use of one or two small intramedullary pins that are driven from the nonarticular edge of the radial head into the cortex of the opposite fragment. These pins should be bent over before cutting them off to prevent migration and allow for easy removal, if that becomes necessary. Shaft fractures of the radius can be reconstructed with individual wires or screws; however, this will only align individual fracture fragments and will not provide a mechanically strong fixation. Intramedullary pins are not commonly used in fractures of the radius, because the radius articulates proximally with the humerus and distally with the carpal bones. Also, the oval shape of the radial marrow cavity makes it difficult to achieve stable medullary fixation points with intramedullary pinning. If an intramedullary pin is to be used in the radius, it should never be placed retrograde in either direction. The pin should always be driven normograde from the distal segment proximally. The pin should be introduced in such a fashion that it does not interfere with carpal-joint motion or muscle action. It may be necessary to start the pin at a steep angle at a point just above the articular surface, and, as soon as the pinpoint has penetrated the bone, the angle should be reduced, allowing the pin to be driven proximally in the medullary canal. Flexing the carpus while driving the pin will help identify the best position for pin placement. An external fixator may be used as the primary method of fixation in the radius. Driving the fixation pins from medial to lateral and using either a Type I or Type II fixation configuration is preferable. Auxiliary fixation with orthopedic wire or lag screws may be employed in addition to the external fixator device. This will result in better anatomic reduction and more stable fracture fixation.

Radial fractures are very amenable to fixation with bone plates. Bone plates may be applied along the cranial surface of the radius no matter where the fracture is, or along the medial side of the radius in fractures that involve the distal two thirds of the radial shaft. If the articular surface of the radius is involved, then lag screws can be used to reestablish the anatomic configuration of the joint surface. A fracture of the styloid process of the radius may be repaired with either lag-screw or tension-band technique.

In very young animals where the fractures are nondisplaced or can be reduced externally, casts and splints properly applied are sometimes used for fracture stabilization. In the very young animal, fracture healing may occur in 10 to 28 days, and thus the cast or splint can be removed in a relatively short period of time.

Most fractures of the radius and ulna result in a very good to excellent prognosis. In very immature animals, owners should be warned about the likelihood of premature closure of growth plates and the possibility of growth deformity.

Fractures of the Carpus, Metacarpus, and Phalanges

Fractures of the carpal bones are most commonly encountered in working dogs, such as racing greyhounds. The fractures often are created by a combination of compression and sheer forces. This results in either severe comminution or slab fractures of individual bones. In the face of severe comminution, primary arthrodesis should be considered, if the fracture cannot be reconstructed. Untreated fragments generally will not heal and often will result in osteoarthritis. Persistent lameness is the sequela to an untreated fracture in this area.

If the fragments are large enough, a lag screw should be used to stabilize the fracture segments. The screw should be positioned so that its head does not interfere with joint motion. Additional stability is sometimes achieved by driving Kirschner wires across the fragments. Following surgery, a cast or splint is recommended to support the limb for 3 or 4 weeks while callus is forming at the fracture site. Limited activity should continue until there is radiographic evidence of fracture healing, generally at 6 to 8 weeks.

Fractures of the metacarpal bones are often treated with only splints or casts, if only one or two of the metacarpals are involved. If all four of the bones are involved, then at least the third and fourth metacarpal bones should be repaired with the use of intramedullary pins or bone plates, because these are the major weight-bearing bones. Intramedullary pins should be driven normograde from the most distal end proximally. The metacarpal phalangeal joints are flexed during this process, and the pins are not started within the joint surface. Bending the pins away from the joint surface will help prevent irritation to the metacarpal phalangeal joint. Mini bone plates may be applied to the dorsal surface of the metacarpal in large dogs. If the fracture is oblique, small lag screws may be the only means of internal fixation employed, but a cast or splint should be applied as auxiliary support. If the trauma to the foot is severe, then care must be taken when performing surgery to avoid compromising the blood supply further.

Fractures of metacarpal bones invariably carry a good to excellent prognosis. Malunion or nonunion is extremely rare.

Fractures of the phalanges are generally managed by external fixation with a cast or splint. In severe cases where the tissue trauma is great, amputation of the digit may be considered. In most cases, 4 to 6 weeks of support is adequate to achieve functional healing.

Fractures of the Pelvis

Pelvic fractures comprise about 25% of all fractures seen in small animal practice. Indications for surgical treatment include:

- Fractures that cause moderate to severe pain
- Fractures that are unstable based on palpation and rectal examination
- Fractures that involve the force transfer surfaces of the pelvis (sacroiliac junction)
- Fractures that compromise the pelvic canal resulting in marked narrowing
- Fractures that involve the weight-bearing surface of the articular cartilage of the acetabulum

Fractures or dislocations that involve the sacroiliac junction occasionally require surgical stabilization. Fractures of the acetabulum and the ilium usually require surgical intervention. Fractures of the pubis and ischium infrequently need surgical stabilization.

A patient to be treated without surgery should be confined to a cage for 3 to 8 weeks depending on the nature of the fracture and the age of the animal. This animal may need extensive nursing care in the form of hygiene, physical therapy, and bowel and bladder management until such time as the animal is able to walk adequately on its own. While these animals are recumbent, they must be protected from the development of decubital ulcers. Thus, soft padding and a clean environment are essential.

Bone plate and screw techniques have proven to be the most successful for most pelvic fractures. Intramedullary pins and orthopedic wire have limited application when treating pelvic fractures. Ideally, pelvic fractures should be repaired within a few days after the trauma.

The fracture or dislocation of the sacroiliac joint should be surgically stabilized, if the displacement of the ilium is great, or if the instability or pain associated with the fracture or dislocation prevents the animal from ambulating.

A dorsal approach is generally used to expose the sacroiliac area. The displaced wing of the ilium is reduced through caudal traction. Stabilization is achieved by placing one or two lag screws through the ilium into the body of the ischium. Either cancellous or cortex screws may be used for this purpose. Sometimes a single screw and an intramedullary pin are used to provide two points of fixation and, thus, rotational stability. Care must be taken to see that the screws do not penetrate too far, violating the neurocanal. Measurements taken from the radiographs can assist the surgeon in avoiding this complication.

Fractures of the ilium may be approached by elevation of the middle and deep gluteal muscles. These fractures, which are usually oblique, often are displaced medially and may bruise the sciatic nerve. Once the fragment has been elevated laterally away from the sciatic nerve, it is usually necessary to move the distal fragment caudally. This can be achieved by direct traction on the fragment or by manipulation with bone clamps placed into the greater trochanter or tuber ischii (and distracted caudally). The plate is placed on the lateral surface of the ilium. It is extremely important to contour the plate to fit the concave shape of the iliac shaft. The dog's ilium is much more concave than the cat's ilium and, thus, requires much more contouring of the plate. The plate is first fixed to the free caudal fragment of the ilium with the use of bone screws. Insertion of the screws in the proximal segment, starting with the screw closest to the fracture line and working cranially, will help elevate the caudal segment if the plate has been properly contoured.

Fractures of the acetabulum are exposed either through a trochanteric osteotomy or a caudal approach. Care must be taken to protect the sciatic nerve, which courses near the caudal aspect of the acetabulum. Once the fragments are exposed, they are reduced through elevation, traction, or rotation of the free fragments. It is generally easiest to manipulate the caudal fragment, if it is continuous with the ischium, by grasping the ischium with a toothed bone clamp, such as a Kern bone clamp, or inserting an intramedullary pin through the ischium to act as a handle on the fragment. Once reduction is achieved, a bone plate is placed over the dorsal rim of the acetabulum. Care must be taken to see that the screws of the bone plate do not penetrate the articular surface of the acetabulum. To maintain the anatomic shape of the acetabulum, the bone plate must be contoured to match the normal anatomy of the acetabulum. Generally, either mini-plates or a C-plate are used in acetabular repair. If there are multiple comminuted fragments of the acetabulum, then the small fragments are held in position with the use of two or more Kirschner wires. In severely comminuted fractures that cannot be reconstructed, or in fractures where damage to the articular surface of either the acetabulum

or the femur is extensive, excision arthroplasty may be considered as a salvage procedure. If an iliac shaft fracture and an acetabular fracture are present on the same side, the iliac shaft fracture should be stabilized first.

Fractures involving the ischium are seldom stabilized. Those fractures lying just behind the acetabulum are difficult to approach surgically without risk to the sciatic nerve. If the ischial tuberosity is fractured and displaced distally, it can be stabilized with the use of either two lag screws or intramedullary pins.

Fractures of the sacroiliac joint, iliac shaft, ischium, and pubis carry an excellent prognosis, unless there is also neurologic trauma.

Acetabular fractures may have an excellent to poor result depending on the perfection of reduction and the amount of degenerative joint disease which follows.

Fractures of the Femur

The femur is the most frequently fractured long bone in veterinary medicine. About 20% of all fractures involve the femur. Because external fixation of femoral fractures usually results in a poor outcome, essentially all fractures of the femur are best repaired surgically.

Fractures of the proximal femur are most frequently encountered in young animals, because the growth plates are relatively weaker than the ligament of the head of the femur and the joint capsule surrounding the developing bone. Avulsion fractures appear at the proximal femoral physis and are usually associated with a dislocation of the femoral head. Very small fragmented chips of the bone are removed. Chips of one fourth of the femoral head or bigger can be reattached with a lag screw and a small intramedullary pin for rotational stability. Fractures of the proximal femoral epiphysis are more commonly seen and should be repaired relatively quickly to avoid further damage to the soft tissues and osseous structure of the femoral head and neck. A fractured femoral physis is exposed via a craniolateral approach. Before the fracture is reduced, three small Steinmann pins or Kirschner wires (depending on the size of animal) are driven from a point distal to the third trochanter and in a line parallel with the femoral neck. All three pins are inserted prior to reduction of the fracture, so that their emergence point in the distal fragment can be ascertained. These steps will insure that proper pin placement is achieved. The fracture is reduced by traction on the greater trochanter and gentle manipulation of the proximal epiphyseal fragment. Each pin is driven into the femoral epiphysis just far enough to place the point of the pin below the articular cartilage. After each pin is inserted, the joint is placed through a range of motion to determine if the pin has been driven too far. If the pin has penetrated the articular cartilage, it will either be seen or its scraping (the pin engaging the bone of the acetabulum) will be felt. If the pin has been driven too far, it should be withdrawn until the tip is below the cartilage surface. After each pin has been seated in the bone, it should be bent 90° to the lateral surface of the femur, then cut off, leaving 2 to 3 mm of pin exposed. This achieves three-point fixation in the femoral epiphysis. If the animal is near the end of its growth phase at the time of fracturing, then an optional procedure using a lag screw in the epiphysis may be considered. An intramedullary pin should be inserted parallel to the lag screw to add rotational stability to the fragments.

Fractures involving the greater trochanter may be observed singularly or in combination with a fracture of the epiphysis. In either case, the appropriate treatment is fixation of the trochanter with two small intramedullary pins or Kirschner wires and a tension band of orthopedic wire. Remember, if the animal is very young, placement of the tension-band wire will close the physis, and in such cases, this wire should be removed in 2 to 3 weeks if there is considerable remaining growth potential.

Fractures of the femoral neck are best fixed using a lag screw. If the animal is less than 9 months (or if the growth plate is still visible radiographically), then the tip of the screw should not cross the physis of the femoral head. A Steinmann pin should be inserted parallel with the lag screw to provide rotational stability to the fragment. The lag screw should be inserted to about perpendicular to the fracture line and parallel with the neck of the femur. This means that the point of insertion of the screw is distal to the level of the third trochanter.

In older animals, fractures of the proximal femur may be quite severe, because the bony structure gains strength after the physis is closed, and, thus, it takes a greater force to create a fracture. When there is comminution in the area of the proximal femur, it may be desirable to repair the fracture with the use of a bone plate. The bone plate must be contoured to the shape of the greater trochanter and the femoral shaft throughout the distance it is to cover. At least two (and, if possible, more) screws are inserted in the proximal fragment. If the femoral neck is fractured, then a lag screw may be placed either through the plate or next to the plate into the femoral head and neck. It may also be necessary to place a Steinmann pin for rotational stability parallel with the lag screw in the femoral neck. It is sometimes possible to repair proximal femoral fractures with the use of intramedullary pins or orthopedic wire and, if necessary, external fixators. Although this type of fixation is not as stable as bone plate fixation, if the principles of application are adhered to, fractures can be successfully treated using these techniques.

Fractures of the femur are most commonly approached laterally. To avoid damaging the sciatic nerve, the hip should be extended and the limb adducted and internally rotated when pins are inserted. Fractures of the shaft of the femur are repaired through correct application of any of the methods used for internal fixation. Intramedullary pins are inserted either retrograde or normograde through the greater trochanter. Retrograde pins should exit the trochanteric fossa along the medial side of the greater trochanter. Either single or multiple intramedullary pins can be used in repair of femoral fractures.

If an external fixator is to be used, it is

applied to the lateral side of the bone. The most distal pin should be placed at the level of the femoral condyle and the most proximal pin at or just below the level of the greater trochanter. Most external fixators are Type I. The Type II fixator is not used, because the medial bar would be placed in the groin area. Type I half-pin splints can be combined with intramedullary pinning in cases that are rotationally unstable or have a considerable potential of collapse (*i.e.*, comminuted). Long oblique fractures or comminuted fragments can be stabilized with the use of either full cerclage, hemicerclage, or figure-8 skewer pins.

If a bone plate is to be applied to the femur, it should be positioned on the lateral side of the bone (Fig. 22-6), the tension side. Because of the bone's eccentric loading pattern, the lateral side is the best place for the plate. Comminuted fragments and spiral or oblique fractures of the femoral shaft can be reconstructed with the use of lag screws. The lag screws may be inserted before the plate is applied, or they may be positioned through the plate to help provide stabilization and compression at the fracture line. If the lag screws are applied before plate application, then they

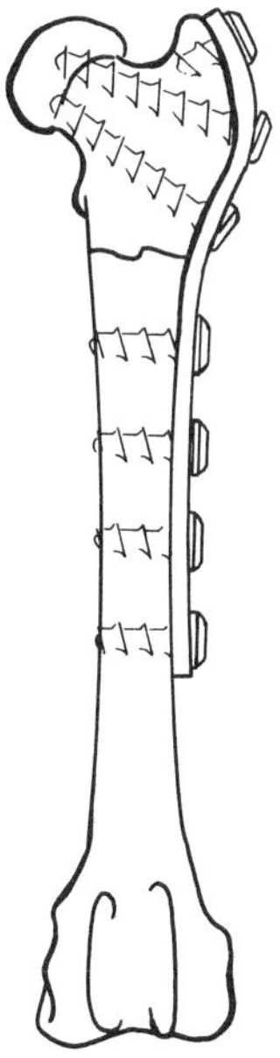

Figure 22-6. *Typical plate and screw placement for fixation of a subtrochanteric femoral fracture. (Newton CD, Nunamaker DM, eds. Textbook of small animal orthopaedics. Philadelphia: JB Lippincott, 1985:419.)*

must be positioned in a manner that will not interfere with positioning of the plate.

The prognosis for diaphyseal fractures of the femur is good to excellent.

The most common fracture seen in the distal femur is a supracondylar fracture or a Salter–Harris Type II fracture. This fracture is approached through a lateral arthrotomy incision. Because the femoral condyles are generally displaced caudally, care must be taken to establish appropriate landmarks—including the patella, the straight patellar ligament, and the tibial tuberosity—before an incision is made into the joint capsule. Several different methods have been described for fixation of this type of fracture. Generally, intramedullary pins are used in these different techniques. In the young animal, bone plating is contraindicated, because it would act as a bridge across the growth plate, and usually the fragment is too small to allow two screws to be placed in the distal fragment. The fracture segments should be reduced anatomically before the fixation is applied. Care must be taken in reducing the fracture, because the bone of the epiphysis is soft in young animals. Gentle traction and manipulation of the fragments is necessary to achieve successful reduction. Excessive force will result in a new fracture developing. Once the fracture is reduced, it may be stabilized by one of the following methods. A single intramedullary pin can be introduced at a point just cranial to the origin of the caudal cruciate ligament. This pin is then driven proximally along the medullary canal, aiming slightly laterally to cause the pin to exit the trochanteric fossa on the lateral side. The pin exits the skin proximally. The distal end is cut flat, and the pin is withdrawn until the distal end is 1 or 2 mm below the cartilage surface. The proximal end can then be cut off just below the skin level, leaving enough pin above the trochanter so that the pin can be removed at a later date. This pin should not be greater than one half the diameter of the medullary canal. When the pin is inserted, the hip should be placed in an adducted and extended position to avoid damaging the sciatic nerve with the pin. If the fracture segments are found to be rotationally unstable, then a small intramedullary pin can be driven from lateral to medial between the two fragments at the level of the metaphysis. Another method of repairing this type of fracture is to insert two relatively small Steinmann pins or Kirschner wires in a crossing fashion. One pin is inserted from the medial side and exits laterally, while the other is inserted from the lateral condyle and exits in the medial metaphysis. Generally, it is not possible to retrieve these pins following fracture healing.

Supracondylar fractures usually heal uneventfully and have a very good prognosis. The most common complication is a medial patellar luxation if the surgical approach is not properly closed.

Occasionally, the fracture of the condyles is in the form of a "T" or "Y" fracture. In these cases, lag screws are placed perpendicular to the fracture lines to achieve stabilization of the fracture. Care must be taken with the placement of these lag screws so that the heads of the screws do not interfere with joint motion. Once the intercondylar fracture is reduced,

then Steinmann pins or Kirschner wires can be placed in a cross fashion or from each condyle proximally along the femoral shaft to provide additional stabilization to the fracture site. If only one condyle is fractured, then a lag screw can be placed perpendicular to the fracture surface. If the head of that screw is located in the condylar fragment, care must be taken to be sure that the screw's position does not interfere with joint motion. Additional lag screws or intramedullary pins may be placed for rotational stability.

Results of condylar fractures are very good unless a fracture line compromises the trochlea and results in degenerative joint disease.

Fractures of the Patella

Patellar fractures are uncommon in dogs and cats. If they do occur, tension-band wires, with or without intramedullary pins, are used to repair the patellar fracture (Fig. 22-7). The intramedullary pin may be driven through the two fragments of bone and a wire placed around

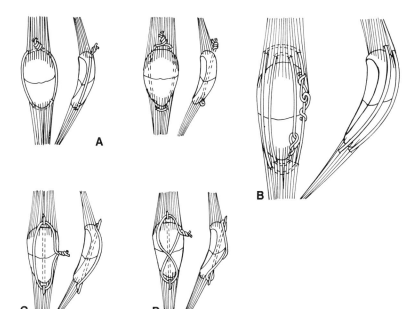

Figure 22-7. *Four methods of internal fixation of the canine or feline patella:* **A,** *Circumferential wiring cranial to the patellar axis;* **B,** *Two cranial wires;* **C** and **D,** *Two methods of tension-band wire placement. (Weber MJ, Janecki CJ, McLeod P, et al. Efficacy of various forms of fixation of transverse fractures of the patella. J Bone Joint Surg 1980;62(A):215.)*

the intramedullary pin, as is done with the figure-8 skewer wire.

Fractures of the Tibia

Fractures of the proximal tibia are uncommon. Fractures in this area, when they occur, usually involve an avulsion of the tibial tuberosity or a Salter–Harris I or II fracture of the tibial plateau. These fractures occur in young animals due to the relative weakness of the physis. Avulsion fractures of the tibial tuberosity in animals with limited growth potential are repaired with the use of two intramedullary pins or Kirschner wires placed cranial to caudal through the tibial tuberosity into the distal segment of tibia. A tension-band wire is anchored in the distal segment and secured around the two pins. If the tibial growth plates are not yet closed radiographically, then two slightly divergent Steinmann pins are used for the fracture fixation. Additional stabilization can be achieved by suturing the soft tissues across the fracture site. Premature closure of this physis can cause a marked deformity of the tibial plateau. If a tension-band wire is used in a young animal, it must be removed within 2 to 4 weeks of placement to prevent premature closure of this physis.

Fractures involving the proximal tibial physis can be stabilized by several methods. The fracture is reduced anatomically before it is stabilized by any method. Once reduced, a single intramedullary pin may be introduced from the medial side at a point halfway between the tibial tuberosity and the medial condyle of the tibia. This pin is inserted at least halfway down the tibial shaft. In another method, two or three small cross pins may be placed from the very caudal aspect of the medial and lateral condyle of the tibia. If there is a metaphyseal segment, as would be found in a Salter–Harris Type II fracture, a lag screw may be placed from the distal fragment into the metaphyseal segment of the proximal fragment. There is rarely enough room in these types of fractures to apply a bone plate.

Fractures involving the proximal end of the tibia are often simple in nature and can be reduced. If the fracture is stable following this reduction, either cast fixation or closed intramedullary pinning can be considered. If a cast is applied, the leg should be placed in a slightly flexed, standing, position. Intramedullary pins, used in open or closed fracture repair, should always be driven normograde and are inserted at a point halfway between the tibial tuberosity and the medial condyle of the tibia just adjacent to the edge of the joint capsule. These pins should be inserted until they embed into the cancellous bone at the distal end of the tibia. To prevent excessive straightening of the bone, these pins should be no larger than two thirds the diameter of the medullary cavity.

If open reduction is to be used, the fracture site can be approached medially or cranially where the skin is reflected medially. Bone plates are applied to the medial surface of the tibia, because such an approach is easy, and no muscle in found in this area. Type I external fixators may be inserted from the medial or lateral side of the tibia. Type II external fixators can be applied to the tibia as the sole means of fracture stabilization. Fractures in the tibia are often oblique or spiral, and intramedullary pinning with cerclage wires or figure-8 skewer pins is an effective method of treating this type of fracture. Fractures of the distal tibial epiphysis are repaired with the use of two cross pins, one inserted mediolaterally from the physis to the metaphysis and the other inserted from lateral to medial. Avulsion fractures of the medial malleolus are stabilized with the use of one or two intramedullary pins and a tension-band wire.

Fractures of the Tarsus, Metatarsus, and Phalanges

Fractures of the bones of the tarsus are rare in most pet animals. They are more commonly encountered in racing dogs.

A fracture of the tuber calcanei will cause dorsal displacement of the proximal fragment because of the pull of the gastrocnemius and the superficial digital flexor muscles. Fractures in this area are repaired with the use of tension-band wiring. The tension-band wire may be placed either around the two pins that have been driven down the shaft of the cal- caneus or through holes that are drilled in the calcaneus on either side of the fracture line. Slab fractures of the talus may be repaired by placing two small divergent Kirschner wires from the articular surface into the body of the talus. These Kirschner wires must be counter- sunk below the articular cartilage. If the frag- ment is large enough, it may be possible to place a lag screw from caudocranially to pro- vide compression across the fracture line. Care must be taken that the tip of the lag screw does not penetrate the articular cartilage. Fractures involving the numbered or central carpal bones can be repaired with the use of small lag screws if the fragments are large enough. If the fragments are too small or are greatly comminuted, then arthrodesis of the involved area should be considered. It is nec- essary to remove the bone fragments and fill the void with cancellous graft. The area must then be stabilized until the arthrodesis is com- pletely healed.

Fractures of the metatarsus and phalan- ges are treated in an identical fashion to frac- tures of the metacarpus and phalanges of the front foot (see "Fractures of the Carpus, Meta- carpus, and Phalanges," p. 593).

Fractures of the Coccygeal Vertebrae

Fractures of the coccygeal vertebrae are usually not treated surgically. If the fracture is close to the sacrum, and the tail is not func- tional and is becoming soiled with urine or feces, then amputation of the tail may be con- sidered. The amputation should be performed between the vertebrae that are just dorsal to the anus.

Traumatic Joint Dislocations

Dislocation or luxation of a joint is classified in relationship to the position of the most distal bone of a given joint, because it is that bone which is out of normal position. For example, a lateral luxation of the scapulohumeral joint in- dicates that the humerus is laterally displaced relative to the scapula. A thorough physical examination will help isolate which joint is dislocated. Knowledge of proper anatomic re- lationships and bone positions during range of motion evaluations is necessary when diag- nosing a dislocation. Radiographic evaluation should always be performed on a dislocated joint to confirm the diagnosis and to evaluate for possible avulsion fractures that may ac- company the dislocation. Treatment of dislo- cations is dependent on their initiating cause, the presence or absence of avulsion fractures, and the duration of the dislocation. Some dis- locations are developmental in nature and will need surgical intervention to preserve normal joint function. Traumatic dislocations are sometimes treated nonsurgically. The best chance of success with a nonsurgical treatment occurs if the dislocation is treated relatively early in the course of events. Delay in treat- ment allows the muscles to shorten and the support structures to be further damaged by the malpositioned bone segment.

Dislocations of the Scapulohumeral Joint

Although they do not occur frequently in small animals, dislocations of the scapulohu- meral joint are usually medial in position. Lat- eral luxations are the next most frequent in occurrence; cranial and caudal luxations occur rarely. Toy poodles and Shelties have a breed predisposition for nontraumatically induced medial dislocation of the scapulohumeral joint (see Chap. 24, Diseases Affecting Joints).

If a traumatic dislocation can be reduced and seems to be stable following reduction, then a non-weight-bearing flexion sling (Vel- peau sling) is the indicated treatment of choice. The animal should remain in the sling for 10 to 14 days. However, if the joint is unstable fol- lowing reduction, or another dislocation occurs after the leg has been removed from the sling, surgical treatment is indicated.

Medial Dislocations of the Scapulohumeral Joint

The most effective surgical method of treating medial dislocations of the scapulohumeral joint is caudal medial transposition of the biceps brachii tendon of origin. (For a detailed discussion of this procedure, see Chap. 24.)

Lateral Dislocations of the Scapulohumeral Joint

Lateral dislocations tend to be traumatically induced and appear most frequently in large breed dogs. The surgical treatment of choice for lateral dislocations is lateral transposition of the biceps tendon. The biceps tendon is approached through a cranial exposure, and the transverse humeral ligament is transected. An osteotomy of the greater tubercle is performed, and a trough is made in the bed of cancellous bone under the tubercle. The biceps tendon is placed within the trough, and the greater tubercle is reattached using two Kirschner wires and a tension-band wire (Fig. 22-8). Imbrication of the joint capsule will add stability to the joint. Limited activity should be enforced for 4 to 6 weeks following this surgery.

Dislocations of the Elbow

Almost all dislocations of the elbow are lateral. The relatively large caudal distal end of the medial condyle of the humerus does not allow the radius and ulna to be displaced medially except when there is severe damage to the ligamentous support structures. The normal relationship between the lateral epicondyle and the lateral radial head will not be present in a laterally dislocated elbow. There may be pain on flexion or extension of the elbow joint, as well as swelling or an apparent thickness to the elbow joint, caused by the lateral position of the radius and ulna. Early closed reduction of all elbow fractures should be attempted. If the dislocation persists for several days or more, part of the lateral condyle of the humerus is worn away by the radius and ulna, preventing normal articulation from being achieved. To reduce the elbow closed, the animal should be placed under general anesthetic, and the elbow should be flexed. The anconeal process is manipulated through internal rotation of the antebrachium, until it is located in the supratrochlear fossa medial to the lateral epicondyle. Medial pressure is applied to the radial head while the leg is extended slightly. Inward rotation and adduction of the antebra-

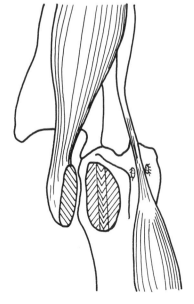 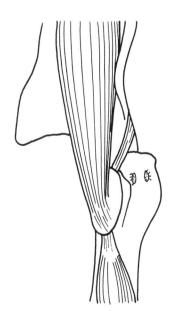

Figure 22-8. *Cranial view of the shoulder joint.* **Left,** *preparation for transposition of the brachial biceps tendon into a groove beneath the osteotomized greater tubercle.* **Right,** *reattachment of the greater tubercle with the tendon trapped beneath. (Newton CD, Nunamaker DM, eds. Textbook of small animal orthopaedics. Philadelphia: JB Lippincott, 1985:353.)*

chium usually results in reduction of the dislocated elbow. Following reduction, the limb should be held in extension for 10 to 14 days using a bandage with lateral reinforcement.

If open reduction of the elbow is required, a medial approach is used to expose the elbow joint. It may be necessary to lever the radius and ulna back into normal position with the use of a smooth-surfaced instrument. Care should be taken to minimize the amount of damage that this will cause to the cartilage surface. Generally, the medial collateral ligament will be ruptured in elbow dislocations, and repair of this ligament, if possible, will help restabilize the elbow. Following surgery, the elbow should be again stabilized in an extended position for 7 to 10 days. Limited activity should be enforced for a 4 to 6 week period.

The results of open or closed reduction are very good, although degenerative joint disease can be expected as the animal ages, as a result of the original trauma.

Dislocations of the Carpus

Dislocations of the carpus are usually traumatic in origin except in those cases that are caused by erosive immunomediated osteoarthritis. Stress-view radiographs should be taken of the carpal joint to accurately diagnose the area of damage. Nonsurgical treatment of carpal dislocations is generally ineffective. Surgical treatment should consist of either direct repair of the torn ligaments or replacement of the ligaments with artificial stabilization. Anchor screws at the origin and insertion points of the ligaments with figure 8-wires between these screws can be used to replace ligament function. In some cases, it is also possible to pass the wire through holes that have been drilled through the bone at the site of origin and insertion of the ligaments. In very severe cases, either total arthrodesis or partial arthrodesis should be considered as a primary option. Following surgical stabilization of the joint, the limb should be protected with the use of a metasplint on the palmar surface for 14 to 21 days. Following the removal of this splint, a padded bandage will provide additional protection during the next 4 to 6 weeks. Limitation of activity should be enforced for at least 8 weeks following surgical repair.

Dislocations of the Hip

The most common dislocation in small animals is that of the hip joint, with craniodorsal dislocations being the most frequently reported. Caudal–dorsal and ventral dislocations are infrequently encountered. If hip dysplasia is excluded, the most common cause of hip dislocations is trauma. Most of these patients will be non-weight bearing and painful when the hip is manipulated. The normal anatomic relationship between the ischiatic tuberosity and the greater trochanter is lost when the hip is dislocated. With craniodorsal dislocations, the distance between the trochanter and the ischiatic tuberosity is greater; with ventral dislocations, it is decreased. Radiographic evaluation of dislocated hips should always be performed to establish the diagnosis and to look for avulsion fractures of the femoral physis. If a fragment of the femoral physis remains attached to the ligament of the head of the femur, surgical treatment is indicated, and closed reduction should not be attempted.

Closed reduction of the hip should be performed soon after the dislocation occurs. Delay in reducing the hip will allow the femoral head to wear away the dorsal rim of the acetabulum and the adjacent joint capsule. The hip is reduced under general anesthesia. The person reducing the hip can stabilize the pelvis and apply counterpressure by placing a hand in the groin over the area of the pubis. The limb is grasped just proximal to the hock and externally rotated while traction is applied. When the femoral head has cleared the acetabulum, the limb is internally rotated, which should reduce the dislocation. While medial pressure is maintained on the trochanter, the hip is put through repeated range of motion maneuvers to help extrude soft tissues and blood clots that may have filled the acetabular cup. Range of motion without pressure is then checked, and if the hip seems stable, a non-weight-bearing sling is applied. If reluxation occurs, then open reduction should be performed. A non-weight-bearing sling (Ehmer sling) should be left in place for 7 to 10 days (Fig. 22-9).

If the animal has a ventral dislocation, then the leg should be abducted until the femoral head is above the ventral acetabular rim. The femur is then externally rotated, allowing the femoral head to relocate in the acetabulum. Following reduction, the animal should be placed in hobbles to prevent abduction of the limb, which promotes ventral dislocation. The hobbles should be left in place for 7 to 14 days.

If a hip cannot be reduced, or stabilized closed, then a surgical repair is indicated. Most dislocated hips are approached surgically through the craniolateral exposure or a trochanteric osteotomy. The acetabulum should be inspected and cleaned prior to relocation of the femoral head within the cup. Once the femoral head is reduced, the tears in the joint capsule can be assessed. It is sometimes possible to maintain reduction of the femoral head through suture imbrication of the joint capsule. Heavy-gauge, absorbable mono-filament suture should be used to suture the joint capsule. In those cases where the joint capsule has torn, either at its origin or insertion, or is too severely shredded to hold suture material, then artificial anchors must be provided for the suture. This can be done by placing two or three screws dorsal to the acetabulum and passing the suture around the screws. On the femoral side the suture may be anchored in tendons, joint capsule, or holes that have been drilled through the bone. Stainless steel wire may also be used in place of synthetic sutures. The sutures are tightened with the leg held in a normal standing position. If support for the hip cannot be achieved by the previously described methods, then a transacetabular pin may be used. To place this, a Steinmann pin is driven on a line parallel to the femoral neck in such a manner that it penetrates the nonarticular surface of both the femoral head and the acetabular cup. This pin should penetrate no more than 1 or 2 mm beyond the medial acetabular wall. The pin should be bent over on the femoral side, and a long enough portion of pin should be left so that the pin can be easily removed 7 to 14 days later. Following surgery, the leg should be placed in a non-weight-bearing sling, if there is any doubt about the security of the surgical repair. When a transacetabular pin is used, the leg should be put in a sling until the pin can be removed. Ten to 14 days is usually an adequate amount of time to have the leg in a sling. The animal should have restricted activity for 3 to 4 weeks following the surgery.

Hip luxations have a very good to excellent prognosis. Degenerative joint disease will become progressive as the animal ages; this is a result of the original trauma.

Dislocations of the Stifle

Dislocations of the stifle are rare and are almost always associated with a traumatic event. Because of the amount of force necessary to cause a dislocation of the stifle, it can be as-

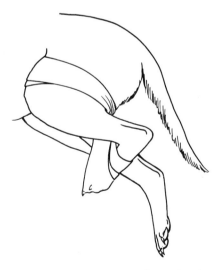

Figure 22-9. *An Ehmer sling is shown in place. (Newton CD, Nunamaker DM, eds. Textbook of small animal orthopaedics. Philadelphia: JB Lippincott, 1985:251.)*

sumed that all or nearly all ligament structures of the stifle joint have been torn and that the joint capsule is disrupted. Such cases are always treated surgically. The objective of surgical repair is to reestablish the function of the collateral ligaments and the cranial cruciate ligament. Whenever possible, the collateral ligaments should be repaired primarily. If the damage to the ligaments is too great to allow their repair, then the stifle can be stabilized by placing a screw at the origin of the ligament and another at the insertion of the ligament. Stainless steel orthopedic wire is then placed between the two screws in a figure-8 pattern and tightened until it allows normal range of motion of the joints. Care must be taken not to tighten this wire too much, because such excessive tightening will interfere with normal joint motion and increase the pressure on articular cartilage. Functions of the cranial cruciate ligament can be replaced with either intracapsular or extracapsular techniques (see Chap. 24, Diseases Affecting the Joints). Following surgery, the leg should be placed in a padded bandage with lateral reinforcement for 10 to 14 days.

The prognosis can be poor to excellent, although most have a poor end result with a severe compromised range of motion.

Dislocations of the Hock

Most dislocations of the hock (talocrural joint) occur because of scraping injuries that have torn or obliterated one or both of the collateral ligaments. If the dislocation is closed, and the joint can be reduced and is felt to be stable, then a short leg cast may be used for the treatment of this dislocation.

Most dislocations of the hock will require surgical intervention. When possible, the collateral ligament should be sutured primarily. If it is not possible to reestablish the collateral ligaments, then screws placed at the origin site

and the insertion site of the collateral ligaments and a wire placed in a figure-8 pattern between the screws can be used as replacement ligaments.

If the dislocation occurs within the numbered bones of the tarsus or at the tarsal–metatarsal joint, then the dislocation can be reduced and stabilized with the use of intramedullary pins driven from medial to lateral and lateral to medial across the point of dislocation. In large dogs, it may be advisable to add a tension-band wire anchored in holes drilled through the ischiatic tuberosity and the metatarsus. This must be coupled with arthrodesis of the affected joints.

Dislocations of the Tail

Dislocation of the coccygeal vertebrae occurs rarely and usually requires no treatment. If the dislocation can be reduced under anesthesia, then a reinforced bandage may be applied to the tail. Care must be taken not to compromise the blood supply to the tail. If there is severe tissue trauma or a marked displacement of the vertebra, amputation of the tail may be considered.

Suggested Readings

Bojrab MJ, ed. Current techniques in small animal surgery. Philadelphia: Lea & Febiger, 1983.
Brinker WO, Hohn RB, Prieur WD. Manual of internal fixation in small animals. Berlin: Springer-Verlag, 1984.
Brinker WO, Piermattei DL, Flo GL. Handbook of small animal orthopedics and fracture treatment. Philadelphia: WB Saunders, 1983.
Newton CD, Nunamaker DM, eds. Textbook of small animal orthopaedics. Philadelphia: JB Lippincott, 1985.
Piermattei DL, Greely RC. Atlas of surgical approaches to the bones of the dog and cat. 2nd ed. Philadelphia: WB Saunders, 1979.
Slatter DH, ed. Textbook of small animal surgery. Philadelphia: WB Saunders, 1985.

23

Charles D. Newton
Marvin L. Olmstead

Reconstructive Surgery

Principles and Techniques of Osteotomy

Definition and Indications

Osteotomy is an elective surgical procedure wherein bone is cut in an attempt to correct an abnormality that has resulted from trauma or disease. Correction can be made in six different planes: valgus–varus, flexion–extension, internal–external rotation, lengthening–shortening, medial–lateral displacement, or dorsal-ventral displacement.

Osteotomy is used for several specific indications:

- Variation in growth of paired bones
- Eccentric epiphysiodesis
- Diaphyseal angulation due to malunion fractures or growth anomalies
- Torsional deformities
- Limb length discrepancy
- Correction of disease requiring osteotomy of normal bone

Principles of Osteotomy

The basic principles of osteotomy and subsequent fixation of the osteotomy site are the same as for any internal fixation. Accurate alignment and reduction of the osteotomy gap must be accomplished, soft tissues must be carefully protected from the saw or osteotome during osteotomy, and early exercise should be encouraged postoperatively.

It is imperative to preplan an osteotomy procedure to minimize any chance for error. Preoperative radiographs in at least two views should be taken of both the affected bone or bones and the unaffected contralateral limb. Radiographs must include the entire joint above and below the deformed bone.

When performing osteotomy, attempt to perform the correction at the site of greatest deformity to allow for optimal cosmetic, as well as functional, results.

When performing the osteotomy with an osteotome, hand saw, or power saw, protect all surrounding tissues from saw trauma by placing an encircling retractor around the bone.

When using power equipment, lubricate the bone surfaces and the saw blade with room temperature saline to prevent thermal burn to the bone ends or surrounding soft tissues.

The end point of any osteotomy is to return the cut bone pieces to a position of optimum function. This necessitates correctly aligning the joints above and below the deformity. Following realignment, use rigid internal or external fixation to assure bone fragment stability.

Techniques of Osteotomy

Three basic techniques of osteotomy are used singly or in combination to correct bony deformity.

Transverse Osteotomy. This technique is used for rotational deformity. The osteotomy is performed at the area of major rotation by cutting a transverse plane through the bone. By using wires or scoring the bone, the surgeon derotates the bone to the predetermined correct alignment (Fig. 23-1).

Cuneiform (Wedge) Osteotomy. The techniques below are used primarily to correct angular deformity, but may be used for angular and rotational problems if both exist simultaneously.

Opening Wedge Osteotomy. This technique is accomplished using a single transverse cut. The cut is then opened on the concave surface. The resulting wedge must be packed with cancellous bone following rigid internal fixation (Fig. 23-2).

Closing Wedge Osteotomy. This technique is accomplished by removing a wedge of bone of predetermined size from the point of maximal deformity (Fig. 23-3). The base of the wedge is at the convex surface of the deformity.

Combination Opening–Closing Wedge Osteotomy. This technique is used where angulation needs correction, but limb length cannot suffer further loss. The predetermined wedge of correction is divided in half, removed from the convex surface, and reinserted from the concave surface (Fig. 23-4).

Oblique Osteotomy. Oblique osteotomy can be used to correct multiparameter abnormali-

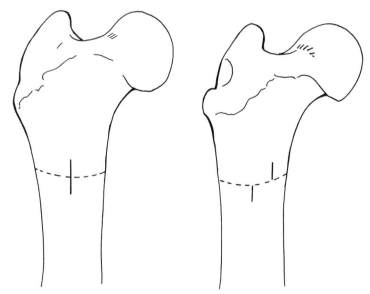

Figure 23-1. *Transverse osteotomy. (Newton CD, Nunamaker DM, eds. Textbook of small animal orthopaedics. Philadelphia: JB Lippincott, 1985:531.)*

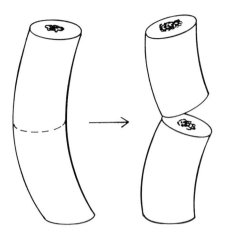

Figure 23-2. *Opening wedge osteotomy. (Newton CD, Nunamaker DM, eds. Philadelphia: JB Lippincott, 1985:531.)*

ties (Fig. 23-5). In rotational and varus or valgus deformity, it can be used to provide total correction by placing the proximal obliquity into the medullary cavity of the distal fragment, thus providing a pivotal point for derotation and varus or valgus realignment (Fig. 23-6).

Methods of Osteotomy

The methods of actual osteotomy will be determined by the type of correction needed, the abilities of the surgeon, and the equipment available.

Closed Osteotomy. Osteotomy can be performed with minimal surgical exposure. Closed techniques involve multiple bony perforation performed with a Steinmann pin, followed by connecting the perforations using an osteotome.

Open Osteotomy. Surgical exposure of the bone to be cut allows for complete visualization of the affected area and provides for a safer surgery.

Osteotomy is best performed using an oscillating or reciprocating saw that permits rapid and exact osteotomy; these saws require intraoperative irrigation with saline to prevent thermal injury to bone.

Osteotomes are very useful for cutting small bony prominences but rarely are used to cut diaphyses. An osteotome is most useful for cutting through cancellous bone and, therefore, is used primarily in osteotomy aimed at providing surgical exposures.

Fixation of Osteotomy

Osteotomies can be stabilized using all conventional forms of internal or external fixation. Choose a type of fixation that best protects the osteotomy site from forces that tend to return the fragments to their original positions. The selection of fixators will also reflect the equipment available to the surgeon.

Principles and Techniques of Arthrodesis

Definition and Indications

Arthrodesis is an elective surgical procedure that eliminates motion in a joint by providing a bony fusion. The procedure is used for several specific purposes: to relieve pain, to provide stability, to overcome postural deformity resulting from neurologic deficit, and to halt advancing disease.

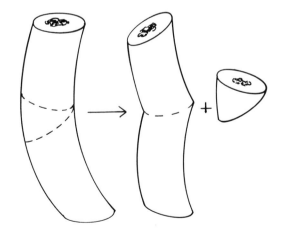

Figure 23-3. *Closing wedge osteotomy. (Newton CD, Nunamaker DM, eds. Textbook of small animal orthopaedics. Philadelphia: JB Lippincott, 1985:531.)*

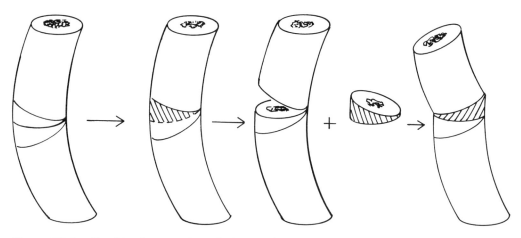

Figure 23-4. *Combination opening–closing wedge osteotomy. (Newton CD, Nunamaker DM, eds. Textbook of small animal orthopaedics. Philadelphia: JB Lippincott, 1985:531.)*

Principles of Arthrodesis

Preplanning an arthrodesis is as important as preplanning an osteotomy and must include observation of the patient standing and walking to determine the best angle for arthrodesis of a particular joint, because the angle varies from breed to breed.

To best accomplish arthrodesis of a joint, all articular cartilage must be removed to expose bleeding cancellous subchondral bone. If bone ends are sclerotic as a result of disease, they must be removed.

Where possible, flat surfaces should be cut on opposing joint ends to assure optimal bony contact for the bony union. Joints with

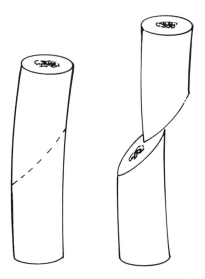

Figure 23-5. *Oblique osteotomy used for bone lengthening. (Newton CD, Nunamaker DM, eds. Textbook of small animal orthopaedics. Philadelphia: JB Lippincott, 1985:532.)*

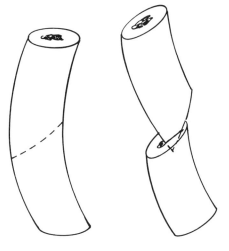

Figure 23-6. *Oblique osteotomy used for rotational correction as well as correction of varus or valgus. (Newton CD, Nunamaker DM, eds. Textbook of small animal orthopaedics. Philadelphia: JB Lippincott, 1985:532.)*

deep joint contours may be debrided of carti-lage and allowed to remain with naturally stable geometry.

The angle of arthrodesis must approxi-mate the normal anatomic position; however this normal position may differ from animal to animal because of other underlying disease of the limb or contralateral normal limb. It is pref-erable to err by making the angle of arthrode-sis too flexed, rather than too extended.

Following proper joint positioning, the internal fixation should be applied to assure joint stability during the period of bone heal-ing. Cancellous bone should be placed around and over the arthrodesis site.

Following completion of surgery, the limb must be placed in a rigid external fixation de-vice until there is radiographic evidence of bony union.

A limb with an arthrodesed joint is more prone to subsequent injury than a normal limb.

Techniques and Methods of Arthrodesis

Two types of arthrodesis procedures are rou-tinely performed in veterinary medicine: intra-articular and extra-articular. Intra-artic-ular arthrodesis is used to fuse peripheral joints, and includes debriding the joint carti-lage, grafting, and stabilizing. Extra-articular arthrodesis is performed on the spine to bridge short or long segments of spine with bone, thereby providing stability to entire segments of the spine. Generally extra-articular ar-throdesis is performed without destroying each spinal facet or the intervertebral joints prior to bridging (see Chap. 19, The Spine).

The technique used for articular cartilage removal depends on the available instruments and the surgeon's desires. The most efficient and fastest method is to use a power bur or similar cutting tool. Equally effective, al-though slower, is the use of a sharp bone curet, rasps, or gouges.

Because cancellous bone is such an inte-gral part of arthrodesis, the surgeon must pre-plan what sites to use and estimate how much bone is necessary.

Fixation Used in Arthrodesis

All types of conventional internal and external fixation can be used in arthrodesis. The de-sired end result is rigid fixation regardless of the fixation type used.

Arthrodesis Techniques for Specific Joints

Arthrodesis of the Shoulder

Shoulder arthrodesis is not commonly per-formed. It may be indicated for severe degen-erative arthritis secondary to fracture, osteo-chondritis dissecans, or chronic shoulder luxation. Occasionally, in the presence of a severe articular fracture, arthrodesis may be used as a primary procedure if fracture repair is not possible.

The shoulder can be adequately fixed using plate and screw fixation. The plate is contoured to lay over the lateral surface of the scapula, cranial to the scapular spine, and to lie on the cranial or craniolateral humeral sur-face. This requires bending and torquing the plate.

Arthrodesis may also be accomplished using pin and tension band wire techniques. Following joint debridement and cancellous grafting, two pins are driven from the cranial proximal humerus obliquely across the ar-throdesis site into the scapular neck. Likewise, two pins are driven from the cranial scapular neck obliquely into the humeral head. A fig-ure-8 or tension-band wire is applied around the pins over the cranial surface of the shoulder.

Arthrodesis of the Elbow

Arthrodesis of the elbow is necessitated by se-vere degenerative arthritis that is secondary to primary fracture of the elbow, ununited an-coneal process, ununited coronoid process, osteochondritis dissecans, or traumatic recurrent luxation. Plate and screw fixation is used most commonly.

Surgical exposure for elbow arthrodesis is best accomplished via olecranon osteotomy to expose the caudal surface of the distal humerus.

An eight- or ten-hole plate should be contoured to the caudal surface of the joint, and positioned so that at least three screws seat completely into the humerus and three into the ulna. If needed, additional interfragmentary screws may be placed across the arthrodesis site.

Following plate placement the olecranon must be retracted to preserve the triceps attachment. The olecranon is usually attached with a single screw to the lateral surface of the arthrodesis site.

Arthrodesis of the Carpus

Carpal arthrodesis is often required following severe internal derangement that results in dislocation. Generally all supporting ligaments are torn, and nonsurgical methods of repair prove unsuccessful. Subluxation or dislocation may involve all three levels of the carpal joint and require pancarpal arthrodesis. If injury involves only the antebrachiocarpal, middle carpal, or carpometacarpal joint, then only the affected joint is fused via arthrodesis.

Flexion deformities resulting from radial nerve paralysis may be treated by pancarpal arthrodesis if the level of paralysis is below the elbow. Carpal arthrodesis is also used to treat end-stage degenerative joint disease resulting from fracture or sepsis.

Pancarpal Arthrodesis

Plate and screw fixation is used most frequently. All three joints of the carpus are opened transversely to expose the articular surfaces. The articular cartilage is debrided from all surfaces to the depth of bleeding subchondral bone. The carpus is fixed either straight (0° flexion) or in 5° extension. An eight-hole plate should be placed over the cranial surface of the joints.

Transfixation pins have been used very successfully in carpal arthrodesis. Following joint debridement and graft placement, two or more Steinmann pins are placed through the joint surfaces. The pins should be placed as widely apart as possible to prevent rotational instability.

Antebrachiocarpal Arthrodesis

This procedure is indicated if only the antebrachiocarpal joint is diseased or unstable. Its advantage over pancarpal arthrodesis is that some motion (15–25°) will be preserved by not fixating the middle carpal or carpometacarpal joints.

Plate and screw fixation using an inverted T-plate has been used successfully. Transfixation pinning of these joints is also successful.

Middle Carpal–Carpometacarpal Arthrodesis

This procedure is required only if one or both of the distal two joints of the carpus is damaged. Its obvious advantage is that antebrachiocarpal motion can be preserved. Animals with middle carpal and carpometacarpal arthrodesis have a near-normal range of motion in the carpus because of the normal antebrachiocarpal joint.

Transfixation pinning may be accomplished in middle carpal–carpometacarpal arthrodesis using two or more crossed pins, or pins may be introduced at metacarpal bones II and V and across one or both joints.

Arthrodesis of the Stifle

Arthrodesis of the stifle is not commonly performed. Usually only very severe end-stage disease or instability requires such a procedure.

Plate and screw fixation is used most commonly. The stifle is positioned at the desired angle of arthrodesis, and flat surfaces are cut from the femoral condyles and the proximal tibia using a saw. An eight- to ten-hole plate should be bent to fit the cranial surface of the femur, stifle, and tibia.

Transfixation pins or screws may be used in very small animals where plates are considered too large.

Dogs manage well with arthrodesis of the knee; most learn to walk well and can resume normal nonathletic activity.

Arthrodesis of the Talocrural Joint

Most injuries to the ligamentous structures of the talocrural joint are amenable to repair. Occasionally when repairs fail, or secondary degenerative joint disease is severe, arthrodesis becomes necessary.

Plate and screw fixation is used successfully. A six- to eight-hole plate is bent to fit the caudal surface of the tibia, tarsus, and metatarsal III.

Another technique, requiring less surgical exposure, uses a transfixation screw. Following joint debridement and grafting, a single cancellous screw is placed from a caudal insertion point through the tibial tarsal bone, across the arthrodesis site and is seated in the distal tibia. An additional tension-band wire is placed between the tuber calcis and the tibia to protect the screw.

Arthrodesis of the Intertarsal Joint

Intertarsal arthrodesis is usually necessary in cases of traumatic luxation or subluxation of the intertarsal joint.

Plate and screw fixation may be used for intertarsal arthrodesis but is rarely the method of choice, because extensive surgical exposure is needed.

The tension-band wire is the preferred method of fixation for intertarsal arthrodesis. Following joint debridement and grafting, two Steinmann pins are placed through the length of the fibular tarsal bone, across the arthrodesis site, and seated into the metatarsal bones. A tension wire is placed over the caudal surface of the fixation.

Arthrodesis of the Tarsometatarsal Joint

Tarsometatarsal arthrodesis is commonly performed when trauma and subsequent luxation or subluxation is not improved with conservative treatment.

Similar to intertarsal arthrodesis, tarsometatarsal procedures are successfully performed with plate and screw fixation. The substantial surgical exposure required may be a drawback. The plate is placed either laterally or caudally over the arthrodesis site.

Transfixation pins seem to be the method of choice due to their ease of application. Following debridement and grafting, one large pin is placed through the fibular tarsal bone, through the tarsal bones, and into metatarsal bone III. This provides the primary fixation. Two additional Steinmann pins are placed, beginning at the base of metatarsal II and metatarsal V and crossing through the arthrodesis site. This method of fixation provides excellent stability.

Amputation

Amputation is the surgical cutting off or resection of a body part. The procedure is usually used only in cases of severe trauma or mangling of a body part, end-stage osteomyelitis, gangrene, neoplasia, or cases where total loss of neurologic function results in limb dysfunction. Amputation of ears or tails are also performed for cosmetic purposes to make an animal match a breed standard.

Several basic principles must be adhered to:

- Be sure the end result will be cosmetic.
- Remove limbs as near to the trunk as possible.
- Hemostasis is critical; replace fluid or blood lost during the surgery.
- Strive for speed in the surgery to prevent excessive hemorrhage and soft tissue drying.
- Never ligate large arteries and veins together, because an arterio-venous fistula may develop.
- Be certain that the animal's general condition can tolerate such a traumatic procedure.
- Never amputate a limb in the face of thoracic metastasis, unless the pain is excessive.

(text continues on page 619)

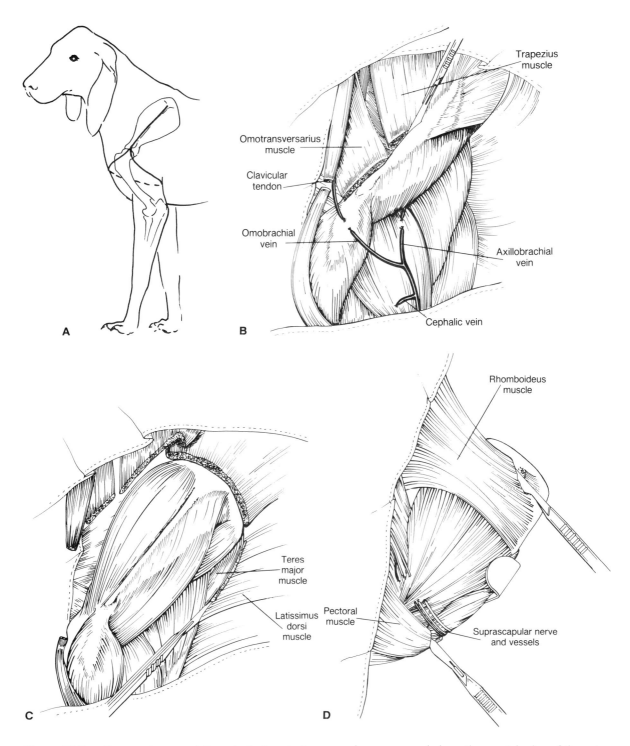

Figure 23-7. *Forequarter amputation.* **A,** *An inverted Y-shaped skin incision is made extending along the spine of the scapula to the greater tubercle and half way to the elbow. The incision is extended medially from the fold of the axilla to the greater tubercle.* **B,** *Lateral view. The axillobrachial and omobrachial veins are ligated and severed proximal to the greater tubercle. The cephalic vein is ligated and severed distal to the cleidobrachialis muscle. The location and size of these veins are variable. The brachiocephalicus muscle is transected through the clavicular tendon. The omotransversarius and trapezius*

muscles are severed along the cranial edge of the spine of the scapula. **C,** *Lateral view. The latissimus dorsi muscle is separated from the teres major and severed close to its insertion on the humerus.* **D,** *Cranial–medial view. The cranial edge of the scapula is rotated externally. The insertions of the rhomboideus and serratus ventralis muscles are severed. The suprascapular artery and vein are ligated and severed. The suprascapular nerve is severed. The superficial and deep pectoral muscles are transected at their attachment on the humerus.*

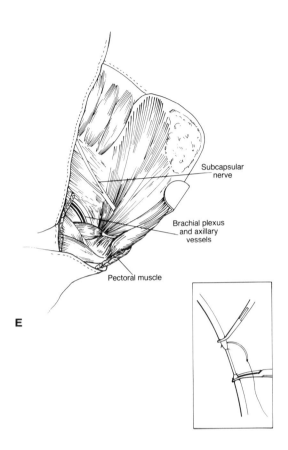

E

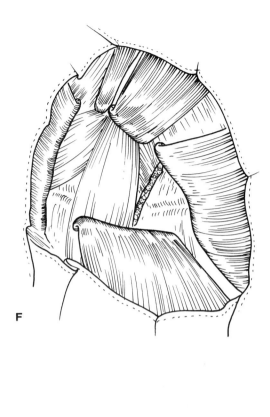

F

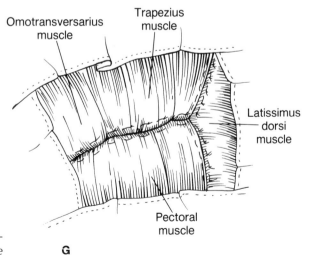

G

E, Cranial–medial view. The subscapular nerve is severed. The nerves of the brachial plexus are severed. The axillary artery is doubly ligated, transfixed, and severed (see inset). The axillary vein is ligated and severed. F, Closure. The cut ends of the muscle bellies are turned inward. G, The lateral fascial sheaths of the latissimus dorsi muscle, omotransversarius muscle, and the trapezius muscle are sutured to the lateral fascial sheaths of the pectoral muscle. (Newton CD, Nunamaker DM, eds. Textbook of small animal orthopaedics. Philadelphia: JB Lippincott, 1985:580.)

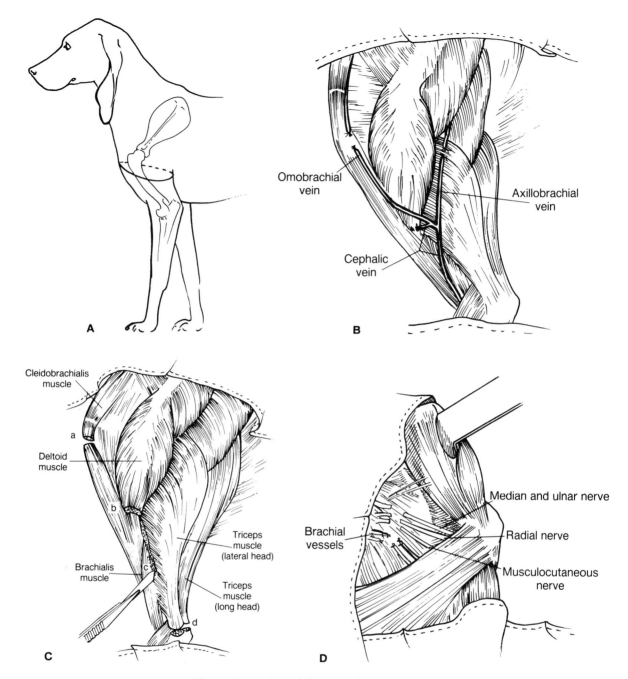

Figure 23-8. *Scapulohumeral disarticulation. **A,** A lateral semilunar skin incision is made from the point of the shoulder to the caudal angle of the axilla. A straight medial skin incision connects the sides of the lateral incision. **B,** Lateral view. The axillobrachial and omobrachial veins are ligated and severed just proximal to the greater tubercle. The cephalic vein is ligated and severed distal to the cleidobrachialis muscle. The size and location of these veins are variable. **C,** Lateral view: (a) The cleidobrachialis muscle is transected distal to the clavicular tendon; (b) The deltoid is severed at its insertion on the deltoid tuberosity of the humerus; (c) The lateral and long heads of the triceps muscle are separated from the caudal border of the humerus and the brachialis muscle; (d) The tendon of insertion of the triceps muscle is severed at its insertion on the olecranon. **D,** Medial view. The scapula and humerus are elevated to expose the medial surface. The branchial artery is doubly ligated, transfixed, and severed. The median, ulnar, radial, and musculocutaneous nerves are severed.*

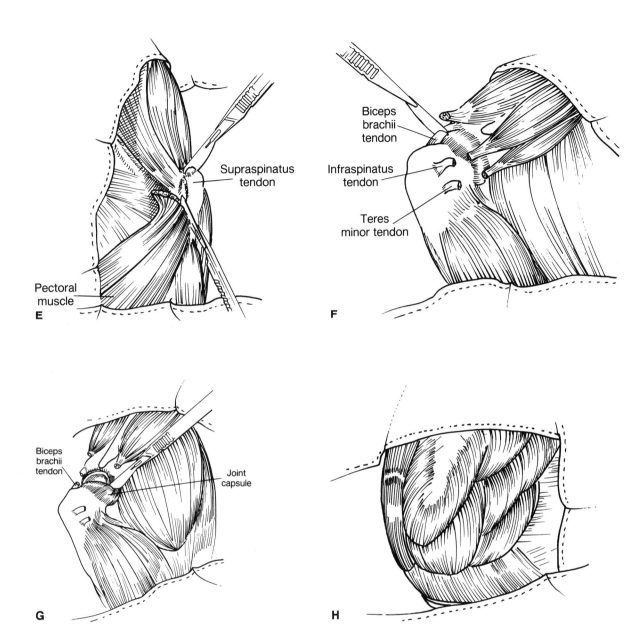

E, Cranial view. The pectoral muscles are transected through their insertions on the humerus. The supraspinatus tendon is severed at its insertion on the greater tubercle. F, Lateral view. The tendons of the biceps brachii infraspinatis, and teres minor are severed. G, Disarticulation. Beginning cranially and proceeding caudolaterally, the joint capsule is incised. The medial joint capsule is incised, and the coracobrachialis tendon is severed. H, Closure. The fascial sheaths of the triceps brachii and the deltoid muscles are sutured to the brachiocephalic and pectoral muscles. (Newton CD, Nunamaker DM, eds. Textbook of small animal orthopaedics. Philadelphia: JB Lippincott, 1985:582.)

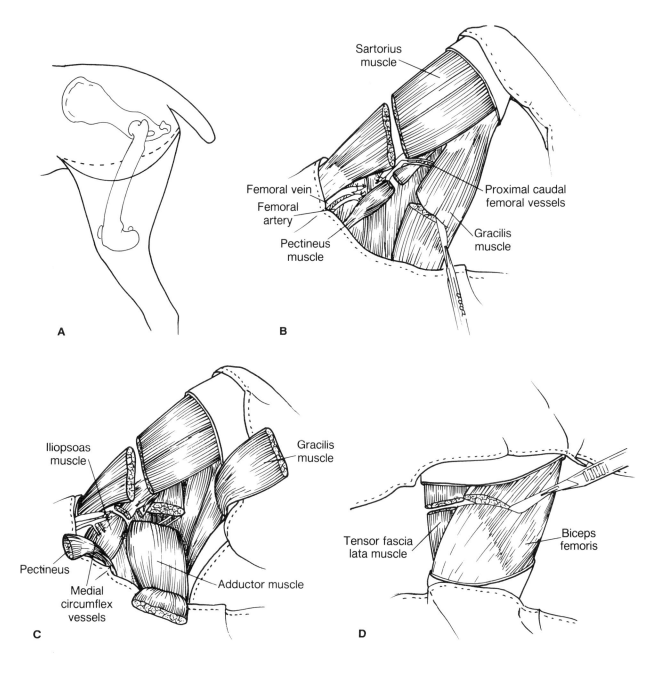

Figure 23-9. *Coxofemoral disarticulation.* ***A,*** *The lateral skin incision extends from the fold of the flank across the midshaft of the femur to the ischial tuberosity. The medial skin incision is made 1 cm distal to the inguinal crease.* ***B,*** *Medial view. The leg is elevated. The femoral artery is doubly ligated, transfixed, and severed proximal to the proximal caudal femoral artery. The femoral vein is ligated and severed at the same position. The sartorious, pectineus, and gracilis muscles are severed through their muscle bellies 2 cm from the inguinal crease.* ***C,*** *Medial view. The proximal part of the pectineus muscle is reflected proximally, exposing the medial circumflex femoral artery and vein. The vessels are ligated and severed. The iliopsoas and adductor muscles are transected.* ***D,*** *Lateral view. The tensor fascia lata and biceps femoris muscles are transected at the level of the midshaft femur.*

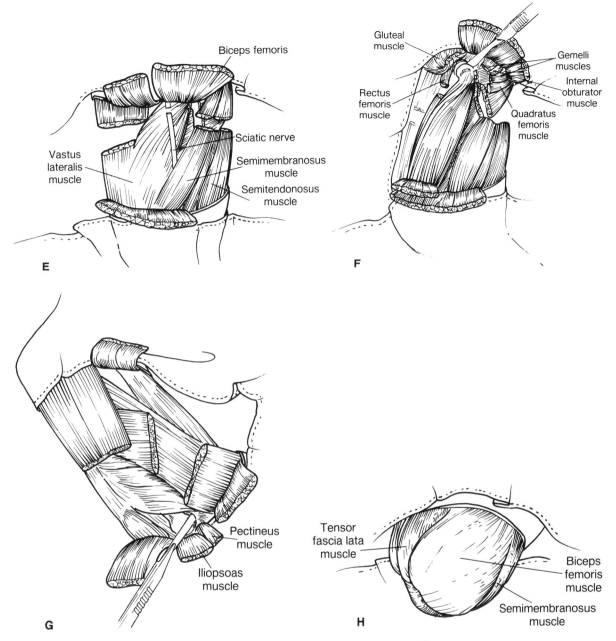

E, Lateral view. The biceps femoris muscle is reflected proximally to expose the sciatic nerve. The sciatic nerve is severed. The semimembranosus and the semitendinosus muscles are transected at the level of the proximal one third of the femur. The vastus lateralis, medialis, and intermedius are not severed and are removed with the femur. F, Lateral view. The semimembranosus and semitendinosus muscles are reflected proximally to reveal the gemelli, internal obturator, and quadratus femoris muscles. These muscles are transected at their insertions on the femur. The gluteal muscles are transected at their insertions on the femur. The rectus femoris muscle is transected at the level of the greater trochanter. The lateral joint capsule is incised cranially, dorsally, and caudally. G, Medial view. The leg is elevated. The pectineus and iliopsoas muscles are reflected proximally. The medial joint capsule is incised, and the round ligament is severed. H, Closure. The biceps femoris muscle is sutured to the gracilis, semimembranosus, and semitendinosus muscles. The tensor fascia lata muscle is sutured to the sartorius muscle. (Newton CD, Nunamaker DM, eds. Textbook of small animal orthopaedics. Philadelphia: JB Lippincott, 1985:584.)

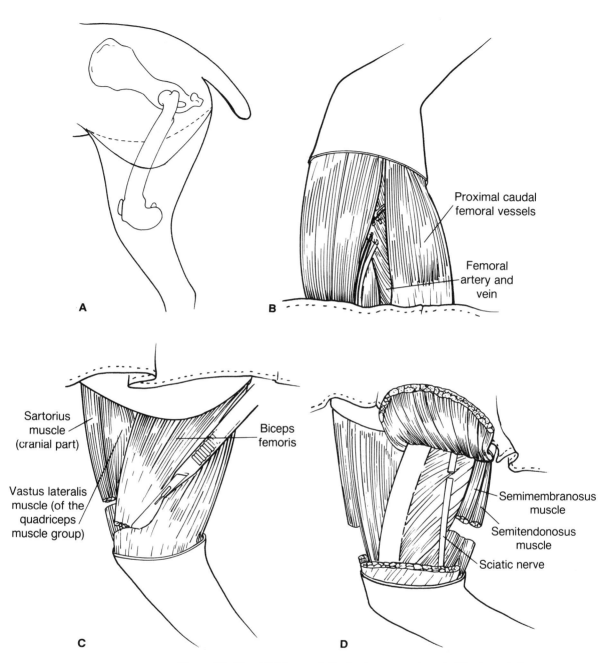

A

B

Proximal caudal
femoral vessels

Femoral
artery and
vein

C

Sartorius
muscle
(cranial part)

Vastus lateralis
muscle (of the
quadriceps
muscle group)

Biceps
femoris

D

Semimembranosus
muscle

Semitendonosus
muscle

Sciatic nerve

Figure 23-10. *Mid-femoral diaphysis amputation.* **A,** *The lateral skin incision extends from the fold of the flank across the junction between the proximal two thirds and distal one third of the femur. The medial skin incision is made 2 cm distal to the inguinal crease.* **B,** *Medial view. The femoral artery is doubly ligated, transfixed, and severed just proximal to the proximal caudal femoral artery. The vein is ligated and severed at the same position.* **C,** *Lateral view. The tensor fascia lata, cranial part of the sartorius, quadriceps, and biceps femoris muscles are transected at the level of the distal femur.* **D,** *Lateral view. The biceps femoris and quadriceps muscles are reflected proximally. The sciatic nerve is severed. The semimembranosus and semitendinosus muscles are transected at the level of the midshaft femur.*

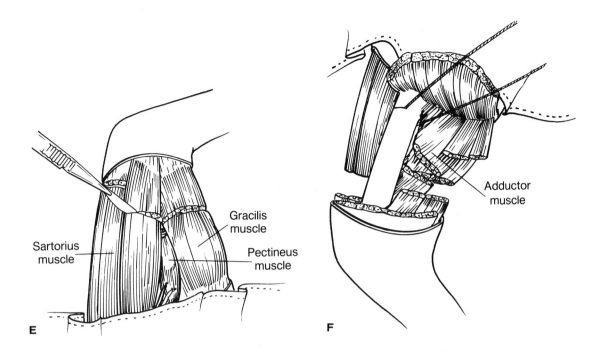

E, Medial view. The leg is elevated. The gracilis and pectineus muscles and caudal part of the sartorius muscle are transected at the level of the midshaft femur. **F,** Lateral view. The adductor muscle is severed at the level of the midshaft femur. It is elevated subperiosteally from the femur to the level of the proximal one third of the femur. The femur is transected between the proximal one third and distal two thirds. **G,** Closure. The cranial part of the sartorius, quadriceps, and biceps femoris muscles are sutured to the semimembranosus, semitendinosus, and gracilis muscles, and caudal part of the sartorius muscle. (Newton CD, Nunamaker DM, eds. Textbook of small animal orthopaedics. Philadelphia: JB Lippincott, 1985:586.)

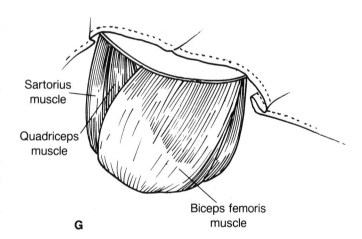

Three different techniques can be used in the process of amputation. Most surgeons prefer one technique over the other two and will use it exclusively during the procedure. However, all three can be used simultaneously, if desired.

Crushing Technique. Individual muscles are subdivided and held in hemostatic forceps prior to cutting to decrease the extent of hemorrhage.

Ligation Technique. All major arteries and veins are ligated near the trunk before any muscles are cut. This technique risks the possibility of leaving devitalized tissue within the animal.

Sharp-Cutting Technique. Muscles are transected with a scalpel, and hemostasis is accomplished by ligating vessels as they are encountered. The last ligation is the large arteries and veins near the trunk.

Pectoral Limb Amputation

The pectoral limb is amputated using one of two specific techniques: forequarter amputation, which includes scapulectomy (Fig. 23-7), or a scapulohumeral disarticulation (Fig. 23-8).

Pelvic Limb Amputation

The pelvic limb is amputated using one of two specific techniques: coxofemoral disarticulation (Fig. 23-9) or a mid-diaphyseal femoral amputation (Fig. 23-10). There is no inherent advantage in one technique over the other; however, the midshaft technique may be considered more cosmetically acceptable by the owners of male dogs, because it will cover the genitals. Hemipelvectomy, a heroic method used in people with extensive pelvic cancer, is not practical in the dog or cat and will not be described.

Dewclaw Amputation

Dewclaws are routinely removed from certain breeds of show dog to meet a breed standard or from hunting breeds to prevent traumatic laceration or amputation while in the field.

During the first few days following birth, the dewclaws are removed using a scissors, amputating the digit and metacarpal or metatarsal bone I. The resulting incision is either

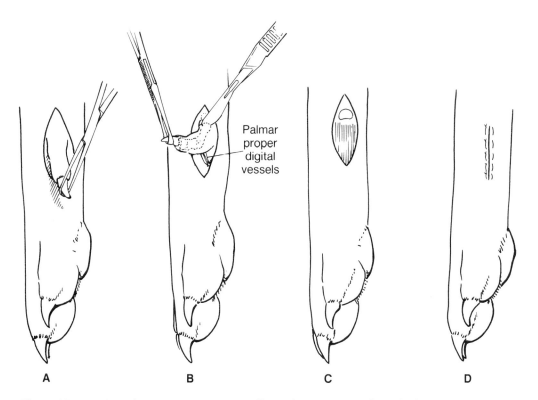

Figure 23-11. *Dewclaw amputation.* **A,** *An elliptical incision is made at the base of the digit and extended distal to the carpometacarpal (or tarsometatarsal) joint.* **B** *and* **C,** *The tissues between the dewclaw and the second metacarpal bone are severed. The palmar proper digital artery and vein are ligated individually and severed. The carpometacarpal (or tarsometatarsal) joint is disarticulated, and the dewclaw is removed.* **D,** *Skin closure is routine. (Newton CD, Nunamaker DM, eds. Textbook of small animal orthopaedics. Philadelphia: JB Lippincott, 1985:587.)*

sutured with a single suture or bandaged. In older dogs an elliptical incision around the base of the dewclaw is needed (Fig. 23-11). Removing the digit at the level of the carpometacarpal joint or the tarsometatarsal joint is preferable, because this technique will provide a better cosmetic result than an amputation through the center of the metacarpal or metatarsal bone.

Digital Amputation

Individual toes often have to be amputated due to trauma, infection, or neoplasia. It is always preferable to leave the digital pad if possible when amputating a third phalanx. When removing the entire digit, do not damage the large metacarpal or metatarsal pad. In instances of mangled feet, amputate only the toes which cannot be reconstructed. However, if all toes must be amputated, the animal will still be able to use the foot, if the large metacarpal or metatarsal pad remains.

In digital amputation an incision should start dorsally and course from 1 cm above the

appropriate metacarpophalangeal or metatarsophalangeal joint to 1 cm below the joint, and then encircle the digit, avoiding the main metacarpal or metatarsal pad. Following ligation of the large arteries and veins on the lateral sides of the digit, the joint is disarticulated. The resulting effect can be sutured closed in a straight line or in an inverted "T".

Tail Amputation

Amputation of the tail is performed in certain breeds of show dogs to match a breed standard. Other reasons for amputation include trauma, osteomyelitis of a vertebra, severe deformity, loss of sensation, severe soft-tissue infection, or neoplasia.

In the very immature dog, amputation can be accomplished by amputating the tail with a scissors. The resulting incision will require one or more sutures to close. In the mature dog the tail is removed by making dorsal and ventral semilunar skin incisions, ligation of the lateral caudal vessels and the median caudal vessels, transection of the coccygeal

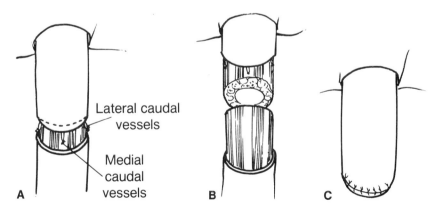

Figure 23-12. *Tail amputation.* **A,** *A tourniquet can be applied at the base of the tail to reduce hemorrhage. Semilunar skin flaps are made dorsally and ventrally. The skin flaps extend beyond the point of disarticulation. The two lateral caudal vessels and the median caudal vessels are ligated and severed just proximal to the joint.* **B,** *The skin flaps are retracted cranially. The coccygeal muscles are transected, and the coccygeal vertebrae are disarticulated.* **C,** *The dorsal skin flap is pulled over the stump and sutured to the ventral skin flap. (Newton CD, Nunamaker DM, eds. Textbook of small animal orthopaedics. Philadelphia: JB Lippincott, 1985:587.)*

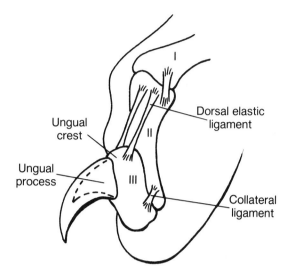

Figure 23-13. *Normal anatomy of feline claw. (Redrawn after Herron MR. Declawing the cat. Mod Vet Pract 1967;48:40.)*

muscles at the same level, and finally disarticulation of the coccygeal vertebrae at the desired level. Routine closure requires subcutaneous sutures and skin sutures (Fig. 23-12).

Feline Onychectomy

Cat declaw is a procedure performed to prevent cats from destroying household furnishings with their claws. The procedure is usually performed on the forepaws only.

Declaw is the amputation of the third phalanx of each digit on the paw. Before beginning, a tourniquet should be placed on the limb above the elbow to help control hemorrhage. The procedure is accomplished by careful dissection with a #11, #12, or #15 scalpel blade, or the use of a Resco nail trimmer (Figs. 23-13, 14, 15). Both ways can be equally effective in the complete removal of the third phalanx. During the amputation, be careful not to cut or damage the individual digital pad. Post-amputation, the resulting small incision may be sutured or simply bandaged. Usually a constrictive bandage is applied over the paw and

forearm and left in place for the next 12 hours to help control hemorrhage.

If drainage or regrowth of any toenail occurs at a later time following the surgery, it is probably the result of regrowth of nail from germinal epithelium at the base of the third phalanx that was not completely removed at the first surgery. Removal of the remainder of the third phalanx should eliminate the problem.

Prosthetics

The use of prosthetic joint replacements in clinical veterinary medicine has, for the most part, been very limited. Except for the canine hip, no commercial prosthetic joint implants have been designed specifically for the veteri-

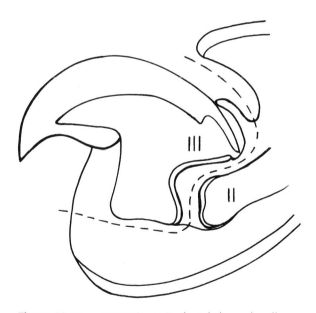

Figure 23-14. *A tourniquet is placed above the elbow. A #11 Bard–Parker blade or a Resco nail trimmer can be used to remove the third phalanx. Severing the dorsal elastic ligament and the collateral ligaments with a scalpel permits complete removal of the third phalanx. The digital pad should not be lacerated. (Redrawn after Herron MR. Declawing the cat. Mod Vet Pract 1967;48:40.)*

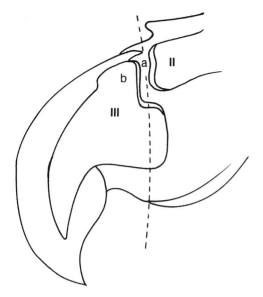

Figure 23-15. *If a Resco nail trimmer is used, the nail should be grasped with a forceps and extended. The nail trimmer is placed in the space between the second and third phalanx (a). The pad should be retracted caudally. The dorsal part of the ungual process must be removed to prevent regrowth of the nail (b). An absorbable suture may be placed to close the skin defect. After removal of all claws on one foot, a snug foot bandage is applied and the tourniquet is removed. The bandages are removed the following day. (Redrawn after Herron MR. Declawing the cat. Mod Vet Pract 1967;48:40.)*

nary patient. The few isolated reports in the literature of joint replacements other than the hip have been in cases where a prosthetic implant intended for a human joint was adapted to a veterinary situation. The lack of joint replacements specifically designed for veterinary patients is primarily economic from the standpoint of both the manufacturing company and the veterinarian. The varying joint sizes of veterinary patients and the relatively low number of cases where a joint replacement would be indicated has made development of prostheses for most joints impractical.

However, in the canine hip, disabling conditions are frequently encountered; the primary one of these is hip dysplasia. Because this generally affects large dogs in which exci-

sion arthroplasty gives highly variable results and is usually not as successful as when performed in small breed dogs, a need for a prosthetic device has developed. The Richards Canine II Total Hip Prosthesis has proven to be an implant that effectively reestablishes a pain-free ball and socket joint for the dog (Fig. 23-42). The implantation of this device requires strict aseptic technique, meticulous surgical detail, and the use of polymethylmethacrylate for stabilization of the implant. In this procedure the acetabular cup is replaced with a high density polyethylene plastic cup, and the femoral head is replaced with a cobalt chrome endoprosthesis. Because of the highly specialized nature of this procedure, it is usually only performed at university teaching hospitals or private practices that specialize in surgery.

A 95% success rate has been established for this procedure. A successful case is one in which the dog is considered to be full weight bearing with a normal clinical range of motion, normal muscle mass, pain-free joint function, and normal levels of exercise tolerance. A successful dog may have periodic episodes of stiffness following heavy exercise or rest but should not show any signs of overt lameness or pain.

A dog is considered a candidate for a total hip replacement if it has disabling disease of the coxofemoral joint, is 10 months of age or older, and weighs over 18 kg. These dogs must be evaluated for the presence of neurologic dysfunctions, pathology in joints other than the hip, neoplasms, systemic or local infections, and systemic disease. If any of these conditions are found to be present, they must be fully resolved before the dog should be considered a candidate for a total hip replacement.

The complications encountered with total hip replacement are infrequent but include dislocations of the prosthesis, osteomyelitis, fractures, sciatic neuropraxia, and implant loosening. Meticulous surgical technique and controlled, monitored convalescence will minimize the potential for any of these complica-

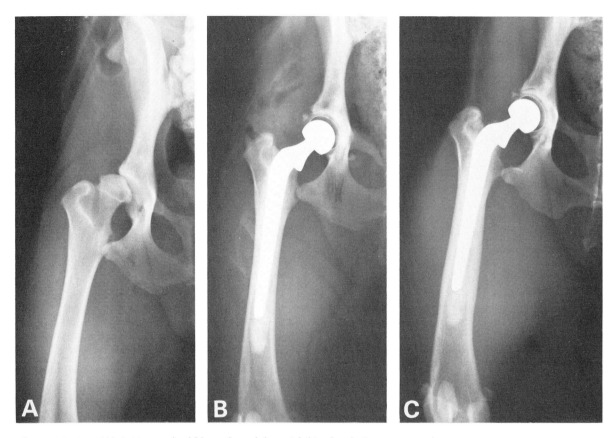

Figure 23-16. *(A) A 14-month old large breed dog with hip dysplasia was treated by total joint replacement (B). The dog is seen again in this 164-week follow-up radiograph (C). Note the increased bone stock around the stem of the prosthesis, indicating some interaction between the implant and bone. The bone remodeling is thought to be related to weight-bearing stresses; at times it causes hypertrophy, at other times, resorption. (Courtesy of M. L. Olmstead, Ohio State University. Newton CD, Nunamaker DM, eds. Textbook of small animal orthopaedics. Philadelphia: JB Lippincott, 1985:558.)*

tions to develop. Except for infection, if one of these complications does occur, it frequently can be successfully treated and the prosthesis preserved. Infected patients should have all of the implant material removed.

The total hip replacement has proved to be an effective long-term treatment for disabling conditions of the dog's hip. In some cases, dogs have functioned normally for over 10 years with a prosthesis in place. The total hip replacement can be used to return the working dog to its intended use or to improve the quality of life for the pet dog by providing a pain-free, mechanically sound hip joint.

Suggested Readings

Brinker WO, Piermattei DL, Flo GL. Handbook of small animal orthopedics and fracture treatment. Philadelphia: WB Saunders, 1983.

Duff, R, Campbell JR. Long-term results of excision arthroplasty of the canine hip. Vet Res 1977;101:181.

Herron MR. Declawing the cat. Mod Vet Pract 1967;48:40.

Moore RW, Withrow SJ. Arthrodesis. Compend Contin Ed Pract Vet 1981;3:319.

Newton CD. Principles and techniques of arthrodesis. In: Newton CD, Nunamaker DM, eds. Textbook of small animal orthopaedics. Philadelphia: JB Lippincott, 1985:561.

Newton CD. Principles and techniques of osteotomy. In: Newton CD, Nunamaker DM, eds. Textbook of small animal orthopaedics. Philadelphia: JB Lippincott, 1985:529.

Newton CD, Nunamaker DM. Osteotomy and arthrodesis. In: Brinker WO, Hohn RB, Prieur WD, eds. Manual of internal fixation for small animals. New York: Springer-Verlag, 1984:255.

Olds RB. Arthrodesis of elbow, carpus, stifle and hock. In: Bojrab MJ ed. Current techniques in small animal surgery. Philadelphia: Lea & Febiger, 1975:549.

Olmstead ML. Total hip replacement in the dog. Sem in Vet Med and Surg (Sm Anim) 1987;2:131.

Olmstead ML, Hohn RB, Turner TM. A five year study of 221 total hip replacements in the dog. J Am Vet Med Assoc 1983;183:191.

Stone EA. Amputation. In: Newton CD, Nunamaker DM, eds. Textbook of small animal orthopaedics. Philadelphia: JB Lippincott, 1985:577.

Weigel JP. Amputations. In: Slatter DH, ed. Textbook of small animal surgery. Philadelphia: WB Saunders, 1985:2276.

24

Donald A. Hulse

Diseases Affecting the Joints

Shoulder Joint

The shoulder joint is a true diarthrodial joint. The ball and socket configuration of the joint allows for flexion, extension, adduction, abduction, and rotation. The joint capsule attaches to the periphery of the glenoid and extends distally for several millimeters beyond the articular margins of the humeral head. Medially, the joint capsule surrounds the biceps brachii tendon where it crosses the joint to attach to the supraglenoid tuberosity. The encircling muscles give dynamic stability to the joint, and the glenohumeral ligaments and cartilaginous glenoid labrum lend static support to the joint.

Osteochondrosis

Articular cartilage serves as a protective surface during normal joint motion and as the growth center of the epiphysis. As such, the articular cartilage cells proliferate and undergo endochondral ossification for enlargement and development of the normal anatomic shape of the epiphysis. Osteochondrosis is a pathologic condition of maturing cartilage. Normal cell differentiation, hypertrophy, and ossification fail to occur. With continued growth of cartilage from the epiphyseal side and a lack of ossification on the metaphyseal side of the articular cartilage, a thickened zone of cartilage occurs. Physiologic load creates shear stress, which is concentrated at the periphery of the thickened cartilage because of the difference in stiffness between peripheral cartilage and adjacent cancellous bone. Also, nutrition is impaired in the basal layers of the thickened cartilage, resulting in necrotic areas that are more susceptible to the normal shear stress at the cartilage–bone interface. The zones of stress concentration and necrosis are starting points for development of fissures. The fissures will propagate and eventually reach the articular surface, creating a cartilage flap. This cartilage flap opens a pathway for synovial fluid to reach the basal layer of thickened cartilage and subchondral bone. When osteochondrosis has reached this stage, the condition is referred to as osteochondritis dissecans (OCD—a dissecting lesion). Painful synovitis results from the necrotic debris and inflammatory products released into the joint cavity. The cartilage flap may remain in place overlying the defect or dislodge and become a loose joint body. In either situation, disruption of the joint surface will lead to osteoarthrosis.

The cause of osteochondrosis is not precisely known, but several theories have been postulated. Dogs with a genetic capacity for rapid growth have been shown experimentally and clinically to be predisposed to the development of osteochondrosis. The condition is rarely reported in dogs weighing less than 20 to 25 kg and has not been seen in miniature and toy breeds. Osteochondrosis is seen twice as frequently in male dogs as in female dogs, which grow at a slower pace than male dogs. A second theory is that overnutrition, a free-choice diet, can cause rapid growth and contribute to the development of osteochondrosis. In addition to rapid growth, overnutrition may lead to excessive calcium intake, which causes hypercalcitonism. Hypercalcitonism may cause a delay in cartilage maturation, which increases cartilage thickness in predisposed areas.

The sites of predilection of osteochondrosis in order of decreasing frequency are: the caudocentral part of the humeral head, the medial ridge of the talus, the medial condyle of the humerus, and the lateral condyle of the stifle. Osteochondrosis frequently occurs in the same joint of the opposite limb and may involve more than one joint in the same limb.

OCD of the Shoulder

OCD is seen most frequently in the large and giant breeds of dogs between the ages of 4 and 12 months, but may be diagnosed later in life as degenerative joint disease. The onset of lameness is gradual and generally first noticed fol-

lowing periods of strenuous exercise or when first rising in the morning. At this time, if the patient is rested for 3 to 7 days, the lameness will subside, and the patient may return to normal function. However, exercise aggravates the problem and lameness recurs. The problem may be present in both limbs, but the patient is generally more lame in one limb than the other. The degree of lameness will vary from a mild weight-bearing lameness to moderate weight-bearing lameness. With time the lameness worsens and will not subside with enforced rest. The older patient with severe secondary degenerative joint disease may present with a non-weight-bearing lameness.

On physical examination it may be difficult to detect a lameness upon first observation. The patient may have been rested prior to examination, which reduces the patient's discomfort. Also, most of these patients are active young dogs—excitement of being in a strange environment may mask an underlying subtle lameness. Movement of the shoulder through a normal range of motion usually elicits pain. However, the degree of pain is dependent upon the severity of joint inflammation. The patient with mild synovitis exhibits little or no pain upon manipulation of the shoulder. Joint inflammation is advanced sufficiently in most patients, so that flexion and extension of the shoulder joint will elicit discomfort.

Differential Diagnosis

The primary differential for shoulder pain is trauma to the shoulder region. The young patient has cartilaginous growth plates that are subject to injury from minimal trauma. Avulsion of the biceps tendon or injury to the proximal physis should be considered as part of the differential diagnosis. Patients prone to develop OCD are very active working dogs; they may sustain muscle strains or ligament sprains. The most important consideration in formulating a differential diagnosis is the inclusion of juvenile orthopedic conditions that may occur simultaneously. Osteochondrosis or ununited anconeal process may occur concurrently in the elbow joint, and panosteitis or hypertrophic osteodystrophy may involve the long bones of the forelimb.

Diagnosis

Craniocaudal and lateromedial radiographs are used to confirm the presence of OCD. It may be necessary to take slightly oblique lateral views to see the lesion early in the course of the disease. Initially, the area of thickened cartilage shows as a radiolucent zone, causing a slight flattening of the caudal margin of the humeral head (Fig. 24-1). Both shoulder joints should always be radiographed, because the lesion occurs bilaterally in a high percentage of cases. As the condition progresses, the dissected section of cartilage mineralizes and is

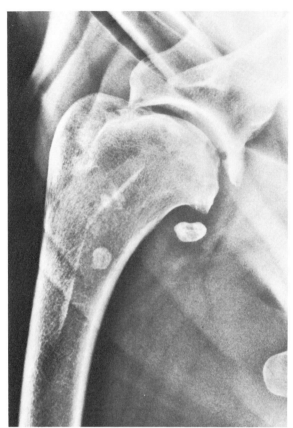

Figure 24-2. *Lateromedial radiograph of a patient who has severe degenerative joint disease secondary to osteochondritis dissecans.*

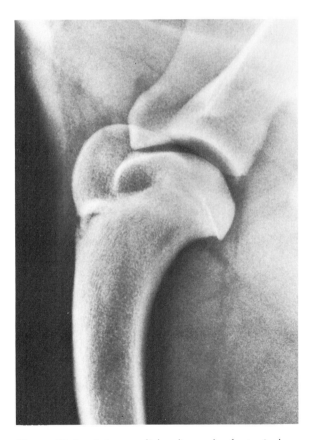

Figure 24-1. *Lateromedial radiograph of a typical osteochondritis dissecans lesion. There is a radiolucent zone and slight flattening of the caudal margin of the humeral head.*

visible radiographically as a thin line overlying the cartilage defect (Fig. 24-2). If left untreated, moderate to severe degenerative joint disease occurs. The dissected cartilage may dislodge and become a free joint body. It may then be resorbed or, as in most cases, remain in the caudal pouch of the joint. If a radiographic lesion persists, but the cartilage does not mineralize, an arthrogram can be used to outline a free section of cartilage.

Treatment

Conservative therapy consisting of enforced rest and nonsteroidal anti-inflammatory drugs can be used if osteochondrosis has not progressed to OCD. Buffered aspirin (10 mg/kg), administered 3 times each day is the drug used initially. Drug therapy is maintained during the inflammatory period and need not continue for more than 7 to 10 days. Osteochondrosis and OCD are difficult to diagnose. Conservative treatment is chosen if there is minimal discomfort and the radiographic lesion is small with no demonstrable mineralized cartilage flap or free joint body. These patients must be evaluated monthly for radiographic signs of healing. If the lesion persists for 2 months or the patient worsens clinically, then an arthrogram or surgical intervention is indicated.

Surgery is indicated in those patients who have moderate to severe clinical signs or radiographic evidence of OCD. This is especially true if evidence of a cartilaginous flap is present. Surgery involves exposure of the lesion, removal of free cartilage, and penetration of the subchondral bone plate by drilling or curettage of the base of the lesion.

The patient is anesthetized and prepared for aseptic surgery using standard methods. The patient is placed in lateral recumbency with the affected limb draped for aseptic surgery (Fig. 24-3). The joint may be approached

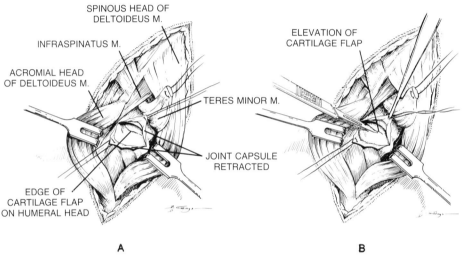

A

B

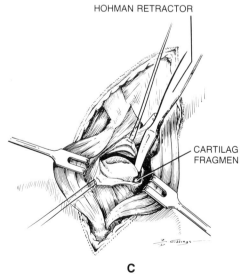

C

Figure 24-3. *Osteochondroplasty of the humeral head for osteochondritis dissecans. **A,** The left shoulder has been exposed by a caudolateral approach. The lateral edge of the cartilage flap is visible after retraction of the joint capsule by stay sutures. **B,** The cartilage flap is elevated from the humeral head by sharp dissection. When the flap has been sufficiently elevated, it can be cut free along its cranial border. **C,** The caudal cul-de-sac of the joint capsule is retracted with a small Hohman retractor to allow removal of any free cartilage fragments. (Brinker WO. Handbook of small animal orthopedics. Philadelphia: WB Saunders, 1983:368.)*

cranially, laterally by separation of the acromial head of the deltoid muscle, or caudally as described below. A craniolateral incision is made from the midpoint of the scapular spine to the proximal one third of the humeral shaft. The subcutaneous tissue is incised to expose the acromial and spinous part of the deltoid muscle. The fascial plane of the two muscle bellies is separated allowing the teres minor muscle and infraspinatus muscles to be seen. These two muscles are undermined and retracted craniodorsally. The insertion of the teres minor muscle can be incised to allow greater retraction. Care must be taken to identify and preserve the muscular branch of the axillary nerve. The joint capsule is incised parallel to the glenoid rim. The limb is rotated internally and adducted to expose the caudal humeral head. If a cartilage flap is overlying the lesion, it is usually attached medially. The attachment is incised and the cartilage removed. The cartilage edges are trimmed perpendicular to the base of the defect and checked to assure that cartilage is attached to the cancellous bone. Multiple holes are drilled in the base of the lesion or the base is scraped with a curette to allow pluripotential cells located in the marrow of the cancellous bone to gain access to the defect. This technique will accelerate healing with functional fibrocartilage. Before closure the joint is flushed thoroughly with sterile saline to remove cartilage fragments. This flushing is particularly important if, upon opening the joint, the cartilage flap is seen to have separated from the defect. The joint capsule is sutured with an absorbable suture using a simple interrupted pattern. The fascial plane between the deltoid group and subcutaneous tissue is sutured with an absorbable suture using a simple continuous pattern. The skin is sutured with a nonabsorbable suture using a simple interrupted pattern.

Postoperative care includes enforced rest; activity is supervised and restricted to leash walking for 6 weeks. The most common postoperative complication is seroma formation, which is usually associated with excessive postoperative activity. The prognosis with surgical therapy when performed early is good. Patients with degenerative joint disease at the time of diagnosis benefit from surgery but may continue to have periodic lameness associated with arthritis.

Congenital Shoulder Joint Luxation

The breeds of dogs most commonly diagnosed as having congenital shoulder luxation are the toy breeds. These breeds have conformational defects characterized by a shallow glenoid cavity and a flattened humeral head (Fig. 24-4). Medial luxation is the most common

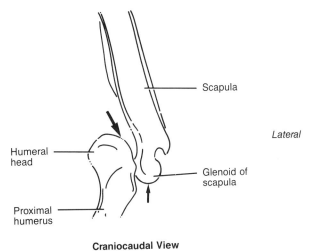

Figure 24-4. *Congenital humeral joint luxation. (Puglisi A. Canine humeral joint instability, part I. Compend Contin Ed Pract Vet 1986;8:596.)*

Craniocaudal View

congenital luxation diagnosed. Historically, the patient has a mild periodic weight-bearing lameness. Presentation for evaluation usually follows a mild traumatic episode that has exacerbated the lameness. Clinically, joint laxity can be palpated during abduction and internal rotation of the shoulder joint. There is medial displacement of the greater tubercle of the humerus, and the elbow is carried flexed and abducted. The condition usually occurs bilaterally.

Diagnosis

Differential diagnosis includes traumatic luxation, physeal injury, muscle strain, or joint sprain. The diagnosis is confirmed radiographically; a flattened humeral head and abnormally shallow glenoid are seen radiographically. The medial labrum of the glenoid will be eroded, and soft tissue proliferation is noted medially.

Treatment

Treatment may be conservative or surgical. Conservative treatment may be used in a patient exhibiting no clinical problems until a traumatic episode results in acute lameness. As seen radiographically, the deformity of the joint is such that surgical reconstruction is not feasible. Conservative therapy includes rest and nonsteroidal anti-inflammatory medication (buffered aspirin, 10 mg/kg, 3 times a day for 7 days). The purpose in using conservative treatment is to allow the soft-tissue injury associated with trauma to heal. Once healed, return of function to the pre-injury level is expected. If this does not occur, then surgical intervention is recommended. Surgical procedures may be categorized as reconstructive procedures, excision arthroplasty or arthrodesis.

Reconstructive procedures should only be used if there is a reasonable chance of maintaining reduction and of having a pain-free articulation. This decision is based on careful assessment of preoperative radiographs, the appearance of joint cartilage at

surgery, and the appearance of joint conformation at surgery. If the conformation of the joint precludes maintaining reduction, or if the articular cartilage is degenerative, then excision arthroplasty is the procedure of choice in the small breed dogs.

The patient is anesthetized, clipped, and prepared for aseptic surgery. The dog should be positioned in lateral recumbency and the limb draped to allow manipulation during surgery. A craniomedial incision is made from the midpoint of the scapular spine distally to the level of the proximal one third of the humeral shaft. The fascial plane along the lateral border of the brachiocephalicus muscle is incised to allow medial retraction of the muscle belly. The insertions of the superficial and deep pectoral muscles are released from the proximal humerus. Proximally the bicipital groove and medial head of the supraspinatus muscle are identified. The tendinous insertion of the subscapularis muscle is incised at the lesser tubercle and the muscle belly retracted to expose the medial joint capsule. The joint capsule is incised to gain access to the medial compartment of the shoulder joint. The joint is inspected, and a decision is made whether surgical reconstruction or excision arthroplasty is performed.

Reconstruction may be accomplished by biceps tendon transposition or transposition of the medial head of the supraspinatus muscle. The luxation is reduced, and the joint capsule is sutured using an imbrication technique. Bicipital tendon transposition relocates the biceps tendon medial to the joint to function as a medial collateral ligament. A section of cancellous bone is elevated in the lesser tubercle of the proximal humerus as a site for the biceps tendon relocation. One edge of the osteotomy is left attached to the underlying bone to create a hinge that allows replacement of the osteotomy when securing the biceps tendon within the osteotomy site. The transverse ligament overlying the bicipital groove is incised to allow mobilization of the bicipital tendon. The tendon is then translocated medially and positioned within the bed of the osteotomy site.

The tendon is covered with the cut piece of bone, and the latter is secured with two small Kirschner wires (Fig. 24-5). Partial transposition of the supraspinatus tendon is accomplished by isolating the tendinous insertion of the medial section of the muscle as it inserts onto the greater tubercle. A partial osteotomy of the greater tubercle is performed at the site of the insertion. A site is prepared for attachment of the osteotomy and attached tendon at the lesser tubercle. The bone and tendon are translocated and secured with two small Kirschner wires. The released insertions of the subscapularis muscle and pectoral muscles are sutured. The fascial plane of the brachiocephalicus muscle, subcutaneous muscle, and skin are sutured using standard methods. Postoperatively, the limb is placed in a Velpeau sling for 10 to 14 days. After bandage removal, supervised exercise on a leash is necessary for 3 weeks. Prognosis depends upon the conformation of the joint. With adequate medial labrum and joint conformation, the prognosis is good. Otherwise, the prognosis is poor, and the most common complication, reluxation, is

likely to occur. If reluxation occurs, excision arthroplasty is indicated.

Excision arthroplasty is performed if reconstruction is not deemed feasible or if previous reconstructive surgery has failed. Failure is usually due to wear of the medial labrum as a result of chronic medial luxation. The joint is exposed via an osteotomy of the acromial process and release of the insertions of the infraspinatus muscle and teres minor muscle. If the joint has been exposed for medial reconstruction, that exposure is combined with the lateral acromial osteotomy. The tendon of the biceps brachii muscle is detached from the supraglenoid tuberosity, and the suprascapular nerve is identified and protected. Ostectomies of the humeral head and glenoid are made with an oscillating saw or high-speed surgical bur. A notch is made at the base of the spine of the scapula to accept proximal translocation of the suprascapular nerve. The teres minor muscle is translocated and sutured to the biceps tendon to lie between the cut surfaces of the two osteotomy sites. The infraspinatus muscle is sutured to its insertion site, and the acromial

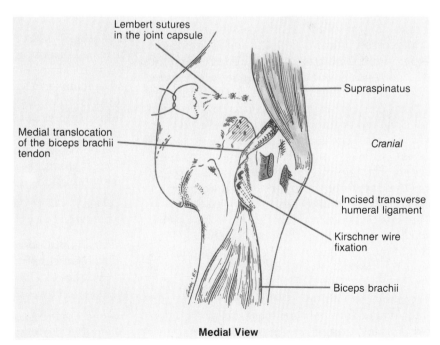

Figure 24-5. *Medial translocation and fixation of the biceps brachii tendon using two small Kirschner wires. (Puglisi A. Canine humeral joint instability, part I. Compend Contin Ed Pract Vet 1986;8:743.)*

Lembert sutures in the joint capsule

Supraspinatus

Cranial

Medial translocation of the biceps brachii tendon

Incised transverse humeral ligament

Kirschner wire fixation

Biceps brachii

Medial View

process is wired to the scapular spine. The subcutaneous tissue and skin are closed using standard methods. The limb is not immobilized postoperatively. Passive physical therapy is begun as soon as the patient will tolerate movement of the shoulder joint. Ten days after surgery, swimming and leash walking are encouraged to maintain a good range of motion during healing. The prognosis is good for normal, daily, nonathletic activity.

Arthrodesis of the shoulder joint is an alternate salvage procedure when reconstruction of the shoulder joint has failed or is not feasible. However, the postoperative function with excision arthroplasty is superior to that with arthrodesis in the small patient. Therefore, arthrodesis is not indicated in toy breeds with congenital medial shoulder luxation.

Tenosynovitis of the Biceps Brachii Tendon

The biceps brachii muscle originates from the supraglenoid tuberosity by a long tendon that passes through the intertubercular groove of the proximal humerus. The scapulohumeral joint space is continuous through the intertubercular groove to a point just distal to the transverse ligament. Bicipital tenosynovitis is a painful inflammatory condition involving the biceps tendon and its accompanying tendon sheath. The causes of bicipital tenosynovitis have been reported as trauma, strain of the tendon, and entrapment of loose bodies within the sheath. The associated lameness characteristically is weight bearing and is exacerbated with exercise. Physical findings depend on the nature of the injury. With acute injuries, the patient shows pain on palpation over the intertubercular groove. However, with chronic injury no discomfort can be elicited. Slight muscle atrophy of the shoulder muscles will be present with chronic inflammation of the tendon. The differential diagnosis includes neurologic conditions that cause root pain and subsequent forelimb lameness. Also included are sprains, strains, neoplasia, arthropathies,

and trauma of the forelimb. The diagnosis is difficult and may be based on elimination of other causes and response to treatment. In acute cases, pain may be obvious, leading to the correct diagnosis. In chronic cases, radiographs may reveal dystrophic calcification in or around the tendon sheath. Contrast arthrograms may reveal irregularities in the area of the tendon sheath. Treatment includes enforced rest and administration of anti-inflammatory drugs. Steroids can be injected directly into the inflamed tendon sheath, and, if the lameness improves dramatically, the diagnosis is substantiated. Surgery may be necessary, in some cases, to release adhesions and remove osteophytes or free bodies in the synovial sheath. The movement of the tendon can be stabilized by transposing the tendon of origin from the scapular tuberosity to the proximal humerus. The tendon can be secured to the humerus by drilling a tunnel through the humerus, passing the tendon through the tunnel, and then suturing the tendon to itself. The prognosis is good for a return to normal function.

Elbow Joint

The elbow is a compound synovial joint. The primary direction of motion is flexion and extension. There is a limited range of rotational movement and varus–valgus movement. The joint is composed of three distinct articulations: humeroradial, humeroulnar, and radioulnar. The joint is stabilized by the articulation of the semilunar notch of the ulna with the conical trochlea of the humerus, the collateral ligaments, and the annular ligament.

Congenital Elbow Luxation

Alteration of osseous physeal development or soft tissue constraints during growth can lead to congenital elbow luxation. There are three types of elbow luxation:

Type I. Proximal luxation of the radial head
Type II. Proximolateral luxation of the ulna

Type III. Luxation of both the radius and ulna

Breeds most commonly afflicted with congenital elbow luxation are the English bulldog, sheepdog, dachshund, Yorkshire terrier and Pekingese. Historically, the patient with congenital elbow luxation is first noted to have difficulty ambulating at 4 to 6 weeks of age. The lameness is nonpainful, does not have an acute onset, and is not associated with trauma. The lameness seen on physical exam is mild to moderate with Type I luxation but severe with Types II and III. The patient with Type II or Type III luxation may be able to ambulate but does so with the elbow flexed and the paw pronated. The front limbs are advanced in a creeping or paddling motion, with most of the body weight placed on the rear limbs. Flexion and extension are pain-free, but the elbow cannot be extended to a normal position. The condition most often occurs bilaterally, but may be present in only one limb.

Differential diagnoses include traumatic luxation, elbow fracture and elbow luxation secondary to growth-plate abnormalities. Radiographic findings associated with congenital elbow luxation are dependent upon the type of luxation present. With Type I luxations, the proximal radius is displaced laterally and caudally (Fig. 24-6). The radial epiphysis is underdeveloped and shows a convex outline of the articular surface. The humeroulnar articulation appears normal, but the ulna may be more centered relative to the humeral condyles. With Type II luxations, the proximal part of the ulna is displaced laterally and tilted, so that the caudal part of the olecranon faces laterally (Fig. 24-7). The radial head remains in a relatively normal position, but the humerus is subluxated medially with the medial humeral condyle possessing no articulation. With Type III luxations, both the radius and ulna are displaced and dislocated laterally.

Treatment is directed towards reestablishing normal elbow articulation as much as is feasible and directing the force of the triceps muscle mass in a more normal direction. In

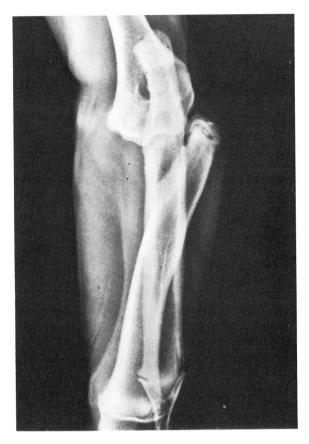

Figure 24-6. *Craniocaudal radiograph of a patient having a Type I congenital elbow luxation.*

mild cases, this may be accomplished by closed reduction and stabilization with an external fixation device. However, most cases require open reduction and stabilization. The elbow is approached through a caudomedial or transolecranon approach. With Type I luxations, the radius is shortened by ostectomy, which facilitates radial head reduction. The radius is held in position by transfixation to the proximal ulna. If the proximal radial physis is active, it must be surgically fused. With Type II luxations, reduction is maintained by plication of the medial joint capsule, transposition of the olecranon process distally on the ulna, and fixation of the proximal part of the ulna to the radius with small Steinmann pins. With Type III luxations, arthrodesis or

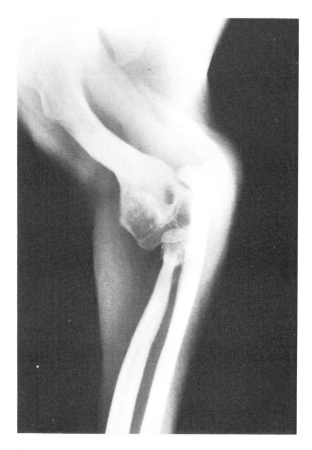

Figure 24-7. *Craniocaudal radiograph of a patient having a Type II congenital elbow luxation.*

radial head ostectomy is indicated when limb function is not acceptable. The prognosis with Type I or II luxations is good for return to function but guarded for Type III luxations.

Subluxation of the Elbow Joint Secondary to Physeal Injury

Subluxation of the elbow joint in the immature patient occurs most commonly secondary to abnormal physeal development resulting from injury. The most common abnormality seen is premature closure of the distal ulnar physis. The result is distal displacement of the medial and lateral coronoid processes of the ulna relative to the radial head. Abnormal or iatrogenic synostosis of the proximal radius and ulna will

also result in distal displacement of the ulnar coronoid processes relative to the radius. This displacement is due to the rapid growth of the proximal radius compared to the slow or zero growth of the proximal ulna. As the proximal radius grows in length, the radial head forces the humeral condyles proximally away from the ulnar articular surface. Distal or proximal radial physeal injury will result in distal subluxation of the radial head from the humeral condyles. In severe cases, the ulna may subluxate proximally. Treatment is aimed at restoring articular congruency and preventing further deformity. In the basset hound, separation of the anconeal process can occur secondary to retardation of growth of the ulna.

Fragmented Medial Coronoid Process

Fragmented medial coronoid process is often considered to be part of the osteochondrosis syndrome but trauma and growth disparity between the radius and ulna have also been incriminated as etiologic factors. The condition is most frequently seen in the large rapidly growing breeds of dogs. There is a predilection for this syndrome in yellow Labradors, golden retrievers, rottweilers, Newfoundlands, and German shepherds. The lameness is usually first noticed between 5 and 8 months of age but is intermittent and may only be visible after prolonged exercise. However, the client may not seek veterinary care until the lameness is noticed more consistently. For this reason, the patient may be 1 year old or more at presentation. The problem frequently occurs bilaterally but may present as a unilateral lameness. Physical examination may be unrewarding in that the patients normally afflicted with the syndrome are the sporting breeds, which are usually stoic. In some patients, extension of the elbow or slight pressure over the medial coronoid may elicit discomfort. When the patient is bearing weight, joint distension from synovial effusion may be palpable in the space between the lateral olecranon and epicondyle of the humerus. Periarticular proliferation may

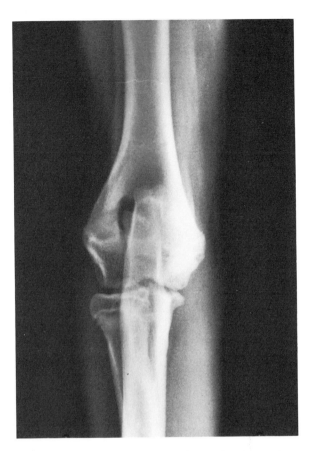

Figure 24-8. *Craniocaudal radiograph of a patient with a fragmental medial coronoid process.*

be palpable in the older patient with secondary degenerative joint disease.

The differential diagnoses include other juvenile orthopedic conditions, such as OCD of the shoulder or medial condyle of the elbow, ununited anconeal process, panosteitis, or hypertrophic osteodystrophy. Physeal trauma, muscle strain, or ligament sprain also should be considered. Importantly, these problems may occur concurrently with fragmented medial coronoid process. The diagnosis is based on signalment, history, and clinical signs. The separation of the medial coronoid process is difficult to visualize radiographically because of superimposition of the radial head and medial coronoid process. The detached process may be visible on a 25° craniocaudal–lateromedial projection. As degenerative changes develop, radiographs will show osteophytes on the dorsal border of the anconeal process, lateral coronoid process of the ulna, and distal border of the medial condyle (Fig. 24-8). Although radiographic changes may be suggestive, definitive diagnosis often depends upon arthrotomy.

The only effective treatment is excision of the fragmented medial coronoid (Fig. 24-9). The elbow is approached through a medial incision located over the medial epicondyle and extending from 3 cm above the epicondyle to 4 cm distal to the joint line. In the patient with little or no periarticular proliferation, separation and partial tendinotomy of the pronator teres muscle and flexor carpi radialis muscle allows adequate access to the medial compartment of the joint. The medial coronoid in a patient with periarticular fibrosis is more readily

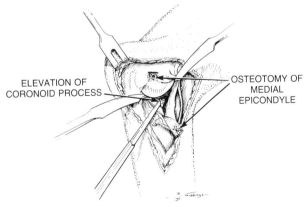

ELEVATION OF CORONOID PROCESS

OSTEOTOMY OF MEDIAL EPICONDYLE

Figure 24-9. *Surgical treatment of a fragmented medial coronoid process. The left elbow has been exposed by a medial approach with osteotomy of the epicondyle. The coronoid process is being elevated with a small osteotome. (Brinker WO. Handbook of small animal orthopedics. Philadelphia: WB Saunders, 1983:383.)*

accessible through an osteotomy of the medial epicondyle. This approach allows distal retraction of the muscle group and medial collateral ligament. The fragmented coronoid may be a free body lying alongside the articular surface of the ulna or attached by fibrous tissue and require sharp excision for removal. Once removed, the medial condyle should be inspected for the presence of an OCD lesion or a "kiss" lesion. The latter is an area of cartilage eburnation directly overlying the fragmented coronoid. If an OCD lesion is present, loose cartilage is removed and the base of the lesion drilled. If a zone of cartilage eburnation is noted, the base of the lesion should be drilled. The epicondylar osteotomy is reduced and stabilized with a cancellous bone screw, and the soft tissues are sutured using standard technique. Postoperatively, the patient should have only supervised activity on a leash for 6 weeks. A possible complication is loosening of the screw. If this occurs, removal of the screw is indicated. The prognosis is good if the fragment is removed before secondary degenerative joint disease occurs. If the patient has degenerative joint disease, removal of the fragment is helpful, but the patient may not return to the previous level of athletic performance.

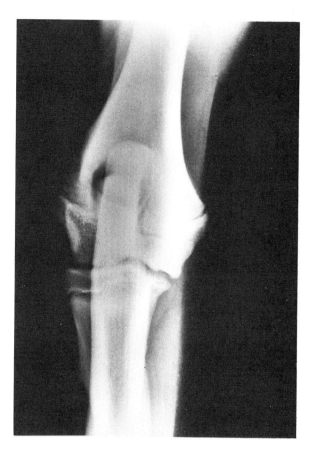

Figure 24-10. *Craniocaudal radiograph of a patient who has osteochondritis dissecans affecting the medial humeral condyle.*

Osteochondrosis of the Medial Condyle of the Elbow

OCD affects the articular surface of the medial humeral condyle; it may occur alone or in conjunction with a fragmented coronoid. The breeds of animals affected, clinical manifestations, and etiopathology are the same as for fragmented coronoid process. Radiographically, a saucer-shaped defect can be seen at the articular surface of the medial humeral condyle on the craniocaudal projection (Fig. 24-10). Osteophytes form on the medial epicondyle, coronoid process of the ulna, and ridge of the anconeal process. Treatment is directed at removal of free cartilage flaps and curettage or drilling of the base of the lesion.

The surgical exposure is the same as that described for fragmented coronoid process. Postoperatively, the limb is placed in a padded bandage for 3 to 4 days. The prognosis is dependent upon the degree of degenerative changes present at the time of surgery. The return to function is good with mild or no degenerative changes.

Ununited Anconeal Process

Ununited anconeal process (UAP) is a failure of the ossification center of the anconeal process to unite with the proximal ulnar metaphysis by 5 months of age. It may be an expression of osteochondrosis, that is, a failure of endochondral ossification. Ultimately, the un-united process fractures through the zone of cartilage. It is primarily seen in the large breeds of dogs such as the German shepherd and Saint Bernard. Separation of the anconeal process may occur in the basset hound but is secondary to growth disparity between the radius and ulna and is not considered part of this syndrome. The lameness associated with UAP is intermittent and is exacerbated with exercise. Clinical signs are not generally seen before 7 or 8 months of age and, in some cases, may not be apparent until degenerative joint disease occurs later in life. The patient will exhibit discomfort with manipulation of the elbow. Crepitus and joint effusion are present in older patients with secondary degenerative joint disease. When walking, these patients tend to circumduct the elbow laterally during the swing phase of gait and may sit with the paw externally rotated.

Diagnosis of UAP is based on radiographic findings, clinical signs, age, and breed of the patient (Fig. 24-11). Both elbows should be examined radiographically with standard craniocaudal and mediolateral views. In addition, a mediolateral view of the elbow in acute flexion facilitates visualization of the anconeal

process. Differential diagnoses include panosteitis, fragmented coronoid process, OCD, ligamentous injury, and muscle strain.

The recommended treatment is surgical removal of the ununited anconeal process. The anconeal process is important to the stability of the elbow joint, and its removal will initially result in a mildly unstable joint. However, it is much better to remove the free-joint body, which will cause severe arthritis if left in place. Also, with time, fibroplasia of the joint capsule stabilizes the joint sufficiently to prevent long-term instability. The patient is prepared for aseptic surgery and positioned in lateral recumbency. The elbow is approached through a caudolateral incision (Fig. 24-12). A skin incision in made midway between the lateral epicondyle of the humerus and olecranon. The incision is started 6 cm above the joint and extends distally the same distance below the joint line. A similar incision is made along the cranial border of the deep brachial fascia and the lateral head of the triceps muscle. The triceps muscle is retracted caudally to expose the anconeus muscle, which is incised at its origin along the crest of the epicondyle. The joint capsule is very thin in this region and tightly adherent to the deep surface of the anconeus

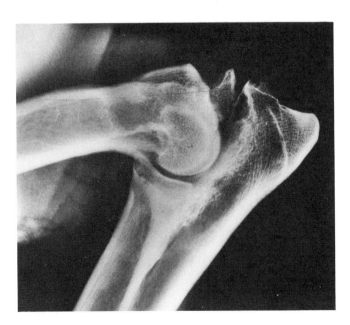

Figure 24-11. *Lateromedial radiograph of a patient who has an ununited anconeal process.*

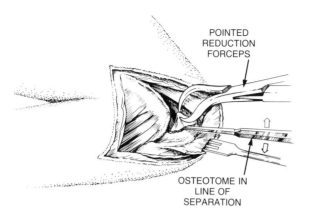

POINTED
REDUCTION
FORCEPS

OSTEOTOME IN
LINE OF
SEPARATION

Figure 24-12. *Surgical removal of ununited anconeal process. The left elbow has been exposed by an approach to the caudal compartment of the elbow joint. With the anconeus muscle retracted, the anconeal process is visualized. A narrow osteotome is being used to free the anconeal process from the ulna. Grasping the process with a small pointed bone forceps aids in removing the process. (Brinker WO. Handbook of small animal orthopedics. Philadelphia: WB Saunders, 1983:379.)*

muscle. Subperiosteal reflection of the anconeus muscle and flexion of the elbow joint exposes the anconeal process. Generally, the anconeal process is still firmly attached to the ulna through a fibrous union in the younger patient and must be removed by sharp dissection. Finding the point of union and removal are facilitated by grasping the anconeal process with a small bone-holding forceps or towel clamp. In the older patient, the anconeal process may be separated from the ulna and displaced to the proximal part of the joint. In chronic cases, osteophytes that impinge during normal extension of the elbow should be removed, if present. The anconeus muscle is apposed with absorbable suture using a simple interrupted pattern. The subcutaneous tissue is sutured with a simple continuous pattern using absorbable suture. The skin incision is closed with nonabsorbable suture using a simple interrupted pattern. A soft padded bandage is placed on the limb for 3 to 4 days after surgery, and patient activity is limited for 3 weeks. Although the anconeal process lends

stability to the elbow joint, and removal of the process results in a mild degree of instability, clinical function is improved following surgery. This is because removal of the loose process reduces joint inflammation. Prognosis is dependent upon the degree of degenerative changes present at the time of surgery but is usually regarded as favorable.

Carpal Joint

The carpal joint in the dog is composed of four separate joints: antebrachiocarpal (radiocarpal), middle carpal, intercarpal, and carpometacarpal joints. The normal standing angle of the carpal joint is 2° to 10° of hyperextension, and most movement occurs at the antebrachiocarpal articulation. The main supporting ligaments are located on the palmar aspect of the joint. In addition, the flexor carpi ulnaris muscle, superficial and deep flexor muscles, and ulnaris lateralis muscle lend support to the palmar surface of the joint.

Carpal Laxity Syndrome in Young Dogs

Carpal laxity syndrome occurs in dogs under 4 months of age. A common observation is that affected dogs have been raised on a smooth surface and confined to a small area with limited exercise. Two syndromes have been recognized: hyperextension of the antebrachiocarpal joint (caudal bowing—Fig. 24-13) and hypoextension of the antebrachiocarpal joint (cranial bowing). Generally both forelimbs are involved, but one carpus tends to be worse than the contralateral one. Radiographically no abnormalities are seen. Diagnosis is based on age, history, and lack of abnormal radiographic findings. Differential diagnoses include growth-plate injury, injury to the superficial and deep flexor muscle-tendon unit, and injury to the palmar supporting ligaments. Treatment depends upon the degree of the deformity. All patients should be housed in an area with a floor surface that provides good

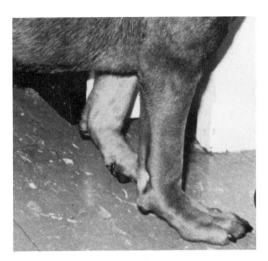

Figure 24-13. *An 8-week-old pup with carpal hyper-extension. The range of motion was measured as 245° using a goniometer. (Shires P. Carpal hyperextension in two-month-old pups. J Am Vet Med Assoc 1985;186:51.)*

footing and should be provided with a moderate, controlled exercise program. Patients with hypoextension or severe hyperextension need temporary external support for 2 to 3 weeks. This is followed by passive physical therapy and a controlled exercise program. Due to the similarities between this syndrome and injury to the radial or ulnar growth plates, patients with carpal laxity syndrome must be followed closely and examined weekly. Radiographs should be taken every 2 weeks to assure normal development of the radial and ulnar growth plates. Most patients will respond to treatment rapidly, but a small percentage will need continued physical therapy and periodic external coaptation. Although some patients may need treatment for 2 to 3 months, the prognosis for return to normal appearance and function is good.

Hip Joint

Hip Dysplasia

Hip dysplasia is an abnormal development of the coxofemoral joint. The syndrome is characterized by subluxation or complete luxation of the femoral head in the younger patient; in the older patient, mild to severe degenerative joint disease is present. The cause is multifactorial with both hereditary traits and environmental factors playing a part in the disease process. Rapid weight gain and growth through excessive nutritional intake can lead to hip dysplasia by causing a disparity in development of the supporting soft tissues and bony skeleton. Factors that cause synovial inflammation, such as mild repeated trauma and viral or bacterial synovitis, may be important in the pathogenesis of hip dysplasia. Synovitis leads to increased joint fluid volume, which abolishes the joint stability associated with the negative suctionlike action produced between the articular surfaces by a thin layer of normal synovial fluid. Although many factors may contribute to the development of hip joint laxity, it is the resulting laxity that is responsible for the early clinical signs and joint changes. Subluxation stretches the fibrous joint capsule, producing pain and lameness. Also, the surface area of articulation is decreased, which concentrates the stress of weight bearing over a small area through the hip joint. Subsequently, fractures of the trabecular cancellous bone of the acetabulum occur, causing pain and lameness. The cancellous bone of the acetabulum is easily deformed by the continual dorsal subluxation of the femoral head. This pistonlike action causes a tilting of the acetabular articular surface from a horizontal plane to a more vertical plane. The physiologic response to joint laxity is proliferative fibroplasia of the joint capsule and increased thickness of the trabecular bone. This relieves the pain associated with capsular sprain and trabecular fractures. However, the surface area of articulation is still decreased, which causes premature wear of articular cartilage, exposure of subchondral pain fibers, and lameness.

History and Clinical Signs

The incidence of hip dysplasia is greatest in the Saint Bernard and German shepherd, but most sporting breeds are affected. History and clinical signs vary with the age of the patient. There are two general recognizable clinical syndromes associated with hip dysplasia: (1) patients 5 to 16 months of age, (2) patients with chronic degenerative joint disease. Patients in the first group present with lameness between 5 to 8 months of age. Clinical signs in these young dogs include difficulty when rising after periods of rest, exercise intolerance, and intermittent or continual lameness. Some patients will present with an acute non-weight-bearing lameness of one rear leg. This latter group of patients have torn the round ligament of the affected hip joint and severely sprained the fibrous joint capsule. Some patients will spontaneously improve clinically at 15 to 18 months of age. This clinical improvement results from relief of pain, because proliferative fibrous tissue prevents further capsular sprain, and increased thickness of the subchondral bone prevents trabecular fractures. However, these patients are still afflicted with hip dysplasia and have a decreased surface area of hip joint articulation. Depending on the degree of wear on articular cartilage and progression of degenerative joint disease, this group of patients may develop clinical signs later in life, including difficulty in rising, exercise intolerance, lameness following exercise, atrophy of the pelvic muscle mass, and a waddling gait in the hindquarters.

Physical findings in the younger group of patients include pain during external rotation and abduction of the hip joint, poorly developed pelvic muscle mass, and exercise intolerance. Hip examination performed under general anesthesia will reveal abnormal angles of reduction and subluxation, reflecting excessive joint laxity (Fig. 24-14). Physical findings in the older group of patients include pain during extension of the hip joint, reduced range of motion, atrophy of the pelvic muscu-

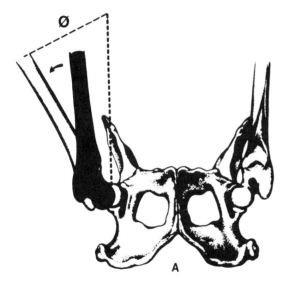 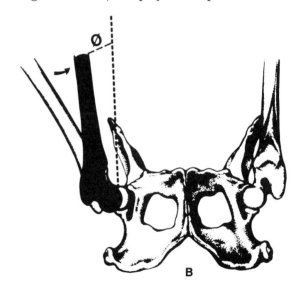

Figure 24-14. **A,** *Measurement of the maximal amount of axial rotation of the pelvis. The leg is abducted* (arrow) *to the position where the hip relocates into the acetabulum. This angle θ is measured from the vertical using a goniometer. This represents the maximal angle needed for bony stability and the maximal angle needed for twisting the plate used in the pelvic osteotomy technique.* **B,** *Measurement of the minimal amount of axial rotation of the pelvis. The leg is adducted slowly* (arrow) *until the hip reluxates from the socket. The angle θ is measured from the vertical and represents the minimal angle needed for twisting the plate used in the pelvic osteotomy technique. (Slocum B. Pelvic osteotomy technique for axial rotation of the acetabular segment in dogs. J Am Anim Hosp Assoc 1986;22:333)*

lature, and exercise intolerance. There is generally no joint laxity, but crepitus may be detected on joint manipulation.

Differential Diagnosis

Differential diagnoses include panosteitis, osteochondrosis, physeal separation, and ligament injury in the younger patient. In the older group of patients, it is extremely important to rule out neurologic problems as a cause of the clinical symptoms. Orthopedic conditions, such as ruptured cranial cruciate ligament, polyarthritis, and bone neoplasia, must be considered before attributing clinical signs to hip dysplasia. Radiographically, there are seven grades of variation in the congruity between the femoral head and acetabulum, established by the Orthopedic Foundation for Animals. Excellent, good, fair, and near normal are considered within a range of normal. Dysplastic animals fall into the categories of mild, moderate, and severe (Fig. 24-15). It is important to note that clinical signs do not always correlate with radiographic findings. A correct diagnosis of hip dysplasia as the cause of clinical problems is based on age, breed, history, physical findings, and radiographs.

Treatment

Treatment is dependent upon the age of the patient, the degree of patient discomfort, physical and radiographic findings, client expectations of patient performance, and financial capability of the client. Conservative treatment is beneficial in a large number of patients in both the young and older patient groups. During episodes of acute pain, rest and nonsteroidal analgesics will relieve signs in most of patients. Aspirin is generally the first choice at a dosage rate of 10–25 mg/kg 3 times a day. Other nonsteroidal anti-inflammatory drugs can be used, but the more potent the anti-inflammatory property, the more likely gastric or intestinal irritation will occur. Once the clinical signs are under control, maintaining a lean body weight and a moderate exercise program are helpful. Exercise programs aimed at

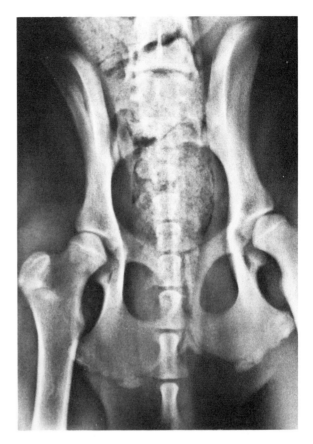

Figure 24-15. *Ventrodorsal radiograph of a patient who has mild radiographic changes associated with hip dysplasia.*

developing the pelvic muscles should be gradually started; swimming and walking (trotting) uphill will increase pelvic muscle strength. Signs in young patients may resolve as the physiologic proliferation of the fibrous joint capsule stabilizes the hip joint. Signs in the older patient may be controlled for years with the aid of weight control and intermittent administration of nonsteroidal analgesics. Surgery is indicated when conservative treatment is not effective, when an athletic performance level is desired, or, in the young patient, when the client wishes to arrest or slow the progression of degenerative joint disease. There are four surgical procedures commonly used for treatment of hip dysplasia:

Pelvic osteotomy
Femoral osteotomy
Total hip prosthesis
Femoral head ostectomy

Pelvic osteotomy is used in the group of younger patients to axially rotate and lateralize the acetabulum in an effort to increase dorsal coverage of the femoral head. This procedure is indicated in patients that will lead athletic lives, such as the working breeds, or in those patients in which the client wishes to arrest or slow the progress of osteoarthritis associated with hip dysplasia. The most favorable prognosis is in patients having minimal existing radiographic degenerative changes and an angle of reduction less than 45°. The prognosis is less favorable in patients with existing degenerative changes and angles of reduction greater than 45°. The procedure is not indicated in patients with dislocated hip joints. Of the procedures described, the transverse pelvic osteotomy (Slocum technique) is the most effective method of obtaining axial rotation and lateralization of the acetabulum (Fig. 24-16). The details of the technique are beyond the scope of this book. Briefly, the degree of axial rotation of the acetabulum is set by the previously determined angles of reduction and subluxation. The angle of reduction is the maximum degree of rotation, and the angle of subluxation is the minimum degree of rotation. The most commonly used angle of acetabular axial rotation is slightly less than the measured angle of reduction. The pelvis is cut through the pubic brim, ischial floor, and body of the ilium. The acetabulum is rotated axially, lateralized, and stabilized with the appropriate Slocum osteotomy plate. Postoperatively the patient is restricted to exercise on a leash until radiographic healing of the osteotomies is complete. If the contralateral side is to be operated, the second surgery can be performed as soon as the patient is clinically functional with the limb initially operated. Reported complications include implant failure, loss of limb abduction, and pelvic outlet narrowing. However, the incidence of complications is

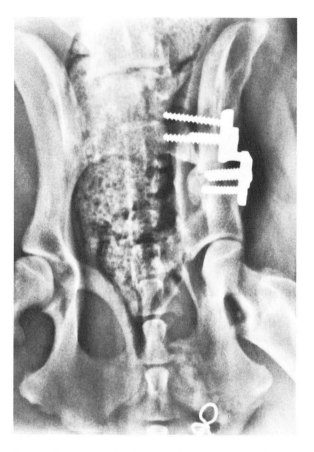

Figure 24-16. *Ventrodorsal radiograph of a patient 5 weeks following a pelvic osteotomy.*

very low, and the reports of long-term clinical function are good to excellent.

Proximal femoral varus osteotomy, derotational osteotomy, or a combination of the two also results in increased joint stability. Varus osteotomy involves an intertrochanteric osteotomy with removal of a wedge-shaped piece of bone. Removal of the correct amount of predetermined wedge of bone decreases the angle of inclination and elevates the height of the greater trochanter. This reorientation of both the femoral neck angle and mechanical force of the gluteal muscles results in a more stable hip. Large femoral anteversion angles have been reported in dogs with hip dysplasia. If present, a derotational femoral osteotomy may be combined with varus osteotomy to increase hip joint stability.

A total hip prosthesis involves the replacement of the dysplastic hip joint with a plastic acetabular cup and stainless steel femoral component. This procedure is used in older patients, in which conservative treatment is not effective. Total hip replacement is also indicated in younger patients with severe subluxation, in which conservative treatment is unrewarding, and a pelvic osteotomy is not advisable. The success rate is very good to excellent but is directly dependent upon the experience of the surgeon. Therefore, this procedure should only be performed by a trained and experienced surgeon (see Chap. 23, Reconstructive Surgery).

Femoral head and neck excision prevents bony contact between the femoral head and acetabulum and allows formation of a fibrous false joint. This technique can be used in both the younger group of patients (as a primary method of treatment) and in the older group of patients (when conservative treatment has failed). A fibrous pseudoarthrosis is an unstable joint; therefore, the clinical function postoperatively is somewhat unpredictable. For this reason most surgeons consider the technique a salvage procedure. However, many patients with painful arthritic hips, undergoing femoral head and neck excision, have improved limb function and quality of life postoperatively. In fact, most patients function with only a slight gait abnormality or no detectable gait abnormality.

The patient is anesthetized, prepared for aseptic surgery, and positioned in lateral recumbency. It is desirable to drape the patient in a manner that allows manipulation of the limb during surgery. A craniolateral skin incision is centered over the hip joint (Fig. 24-17). The incision begins 5 cm above the joint, courses slightly cranial to the greater trochanter, and extends distally 5 cm below the joint. The subcutaneous tissues are incised along the same line, exposing the tensor fascia lata muscle and cranial border of the biceps femoris muscle. An incision is made through the fascia lata along the cranial edge of the biceps muscle. At the region of the greater trochanter, the incision curves cranially to follow the cranial border of the superficial glu-

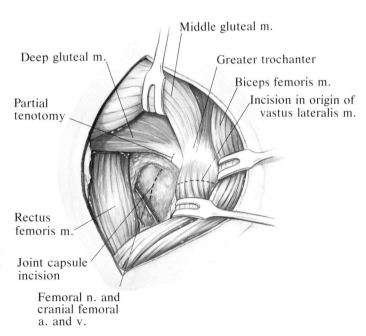

Figure 24-17. *Approach to the hip joint through a craniolateral incision. (Piermattei D, Greely RC. An atlas of surgical approaches to the bones of the dog and cat. 2nd ed. Philadelphia: WB Saunders, 1979:133.)*

Middle gluteal m.

Deep gluteal m.

Greater trochanter

Biceps femoris m.

Incision in origin of vastus lateralis m.

Partial tenotomy

Rectus femoris m.

Joint capsule incision

Femoral n. and cranial femoral a. and v.

teal muscle. Dorsal reflection of the superficial gluteal muscle and caudal retraction of the biceps femoris muscle exposes the middle gluteal muscle. With dorsal retraction of this muscle, the tendon of insertion of the deep gluteal muscle can be seen. A periosteal elevator is used to separate the deep gluteal muscle from the coxofemoral fibrous joint capsule, and a partial tendinotomy of the deep gluteal muscle is performed near the greater trochanter. An incision through the fibrous joint capsule is made parallel to the longitudinal axis of the femoral neck. The incision is begun medially at the lateral rim of the acetabulum and extended laterally through the origin of the vastus lateralis muscle. The vastus lateralis muscle is reflected distally to expose the site where the femoral neck joins the femoral metaphysis. If the round ligament is intact, it must be incised. Incision is facilitated by placing lateral traction on the greater trochanter with bone-holding forceps, which will subluxate the femoral head, allowing for placement of curved scissors into the joint to cut the round ligament. The osteotomy is most easily accomplished by externally rotating the limb to where the joint line of the stifle is parallel to the operating table. The line of osteotomy is then perpendicular to the operating table and located at the junction of the femoral neck and femoral metaphysis. The accuracy of the bony cut can be assured by predrilling a series of three or more holes along the line of the osteotomy. An osteotome and mallet are used to complete the cut. Once the femoral neck and head are removed, the cut surface of the femoral neck is palpated for irregularities. The most common finding is a shelf of femoral neck left on the caudal surface of the femur. Rough edges are removed with rongeurs. Clinical studies have not indicated improved postoperative function when soft tissue is interposed between the cut surface of the femoral neck and acetabulum. The joint capsule may be closed over the acetabulum, if possible. Alternatively, a proximally based biceps femoris muscle pedicle can be fashioned and passed from caudal to cranial across the excision site. The vastus lateralis

and deep gluteal muscles are repositioned and sutured with absorbable suture using a simple interrupted pattern. The fascia lata is sutured with absorbable suture using a simple continuous pattern, and the skin is sutured with nonabsorbable suture using a simple interrupted pattern. Postoperatively, early active use of the limb is beneficial. Passive flexion and extension of the hip joint is encouraged two to three times daily. Frequent leash walking is begun immediately and continued until sutures are removed. After suture removal, more active running and swimming exercises are encouraged. Good return of active limb function is dependent upon the length of time the hip joint pathology was present and the severity of the degenerative changes. Patients having chronic disease with muscle atrophy and proliferative degenerative joint disease are slower to return to function than patients with acute problems.

Legg–Perthes Disease

Legg–Perthes disease is a noninflammatory aseptic necrosis of the femoral head occurring in young patients prior to closure of the capital femoral physis. The peak incidence of onset is 6 to 10 months, and the syndrome is seen only in the small breeds of dogs. Males and females are equally affected, and the problem occurs bilaterally in 12% to 17% of the patients. The reason for the bone necrosis is not known for certain, but several theories have been proposed. The vascular supply to the femoral head in a patient with an open proximal femoral physis is derived solely from the epiphyseal vessels. Metaphyseal vessels do not cross the physis to contribute to femoral head vascularity. Epiphyseal vessels course extraosseously along the surface of the femoral neck, cross the growth plate, and then penetrate the bone to supply nourishment to the femoral epiphysis. Synovitis or sustained abnormal limb position may cause sufficient increased intra-articular pressure to collapse the fragile veins and inhibit blood flow. Also, an autosomal recessive gene has been proposed as a genetic cause for the development of aseptic necrosis of the femoral head. Once cell death has occurred, the reparative processes begin. The bone substance is weakened mechanically during the revascularization period, and normal physiologic weight-bearing forces can cause collapse and fragmentation of the femoral epiphysis. When this happens, incongruence of the femoral epiphysis and acetabulum results in degenerative joint disease. Fragmentation (fractures) of the femoral epiphysis and osteoarthrosis cause pain that leads to clinical lameness.

Lameness usually presents as a slow-onset, weight-bearing lameness that continues to worsen over a 6- to 8-week period and may progress to non-weight bearing. Some clients report acute onset of clinical lameness. In these patients, sudden collapse of the epiphysis may have caused acute exacerbation of already present, but imperceptible, clinical lameness. Other clinical signs can include irritability, reduced appetite, and chewing at the hip area. Manipulation of the hip joint at physical examination consistently elicits pain. With advanced disease, limited range of motion, muscle atrophy, and crepitus may be present.

Differential diagnoses include physeal trauma, medial patellar luxation, and Legg–Perthes disease. Small breeds of dogs may have bilateral medial patellar luxation, and care must be taken to examine the hip joint carefully. Diagnosis is based on age, breed, physical findings, and radiographic signs. Radiographs show deformity of the femoral head, shortening of the femoral neck, and foci of decreased bone density within the femoral epiphysis (Fig. 24-18). Excision of the femoral head and neck is the treatment of choice. Patients weighing less than 10 kg have an excellent prognosis for full recovery.

Stifle Joint

Injury of the stifle joint restraints or abnormalities of the extensor mechanism are frequently encountered in veterinary practice. Primary restraints include the cranial and caudal cruciate ligaments, which resist abnormal cranio-

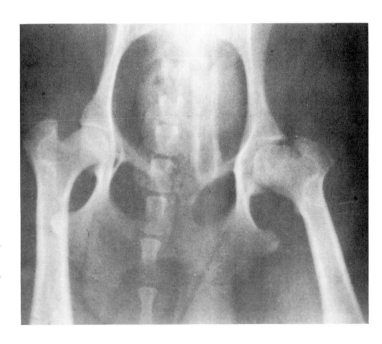

Figure 24-18. *Ventrodorsal radiography depicting the radiograph changes associated with Legg–Perthes disease in the dog. (Newton CD, Nunamaker DM, eds. Textbook of small animal orthopaedics. Philadelphia: JB Lippincott, 1985:951.)*

caudal movement of the tibia relative to the femur, and the collateral ligaments, which prevent excessive varus–valgus movement. Secondary restraints include: the menisci, which give rotational and craniocaudal stability; the fibrous joint capsule; and the dynamic muscular restraint of the extensor mechanism, popliteal muscle, long digital extensor muscle, and the hamstring muscles.

Cranial Cruciate Ligament Injury

Rupture of the cranial cruciate ligament is the ligament injury most frequently seen in veterinary medicine. The ligament originates from the medial surface of the lateral femoral condyle and courses distomedially to insert into the craniomedial tibial plateau. The ligament is divided into two anatomic bands, craniomedial and caudolateral, which are named for their point of insertion onto the tibial plateau. The function of the cranial cruciate ligament is to prevent abnormal craniocaudal movement of the tibia relative to the femur. The craniomedial band is taut during both flexion and extension, although the caudolateral band is seen to relax slightly upon flexion. The mechanism of injury is hyperextension of the stifle or forceful twisting of the stifle during weight bearing. Histologic evidence of cranial cruciate ligament degeneration coupled with weakened biomechanic material properties has been described as an aging phenomenon in the dog. Most cranial cruciate tears are "mop end" mid-ligament tears. However, in young patients, a bony avulsion failure at the point of insertion onto the tibial plateau is common.

History and Clinical Signs

There are three clinical presentations associated with cranial cruciate ligament injury: acute injury, chronic injury, and partial tears of the cruciate ligament. Patients with acute tears will present with an acute non-weight-bearing or partial weight-bearing lameness. The patient will be apprehensive during examination of the stifle joint, but pain, if present, is usually mild. Joint effusion may be palpable adjacent to the patellar tendon. Muscle contraction and an apprehensive patient make instability difficult to elicit. Patients with more chronic injury will have a history as described above, but, in which lameness improved with time. Three to 4 weeks after injury, the lameness may appear to be resolving without treatment. This is particularly true in patients weighing less than 10 kg. Long-term follow-up studies of this population of patients indicate that they may have normal clinical function with conservative treatment. In patients weighing greater than 10 kg, the lameness improves but the patient never returns to pre-injury activity without evidence of recurring periodic lameness. Thigh muscle mass measurement will show muscle atrophy in the injured leg. Crepitus may be evident with flexion and extension due to soft tissue proliferation and osteophyte formation. A clicking or popping sensation may be felt or heard when extending the joint from a starting point of 90° or more of flexion. Osteophytes are present along the medial and lateral trochlear ridges, and a palpable enlargement of the medial joint capsule is evident. Craniocaudal instability is difficult to elicit in this group of patients because of the proliferative response of the fibrous joint capsule. Patients with partial tears of the cranial cruciate ligament are difficult to diagnose. Historically, they have a mild weight-bearing lameness associated with exercise. Initially, instability of the stifle joint is difficult to detect. There is no pain, detectable synovial effusion, or crepitus. As time progresses, signs of instability and degenerative joint disease become evident. Some patients tear the remaining ligament tissue abruptly and present clinically, as do the patients with acute tears.

Differential Diagnosis

Differential diagnosis includes mild ligament sprains or muscle strains, patellar luxation, caudal cruciate ligament injury, long digital extensor tendon avulsion, and primary or secondary arthritis. Cranial drawer (excessive craniocaudal movement) is diagnostic of cranial cruciate ligament injury. The cranial drawer test is performed with the patient in lateral recumbency. General anesthesia or heavy sedation is required to negate the influence of muscle tension. Lack of adequate patient relaxation is the most common cause of failure to elicit cranial drawer movement. The examiner stands to the patient's rear and positions the thumb and forefinger of one hand on the femur (Fig. 24-19). The thumb is placed directly behind the fabella and the forefinger over the patella. The other hand is placed on the tibia with the thumb directly behind the fibular head and the forefinger over the tibial crest. The femur is stabilized with the one hand, while the tibia is moved forward and backward with the second hand. A positive test is craniocaudal movement beyond the 1 to

2 mm found in normal stifle joints. The tibia must be held in neutral position, as determined by the position of the fingers on the patellar and tibial crest, and not be allowed to internally rotate. If internal rotation of the joint is allowed to occur, it may appear as cranial drawer movement. When testing for partial cruciate tears, the examiner must test for signs of instability with the stifle joint in extension, normal standing angle, and 90° of flexion. If the degree of movement is questionable, comparison with the opposite limb is helpful. Abnormal popping or clicking during flexion and extension, in association with a positive cranial drawer test, is indicative of meniscal injury. Craniocaudal and mediolateral radiographs should be taken. With acute tears, radiographs are helpful to rule out other causes of stifle joint lameness. Radiographic findings in patients with chronic ligament tears include osteophyte formation along the trochlear ridge, caudal surface of the tibial plateau, and distal pole of the patella (Fig. 24-20). Also, thickening of the medial fibrous joint capsule and subchondral sclerosis are evident. Joint centesis and synovial fluid examination are helpful in cases of partial ligament tears to identify stifle joint involvement. Increased amounts of joint fluid and a two- to threefold increase in the number of cells (6000 to 9000/ ml) indicate the presence of secondary degenerative joint disease.

Patients with cranial cruciate ligament tears should undergo surgical reconstruction of the injured stifle joint. Although patients weighing less than 7 to 10 kg appear to function very well clinically following conservative treatment, they may have problems in the future. Following conservative treatment, the lameness resolves within 6 weeks, and the patient appears to function normally on the injured leg, despite persisting instability and developing secondary degenerative joint disease. However, this population of patients will likely injure the cruciate ligament of the opposite limb 12 to 18 months later. When both limbs have ruptured cruciate ligaments, the patient may be nonambulatory and appear to

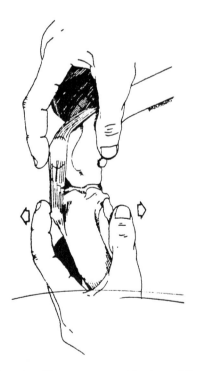

Figure 24-19. *The proper positioning of the examiner's hands when performing a cranial drawer test. (Hulse DA, Shires PK. The stifle joint. In: Slatter DH. Textbook of small animal surgery. Philadelphia: WB Saunders, 1985:2196.)*

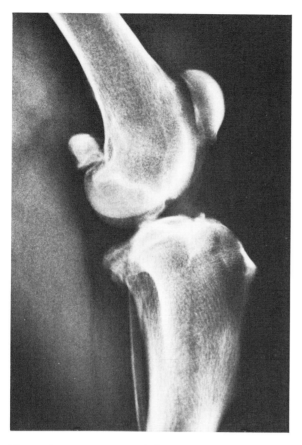

Figure 24-20. *Lateromedial radiograph showing typical degenerative changes associated with chronic stifle joint instability.*

have an acute neurologic problem. With accurate historical information and physical examination, it becomes evident that the patient's problem is bilateral cruciate ligament injury. Although the patient appears to function normally following injury to the first limb, its body weight is merely shifted to the uninjured limb. Abnormal stress, coupled with the increasing mechanical weakness of the cruciate ligament associated with aging, lead to rupture of the cruciate ligament in the opposite stifle joint. Successful treatment of patients with bilateral cruciate ligament ruptures is not as good as the success in patients with only one injured stifle joint. For this reason, surgical reconstruction is recommended in all patients with cranial

cruciate ligament injury. Surgical therapy is divided into reconstruction techniques and primary repair with augmentation.

Treatment

Intracapsular and extracapsular reconstruction of the cranial cruciate ligament are techniques that share equal popularity among veterinary surgeons. Intracapsular reconstructions consist of passing autogenous tissue through the joint using the "over the top" method (see below) or passing the tissue through predrilled holes in the femur and tibia. More recently, the "over the top" techniques have been more popular. Extracapsular reconstructions involve the placement of sutures outside the joint or redirection of the lateral collateral ligament. It is often useful to combine intracapsular and extracapsular reconstructions in the large and giant breeds of dogs.

The most frequently used intracapsular reconstruction is the "over the top" placement of an autogenous fascia lata graft. The limb is surgically prepared to allow manipulation during surgery, and the patient is placed in lateral recumbency with the limb to be operated uppermost. The skin incision is begun from a point proximally midway between the greater trochanter and proximal pole of the patella. From this point the incision courses craniolaterally along the thigh and extends distally to the level of the tibial plateau. The subcutaneous tissue and loose connective tissues are reflected from the fascia lata medially to the border of the cranial sartorius muscle and laterally to the biceps femoris muscle. The superficial surface of the patellar tendon is freed of loose connective tissue. The leg is flexed to tighten the patellar tendon and lateral retinacular tissue. An incision is made beginning at the lateral edge of the distal pole of the patella and extending distally through the lateral one third of the patellar tendon and retinaculum to the tibial crest. The leg is then extended to slacken the retinacular tissues lateral to the patella. Blunt scissors are placed deep into the incision made through the retinaculum and patellar tendon at the distolateral pole of the patella. The scissors are forced proximally along the lateral surface of the patella, separating the fascia lata and retinaculum from the fibrous joint capsule. The scissors are then used to incise the tissue along the predetermined course lateral to the patella. It is important to follow a line medially to the cranial sartorius muscle when the proximal extent of the patella is reached. The incision through the fascia lata is carried proximally the full length of the skin incision along the cranial border of the sartorius muscle (Fig. 24-21). When the proximal extent of the incision is reached, the fascia lata is incised caudally to the reflection of the biceps femoris muscle. The incision is continued distally along the cranial edge of the biceps muscle to

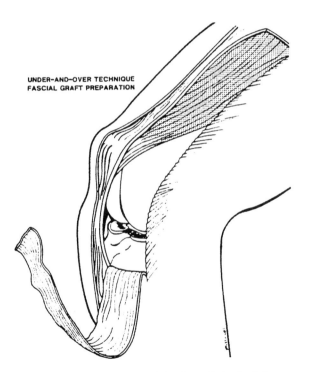

UNDER-AND-OVER TECHNIQUE
FASCIAL GRAFT PREPARATION

Figure 24-21. *Isolation of the lateral third of the patella tendon and fascia lata for intracapsular reconstruction of cranial cruciate ligament insufficiency. (Hulse DA, Shires PK. The stifle joint. In: Slatter DH. Textbook of Small Animal Surgery. Philadelphia: WB Saunders, 1985:2206.)*

the tibial plateau. When carrying the fascial incision distally, it is extremely important to maintain equal width of the fascial graft along its entire length. The graft needs to be undermined from proximal to distal points and freed from the loose connective tissue attachments. This process is stopped midway between the patella and tibial crest to insure vascularity of the graft. The joint capsule is incised from the distal pole of the patella to the tibial crest. At the level of the patella, the capsule incision is directed proximally and caudally along the border of the vastus lateralis to the region of the lateral fabella. The patella is dislocated medially, exposing the cranial view of the stifle. Remnants of the torn cruciate are excised, and the internal structures of the joint are examined. To inspect the caudomedial compartment of the joint, a Hohman retractor is used. The tip of the retractor is placed on the caudal tibial spine, and the body of the retractor is set against the distal trochlea. Caudal pressure on the retractor handle forces the tibia forward and down, exposing the medial meniscus. A bucket handle tear of the caudal body of the medial meniscus is seen in 50% to 75% of patients with a torn cranial cruciate ligament. In patients with bucket handle tears of the medial meniscus, the torn section of meniscus is excised. The fascial graft is passed beneath the intermeniscal ligament with right-angle forceps. The "over the top" maneuver is completed by passing Adson curved hemostatic forceps over the top of the fabella and, by gliding next to the lateral condyle, penetrating the caudal joint capsule. The free end of the graft is grasped and pulled through the joint. A cut is made through the femoral fabellar ligament, and the graft is passed through the ligament. The fascial graft is secured to the lateral femoral condyle with a spiked polyacetyl washer and bone screw or sutured to the femoral fabellar ligament, fibrous joint capsule, and patellar tendon (Fig. 24-22). All but 2 to 3 mm of cranial drawer should be eliminated with the leg held in a normal standing angle. The fibrous joint capsule, cut edge of fascia lata, and subcutaneous tissues are sutured with absorb-

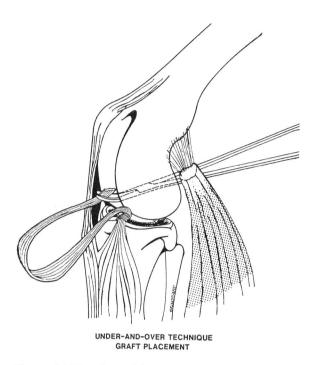

**UNDER-AND-OVER TECHNIQUE
GRAFT PLACEMENT**

Figure 24-22. *Curved forceps are used to penetrate the caudal joint capsule to grasp the free end of the graft. The graft is then pulled through the caudal joint capsule to complete the over-the-top maneuver. (Hulse DA, Shires PK. The stifle joint. In: Slatter DH. Textbook of Small Animal Surgery. Philadelphia: WB Saunders, 1985:2207.)*

able suture using a simple interrupted pattern. The skin is sutured with nonabsorbable suture with a simple interrupted pattern.

Primary repair with augmentation is reserved for a small percentage of patients that have experienced failure of the cruciate ligament at the point of insertion on the tibial plateau or failure from the origin of the ligament on the femur. This mode of ligament failure may occur following trauma to the stifle joint in patients less than 1 year of age. The most frequently seen site of failure is the point of insertion onto the tibial plateau. Surgical exposure and fascial graft isolation are the same as described above. The cranial cruciate ligament is identified. Often a small piece of cancellous bone remains attached at the site of failure. Nonabsorbable suture is passed

through the ligament using a locking-loop pattern. Two small parallel drill holes are made from the medial tibial metaphysis to exit within the joint at the insertion point of the cranial cruciate ligament. Wire loops are used to pass the free ends of the suture through the predrilled holes. The previously isolated fascial graft is passed through the joint and secured to the femoral condyle as described above to eliminate cranial drawer and augment the primary repair. When the joint is stable, the sutures in the ligament are tied outside the joint. The surgical wound is closed using the technique described above.

Postoperatively the limb is placed in a padded soft bandage to prevent overextension and flexion of the stifle joint. The bandage remains and rest is enforced for 3 to 4 weeks postoperatively. Supervised activity on a leash is encouraged for an additional 8 weeks. After this, the patient gradually is permitted to return to normal activity. Prognosis for return of function is good for all breeds of dogs. Possible complications are medial patellar luxation and persistent pain associated with the screw and washer. Medial patellar luxation is rare and can be prevented by careful closure of the lateral retinaculum. If patellar luxation occurs postoperatively, reconstruction of the lateral retinaculum and release of the medial retinaculum will correct the problem. Persistent pain associated with the screw and washer is very common but easily managed by removal of the implants 2 to 3 months after surgery.

A number of surgical techniques have been described for extracapsular suture placement as a method of treatment for the cranial cruciate-deficient stifle joint. The techniques have in common the placement of nonabsorbable sutures that eliminate or reduce cranial drawer. Surgical exposure and inspection of the internal structures of the joint are identical to that described for intracapsular reconstruction. The arthrotomy is then closed with absorbable suture using a simple interrupted pattern. Number 2 polyester suture is passed deeply through the femoral–fabellar ligament. The ligament is located just proximal to the fabella and is the dense fibrous tissue that incorporates the insertion of the fabella and gastrocnemius muscle onto the caudolateral metaphysis of the femur. The suture is then passed through the patellar tendon at its point of insertion or through a predrilled hole through the tibial crest. The tibia is externally rotated, and, while a caudal force is exerted on the proximal tibia to eliminate cranial drawer, the suture is tied (Fig. 24-23). A series of sutures are placed through the fibrous joint capsule with size 0 polyester suture. Each suture passes through the fibrous capsule caudal to the arthrotomy line, crosses superficial to the arthrotomy, and penetrates the fibrous capsule cranial to the arthrotomy. Placement of sutures in this manner imbricates (folds in) the joint capsule. Each suture is preplaced and not tied until the series of sutures are in place. Advancement of the biceps femoris muscle by suturing the cut edge of the fascia lata into the patellar tendon aids in restricting cranial

drawer. The subcutaneous tissue is sutured in a continuous pattern of absorbable material, and the skin is sutured with nonabsorbable material in a simple interrupted pattern. Postoperatively, patient activity is limited to exercise on a leash for 6 weeks. Prognosis for functional limb use is good in the small to medium breeds of dogs. However in the large and giant breeds of dogs the prognosis is less favorable. Persistent instability and progressive degenerative joint disease in this group of patients can lead to varying degrees of lameness.

Static advancement of the lateral collateral ligament is another useful technique for elimination of instability in the cranial cruciate-deficient stifle joint. This is accomplished by advancing the fibular head, which is the point of insertion of the lateral collateral ligament. Surgical exposure and inspection of the joint are the same as described before. The arthrotomy is sutured with absorbable suture using a simple interrupted pattern. The fascia

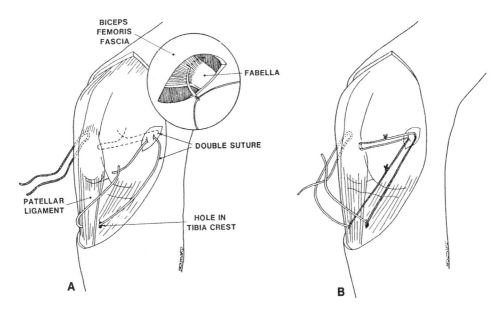

Figure 24-23. *A* and *B,* Lateral view of Flo's extracapsular reconstruction for cranial cruciate ligament insufficiency. One suture is placed through the femorofabellar ligament and a predrilled hole in the tibial tubercle, while a second suture is tied between the lateral parapatellar fibrocartilage and femorofabellar ligament. (Hulse DA, Shires PK. The stifle joint. In: Slatter DH. Textbook of Small Animal Surgery. Philadelphia: WB Saunders, 1985:2202.)

lata is reflected caudally. This is facilitated by a craniocaudal transverse incision of the fascia lata 2 to 3 cm distal to the joint line (Fig. 24-24). Care must be taken to identify and protect the peroneal nerve at this time and throughout the remainder of the procedure. The fibular head is freed cranially and caudally from the tibial epiphysis with a combina-

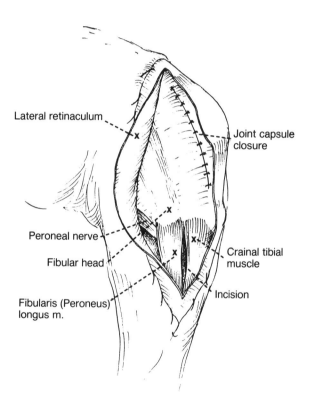

Lateral retinaculum

Joint capsule closure

Peroneal nerve

Fibular head

Craial tibial muscle

Fibularis (Peroneus) longus m.

Incision

Figure 24-24. *Craniolateral view of right stifle, showing closure of synovium after joint exploration and debridement. The lateral retinaculum has been elevated caudolaterally to reveal the peroneal nerve coursing under the flexor hallucis muscle. An incision is made in the thin connective tissue overlying the separation between the fibularis longus muscle and the tibia cranialis muscle and is extended proximally and distally to facilitate complete separation of muscle bellies to the level of the underlying tibia. (Smith GK, Torg JS. Fibular head transposition for repair of cruciate-deficient stifle in the dog. J Am Vet Med Assoc 1985;187:376.)*

tion of sharp dissection and periosteal elevation. An incision is made along the cranial and caudal edges of the lateral collateral ligament. Care must be taken not to injure the popliteal tendon or lateral meniscus, while the deep surface of the ligament is freed from its origin to its insertion onto the fibular head. This is most easily accomplished with a small periosteal elevator. The fibularis longus muscle and lateral digital extensor muscle are incised from caudal to cranial at the joint line and reflected craniodistad to allow redirection of the lateral collateral ligament. The tibia is externally rotated, and the fibular head with the attached ligament is advanced cranially using bone-holding forceps. The fibular head is stabilized with a small Steinmann pin and tension-band wire (Fig. 24-25). The wire is placed through predrilled holes in the tibial crest, deep to the extensor muscles, and around the protruding end of the pin. As the wire is tightened, further advancement of the ligament is obtained. The incised extensor muscles and fascia lata are sutured with absorbable simple interrupted sutures. The subcutaneous tissue and skin incisions are sutured as described before. Postoperatively, the limb is placed in a soft padded bandage for 10 to 14 days. Following this, exercise is limited to leash activity for an additional 3 weeks. Prognosis for return of function is good with all breeds of dogs.

Meniscal injury is a common finding in association with cranial cruciate ligament injury. The caudal body of the medial meniscus is the most common site of injury, because the medial meniscus is relatively immobile owing to attachments of the medial collateral ligament and joint capsule. As the stifle is flexed in the cranial cruciate-deficient joint, the femoral condyles are displaced caudally to rest over the body of the medial meniscus. As the limb extends and bears weight, the medial femoral condyle slides forward over the meniscus, creating an abnormal shearing and crushing force on the meniscal surface. The result is a transverse tear or, more commonly, a "bucket handle" tear of the caudal body of the medial meniscus (Fig. 24-26). The lateral meniscus is

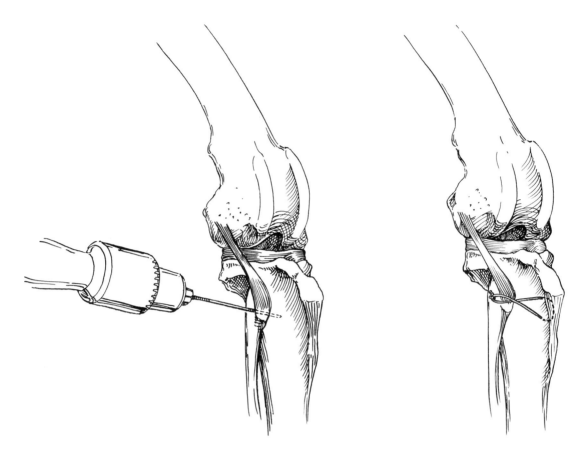

Figure 24-25. *Left,* Two holes large enough for 18-gauge wire are drilled into the tibial crest cranial to the proposed site of fibular head attachment, and a wire is passed (not shown). A Steinmann pin is drilled through the caudal half of the fibular head, providing purchase to transpose the fibular head cranially. With the tibia in complete external rotation and the fibular head maximally advanced, the pin is firmly seated into the tibia. This procedure should be performed with the stifle in a slightly flexed position. **Right,** The wire is looped loosely around the pin in a figure-8 fashion and tightened sufficiently, as shown, to eliminate the potential for cranial drawer movement and to minimize internal tibial rotation. The pin and wire ends are trimmed. Notice the new orientation of the lateral collateral ligament. (Smith GK, Torg JS. Fibular head transposition for repair of cruciate-deficient stifle in the dog. J Am Vet Med Assoc 1985;187:379.)

less commonly injured, because it is more mobile on the tibial plateau and is attached to the femur by the femoral ligament of the lateral meniscus. Therefore, the meniscus is free to move with the lateral femoral condyle, preventing the abnormal shearing injury as described for the medial meniscus. Caudal bucket handle tears of the medial meniscus are often mistaken for peripheral tears at the site of joint capsule attachment. Peripheral separation from the joint capsule attachments occurs infrequently and only in association with multiple ligament injuries. Treatment of meniscal tears depends upon the area of injury relative to the vascular supply. Blood vessels perfuse only the peripheral 20% of the medial and lat-

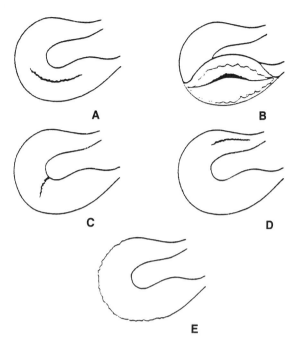

Figure 24-26. *Locations of common meniscal tears.* **A,** *Bucket-handle tear of the caudal body of the medial meniscus.* **B,** *Peripheral capsular tear resulting in a forward folding of the caudal body of the medial meniscus.* **C,** *Transverse tear extending from the free edge toward the peripheral border.* **D,** *Cranial bucket-handle tear.* **E,** *Peripheral capsular tear along the entire border of the meniscus. (Hulse DA, Shires PK. The meniscus: anatomy, function, and treatment. Compend Contin Ed Pract Vet 1983;5:765.)*

eral meniscus. The inner sections of both menisci derive nutrition from synovial fluid diffusion and have little potential for healing. Therefore, bucket handle and transverse tears do not heal, and the damaged meniscus should be removed. Peripheral tears seen with multiple ligament injuries may be repaired by suturing the joint capsule to the meniscus with simple interrupted sutures.

Isolated medial or lateral collateral ligament and caudal cruciate ligament tears are rare in small animals. Injuries that involve one of these ligaments more commonly occur in association with injury to other primary and secondary restraints. These multiple ligament injuries occur following severe trauma directed to the stifle joint. Most commonly these injuries occur following automobile accidents, or more rarely, gunshot wounds. Cranial and caudal cruciate tears, failure of the primary and secondary medial restraints, and peripheral medial meniscal tears are a common triad of injuries. Diagnosis is determined by palpation and radiographs. Combined cranial and caudal cruciate tears are characterized by marked craniocaudal translation of the tibia relative to the femur. Medial or lateral restraint injury is diagnosed by palpation. Medial or lateral restraint injury denotes tears involving both the collateral ligament complex and joint capsule complex. With the leg in extension, a varus stress applied to the distal tibia causes opening of the lateral joint line if the lateral restraints are injured. A valgus stress causes opening of the medial joint line if the medial restraints are injured. Radiographs show subluxation of the stifle joint. Careful assessment of both craniocaudal and mediolateral radiographs may show small bone chips at the origin or insertion of ligaments. Reconstruction of the cranial cruciate ligament is performed as described before. Caudal cruciate ligament reconstruction is performed by extracapsular redirection of the medial collateral ligament and long digital extensor tendon. Alternatively, intracapsular reconstruction may be performed by transposition of the origin of the popliteal tendon. Collateral ligament failure may occur at the origin or insertion of the ligament or interstitially through the substance of the ligament. Bone–ligament failure is managed by fixing the ligament to the failure point with a spiked washer and screw. Interstitial failure is treated by placing screws into the femur and tibia at the point of origin and insertion of the ligament. Next, heavy nonabsorbable suture is passed around the screw heads in a figure-8 pattern. Primary repair of the secondary joint restraints is as important as reconstruction of the collateral ligament complex. Absorbable suture is used in a simple interrupted pattern to carefully repair the joint capsule and meniscocapsular attachments. Postoperative care for patients sustaining multiple ligament injury includes protective bandaging of the stifle joint for 3 weeks. After bandage removal, the patient must have controlled exercise on a leash for a period of 8 weeks. Passive flexion and extension of the stifle joint is recommended to maintain an adequate range of motion. The prognosis for return of good limb function is fair to good. The most common complication is a loss of flexion beyond 110°. However, this loss of motion does not seem to impair the patient's limb function.

Medial Patellar Luxation

Medial patellar luxation is characterized by a hypermobile patella. Patellar luxation is classified as acquired traumatic luxation or congenital luxation. Congenital medial patellar luxation is the more common of the two and is seen most often in small and toy breeds of dogs. Acquired traumatic medial patellar luxation is not common and can be seen in any breed of dog subjected to trauma that tears the lateral retinacular structures. There are four grades of patellar luxation with the least severe, grade 1, exhibiting hypermobility of the patella and the most severe, grade 4, exhibiting permanent and complete luxation. The etiology of congenital medial patellar luxation is unknown, but abnormalities in skeletal development of the hip joint may be the initiating cause. The result is a medial displacement of the quadriceps muscle mass, which in turn alters the physiologic force exerted on the active distal femoral growth plate. Increased force across the medial aspect of the physis retards growth, although decreased force across the lateral part of the physis accelerates growth. An abnormal growth pattern results in angular and torsional deformities of the distal femur and proximal tibia (Fig. 24-27). The normal development of the trochlear groove is dependent upon the physiologic force exerted by the patella on the articular cartilage. The articular cartilage functions as the growth center of the femoral epiphysis and responds to pressure, as does the physis. If the patella remains dislocated,

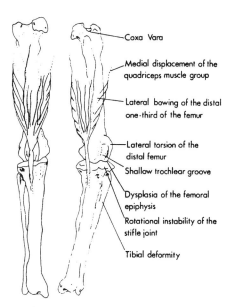

Figure 24-27. *The normal alignment of the extensor mechanism and abnormalities associated with medial displacement of the extensor mechanism. (Hulse DA. Pathophysiology and management of medial patellar luxation in the dog. Vet Med/Small Anim Clin 1981;76:43.)*

normal physiologic pressure is absent, and a shallow trochlear groove develops.

Clinical Signs and Diagnosis

Clinical signs and physical findings are variable and dependent upon the severity of luxation. Patients with grade 1 luxations generally exhibit no lameness, and the diagnosis is made as an incidental finding on physical examination. The patella may be manually luxated but spontaneously reduces when released. Patients with grade 2 luxations exhibit occasional "skipping" when walking or running. On occasion, these patients stretch the lateral retinacular structures and present with a nonweight-bearing lameness. The patella luxates and then spontaneously reduces with flexion and extension of the stifle joint. It may be manually luxated but will reduce when pressure is released. Lameness in patients having a grade 3 patellar luxation varies from an occasional skip to a weight-bearing lameness. The patella easily luxates during manipulation of the stifle joint, can be manually repositioned into the trochlear groove, but will reluxate upon flexion and extension. Patients with grade 4 luxations walk with the rear quarters in a crouched position owing to the inability to extend the stifle joints fully. The patella is hypoplastic and may be found displaced medially adjacent to the medial femoral condyle.

Differential diagnoses include Legg–Perthes disease, coxofemoral luxation, ligamentous sprain, and muscle strain. Diagnosis is based upon the finding of medial patellar luxation during physical examination and the absence of other causes of lameness. Careful examination of the hip joint is essential, because a high percentage of patients with Legg–Perthes disease also have patellar luxation. Craniocaudal and mediolateral radiographs should be taken to assess skeletal deformity.

Treatment

Treatment of medial patellar luxation may be conservative or surgical. The decision as to which method is applicable for a patient is dependent upon physical findings and the age of the patient. An older patient, in which patellar luxation is noted as an incidental finding on physical examination and in which the client reports no clinical lameness, does not warrant surgical intervention. Rather, the client should be told to watch for the clinical signs associated with patellar luxation. Surgery is advised in the young adult patient even though no clinical problem is apparent, because intermittent luxation may prematurely wear the articular cartilage of the patella. Surgery is indicated in any aged patient exhibiting lameness associated with patellar luxation. Also, surgery is strongly advised in a patient with active growth plates, because skeletal deformity may worsen rapidly.

There are numerous surgical techniques aimed at restraining the patella within the trochlear groove. Tibial crest transposition, medial restraint release, lateral restraint rein-

forcement, trochlear groove deepening, femoral osteotomy, and tibial osteotomy all have been advocated. Generally, a combination of techniques are required. The techniques used are dependent upon the severity of luxation, skeletal deformity, and preference of the surgeon. The techniques commonly employed are:

- Lateral reconstruction of the retinaculum and tibial crest transposition in patients with grade 2 luxation.
- Lateral reconstruction, tibial crest transposition, medial release, and deepening of the trochlear groove in patients with grade 3 luxation.
- Lateral reconstruction, femoral osteotomy, tibial osteotomy, and deepening of the trochlear groove in patients with grade 4 luxation.

Tibial Crest Transposition

The dog is placed in ventral recumbency, and the limb is prepared to allow manipulation during surgery (Fig. 24-28). A craniolateral skin incision extends from 6 cm proximal to the patella to 6 cm distal to the tibial crest. The subcutaneous tissue is incised along the same line. A lateral parapatellar incision is made through the fascia lata the length of the skin incision. The fascial incision is carried distally onto the tibial crest 3 cm below the joint line. The cranialis tibialis muscle is reflected caudally from the lateral tibial crest and tibial plateau to the level of the long digital extensor tendon. Careful sharp dissection is used to gain access to the deep surface of the patellar tendon for placement of the osteotome. A medial parapatellar incision is made through the fascia and periosteum to allow lateral movement of the tibial crest. An osteotome is positioned beneath the patellar tendon 3 to 5 mm caudal to the cranial point of the tibial crest. A mallet is used to complete the osteotomy in a proximal to distal direction. The distal periosteal attachment need not be transected to lever the crest laterally. The degree of lateral movement of the tibial crest is subjective but is based on the longitudinal realignment of the

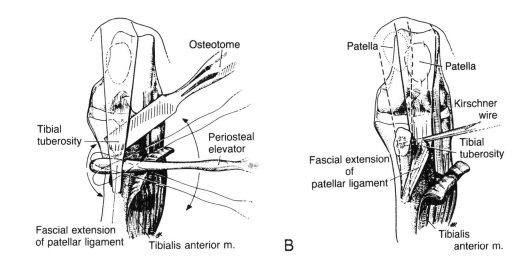

Figure 24-28. *A, A medial patellar luxation is repaired using tibial tuberosity osteotomy and, B, transposition laterally with fixation provided by a Kirshner wire. The soft tissue insertion of the quadriceps has been left intact. This procedure is usually done in conjunction with and at the same time as a capsular overlap repair to help stabilize the patella in the trochlear groove. (DeAngelis M, Hohn RB. Evaluation of surgical correction in 142 cases of patellar luxation in the dog. J Am Vet Med Assoc 1970;156:587.)*

trochlear groove with the crest. Once the site of relocation is chosen, the thin layer of cortical bone at the recipient site is removed with a rasp. The tibial crest is levered into position and stabilized with two small Kirschner wires directed caudally and slightly proximally.

Lateral Reinforcement

Reinforcement of the lateral retinaculum is accomplished with suture placement and imbrication of the fibrous joint capsule or with a graft of fascia lata (Fig. 24-29). For suture reinforcement, polyester suture is passed through the femoral–fabellar ligament and lateral parapatellar fibrocartilage. A series of imbrication sutures are preplaced through the fibrous joint capsule and lateral edge of the patellar tendon. With the limb in slight flexion, the femoral–fabellar suture and imbrication sutures are then tied. The lateral retinaculum may be reinforced through transposition of fascia lata. A section of fascia lata is isolated, which is equal in width to the patella and in length to twice

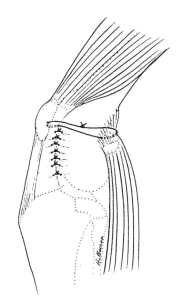

Figure 24-29. *Lateral view showing placement of fabella–patellar suture and imbrication sutures for lateral retinacular reinforcement. (Hulse DA, Shires PK. The stifle joint. In: Slatter DH. Textbook of Small Animal Surgery. Philadelphia: WB Saunders, 1985:2225.)*

the distance from the patella to the fabella. The graft is freed proximally but left attached to the proximal pole of the patella distally. The free end of the graft is passed deep to the femoral–fabellar ligament and back to the lateral parapatellar fibrocartilage. The graft is sutured to itself and the femoral–fabellar ligament with the leg in slight flexion.

Medial Release

The medial joint capsule is thicker than normal and contracted. This tissue must be released to allow lateral placement of the patella. A medial parapatellar incision is made through the medial fascia and joint capsule with a scalpel. The incision is begun at the level of the proximal pole of the patella and extends distally to the tibial crest. The wound is allowed to separate, and the cut edges are not sutured when surgery is completed. Rather, medial subcutaneous tissue is sutured to the cranial cut edge of the incision. If dynamic contraction of the cranial sartorius muscle and vastus lateralis muscle directs the patella medially, the insertions of these muscles at the proximal patella are released. The insertions are redirected and sutured to the vastus medialis.

Deepening of the Trochlear Groove

If the medial and lateral trochlear ridges do not constrain the patella, the trochlear groove must be deepened. This deepening may be achieved with a trochlear wedge recession or a trochleoplasty. A trochlear wedge recession is technically more demanding but preserves the articular cartilage, although a simple trochleoplasty is less demanding but destroys the articular cartilage.

Trochlear wedge recession deepens the trochlear groove to restrain the patella and maintains the integrity of the patellar–femoral articulation (Fig. 24-30). A diamond-shaped outline is cut into the articular cartilage of the trochlea with a scalpel. The width of the cut must be sufficient at its midpoint to accommodate the width of the patella. An osteochondral wedge of bone and cartilage is removed by following the outline previously made. The osteotomy is made so that the two oblique planes

that form the free wedge intersect distally at the intercondylar notch and proximally at the dorsal edge of the trochlear articular cartilage. In larger patients, an oscillating saw is used, but in smaller breeds and toy breeds of dogs a jeweler's saw or the cutting edge of a #20 scalpel blade and mallet are used. The osteochondral wedge is removed, and the recession in the trochlea is deepened by removing additional bone from the sides of the V-shaped groove. When the depth is sufficient to house 50% of the height of the patella, as determined through periodic replacement of the free osteochondral wedge, it is replaced into the trochlea. At times, the apex of the free wedge must be remodelled to fit snugly into the trochlea. The free osteochondral wedge remains in place owing to the net compressive force of the patella and the cohesiveness between the cancellous surfaces of the two cut edges.

Trochleoplasty is a method of deepening the trochlear groove through removal of articular cartilage and subchondral cancellous bone. The width of the articular surface of the patella is measured, and this measurement is used to determine the proper width of the trochleoplasty. Articular cartilage and bone are removed with a bone rasp, power bur, or rongeurs. The length of the trochleoplasty should extend to the proximal margin of articular cartilage and distally to the cartilage margin just above the intercondylar notch. The depth of the groove should be such that it accommodates 50% of the height of the patella and allows the parapatellar fibrocartilages to articulate with the newly formed medial and lateral trochlear ridges. The medial and lateral trochlear ridges are made parallel to each other, and the base of the groove is perpendicular to each trochlear ridge. The advantage of this technique is its' simplicity. The disadvantage of this technique is that it removes the articular cartilage of the trochlea, and articulation of the patella on the rough cancellous surface results in wearing of patellar articular cartilage. Nevertheless, the trochlear groove eventually fills with a combination of fibrous

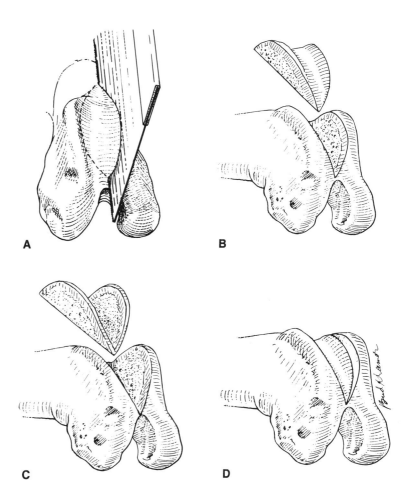

Figure 24-30. **A,** *Using the X-ACTO saw #236, the first diagonal cut is started on the highest point of the lateral trochlear ridge and angles toward the center of the base and the apex.* **B,** *The second cut is started on the highest point on the medial trochlear ridge directed toward the center to intersect the first cut and free the wedge for reimplantation after enlargement of the trochlear cavity.* **C,** *To enlarge the trochlear cavity, the medial and lateral cuts are started on the top of ridges, parallel to the first cuts, to remove a 1- to 1.5-mm thickness.* **D,** *The wedge is replaced in the enlarged trochlear cavity after first removing the distal one fourth of the depth of the feathered edge to permit a deeper seating. (Boone EG. Trochlear recession wedge technique for patellar luxation: An experimental study. J Am Anim Hosp Assoc 1983;19:737.)*

tissue and fibrocartilage, and the patients appear to function normally.

Osteotomy of the Femur

This procedure is only used in patients with severe skeletal deformity, in which it is determined that the success of maintaining patellar reduction is not possible with the techniques described previously. The deformities usually seen are a varus bowing of the distal femur and medial torsional deformity of the proximal tibia. The goal of surgery is to realign the stifle joint in the frontal plane where the transverse axis of the femoral condyles is perpendicular to the longitudinal axis of the femoral diaphysis. This realignment requires accurate preoperative measurement and wedge osteotomy of the femur. Transposition of the tibial crest, lateral retinacular reinforcement, medial restraint release, and deepening of the trochlear groove are also required for success.

Lateral Patellar Luxation

Lateral patellar luxation is seen most frequently in large breeds of dogs but does occur in small and toy breeds. The cause is unknown, but it is thought to be related to abnormal anteversion of the hip joint or coxa valga. Either condition shifts the line of force, produced by the pull of the quadriceps, lateral to the longitudinal axis of the trochlear groove. Clinical signs and physical findings are similar to those seen with medial patellar luxations. One difference is that the lameness associated with lateral patellar luxation usually is more pronounced. As with medial patellar luxations, there are four grades of lateral luxations; grade 1 being the least severe and grade 4 being the most severe.

Differential diagnosis includes hip dysplasia, osteochondrosis dissecans of the stifle or tarsal joints, panosteitis, hypertrophic osteodystrophy, capital physeal injury, cranial cruciate ligament rupture, and muscle strain. Diagnosis is determined by finding lateral patellar luxation on physical examination and eliminating other causes of rear limb lameness. It is important to note that many patients with lateral patellar luxation concurrently have evidence of hip dysplasia. Both conditions may contribute to clinical lameness and require appropriate treatment.

Goals and methods of treatment for lateral patellar luxation are similar to those described for medial patellar luxation. The surgical exposure is the same as for osteotomy of the tibial crest. However, with lateral luxations, the crest is repositioned and stabilized medially. The medial retinaculum is reinforced with suture reconstruction or fascia lata transposition, and the lateral restraints are released. Methods for deepening the trochlear groove are as described for medial patellar luxation.

The stifle joint should be covered with a soft padded bandage for 2 days postoperatively to help prevent swelling and provide patient comfort by immobilizing the soft tissues. The prognosis for full return of limb function is excellent in patients having grade 1, 2, or 3 medial or lateral luxations. The prognosis in patients having grade 4 luxations is fair because of the associated muscle contracture. The most common postoperative complication is a hypermobile patella, that is, one that can be moved beyond the trochlear ridge. However, this hypermobility does not progressively worsen nor does it affect limb function.

Avulsion of the Long Digital Extensor Tendon

The long digital extensor tendon originates from the craniolateral extensor fossa on the lateral femoral condyle. The tendon crosses the joint through a sulcus in the tibial plateau and passes deep to the cranial tibial muscle. This tendon is not important in craniocaudal stability of the joint. Avulsion of the origin of the long digital tendon is not common but can result in moderate to severe degenerative joint disease if not treated. The detached bony fragment rapidly increases in size and acts as a free body within the joint. Osteophytes and joint inflammation rapidly follow. A mild weight-bearing lameness that is exacerbated with exercise is characteristic of the condition. The problem is only seen in immature dogs of large and giant breeds between 5 and 8 months of age. The Great Dane and patients with lateral patellar luxation are more likely to be afflicted. Physical findings include pain and joint effusion occurring early after injury. Pain can be elicited by deep palpation over the craniolateral aspect of the joint. In more chronic cases pain is not easily elicited. Osteophytes, thickening of the joint capsule, and effusion are evident.

Differential diagnosis includes OCD of the stifle, lateral patellar luxation, cranial cruciate ligament failure, and stifle joint sprain. Diagnosis is based on physical findings and radiographs. Flexed mediolateral radiographs reveal an opaque density cranial to the femoral condyles and distal to the extensor fossa.

A craniolateral arthrotomy is made for exposure of the avulsed fragment of bone and tendon. Surgical fixation of the avulsed fragment is the treatment of choice in acute injuries. This fixation is accomplished with a spiked washer and cancellous bone screw. In chronic cases where the section of bone is misshapen and hypertrophied, it is better to resect the hypertrophied bone, fibrous tissue, and cartilage. The tendon is then passed through a predrilled hole in the tibial crest and sutured to itself.

Osteochondrosis of the Stifle Joint

The pathophysiology of osteochondrosis–OCD is discussed in the section above on the shoulder joint. OCD involving the stifle joint is not common but must be considered in patients with hindlimb lameness attributed to the stifle joint. The condition is seen in large breeds of dogs, especially bull mastiffs and retrievers. Lameness is minimal initially but worsens as degenerative changes become more severe. Clinical signs usually become evident between 5 and 8 months of age. Physical findings are nondescript and may include only the presence of joint effusion. As degenerative changes progress, crepitus and joint capsule thickening become apparent.

Differential diagnoses include avulsion of the long digital extensor tendon, lateral patellar luxation, failure of the cranial cruciate ligament, and stifle joint sprain. Diagnosis is confirmed with radiographs. Mediolateral and craniocaudal radiographs are necessary to visualize the lesion on the medial articular surface of the lateral femoral condyle. A radiolucent flattening at the articular surface and subchondral sclerosis are the most common radiographic findings.

Surgical removal of free cartilage and curettage or drilling of the lesion base is the treatment of choice. Craniolateral arthrotomy provides adequate visualization of the lesion. Patients with the least amount of degenerative arthritis have the best prognosis for return to normal function. Patients with moderate or advanced degenerative joint disease will have some degree of clinical lameness postoperatively. In all patients, the radiographic appearance of degenerative joint disease is progressive, but surgery will slow the inflammatory process.

Tarsal Joint

Osteochondrosis of the Talocrural (Tibiotarsal) Joint

The pathogenesis of osteochondrosis is discussed in the section addressing osteochondrosis of the shoulder joint. Osteochondrosis of the talocrural joint is seen in the large breeds of dogs, particularly rottweilers and Labrador retrievers. The medial trochlea of the tibial tarsal bone is most commonly involved, but the lesion has been reported to occur on the lateral trochlea. Osteochondrosis of the talocrural joint often occurs bilaterally. Clinical signs are usually noticed between 7 and 12 months of age. In some patients, clinical signs may not be seen until later in life in association with degenerative joint disease. In the young patient, a weight-bearing lameness is reported. The problem resolves with rest but returns with exercise. In the older patient with degenerative joint disease, intermittent mild lameness is seen. Physical findings are the presence of joint fluid effusion and hyperextension of the talocrural joint. Pain and crepitation may be present on manipulation of the tibiotarsal joint.

Differential diagnosis includes septic arthritis, ligamentous sprain, and fractures of the tarsus. Diagnosis is based on radiographic examination. Radiographic findings are the presence of joint distension and a subchondral defect of the trochlear ridge of the medial or lateral talus (Fig. 24-31). Moderate to severe degenerative joint disease is evident with increasing age of the patient.

Surgical treatment should be considered in the young patient with minimal or no degenerative joint changes and in older patients with loose joint bodies or deteriorating clinical signs. The surgical exposure that causes the least morbidity is craniomedial arthrotomy. If further exposure is needed, the craniomedial arthrotomy is combined with a caudomedial arthrotomy, preserving the medial collateral ligament complex. Osteotomy of the medial malleolus gives the best view of the medial talus but is used only when arthrotomy does not allow adequate exposure. In one study, osteotomy of the medial malleolus resulted in more osteophytosis and morbidity than standard arthrotomy. Free cartilage is removed, and the lesion bed is scraped with a curette to healthy cancellous bone. Care is taken not to remove excessive cancellous bone, which would lead to postoperative instability. An alternative to curettage is drilling multiple holes in the base of the lesion. In patients with de-

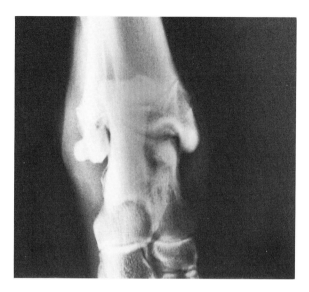

Figure 24-31. *Craniocaudal radiograph of a patient who has osteochondritis dissecans of the medial ridge of the tibial tarsal bone.*

generative joint disease, loose cartilage bodies are removed along with osteophytes that impinge upon normal joint motion.

Prognosis for return to normal clinical function is good if degenerative changes are not present. If significant degenerative changes are present, clinical function is improved with removal of free cartilage joint bodies and curettage of the lesion. In both cases, radiographic degenerative changes are likely to progress, but adequate clinical function will remain.

Congenital Tarsal Luxation

Congenital tarsal luxation is diagnosed occasionally in young kittens and puppies. The time of presentation for treatment ranges from a couple of days to 2 weeks after birth. The limbs are dragged behind the patient with the tarsal joint in hyperextension and the digits flexed. Radiographically no osseous abnormalities are present, although radiographs of patients this age are difficult to interpret because of lack of ossification. Neurologic examination is normal. Treatment consists of manual re-

duction of the luxation and immobilization in normal position with splints, casts, or small Kirschner wires. Prognosis for return of normal limb usage is good if the treatment is begun when the patient is less than 5 weeks of age.

Joint Disease in Companion Animals

The components of a diarthrodial joint are the articular cartilage, synovial membrane, joint capsule, and synovial fluid. Hyaline articular cartilage covers the intra-articular surface of the epiphyses and functions to provide a low friction surface for normal movement. Components of hyaline cartilage are collagen, proteoglycan aggregates, and chondroblasts. Collagen fibrils and their arrangement in the cartilage matrix provide the tensile strength of the matrix. As charged molecules, possessing many ionized sulfate and carboxyl groups, proteoglycans repel each other to exist in an extended form in solution. As such, they occupy a large amount of space in the cartilage matrix. Proteoglycans immobilize and bind water, increasing the resistance to water flow. With application of a load, compression is resisted by arresting the interstitial flow of water and maintaining noncompressible water within the cartilage matrix. Proteoglycans participate in the calcification process through disaggregation. Chondroblasts exist within lacunae and actively participate in the internal remodelling process of cartilage.

The synovial membrane is a highly vascular structure, the function of which is the production of synovial fluid and removal of debris from within the joint. There are two types of cells in the synovial lining. Type A cells are phagocytic and type B cells are secretory. A subintimal layer functions as waste removal via exchange between the capillary bed and joint fluid. The fibrous joint capsule serves as both a protective and supportive layer. It is dense connective tissue rich in proprioceptive and pain fibers. Synovial fluid is a dialysate of plasma combined with a mucoid lubricant. It derives viscosity from hyaluronic acid, which functions as a soft-tissue lubricant. Synovial fluid also provides nutrition to the articular cartilage and maintains metabolic balance.

Arthritis is a very broad disease category that includes many different and discrete types of animal arthritis. The following classification system is the best outline to use when discussing arthritis in animals.

I. Noninflammatory (degenerative joint disease, osteoarthritis, osteoarthrosis, degenerative arthritis)
   A. Primary
   B. Secondary
II. Inflammatory
   A. Infectious
      1. Bacterial
      2. Mycoplasmal
      3. Fungal
      4. Protozoal
      5. Viral
   B. Noninfectious
      1. Immune mediated
         a. Erosive (rheumatoid)
         b. Nonerosive
            (1) Systemic lupus erythematosus
            (2) Idiopathic nonerosive arthritis
      2. Nonimmune mediated
         a. Crystal-induced arthritis
         b. Chronic hemarthrosis

Noninflammatory Arthritis

Noninflammatory degenerative joint disease may be classified as primary or secondary. Primary degenerative joint disease has no known predisposing cause. It is thought to result from wear of the articular cartilage associated with old age. Primary degenerative joint disease is not common in animals but is diagnosed occasionally in the shoulder joints of dogs. Clinically, most patients exhibit signs of stiffness and difficulty when first rising. Rarely, a patient exhibits a non-weight-bearing lameness attributable to primary degenerative joint disease. This condition must be differentiated from secondary degenerative joint disease and inflammatory joint disease. Differentiation is done by means of a thorough orthopedic examination, radiographic evaluation, and joint-fluid analysis. Control of discomfort in patients with primary osteoarthrosis is through the administration of nonsteroidal anti-inflammatory drugs. Curettage of the area of eburnation is helpful in patients who do not respond to administration of nonsteroidal anti-inflammatory drugs.

Secondary degenerative joint disease is the most common cause of noninflammatory arthritis in companion animals. Predisposing causes include congenital or acquired malformations of a joint. Examples are hip dysplasia, osteochondritis dissecans, malunion of intra-articular fractures and ligamentous injury (Fig. 24-32). Secondary degenerative joint disease is characterized by progressive erosion of articular cartilage, osteophyte formation, and proliferation of the fibrous joint capsule and vascular synovial membrane. Decreased proteoglycan aggregation occurs and results in an increased osmotic pressure and inability to arrest the interstitial flow of water. There is a disassociation of collagen fibrils with proteoglycans, which decreases the tensile strength of the collagen matrix. With a loss of normal mechanical properties, minor trauma may create fissures and cell damage. Enzyme release and release of matrix degradation products cause a round-cell synovitis. Synovitis (inflammation of the synovial lining) will result in the production of more synovial fluid, swelling, and pain. Inflammation will also result in thickening of the supporting joint tissues, which reduces the range of motion. At the attachment of the synovial lining tissue to the intra-articular cartilage, small bony projections, called osteophytes, will be formed. Osteophytes can only form in regions away from the weight-bearing force; therefore, they are seen around the perimeter of a joint but will never be found between the weight-bearing surface. Extensive osteophytes can project

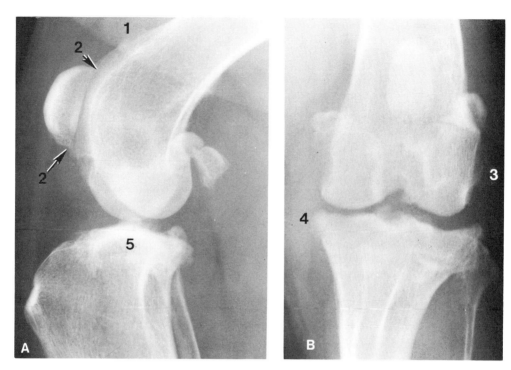

Figure 24-32. *A,* Lateral and *B,* cranial-caudal radiographic views of the stifle of a dog with degenerative joint disease. Osteophytes are present on the proximal aspect of the femoral trochlea (1), proximal and distal aspects of the patella (2), femoral condyles (3), and proximal tibia (4). Sclerosis of the proximal tibia (5) is also present. (Newton CD, Nunamaker DM, eds. Textbook of small animal orthopaedics. Philadelphia: JB Lippincott, 1985:1037.)

out into the periarticular soft tissues causing discomfort and further restriction of joint movement. Fissures in the surface of the articular cartilage result in exposure of pain fibers in the subchondral bone that contribute to the clinical symptoms. Early symptoms are a mild weight-bearing lameness after strenuous exercise, stiffness and difficulty rising after periods of rest, and exercise intolerance. As the condition progresses, the symptoms become more severe. Persistent pain and lameness, as well as reluctance to participate in activity, become evident. Early on, physical examination may not indicate the presence of pain on joint manipulation or other signs of secondary degenerative joint disease. Nevertheless, a thorough physical examination is necessary in all patients with a complaint of lameness. It may be possible to correct the underlying problem at

this time prior to the onset of advanced degenerative changes. Late in the degenerative process, manipulation of the joint will elicit pain and crepitus, and the presence of a thickened fibrous joint capsule will be palpated.

Differential diagnoses include primary degenerative joint disease and inflammatory arthritis. Diagnosis is based on history, physical examination, and radiographic findings. Radiographically, proliferation of the fibrous joint capsule, osteophytes, and subchondral sclerosis are present.

Treatment is directed at relieving pain and correcting the primary cause, if possible. For example, in a patient with secondary degenerative joint disease of the stifle as a result of cranial cruciate rupture, stabilization is necessary as part of the treatment process. Rest is important during acute periods of pain and lameness. Most periods of acute discomfort follow overactivity. For this reason, moderate controlled activity is recommended. Swimming therapy helps maintain muscle tone and a functional range of joint motion without the impact loading that results from walking and running. Most patients with degenerative joint disease are overweight because of a reduction in normal activity and advancing age. Reducing weight reduces the physiologic joint load. Therefore, it is important that these patients loose weight and then maintain a lower body weight. Medications relieve the pain and inflammation associated with degenerative joint changes but do not arrest the underlying cause of the condition. Pain relief without supervised activity may accelerate joint destruction. Therefore, analgesics should be accompanied by enforced rest during treatment of acute lameness and by controlled activity during long-term use. Nonsteroidal anti-inflammatory drugs are the initial drugs of choice. Buffered aspirin at a dose of 10–25 mg/kg given 3 times per day is the first drug of choice. The dose is used continuously for 1 month and then decreased to as low a dose as will still achieve the desired clinical result. Adverse side effects are vomiting and gastrointestinal bleeding. These will generally resolve with discontinuation of the medication. If aspirin is not effective, other more potent nonsteroidal drugs may be tried. However, one must be aware that the more potent the anti-inflammatory effect, the higher the incidence of adverse gastrointestinal effects. Corticosteroids are frequently used by veterinarians for treatment of degenerative joint disease. Although these drugs are tolerated in the short term, long-term use has undesirable systemic effects and should be discouraged. Newer medications aimed at pain relief and slowing of the degenerative process are being investigated. The polysulfated glycosaminoglycans (PSGA) are chief among this group of drugs. PSGAs are claimed to have an anti-inflammatory affect and to promote cartilage healing by increasing the synthesis of hyaluronate.

Surgical methods of treating secondary degenerative joint disease are debridement, arthroplasty, arthrodesis, and amputation. Debridement includes the removal of osteophytes that impede joint movement or cause pain from pinching of soft tissue. Arthroplasty refers to any plastic or reconstructive procedure of a joint. Surface arthroplasty of eburnated cartilage, via drilling the subchondral bone plate with a small Kirschner wire, aids in resurfacing the zone with fibrocartilage. Removal of synovial folds that are impinged between articular surfaces during movement alleviates pain. Excision arthroplasty is the removal of a joint surface and is effective clinically when other methods of treatment have failed. Examples are femoral head or humeral head ostectomy. Arthrodesis is the surgical fusion of a joint surface. This technique is useful when more conventional methods of treatment have failed to relieve pain, and excision arthroplasty cannot be performed on that particular joint. Amputation is a salvage procedure to be used when other methods of treatment have failed.

Inflammatory Arthritis

Inflammatory arthritis may be classified as infectious and noninfectious. Infectious arthritis in small animals is generally caused by bacteria. Other microorganisms such as fungi or virus are rarely involved. Joint infections are caused by bacteria that enter the joint through penetrating wounds or via the blood stream. Penetration of the joint can be through a surgical or traumatic wound. In veterinary medicine, contamination during surgical arthrotomy is the most common method of bacterial entry into the joint. Hematogenous bacterial arthritis is not common but is diagnosed occasionally in juvenile patients. Staphylococcus is the most common organism isolated in joint infections, but all bacteria result in widespread and severe cartilage destruction. Bacteria within a joint elicit an inflammatory response from the animal. Polymorphonuclear leukocytes (PMN) rapidly migrate into the synovial fluid in an attempt to destroy bacteria. Destroyed bacteria and PMNs release degradative enzymes into the synovial fluid; these enzymes then begin to destroy the collagen and proteoglycan structure of articular cartilage. Clinically, the patient has a non-weight-bearing lameness. The joint is swollen, painful, and warm to touch. The patient is pyretic, anorectic, and reluctant to move.

Differential diagnoses are acute trauma and acute exacerbation of immune-mediated arthritis. Diagnosis is based upon clinical signs and joint centesis. Synovial fluid analysis shows a marked increase in total cell count from a normal count of 3000/ml to a high count of 40,000/ml to 300,000/ml. Neutrophils are the predominate cell type. A Gram stain must be performed on the fluid to look for the presence of bacteria. Culture and sensitivity of the synovial tissue will give the most accurate results. Radiographs show joint distension and soft-tissue swelling.

Immediate and aggressive therapy is essential. Evacuation of the exudate from the joint is undertaken by arthrotomy or aspiration. Early infection may respond to aspiration and antibiotics. If accumulation of exudate persists, arthrotomy and instillation of a drain are necessary. The synovial joint capsule is cultured, and a broad spectrum antibiotic is administered. Initially, high levels of intravenous antibiotics are most effective. When clinical signs subside, passive movement of the joint is helpful in promoting healing.

Noninfectious inflammatory arthritis is classified as erosive or nonerosive. Rheumatoid arthritis is erosive, but systemic lupus erythematosus and idiopathic polyarthritis are nonerosive.

Rheumatoid arthritis is a severe, progressive polyarthritis of unknown etiology. It is characterized by severe destruction of the joint cartilage and collagenous structure of the joint. Endogenous IgG protein is altered and subsequently becomes an antigenic stimulus. IgG and IgM antibodies are produced and directed against altered IgG. These factors combine to form immune complexes that are deposited within the avascular collagenous network of the joint. The complexes activate the complement sequence, resulting in leukotaxis. The leukocytes release lysosomal enzymes, which in turn cause cartilage and collagen destruction. Synovial pannus begins to cover the articular surface, which causes further erosion of cartilage.

Clinical signs vary from mild lameness with little joint swelling to severe lameness and marked joint effusion. Clinical signs depend upon the chronicity and stage of the disease. During acute exacerbations, lameness, pain, and joint effusion are evident. The patient may be depressed, anorectic, and pyrexic. During less active stages, lameness, pain, and effusion may not be noticeable. Joint instability can be seen in more chronic cases secondary to ligamentous destruction. Spontaneous exacerbations and remissions occur.

Differential diagnoses include septic arthritis and neoplasia. The diagnosis is based on the presence of criteria set forth by the American Rheumatism Association (Table 24–1). Subcutaneous nodules and their histologic appearance have not been described in the dog. The presence of seven of the nine criteria is highly suggestive of the presence of rheumatoid arthritis. Immunologically, the rheumatoid factor test should be done but is not pathognomonic, because false positive and false negative results have been reported in the dog. The presence of serum or synovial fluid antinuclear antibodies and of immune complexes deposited within the synovial tissue leads to a presumptive diagnosis of immune-mediated disease. However, other conditions, such as drug reactions, can also show positive immunologic tests. Synovial biopsy reveals lymphocytic–plasmacytic infiltration. Radiographic changes include initial soft-tissue swelling and joint effusion. As the disease progresses, joint destruction is evidenced by punctate lytic lesions in the subchondral bone.

Immunosuppressive therapy is essential for control of the disease. There is no absolute cure, but some patients will remain in remission for extended periods of time. The most common causes of treatment failure are the use of an inappropriate dosage of a drug or failure to continue drug therapy for an appropriate time interval. Nonsteroidal anti-inflammatory drugs reduce joint inflammation but do not

Table 24–1. Diagnostic Criteria for Rheumatoid Arthritis

- Morning stiffness
- Pain on motion or tenderness of at least 1 joint*
- Swelling; soft tissue thickening or fluid, not bony alone, in one joint*
- Swelling of at least one other joint; not more than 3 months between signs of one joint and another*
- Symmetrical joint swelling with simultaneous involvement of the same joint on both sides of the body.* Bilateral involvement of proximal interphalangeal, metacarpophalangeal or metatarsophalangeal joints is acceptable without absolute symmetry. Terminal phalangeal joint involvement will not satisfy this criterion
- Subcutaneous nodules*
- Roentgenographic changes typical of rheumatoid arthritis; must include at least bony decalcification localized to the involved joints and not just degenerative changes
- Positive agglutination test; demonstration of the ''rheumatoid factor'' by any method that in 2 laboratories has been positive in not over 5% of normal controls
- Poor mucin precipitate from synovial fluid
- Characteristic histologic changes in the synovium†
- Characteristic histologic changes in nodules

* Observed by a physician
† Must exhibit at least 3 of 5 histologic characteristics
(Primer on Rheumatic Diseases, 7th ed. Atlanta: Arthritis Foundation, 1973)

suppress the immune-mediated disease process. Aspirin is the most commonly used drug and, if administered, must be used at a dosage of 10–25 mg/kg body weight every 8 hours. Therapy must be continued for at least 6 weeks beyond the remission of clinical signs. Immunosuppressive therapy is best initiated with prednisone or prednisolone at a dosage of 1 to 3 mg/kg, beginning with twice daily administration and continuing for 2 weeks. This is reduced to once daily for 2 weeks. If clinical remission occurs, the drug is administered every other day indefinitely. If clinical remission does not occur with prednisolone therapy alone, cyclophosphamide or azathioprine is added to the therapy protocol. Complete blood counts must be performed weekly during the administration of cytotoxic drugs.

Plasmacytic–lymphocytic synovitis is considered to be a form of rheumatoid arthritis. However, the condition involves only a single joint. The most common joint involved is the stifle joint. Patients are usually presented for a non-weight-bearing lameness, and palpation reveals craniocaudal stifle joint instability indicative of cranial cruciate ligament rupture. However, these patients will have significantly more joint effusion than that usually seen with isolated cranial cruciate rupture. Arthrocentesis and fluid analysis shows a moderate to marked increase in cell count, which leads to a suspicion of immune-mediated disease. Treatment should first include drug therapy for remission of immune-mediated complex formation. This treatment should be followed with reconstruction of the cranial cruciate ligament.

Systemic lupus erythematosus (SLE) is an inflammatory nonerosive arthritis of one or more joints. Other symptoms associated with SLE are often present, but these patients are generally presented for evaluation because of lameness. Autoimmunity results in systemic immune complex formation. Immune complexes are deposited in the perivascular tissues of the synovial membrane and activate complement. Activated complement attracts neutrophils, which release lysosomal enzymes and induce severe inflammation. Patients with SLE have moderate to severe lameness. There is polyarticular swelling and pain. Other manifestations of SLE may be present, including fever, anemia, and leukopenia.

Differential diagnosis includes idiopathic polyarthritis, acute trauma, and rheumatoid arthritis. Any chronic disorder that would stimulate immune complex formation and drug reactions must also be considered. Diagnosis is based on clinical signs, joint fluid analysis, immunologic profile, radiography, and synovial biopsy. Synovial fluid analysis shows marked leukocyte infiltration (6000–400,000 cells/ml), poor mucin clot, and occasional LE cells. Serum antinuclear antibody is positive, indicating the presence of immune-mediated disease. Serum rheumatoid factor is generally negative. Synovial tissue immunofluorescence is positive, further substantiating the presence of immune-mediated disease. Radiographs show the presence of joint swelling and no evidence of erosive or proliferative disease. Synovial biopsy findings include a thickened synovium infiltrated with inflammatory cells.

Treatment is aimed at suppression of the immune system to reduce the formation of immune complexes. Prednisolone at an initial dosage of 2 mg/kg twice daily for 2 days is reduced to the same dose administered once per day for 2 weeks. If the patient has improved clinically, prednisolone is administered at 1 mg/kg for 2 months and then discontinued. If relapse occurs, prednisolone should be combined with cytotoxic drug therapy as given for rheumatoid arthritis.

Idiopathic polyarthritis is the most common form of immune-mediated disease seen in companion animals. Clinical findings and results of diagnostic tests are similar to those described for SLE. However, there is no systemic evidence of SLE or chronic disease. Treatment is the same as that of other immune-mediated diseases, but remission after initial therapy is likely.

Suggested Readings

Alexander JW, Richardson DC, Selcer, BA. Osteochondritis dissecans of the elbow, stifle, and hock: A review. J Am Anim Hosp Assoc 1981;17:51.

Brinker WO, Piermattei DL, Flo GL. Small animal orthopedics and fracture treatment. Philadelphia: WB Saunders, 1979.

Milton JL, Horne RD, et al. Congenital elbow luxation. J Am Vet Med Assoc 1979;175:572.

Newton CD, Nunamaker DM, eds. Textbook of small animal orthopaedics. Philadelphia: JB Lippincott, 1985.

Slocum B, Devine T. Pelvic osteotomy in the dog as a treatment for hip dysplasia. Sem in Vet Med and Surg (Sm Anim) 1987;2:107.

Piermattei DL, Greeley RG. Atlas of surgical approaches to the bones of the dog and cat. 2nd ed. Philadelphia: WB Saunders, 1979.

Probst CW, Flo GL. Comparison of two caudolateral approaches to the scapulohumeral joint for treatment of osteochondritis dissecans in dogs. J Am Vet Med Assoc 1987;191:1101.

Puglisi TA. Canine humeral joint instability, part I. Compend Contin Ed Pract Vet 1986;8:593.

Slatter DH, ed. Textbook of small animal surgery. Philadelphia: WB Saunders, 1985.

Smith GK, Torg JS. Fibular head transposition for repair of cruciate-deficient stifle in the dog. J Am Vet Med Assoc 1985;187:375.

Van Sickle DC, Harvey WM. Primary osteoarthritis of the canine shoulder. Proc 4th Kal Kan Sym 1980:53.

Withrow SJ. Transarticular pinning and external splintage for treatment of congenital tarsal abnormalities. J Am Anim Hosp Assoc 1981; 17:469.

Index

Page numbers followed by *f* indicate figures; page numbers followed by *t* indicate tabular material.

ISBN 0-397-50852-2

90000